Vanessa Butler

Equine Medicine, Surgery and Reproduction

Disclaimer

Every effort has been made to check the drug dosages given in this book. However, as it is possible that dosage schedules have been revised, the reader is strongly urged to consult the drug companies' literature before administering any of the drugs listed.

Equine Medicine, Surgery and Reproduction

Edited by

Tim Mair
Bell Equine Veterinary Clinic, Mereworth,
Maidstone, Kent, UK

Sandy Love
University of Glasgow Veterinary School,
Glasgow, UK

Jim Schumacher
College of Veterinary Medicine, Texas A&M University,
College Station, Texas, USA

Elaine Watson
Royal (Dick) School of Veterinary Studies,
University of Edinburgh, UK

WB SAUNDERS COMPANY LTD

London   Philadelphia   Toronto   Sydney   Tokyo

W. B. Saunders
An imprint of Harcourt Brace and Company Limited

© Harcourt Brace and Company 1999

 is a registered trademark of Harcourt Brace and
Company Limited

This book is printed on acid-free paper

First published 1998
  Reprinted 1999

ISBN 0-7020-1725-6

British Library Cataloguing in Publication Data
A catalogue record for this book is available from the
British Library

Library of Congress Cataloging in Publication Data
A catalog record for this book is available from the Library
of Congress.

Note
Medical knowledge is constantly changing. As new
information becomes available, changes in treatment,
procedures, equipment and the use of drugs become
necessary. The editors/authors/contributors and the
publishers have, as far as it is possible, taken care to ensure
that the information given in this text is accurate and up-to-
date. However, readers are strongly advised to confirm that
the information, especially with regard to drug usage,
complies with the latest legislation and standards of practice.

The
publisher's
policy is to use
**paper manufactured
from sustainable forests**

Printed in China
CTPS/02

Contents

Contributors

Alistair RS Barr MA VetMB PhD DVR CertSAO DEO DipECVS MRCVS
Department of Clinical Veterinary Science, University of Bristol, Bristol, UK.

William V Bernard DVMDiplomate ACVIM
Rood & Riddle Equine Hospital, Lexington, Kentucky, USA.

Sheila M Crispin MA VetMB BSc PhD DVA DVOphthal DipECVO MRCVS
Department of Clinical Veterinary Science, Division of Companion Animals, University of Bristol, Bristol, UK.

Robin Duggins DVM
Large Animal Clinical Sciences, College of Veterinary Medicine, University of Tennessee, Knoxville, Tennessee, USA.

G Barrie Edwards BVSc DVetMed FRCVS
Department of Veterinary Clinical Science and Animal Husbandry, University of Liverpool, South Wirral, UK.

Scott Hopper DVM MS
New Veterinary Teaching Hospital, Washington State University, Pullman, Washington, USA.

Leo B Jeffcott MA BVetMed PhD FRCVS DVSc
Department of Clinical Veterinary Medicine, University of Cambridge, Cambridge, UK.

Robert J Kemppainen DVM PhD
Department of Physiology & Pharmacology, College of Veterinary Medicine, Auburn University, Auburn, Alabama, USA.

J Geoffrey Lane BVetMed FRCVS
Department of Clinical Veterinary Science, Division of Companion Animals, University of Bristol, Bristol, UK.

Sandy Love BVMS PhD MRCVS
Department of Veterinary Clinical Studies, University of Glasgow Veterinary School, Glasgow, UK.

Tim S Mair BVSc PhD DEIM MRCVS
Bell Equine Veterinary Clinic, Mereworth, Maidstone, Kent, UK.

Celia M Marr BVMS MVM PhD DEIM MRCVS
Department of Farm Animal and Equine Studies, The Royal Veterinary College, University of London, Hatfield, Hertfordshire, UK.

Elias E Perris DVM
Equine Veterinary Associates, Hamilton Square, New Jersey, USA.

Stuart W J Reid BVMS PhD MRCVS
Department of Veterinary Clinical Studies, University of Glasgow Veterinary School, Glasgow, UK.

Michael C A Schramme DrMedVet CertEO MRCVS DipECVS
Department of Farm Animal and Equine Medicine and Surgery, The Royal Veterinary College, University of London, Hatfield, Hertfordshire, UK.

Jim Schumacher DVM MS DipACVS MRCVS
Department of Large Animal Medicine and Surgery, College of Veterinary Medicine, Texas A&M University, College Station, Texas, USA.

John Schumacher DVM MS DipACVIM DipABVP
Department of Large Animal Medicine & Surgery, College of Veterinary Medicine, Auburn University, Auburn, Alabama, USA.

Debra C Sellon DVM PhD DipACVIM
Department of Veterinary Clinical Sciences, Washington State University, Pullman, Washington, USA.

Joe S Spano DVM PhD
Department of Pathobiology, College of Veterinary Medicine, Auburn University, Auburn, Alabama, USA.

Elaine D Watson BVMS MVM PhD MRCVS

Department of Veterinary Clinical Studies, Royal (Dick) School of Veterinary Studies, The University of Edinburgh, Veterinary Field Station, Midlothian, UK.

Martin P Weaver BVMS DrVetMed(Munich) DVR MRCVS

Department of Farm Animal and Equine Medicine and Surgery, Equine Hospital, The Royal Veterinary College, University of London, Hatfield, Hertfordshire, UK.

Preface

*The art is getting longer and longer, the brain of the
student not bigger and bigger*

Hippocratic aphorism, c. 400 BC

One of the biggest problems facing veterinary
students and practising veterinarians is how to
keep abreast of the rapid and continual advances
in clinical science. Against this background, this
book was produced with the objective of providing within a single volume user-friendly, con-
temporary notes on the wide ranging subjects of
equine medicine, surgery and reproduction.

Each of the authors is highly experienced in
clinical teaching and has presented the material in
a succinct, easily assimilated format suitable for
both undergraduate learning as well as an update

for the practitioner. Undoubtedly some readers
will require greater detail than provided by this
once-over-lightly approach and they are directed
to further reading within each chapter. The book
is largely organised on a body systems basis and
inevitably there are some overlaps which are
cross referenced within the text. For situations
when the book will be used as an aid to diagnosis,
where appropriate, at the end of chapters there
are lists of possible diagnoses of common clinical
presentations.

The substantial clinical expertise of the con-
tributors to this book should ensure that this text
constitutes a useful initial reference point for
those who wish to acquire and apply knowledge
of equine clinical science.

1 *Upper alimentary tract*

CONTENTS

1.1 *Normal upper alimentary tract function: deglutition*

Normal deglutition comprises the prehension and mastication of ingesta followed by its transfer from the oropharynx to the stomach.

Oral, pharyngeal and oesophageal phases of deglutition

Deglutition is divided into three stages:

1. The *oral phase* which includes the gathering of food, movements within the oral cavity, mastication and the formation of boluses of ingesta at the base of the tongue is under voluntary control.
2. The presence of a bolus at the tongue base triggers the sequence of reflexes, collectively known as swallowing, which propel the ingesta from the pharynx – the *pharyngeal phase* – into the oesophagus. The glosso-pharyngeal nerve (IX) and the pharyngeal branches of the vagus (X) innervate the pharynx and larynx and their afferent and efferent pathways are coordinated in the swallowing centre in the brainstem.
3. Waves of peristalsis convey the ingesta along the oesophagus to the stomach – the *oesophageal phase* of deglutition.

Prehension

Prehension in the horse relies on the incisor teeth to grasp and section herbage, and on the lips to pick up smaller pieces of ingesta as well as to contain it within the mouth, and to manipulate food towards the cheek teeth.

Mastication

The molar and premolar teeth are responsible for the mechanical crushing of the fibrous diet.

- The tongue and buccal musculature assist to manipulate the ingesta between the maxillary and mandibular dental arcades.
- Mastication requires free opening and closure of the temporomandibular joints (TMJs) through the action of the masticatory muscles – the masseter, pterygoid and temporal muscles close the jaws, and gravity assisted by the digastric muscles opens them. The masticatory muscles receive their innervation through the mandibular branch of the trigeminal nerve (V).
- The shape of the articular surfaces of the TMJs together with the presence of menisci permit lateral movements by the mandibular teeth across the wearing surfaces of the upper cheek teeth.

Lingual function

- The tip of the tongue assists in prehension and moves the ingesta between the cheek teeth.
- Contraction of the tongue base helps in the formation of boluses and once collected each bolus is driven caudally which triggers the involuntary phases of deglutition by driving food and fluid caudally from the oropharynx.
- The tongue is attached to the hyoid apparatus and free movement at the tympano-hyoid articulation is required for the anteroposterior tongue motion which facilitates bolus formation in the oropharynx.
- The glossal musculature receives its motor supply via the hypoglossal nerve (XII).

Elevation of palate

- The action of the levator palatini muscles draws the soft palate dorsally to close off the naso-pharynx and prevents the nasal reflux of ingesta; this marks the onset of the involuntary stages of deglutition.
- The horse has an intranarial larynx at all times other than during the momentary disengagement for deglutition. (See 5.18 and 5.21.)
- The levator palatini muscles lie parallel with the drainage ostia of the auditory tube diverticula (ATDs) so that when they contract the ostia open to allow exchanges of air for pressure equilibration across the ear drum.

Pharyngeal constriction

The constrictor action of the circular muscles of the pharyngeal walls embraces both oropharynx and nasopharynx. A wave of constriction follows the contraction of the tongue base and passes from rostral to caudal efficiently to empty the oropharynx – the pharyngeal 'stripping' wave – leaving minimal quantities of ingesta at the base of the tongue.

Laryngeal protection

Aspiration of food and fluid through the rima glottidis is prevented primarily by the tight adduction of the vocal folds and arytenoid cartilages, and to a lesser extent by the retroversion of the apex of the epiglottis.

Cricopharyngeal relaxation

The upper oesophageal sphincter is formed by the thyro- and cricopharyngeus muscles and these are maintained in a state of contraction to prevent involuntary aerophagia, especially during forced exercise. Relaxation of the cricopharynx simultaneous with the pharyngeal stripping wave permits the food and fluid boluses to pass caudally into the proximal oesophagus.

Primary and secondary oesophageal peristalsis

- After each bolus has passed through into the proximal oesophagus, primary peristaltic waves are initiated by active closure of the cricopharynx.
- Primary oesophageal peristalsis carries individual boluses to the cardia, but the process is not completely efficient and small quantities of ingesta are left at variable levels in both the cervical and thoracic oesophagus even in normal horses. This ingesta is picked up either in the bolus of a subsequent primary wave or by locally generated secondary peristalsis.

1.2 *Diagnostic approach to cases of dysphagia*

History – signs of dysphagia

The signs of dysphagia include:

- an unwillingness to eat,
- slow, messy feeding,
- halitosis,
- rejection of semi-masticated food onto the ground (quidding),
- productive coughing,
- the nasal reflux of saliva, ingesta and fluids.

Obviously, horses that are unable to eat and swallow food are likely to lose weight rapidly but this process is accelerated if the horse devel-

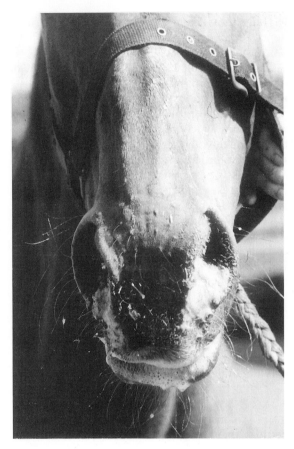

Figure 1 Dysphagic horse, showing nasal reflux of food and saliva.

ops secondary inhalation pneumonia, which is a common sequel to dysphagia. A moist cough is typical of animals aspirating food or saliva into the rima glottidis. In addition to a clear case history, careful observation of the patient's attempts to eat and drink should be made.

- If the horse shows return of ingesta from its mouth, the site of the lesion causing the dysfunction must lie in the oral cavity or oropharynx.
- Nasal reflux of ingesta points to an abnormality of the pharyngeal or oesophageal phase of deglutition (Figure 1).

Physical examination, external and oral inspection

- Evidence of systemic and/or toxic disease, including *Streptococcus equi* infection, botulism, grass sickness, rabies, upper motor neuron disease, lead poisoning and tick paralysis should be sought.

• The external assessment should check for evidence of concurrent neuropathies such as facial paralysis or Horner's syndrome or head tilt.

• Thoracic auscultation should check for signs of inhalation pneumonia.

• Local lymphadenopathies and firm distension of the oesophagus to the left side of the trachea are changes which might be found during palpation of the throat area.

• Useful information can be obtained by attempting to pass a nasogastric tube. This should determine whether pharyngeal swallowing reflexes are still present or whether the upper alimentary tract is physically obstructed.

• Under sedation and with a Haussman gag in place a detailed inspection of the oral cavity (see 1.6, 'Physical examination') should look for evidence of dental malalignment, enamel pointing of the cheek teeth, fractures of the dental crowns, periodontitis, soft tissue lesions of the buccal cleft and palate, oral foreign bodies and lesions of the tongue. The structures involved may require digital manipulation to complete the examination and a tell-tale foul smell points to the presence of stale entrapped ingesta.

• Defects of the palate cannot be appreciated from a conscious examination of the mouth because they are generally restricted to the soft palate.

Endoscopy *per nasum*

Endoscopy *per nasum* is necessary to confirm whether pharyngeal paralysis is present. The usual findings consist of:

• a mixture of saliva and ingesta on the walls of the nasopharynx,

• persistent dorsal displacement of the palatal arch,

• poor constrictor activity during deglutition,

• failure of dilation of one or both ATD ostia during swallowing.

Many cases where functional pharyngeal paralysis is diagnosed are afflicted with pharyngeal hemiplegia, i.e. the glossopharyngeal neuropathy is unilateral, for example in cases of guttural pouch mycosis (see 5.6).

True pharyngeal paralysis may be seen in cases of botulism.

Conchal necrosis may accompany prolonged dental suppuration and may be seen on endoscopy of the nasal chambers (see 5.16).

Provided that an endoscope with a diameter of 8.0 mm or less is available, the diagnosis of a palatal defect by inspection of the floor of the nasopharynx per nasum presents no difficulties even in quite young foals.

Other abnormalities which may cause dysphagia and which can be confirmed by endoscopy of the pharynx and larynx include:

• epiglottal entrapment, with or without a sub-epiglottic cyst (see 5.22),

• epiglottal hypoplasia,

• iatrogenic palatal defects after 'over-enthusiastic' staphylectomy,

• fourth branchial arch defects (4-BAD syndrome) (see 5.25),

• sub-epiglottic foreign bodies, usually in the form of unilateral oedema in the region of the ary-epiglottic folds,

• intrapalatal cysts (see 5.27),

• nasopharyngeal cicatrix,

• arytenoid chondropathy (see 5.24),

• pharyngeal neoplasia (see 5.27),

• pharyngeal distortion by external compressive lesions such as neoplasia or abscesses.

Oesophagoscopy is often unrewarding in the investigation of dysphagia because physical or functional obstructions of the oesophagus invariably lead to a build-up of ingesta and saliva in the lumen which, in turn, inhibits a satisfactory field of view. However, when the patient has been starved prior to endoscopy evidence of conditions such as oesophagitis, megaoesophagus, stricture, rupture, tracheo-oesophageal fistula, diverticulum, intramural cyst, dysautonomia and neoplasia may be found.

Radiography and fluoroscopy

Plain lateral radiographs of the pharynx, larynx and cervical oesophagus are used to investigate the relationships between normal anatomical structures and to identify intraluminal, mural and extramural soft tissue swellings. Contrast media can be helpful to outline these structures. Fluoroscopic studies again using contrast media are required for the dynamic investigation of deglutition.

Lateral radiographs of the chest are a useful aid to monitor the progress of aspiration pneumonia.

Oral examination under general anaesthesia

General anaesthesia is necessary to complete the inspection of the oral cavity. The tendency of the soft tissues to obscure the view particularly towards the base of the tongue can be overcome by the use of an endoscope passed through a polypropylene mare gynaecological speculum. Again, general anaesthesia is required for a more detailed manual examination of the caudal oral cavity, especially in the region of the epiglottis and ary-epiglottic folds.

1.3 Aetiology of dysphagia: oral phase abnormalities

Facial paralysis and lip lesions

• Facial paralysis inhibits the ability of a horse to prehend and retain ingesta in the oral cavity (see Chapter 11).
• Laceration wounds at the commissures of the lips can arise when a horse becomes hooked at the corner of the mouth and a major avulsion injury follows. Careful anatomical reconstruction of the lip margins is required.
• Sarcoids may develop at the lip margins, especially the commissures, and the method of therapy (excision, cryosurgery or chemical cautery) which is used to ablate the lesions must also take regard of the acceptance of a bit after healing.

Temporomandibular joint and hyoid disorders

TMJ disorders are rare in the horse but when they do occur they cause marked pain and a rapid loss of bodily condition. Disuse leads to atrophy of the masticatory muscles, most obviously the masseters. Clinical examination shows resentment of attempts to open the mouth, and even under general anaesthesia the range of opening may be severely reduced. The diagnosis is confirmed by radiography.

Hyoid apparatus involvement usually accompanies otitis media, and ankylosis of the temporohyoid articulation is a likely result. Pathological fracture of the stylo-hyoid bone follows and one of the effects of this is to limit the horse's ability to move the tongue.

Lingual abnormalities

• Hypoglossal nerve injuries with lingual paralysis are rare in the horse and trauma, either in the form of lacerated wounds or tongue-strap strictures, accounts for the majority of tongue lesions in this species.
• A horse with a severely injured tongue may be unable to manoeuvre ingesta around the mouth and is inclined to drop food or to collect it in the buccal cleft.
• Horses that lose the rostral portion of the tongue through incisive wounds can maintain normal bodily condition albeit showing messy feeding patterns.
• Foreign bodies may become buried in the lingual tissues and the painful suppurative response can reduce a horse's inclination to eat.

Dental disorders

Dental disorders are discussed later in this chapter (see 1.6).

Congenital and acquired palatal defects

• The presence of a defect in the soft palate prevents an effective seal between the oral cavity and the nasopharynx during the lingual propulsion of ingesta towards the tongue base and during pharyngeal contraction. The result is that food and fluids are refluxed via the nasal chambers to the nares.
• Simple midline linear defects of the soft palate are the most common cause of nasal reflux of milk in foals.
• Other types of palatal defects include unilateral hypoplasia of the soft palate and pseudo-uvula formation, which can escape confirmation until the patient is considerably older.
• Palatal reconstructive surgery using mandibular symphysectomy has been described, but the results are invariably disappointing.
• Excessive palatal resection (staphylectomy) (see 5.21, 'Treatment') in the treatment of dorsal displacement of the soft palate (DDSP) is irreparable.
• Inadvertent splits in the palate have been reported after the relief of epiglottal entrapment by section with a hooked bistoury passed per nasum in the standing horse (see 5.22, 'Treatment').

Other oral conditions: foreign bodies, neoplasia

The most common foreign bodies in the oropharynx are brambles which become lodged in the sub-epiglottal area or in the lateral food channels causing acute-onset dysphagia. Endoscopy per nasum will show oedema in the ary-epiglottic folds even if the foreign body itself cannot be seen. Such an endoscopic finding is an indication for an oral examination, either by palpation or with a guarded endoscope, under general anaesthesia.

Other foreign bodies such as wire fragments may become wedged between teeth.

Squamous cell carcinomas, lymphosarcoma and connective tissue tumours arise sporadically and they tend to cause dysphagia simply by virtue of space occupation.

1.4 Aetiology of dysphagia: pharyngeal phase abnormalities

Pharyngeal paralysis

Paralysis or paresis of the pharyngeal constrictor muscles arises when the function of the glossopharyngeal nerve (IX) is compromised. When food and fluids are not propelled into the upper oesophagus they may be returned via the nostrils, aspirated into the laryngeal airway or spilled out of the mouth.

The most common causes of pharyngeal paralysis are:

- guttural pouch mycosis (see 5.6),
- ATD diverticulitis (see 5.5),
- botulism (see Chapter 11),
- heavy metal poisoning (see Chapter 22).

It is always correct to investigate the possibility of ATD disease in cases of pharyngeal dysfunction. When there is marked inhalation of ingesta leading to bronchopneumonia or evidence of dehydration, the condition of the patient demands euthanasia on humane grounds. However, some horses with partial pharyngeal dysfunction may survive without distress and simply show an occasional cough and nasal discharge without progress to aspiration pneumonia. Restoration of pharyngeal function may occur, but this may take many months.

Nasopharyngeal cicatrization inhibits the efficiency of pharyngeal constrictor function but horses with this disorder are more likely to present for the investigation of respiratory noises and/or exercise intolerance.

Pharyngeal compression: strangles abscessation

The presence of extramural soft tissue swellings adjacent to the pharynx may cause dysphagia because of external compression of the pharynx and also, in the case of abscessation, because of the pain associated with the movement of food boluses past the lesions (see 19.14).

Pharyngeal cysts, palatal cysts

The origin of pharyngeal cysts is not known but intrapalatal cysts may develop from salivary tissue which is normally distributed widely in the palatal mucosa. Diagnosis of both conditions is by a combination of endoscopy and radiography. While cysts on the pharyngeal walls can be excised, the lesions within the substance of the soft palate are not easily treated because fistulation of the palate is a likely sequel to surgery.

Epiglottal lesions, including sub-epiglottic cysts

Peracute epiglottitis, with oedema and cellulitis, may occur as a complication of upper respiratory tract viral infections and can be so severe that a potentially fatal airway obstruction occurs.

A less severe form of epiglottitis with swelling and distortion of the epiglottis may have a similar aetiology, and causes dysphagia and coughing presumably through discomfort during deglutition. Afflicted horses also produce untoward respiratory sounds at exercise. The diagnosis is established by endoscopy but it can be difficult to differentiate this form of epiglottitis, which is likely to be responsive to vigorous antibiotic therapy, from a para-epiglottic foreign body.

The increased mass of the epiglottis arising in entrapment by the glosso-epiglottal mucosa (see 5.22), or with sub-epiglottic cysts (see 5.23), causes dysphagia because of space occupation and a restriction of the freedom for epiglottal retroversion. Secondary persistent dorsal displacement of the palatal arch may occur. Persistent DDSP is an indication for lateral radiography or oropharyngography using contrast medium. Both conditions are amenable to successful excisional surgery.

Laryngeal abnormalities

Compromised glottic protection leading to the aspiration of ingesta into the lower airways may arise spontaneously in cases of arytenoid chondropathy, or through iatrogenic causes such as complications of prosthetic laryngoplasty or partial arytenoidectomy (see 5.20, 'Treatment'). The precise cause of post-laryngoplasty dysphagia is not known but over-abduction of the arytenoid cartilage, cicatrization associated with reactive implants and nerve injuries may be involved.

Fourth branchial arch defects (4-BAD)

Approximately three Thoroughbreds per thousand born are afflicted with defects of the structures which derive from the fourth branchial arch, specifically the wings of the thyroid cartilage, the cricothyroid articulation, the cricothyroideus muscle and the crico- and thyropharyngeus muscles (see 5.25). When the 4-BAD syndrome includes aplasia or hypoplasia of the crico- and thyropharyngeal muscles, the proximal oesophageal sphincter remains permanently open. Although horses with 4-BAD are more likely to present with abnormal respiratory noises at exercise, some may cough when eating and drinking and show a nasal discharge. They also show bizarre eructation-like noises at rest and may be confused with wind-suckers.

1.5 Aetiology of dysphagia: oesophageal phase abnormalities

Megaoesophagus

Megaoesophagus has been reported sporadically in the horse, sometimes as a primary congenital disorder and sometimes secondary to other conditions causing restriction of oesophageal func-

tion, such as vascular ring strictures. Coughing, nasal reflux of ingesta and distension of the cervical oesophagus may all be features. Confirmation of the diagnosis is achieved by contrast radiography.

Oesophageal obstruction ('choke')

Obstruction of the oesophagus is discussed in greater detail at the end of this chapter (see 1.15). Impaction of dry fibrous material to occlude the lumen of the oesophagus, typically in the cervical segment, is the commonest cause of acute dysphagia in the horse. Older horses seem to be more susceptible but this may relate to the diets offered to animals that are not being fed for competitive exercise. Foals that are beginning to take herbage occasionally plug the oesophagus with a bolus of dry grass.

Oesophageal strictures/stenosis

Oesophageal strictures are thought to be the sequel of episodes of acute obstruction and horses with this condition are presented with recurring 'choke'. Confirmation of the diagnosis is best achieved by contrast radiography. The most common site for stricture development is at the thoracic inlet. Resection of the stenosed segment of oesophagus may be attempted but a guarded prognosis is indicated because recurrence of the stricture at the site of anastomosis is a frequent complication.

Intramural oesophageal cysts

Congenital intramural cysts may be encountered in young horses and cause dysphagia through restricting peristalsis and the passage of oesophageal boluses. The lesions may be seen as swellings in the oesophageal wall at endoscopy or be demonstrated by ultrasonography or contrast radiography.

Oesophageal rupture

Ruptures of the oesophagus may arise through external trauma (kicks or stake wounds) or by trauma from a stomach tube. Regardless of the cause the condition carries a poor prognosis unless cases are presented for treatment soon after the injury has occurred because of the rapid advance of contamination and cellulitis into the surrounding tissues.

Neoplasia

Tumours of the oesophagus are very rare in the horse but squamous cell carcinoma at this site has been reported.

'Wind-sucking'

Horses performing this stereotypy do not swallow air, and deglutition is not part of the sequence of events. The muscles of the upper neck contract to create a pressure gradient across the soft tissues of the throat so that the walls of the pharynx and upper oesophagus are pulled apart. The sudden in-rush of air through the open cricopharynx coincides with the gulping sound which is typically heard during attacks of wind-sucking, but the air is returned from the oesophagus to the pharynx immediately.

Grass sickness

See Chapter 3.

1.6 Diagnostic approach to dental disorders

Normal dental anatomy

The dental formula of the domesticated horse is shown in Table 1. For the purposes of these notes the molars and premolars are collectively termed 'cheek teeth' (CTs), where CTs 1–3 are premolars and 4–6 are molars. The first cheek tooth in both upper and lower jaws has a wearing surface

Table 1 Dentition

Primary dentition	I 3	C 0	PM 3	M 0	Maxilla
	3	0	3	0	Mandible
Secondary dentition	I 3	C 1*	PM 3*	M 3	Maxilla
	3	1*	3	3	Mandible

*Vestigial first premolars are commonly present as the 'wolf' teeth, and the canine teeth are generally either not present or poorly developed in mares.

forming an elongated triangle but all of the other cheek teeth have occlusal surfaces which are almost square in the maxilla and rectangular in the mandible, being narrower in the linguo-buccal dimension. The maxillary cheek teeth have three roots, two simple lateral apices and a larger and more complex medial root. In contrast, the mandibular cheek teeth have only two simple roots except CT6, which has three.

Herbivores, including horses, have long-crowned, short-rooted teeth where much of the crown lies below gum level and the roots are confined to the areas at the apices which are enamel-free.

In the upper jaw the roots of CTs 4–6 lie within the maxillary sinuses and apical suppuration can be a cause of sinus empyema (see 5.11). The reserve crown, roots and alveolar structures of CT3 form the rostral wall of the rostral maxillary sinus and on radiographs may give the false impression that there is a periapical reaction at the site. The close proximity between the roots of CTs 1–3 and the overlying thin bony plate of the maxilla make it more likely that suppurative periapical reactions of these teeth will produce a visible facial swelling.

The incisors of both jaws and the cheek teeth of the upper jaw show folding of enamel and cement from the coronal surfaces to form retention centres known as infundibula. In the incisors the attritional wear of these cups is used as a guide to age. Each upper cheek tooth has two infundibula which are vulnerable to a caries-like process of lysis, but such a change cannot arise in the lower arcades where there are no infundibula.

Development of teeth

Teeth develop from the dental sacs which include ectodermal and mesenchymal elements. Enamel, which forms from ameloblasts, is the only dental tissue with an epithelial derivation. The dental sacs comprise well-defined areas of undifferentiated soft tissue which are readily identifiable on radiographs of the upper and lower jaws as discrete radiolucencies. The reducing dental sacs remain visible on dental radiographs for approximately 4 years after eruption.

Eruption of teeth

Attritional wear is an inevitable consequence of the grinding function of the cheek teeth, and the incisor teeth are also subject to wear through their role in prehension. Equine teeth have a limited formation period. Once the dental sac is exhausted there can be no further formation of reserve crown and the length of a cheek tooth is greatest at the time when the dental sac reaches the limit of its active differentiation. Thereafter the only means to compensate for wear at the coronal surface is progressive eruption with a relentless reduction in the length of the reserve crown. Eruption proceeds at 2–3 mm per year or approximately 1 inch every 10 years. Whenever there is an absent tooth in the occluding arcade an overgrowth develops as eruption continues.

Ageing of horses by dentition

The patterns of eruption and attritional wear of the incisor teeth are used to estimate the age of horses. The age of horses up to 6 six years old can be determined with some confidence based on the sequence of eruption of the incisors, but thereafter the presence or absence of cups, marks and stars, the shape of the occlusal surfaces and the angle of occlusion, and the existence of Galvayne's groove provide no more than clues upon which to base a 'guestimate' which may be in error by many years.

The permanent cheek teeth also erupt in a constant sequence: 4, 2, 5, 1, 3 and finally 6. Thus, CT4 is the oldest tooth in each arcade and for orientation of radiographs has the shortest reserve crown, and CT3 is the last to erupt into the middle of the arcade and has the longest reserve crown.

Clinical signs of dental disease

Enamel pointing of the cheek teeth frequently causes ulceration of the lingual and buccal mucosae which in turn renders mastication and the free movement of ingesta around the mouth painful. Quidding (the rejection from the mouth of semi-masticated ingesta) is the result, and if the horse is unable to sustain an adequate nutritional level, wasting will follow.

Horses with periodontitis characteristically quid when fed hay as opposed to grass, silage and concentrated rations which they can manage satisfactorily until the condition is advanced.

Dental periapical suppuration should be considered when a horse is presented with a swelling at the ventral margin of the lower jaw or a swelling of the maxilla rostral to the facial crest. Discharging sinus tracts may or may not be evident. Swellings of the face rostral to the facial crest imply suppuration at the roots of CTs 1–3. The roots and alveolus of CT3 form the rostral wall of the rostral maxillary sinus.

A foetid unilateral nasal discharge may be caused by periapical dental disease involving CTs 4–6 in the upper jaw with secondary sinus empyema. It is unusual for swellings of the maxillary sinus region to develop as a result of dental suppuration.

Other signs of dental disease in the horse include:

• Reluctance in acceptance of the bit on one or both reins.
• Head shaking when ridden.
• Dorsal displacement of the soft palate (see 5.21).
• Discharging sinus tracts at the rostral margin of the pinna: this is the characteristic site of exit of tracts from a temporal teratoma (dentigerous cyst).

Physical examination of teeth

The examination begins with an external assessment of the face and jaws. External palpation of the cheek areas for pain may be helpful.

Thorough oral inspections of the conscious horse are difficult because of the limited range of opening which can be achieved. The use of Haussman gags in conscious animals is controversial due to potential dangers to attending personnel but will allow a satisfactory view of the dental crowns. A head-lamp can be helpful but it is important to palpate the dental arcades as well as to inspect them.

The intra-oral examination should take account of the following points.

• The overall conformation of the mouth: note any tendency to parrot mouth occlusion of the incisors and shear mouth resulting from an abnormal disparity (anisognathism) between the upper and lower jaws producing a particularly steep angle of wear.
• Evenness or otherwise of the arcades: any steps in the wearing tables may point to the previous total or partial loss of a tooth in the occluding arcade. Note any abnormal spacing where ingesta has gathered.
• The angle of occlusion between the upper and lower incisors is a general guide to age and the

tables should be inspected to make a rough estimation.

• In younger horses check for retention of temporary caps in the premolar dentition and for correct eruption of the permanent cheek teeth.

• Note the presence, size and position of 'wolf' teeth.

• In horses with a history of bit resentment palpate the interdental space of both upper and lower jaws seeking areas of unusual sensitivity, unerupted canine teeth, fractured 'wolf' teeth and evidence of bit trauma, especially in polo ponies.

• Enamel points on the cheek teeth: these form on the buccal aspect in the maxilla and the lingual surface in the mandible; note hooks on maxillary CT1 and mandibular CT6 which arise through superior prognathism.

• Ulceration of the buccal and lingual mucosae and any tendency to periodontitis: pass the fingers around both the lateral and medial gum margins of all four arcades rather than rely on visual examination.

• Displaced or fractured teeth (Figure 2): again, palpation is more accurate than inspection.

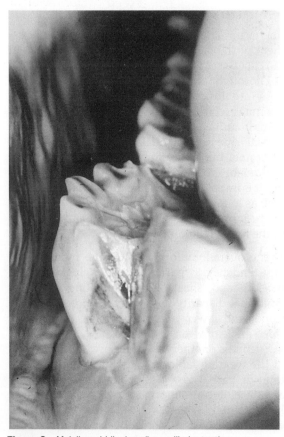

Figure 2 Malaligned (displaced) mandibular tooth.

• Halitosis often points to pocketing of stale ingesta in the clefts of fractured teeth or in periodontal defects. A foetid smell on the hand when it is withdrawn from the mouth is a sign that there is stale ingesta lodged somewhere in the mouth or that there is advanced dental necrosis.

• Abnormal wear on the incisors may point to abrasion in crib-biters.

• An assessment of the soft tissues of the mouth; palpate the tongue, noting motility, and check for ulceration or swelling of the cheeks and palate.

Some clinical circumstances dictate that the oral cavity of a horse should be examined in greater detail, possibly with sedation or even under general anaesthetic. A flexible endoscope can be useful for critical inspections of the least accessible areas of the mouth such as the interproximal spaces between teeth.

Radiography of teeth

Radiography provides information regarding erupted and reserve crowns; unerupted teeth; spacing between teeth; the apical areas; intraoperative progress; and, after extraction, the healing alveolus as well as changes in the associated mandible, maxilla and sinu-nasal structures including fractures and soft tissue masses.

Radiographic signs of dental disease include:

• Periapical 'halo' formation where the zone of rarefaction is surrounded by bone sclerosis. This may extend to a wider endosteitis and divergence of the lamina dura, the dense line of alveolar bone into which the periodontal fibres are imbedded and which normally closely contours the teeth. It is important to note that in immature teeth which have not yet completed formation of the reserve crown, the dental sacs are seen as radiolucencies in the periapical region but without bone sclerosis peripherally. The swellings associated with these dental sacs are often obvious at the ventral aspect of the mandible – so-called '3-year-old bumps', but less frequently prominent dental sacs can distort the facial outline giving some young horses a 'boxed' head conformation.

• Cement production tends to increase in the face of infection and this cementosis may be seen as pearls of density in the adjacent tissues.

• Sinus tracts may be seen passing through the mandibular cortex.

• Occasionally, protracted suppuration from a maxillary cheek tooth extends into the nasal chambers to produce metaplastic calcification of the conchal cartilages, sometimes described as 'coral' formation.

Indications for dental extraction

Incisors

The indications for the extraction of incisor teeth are rare, and include maleruption where the crown of the maldirected tooth impinges onto the gingival or labial soft tissues causing ulceration, or interferes with the position of other teeth, and devitalization through pulp exposure through trauma.

Wolf teeth

The presence of vestigial first premolar teeth is often assumed to be a cause of abnormal bitting behaviour and requests for their routine removal are common. Extraction is performed with the horse standing and sedation is rarely required. Cylindrical or half-curved dental elevators are used but the objective must be to extract the tooth intact and without fracture. Inadvertent damage to the palatal artery which lies immediately medial to the wolf tooth can arise if the instrument slips.

Canine teeth (tushes)

Maxillary canine teeth which fail to erupt, are delayed in eruption or which are positioned abnormally in the interdental space represent a more convincing cause of bit resentment in riding horses. These are large teeth where the erupted crown normally comprises no more than 30% of the total mass; extraction requires a general anaesthetic. The technique depends upon the creation of an osteoplastic flap over the lateral aspect of the tooth. The tooth should only be withdrawn by forceps when it is thoroughly loosened and the edges of the flap should be closed with absorbable sutures.

Cheek teeth

The most frequent indications for dental extraction in horses relate to the cheek teeth in either jaw and include:

- mandibular dental abscessation;

- infundibular necrosis (caries), with or without pathological fracture of the tooth or extension into the maxillary sinus;
- devitalization in fractures of the mandible and maxilla;
- malalignment;
- localized periodontitis.

Options for the extraction of cheek teeth

In order for extraction procedures to be successful it is essential to identify accurately which tooth, if any, is diseased and then to remove the *right tooth*, the *whole tooth* and to damage *nothing but the tooth*. Evidence that a tooth requires extraction is obtained from the external signs, detailed oral examination and radiography.

Extraction by repulsion aims to remove the bone directly over the apex of the diseased tooth before driving it into the mouth with a punch. A trephine may be used to make the osteotomy, but some prefer the greater exposure afforded by a maxillary flap for the more caudal teeth in the upper jaw. The roots of the first three teeth in the upper arcades are approached dorsolaterally through the relatively thin overlying bone plate, but CTs 4–6 can only be reached through the paranasal sinuses. For CT6 repulsion is performed through the frontal sinus with the line of repulsion passing medial to the orbit. In all cases accurate alignment of the instrumentation is essential before repulsion begins and for this radiography can be most useful. Postoperative radiographs should be taken to confirm that no dental fragments have been left *in situ*. Following removal of the tooth, the alveolus is subjected to thorough curettage and provision is made for postoperative irrigation and/or dressing of the site. The oral defect into the alveolus is sealed with a plug of material such as gutta percha or dental impression compound. Postoperative nursing aims to maintain a healthy alveolus as it fills with granulation tissue so that the plugging eventually falls away and the mucosal defect epithelializes. A malodorous discharge at the osteotomy site and the presence of ingesta in the alveolus, or the escape of fluid into the mouth during irrigation, are signs that the oral plug has been lost prematurely.

Complications which can arise from traditional dental repulsion include:

- traumatic fracture of the mandible;
- iatrogenic damage to neighbouring teeth;

- inadvertent disruption of adjacent structures:
  - nasolacrimal duct,
  - parotid salivary duct,
  - branches of linguofacial artery and vein,
  - palatine artery,
  - facial nerve,
  - infraorbital nerve;
- failure to remove the entire tooth – dental sequestration;
- sequestration of alveolar bone fragments;
- loss of the alveolar plugging with contamination of the socket by ingesta;
- oro-antral fistula formation.

Lateral buccotomy extraction comprises an incision through the cheek followed by removal of the lateral bony support of the alveolus and withdrawal of the tooth laterally. When the oral cavity is entered at the dorsal or ventral buccal cleft the tooth to be removed can be positively identified so that the possibility of extraction of the wrong tooth should not arise, and inadvertent damage to a neighbouring tooth is unlikely. The plate of bone lying lateral to the diseased tooth is resected to expose the reserve crown and roots of the tooth. Space for extraction is created by a longitudinal cut in the tooth using a burr. After removal of the tooth, the alveolus is packed with medicated dressing which is withdrawn over the following 14 days. The oral defect is plugged with a cap of dental impression compound and the buccotomy wound is closed in four layers starting with the gingival mucosa. Structures to be avoided during the buccotomy approach include the parotid duct, the buccal venous plexus and the dorsal buccal branch of the facial nerve. Extraction by this route is restricted to maxillary CTs 1–3 and mandibular CTs 1–5 because of the position of the masseter muscle, paranasal sinuses and local vasculature.

1.7   *Odontogenic tumours*

Temporal teratomas (dentigerous cysts) are discussed in Chapter 5, Section 1.

Pathogenesis

Neoplasia may arise from any of the dental tissues, including the cementum and periodontium, although odontomas and ameloblastomas, derived from dentine and enamel respectively, are more common. In general terms the greater the level of differentiation of the tumour tissues the more identifiable mineralized dental material will be present and the better the prospects of successful surgical extirpation. In contrast, poorly differentiated odontogenic tumours have no mineralized elements and are extremely aggressive.

Clinical signs

Although these tumours are rare in horses, the possibility of an odontogenic tumour should be considered whenever an animal develops a localized swelling of either jaw and particular suspicion should be raised when the patient is young coinciding with the time of greatest activity by the primordial dental tissues. However, ameloblastomas are more prevalent in older horses.

Diagnosis

A definitive diagnosis of odontogenic neoplasia can only be made after biopsy of the lesion but histological interpretation is both difficult and confusing. In addition, the result of the biopsy investigation may not be known until long after extirpation surgery has been performed because samples must undergo demineralization before they can be fixed. Thus, the major diagnostic challenge in the case of a horse presented with a swelling of either jaw is to differentiate between dental periapical infection, post-traumatic reaction including sequestration, dental impaction, cysts and tumours not related to dental tissues (see 1.8 below) and odontogenic neoplasia.

Treatment

Some benign well-differentiated lesions are amenable to surgical removal, but this may necessitate the use of an osteoplastic flap through the mandibular cortex or maxilla to expose and withdraw the tumour piecemeal. Postoperative radiographs are advisable to establish that all aberrant dental tissue has been removed. It may be necessary to close defects into the mouth with a sealant such as dental impression compound while closure by granulation takes place.

Prognosis

Some odontogenic tumours are not amenable to surgical removal by virtue of their size or invasive nature and euthanasia may be necessary. The surgical removal of a benign odontogenic lesion may necessitate the loss of a permanent tooth. Although the original lesion may cause considerable swelling, bony remodelling should improve the cosmetic result in the months which follow surgery.

1.8 Other tumours of the jaws

Pathogenesis

The non-dental tumours of the mandible or maxilla include osteoma, osteosarcoma, ossifying fibroma, fibrous dysplasia and juvenile mandibular ossifying fibroma. Horses in any age group may be afflicted by osteomas, and mature animals are more likely to be the subject of malignant bone tumours, but the other three tumours listed occur predominantly in foals. In addition bone cysts may arise in both upper and lower jaws.

Clinical signs

Apart from swelling of the affected jaw, horses with non-dental tumours or cysts may show dysphagia with quidding if there is mechanical interference with mastication, or may not accept the bit if the interdental space is involved. Expansive lesions of the maxilla may obstruct the flow through the nasolacrimal duct leading to an overflow of tears at the medial canthus.

Diagnosis

In the differential diagnosis of swellings of the mandible and maxilla, suppuration at the roots of the cheek teeth predominate, but bone cysts and non-dental neoplasms should be considered. An extensive firm swelling of either jaw of a foal represents an indication for further evaluation particularly by radiography. A definitive diagnosis requires histological confirmation.

Treatment

Localized lesions may lend themselves to excision on similar lines to those described for odontogenic tumours (see 1.7). Bone cysts should be opened and drained before curettage of the lining. Small cysts may be packed with cancellous bone but larger defects are better packed with medicated gauze which is steadily withdrawn in the postoperative period.

Prognosis

Similar prognostic guidelines apply to these lesions as to odontogenic tumours (see 1.7, 'Prognosis').

1.9 Abnormalities of development and eruption of teeth

Pathogenesis

Normal oral conformation comprises matched dental arcades which are of equal length and level in the longitudinal plain, but where the mandible is narrower than the maxilla. This anisognathism is essential to provide transverse shearing forces to crush and break up the ingesta. However, it does lead to enamel pointing through attrition (see 1.10). It follows that malocclusion will arise: (1) if the overall conformation of the jaws is defective, (2) if the full complement of teeth fail to develop, (3) if extra teeth are formed, (4) if any tooth fails to erupt into its normal position in the arcade.

1. Conformational defects of the jaws reflect the absolute length and width of the mandible.
   - Foreshortening of the mandible – brachygnathism – is an inherited defect causing parrot mouth with the upper incisors lying rostral to those in the mandible. Afflicted horses rarely show difficulty in prehension but the abnormal wear of the cheek teeth causes hook formation on the first tooth in the upper jaw and the last in the lower arcade. This latter hook can impinge onto the soft tissues behind CT6 in the maxilla and cause marked discomfort.
   - In normal horses the mandible is 30% narrower than the maxilla but on occasions the disparity is even greater. Such horses are described as 'shear mouthed' because the angle of wear of the cheek teeth is steep and readily produces sharp enamel points.
2. Partial anodontia – oligodontia – is rare in horses and occurs when the dental formula is incomplete. Radiographs show no identifiable

dental tissue where the dental sac of the absent tooth should be. Incisors and cheek teeth may be involved.

3. Supernumerary incisor and cheek teeth are occasionally identified. In the incisor dentition retention of a temporary tooth may confuse the diagnosis and also frustrates an accurate estimation of age. The most common site for a supernumerary tooth is caudal to CT6. The extra tooth often has poor alveolar bone support and ingesta is likely to migrate from the mouth into the caudal maxillary sinus provoking a putrid sinusitis.

4. The precise mechanisms which stimulate dental eruption are not known but the process should be correctly aligned with the eruption pathway clear of obstructions.

• Impactions are most likely to arise when a permanent neighbouring tooth lies across the path of the erupting crown or when the space between the teeth on either side is too narrow. CT3 being the last permanent tooth to erupt is most vulnerable. The result of impaction is that the crown cannot advance into the mouth and therefore the root structures build up aborally. Impactions are more common in the mandible and cause large discrete ventral swellings.

• Malaligned eruption of the mandibular cheek teeth is not uncommon and CT4 or 5 is usually involved. The malalignment consists of medial deviation of the dental crown and is often bilateral; secondary periodontitis causes the discomfort that leads to quidding.

• Malalignments and malformations of the incisor dentition can cause concern for owners because the deformities are so obvious, but the horse is rarely inconvenienced. Radiographs will be required to define the extent of what can be quite bizarre anomalies.

Clinical signs

Defects of oral conformation are likely to lead to progressive dysphagia, the signs of which derive from localized discomfort, i.e. quidding, and reduced efficiency of digestion, i.e. loss of bodily condition and the presence of poorly masticated herbage in faeces. Firm swellings may develop around the roots of impacted teeth.

Diagnosis

A detailed external and intraoral inspection with palpation is required to assess the overall con-formation of a horse's mouth. The absence of a tooth, with or without an external swelling of the jaw, is an indication for radiography which should resolve whether a tooth is present but not correctly erupted, whether a tooth has been present but has been partly or totally lost, or whether a tooth has failed to form. In addition, supernumerary teeth may be identified on radiographs.

Treatment

• Enamel points and hooks on maxillary CT1 and mandibular CT6 are removed by rasping ('float-ing') or resection performed routinely throughout the horse's life (see 1.10, 'Treatment and preven-tion').

• Impacted teeth should be extracted but this cannot be achieved by repulsion without damage to neighbouring teeth. Thus, extraction is likely to entail resection of the overlying bone plate and withdrawal of the affected tooth later-ally.

• Those supernumerary teeth which produce clinical signs should be extracted. In the case of a supernumerary cheek tooth in the maxilla, surgical invasion of the maxillary sinus com-partments may be necessary to achieve the extraction.

Prognosis

Orthodontic techniques to alter oral conforma-tion are as yet not proven in horses, although devices to adjust the incisor occlusion of foals have been used. The prognosis for successful long-term management of developmental dis-orders of the mouth and teeth generally relates directly to how early the anomaly has been identified. Uneven patterns of dental wear through abnormal positioning of teeth lead to overgrowth of some teeth and, less frequently, excessive wear of others so that the plane of occlusion becomes very irregular – 'wave mouth'. Correction of dental projections by rasping or resection becomes progressively more difficult the greater the overgrowths and the consequences may be irreversible in neglected cases. Impacted teeth can usually be removed without damage to the normal teeth on either side.

1.10 *Abnormalities of wear: abrasion and attrition*

Pathogenesis

Abrasion is tooth-against-object-against-tooth wear and in the horse this is typified by the effect of crib-biting on the incisor teeth.

Attrition is tooth-against-tooth wear. An angled plain of wear develops in the equine dental arcades through the skeletal discrepancy which exists between the widths of the maxilla and mandible: anisognathia.

• Even in 'normal' horses the mandible is 30% narrower than the maxilla with the effect that attritional wear leads to the formation of enamel points on the buccal aspect of the upper cheek teeth and the lingual aspect of the lower arcades.
• When the discrepancy is greater than 30% the angle of wear is steeper and the enamel points which form are sharper: such animals are described as 'shear mouthed'.
• In horses with parrot mouths there is an additional discrepancy in the lengths of the jaws so that hooks tend to form on maxillary CT1 and mandibular CT6.
• Enamel pointing of the cheek teeth represents the single most important dental condition of horses because it is the trigger for a group of disorders detrimental to oral health.

Clinical signs

The sharp enamel points cause ulceration of the buccal and lingual mucosae and mastication becomes a painful process. The normal free flow of food around the mouth is inhibited and partially masticated ingesta is either rejected, or becomes impacted at the gingival margins. Enamel pointing is inextricably linked to periodontitis (see 1.11 below), and quidding and poor bodily condition are the dominant signs.

Diagnosis

Confirmation of the presence of enamel pointing is generally straightforward provided that the patient is amenable to a visual and palpation assessment of the wearing surfaces of the cheek teeth (see 1.6, 'Physical examination').

Treatment and prevention

All horses should be subjected to routine rasping (floating) of the outer surfaces of the maxillary cheek teeth and the lingual aspect of the equivalent teeth in the lower jaw. This should commence at around 4 years of age when the permanent teeth have erupted and should be repeated every 6 months throughout life to take account of their continuous eruption and attritional wear. Some practitioners commence routine rasping even earlier in order to displace retained deciduous teeth and to establish a level bite plane.

Dental rasping is performed on standing horses; it may be helpful to have the mouth held open by a Haussman gag. Few patients require sedation for this technique to be performed. The objective of the technique is to maintain a level plain of occlusion by removing irregularities including the enamel points. Over-enthusiastic rasping to lower the bite plain is contraindicated because it renders the occlusal surfaces of the teeth smooth and eliminates the natural grinding action of the enamel ridges.

Hooks on the first upper and sixth lower teeth, particularly the latter, can impinge on the soft tissues of the opposite jaw. They are best resected using purpose-made instruments which guillotine the dental overgrowths without fracture of the remainder of the tooth or damage to neighbouring crowns.

Prognosis

Although enamel points are relatively easily controlled by routine dental care, prolonged neglect leads to periodontitis (see 1.11 below) and irreparable distortions of the occlusal plane of the dental arcades whereby some teeth become overgrown and others are excessively worn. Such horses are said to have a 'wave mouth'.

1.11 *Periodontitis*

Pathogenesis

The periodontium comprises a dense fibrous bridge between the cementum and the alveolar lining. Its function is partly to hold the tooth in the alveolus, partly to provide mechanical tolerance by being able to yield slightly when the teeth are subjected to extreme forces, and partly to provide tactile sensation.

Inflammation of the periodontium, periodontitis, is invariably the immediate sequel to gingivitis. Although neglected enamel pointing is the usual cause of gingivitis, any tendency to malocclusion through dental malalignment will also cause impaction of ingesta at the gum margins. Gingivitis leads to separation of the soft tissue attachments and opens the way for extension of infection into the periodontium. As periodontitis advances, not only does the periodontium itself separate but the alveolar bone is resorbed from the interproximal crests leading to progressive loosening of the tooth.

Clinical signs

A history of spitting out semi-masticated hay (quidding) while still being able to eat grass and other foods without difficulty is highly suggestive of enamel pointing and/or periodontitis. Horses with advanced periodontitis may quid grass as well as hay and there will inevitably be a tendency to loss of bodily condition.

Diagnosis

Confirmation of the presence of periodontitis is not always straightforward because the lesions at the gum margins may well not be visible during a conscious oral examination, but the concurrent presence of enamel pointing, malaligned or overgrown teeth should be detected by inspection and/or palpation. The presence of malodorous material on the fingers after palpation of the gum margins is practically diagnostic of the condition (see 1.6, 'Physical examination'). Periodontitis is a painful condition and this may limit the efficiency of a conscious assessment. A general anaesthetic may be needed to establish the extent of the disorder and the predisposing factors.

Treatment

Once the periodontal attachments between the alveolar lining and the cementum have become separated in the inflammatory process they cannot be re-attached. Thus, the objectives of treatment are to eliminate the factors which precipitated the condition and to provide a diet which the patient can eat more comfortably. The removal of irregularities from the wearing surfaces of the teeth should be followed by regular oral lavage to clear stagnant ingesta from the

periodontal pockets – most horses will accept flushing of the mouth with a hosepipe. Whenever the periodontitis results from the malalignment of a single tooth in an arcade, extraction is the most effective treatment option. However, dental malalignments are frequently bilateral and two extraction operations will be necessary.

Prognosis

Periodontitis is in essence an incurable disease unless the associated teeth can be extracted. When there is multiple dental involvement in one arcade, extraction is likely to be an impracticable or unacceptable option so that the clinical objectives are to limit the advance of the condition by regular dental rasping and by the provision of a manageable diet.

1.12 *Mandibular dental abscessation*

Pathogenesis

Periapical dental suppuration of the permanent mandibular premolar teeth (CTs 1–3) is most common in young horses, between 2 and 6 years of age, although older animals and more caudal teeth are sometimes involved. The cause of this condition is not known but suggestions include haematogenous infection, impaction, traumatic disruption of the blood supply to the tooth and transperiodontal migration of infection.

Clinical signs

The horses present with a swelling at the ventral aspect of the mandible corresponding to the affected tooth root and there are often discharging sinuses. These swellings can be dramatic and painful to palpate. It is likely that the local lymph glands will be enlarged. However, most afflicted horses do not show any reluctance to eat.

Diagnosis

Although the majority of cases of ventral mandibular swelling are caused by dental disease, there are other possibilities such as sequestration of bone fragments from the ventral cortex. Thus, a radiographic confirmation (see 1.6, 'Radiography') is essential before considering extraction. It is unlikely that there will be untoward findings on oral inspection.

Treatment

Treatment of mandibular dental abscessation has traditionally been aimed at extraction of the diseased tooth, and where the more rostral mandibular teeth are concerned the buccotomy technique is preferred (see 1.6). However, in younger patients, where the apical canals are wide and the vascular supply is generous, an intensive course of antibiotics can be effective. Alternatively, it is likely that restoration of the infected tooth by apicectomy and root filling will become the preferred treatment for older patients. For this technique to be successful it is necessary to take measures to check that there is no periodontal route of contamination; otherwise the suppuration will persist.

Prognosis

The prognosis for horses with mandibular dental abscessation is rather better than for animals subjected to extraction of the caudal teeth in the upper jaw (see 1.13 below) and most cases can be brought to a successful conclusion either by extraction or by root filling.

1.13 *Infundibular necrosis/caries*

Pathogenesis

Infundibular necrosis arises by dissolution of the cement and enamel layers which encircle the two infundibular lakes in each maxillary cheek tooth. There are no infundibula in the mandibular teeth and therefore this condition is confined to the upper jaw. It is only when the necrosis reaches the pulp chamber that the tooth becomes devitalized and even then the infection may be contained in some instances. Extension of infection through the apical canal precipitates suppuration in the adjacent tissues but pathological fractures of the teeth along a line of weakness between the infundibular lakes accelerate this process. The suppuration in tissues adjacent to the tooth roots is responsible for some cases of secondary empyema of the maxillary sinuses. On rare occasions the infection may extend into the cartilage of the nasal turbinates provoking conchal metaplasia – 'coral' formation.

Clinical signs

Horses with maxillary periapical dental abscessation, regardless of mode of origin, are likely to present with a facial swelling possibly with discharging tracts when CTs 1–3 are diseased, and secondary maxillary sinusitis with a putrid nasal discharge when CTs 4–6 are involved. Only those patients in whom displaced fragments of tooth irritate the oral mucosa are likely to show evidence of dysphagia.

Diagnosis

The lesions of infundibular necrosis are common but the extension of this disorder to devitalization of teeth and periapical suppuration is much less frequent. Thus, the diagnosis of infundibular necrosis is primarily oriented to the identification of abnormalities at the tooth roots and this is achieved by radiography (see 1.6, 'Radiography') and exploratory surgery. However, although the presence of necrotic infundibular lesions on oral inspection may not be clinically significant on its own, pathological fractures may be confirmed with or without displacement of dental fragments.

Treatment

There is no medical means by which to correct the devitalization of teeth and thus, the treatment of periapical abscessation depends upon the extraction of the offending tooth (see 1.6, 'Options'). The more complex root systems of the maxillary molar and premolar teeth make them less suitable for restorative dentistry by apicectomy and root filling.

Prognosis

In theory the removal of a devitalized tooth and the elimination of local extensions of infection should be an effective means to treat infundibular necrosis. However, the extraction of a maxillary cheek tooth is a major undertaking and protracted nursing may be required, particularly for the more caudal teeth where the roots lie within the paranasal sinuses.

1.14 *Oral trauma, mandibular fractures etc.*

Pathogenesis

Fractures of the teeth and jaws are not unusual and arise from falls, kicks by other horses and by bitting injuries and stick-and-ball trauma in polo. Fractures of the teeth themselves often lead to pulp exposure, devitalization and periapical suppuration. Restoration may be considered but it is rarely a practicable option and thus, extraction becomes the preferred course.

Clinical signs

In many instances, particularly with horses at pasture, the traumatic incident is unwitnessed. Occasionally compound fractures of the mandible or maxilla are sustained with an obvious external wound. Horses with these injuries may present with sudden onset swellings of the facial and mandibular areas, or inability to close the mouth with failure of effective prehension of ingesta and drooling of saliva. Neglected cases of orofacial trauma may show external evidence of suppuration from devitalized tissue and weight loss from an inability to prehend and masticate food.

Diagnosis

Fractures of the mandibular rami should always be considered in cases of acute onset swelling of the jaw. External palpation, a judicious intraoral examination and a careful radiographic investigation are used for damage assessment.

Treatment

Fortunately many fractures of the mandible and maxilla show little displacement of the bone fragments and surgical fixation is often not necessary. However, teeth may be devitalized either by infection through the fracture line or by disruption of their vascular supply. The decision whether or not to extract depends on radiographic findings but such surgery should be delayed at least until a firm fibrous union of the fracture site is present. At this time sequestra may also be located and removed.

• Open wounds over the sinuses may necessitate removal of loose bone fragments and debridement of gross contamination. An implanted irrigation catheter can be a useful measure to flush away blood and debris and should always be used when the sinus wall has sustained a full thickness penetration. The provision of broad spectrum antibiotic cover during the immediate post-traumatic period should be routine.

• Most palpable bone fragments, or those seen on radiographs, retain periosteal or endosteal attachments and heal uneventfully, but occasionally devitalization leads to sequestration with a discharge to the nose or skin surface. These should be dealt with by surgical removal as and when they arise.

• Grossly deforming depression fractures should be treated by elevation as soon as possible after the trauma; otherwise a fibrous union will form in a matter of days.

• Molar and premolar involvement in upper or lower jaw fractures is best managed on a 'wait-and-see' basis because generally it will not be possible to determine whether or not a tooth is devitalized in the acute phase and, in any event, the procedure of dental extraction will simply exacerbate the original trauma.

• Fractures of the incisor quadrants can be repaired effectively by in-and-out wire fixation of the loosened teeth to secure neighbours and/or to the mandible or premaxilla. Alternatively, the canine teeth can be used to anchor the fixation wires.

Prognosis

In general, the outlook for horses which sustain traumatic injuries to the jaws is favourable because there is often little displacement of bone in cases of fracture and the devitalization of soft tissue and teeth is limited.

1.15 *Oesophageal obstruction*

Aetiology

Acute obstruction of the oesophagus by impacted, dry ingesta ('choke') is typically associated with the ingestion of inadequately soaked sugar beet pulp in the United Kingdom. Equivalent offending possibilities occur in other parts of the world. The dry fibrous material swells with the absorption of saliva and an expanding bolus occludes the oesophageal lumen. Subsequent boluses compound the obstruction.

Clinical signs

Horses with 'choke' present in an acutely distressed state with copious reflux particularly of saliva to the nostrils.

Diagnosis

• The initial diagnostic challenge in cases of oesophageal obstruction is to differentiate this condition from other causes of acute dysphagia, most notably pharyngeal paralysis (see 1.4).
• The cervical oesophagus may be palpably distended with firm ingesta and the passage of a stomach tube beyond the pharynx is generally not possible.
• Inhalation tracheitis is invariably present and pneumonia is likely to follow if treatment is not promptly instituted.
• Endoscopy of the pharynx and ATDs may be helpful when the case history convincingly rules out access to the common causes of obstruction.

Treatment

• Many 'chokes' can be relieved by heavy sedation and the repeated administration of spasmolytics. This treatment can be continued for several hours or even days, but the distressed state of the patient and the likelihood of serious respiratory complications demand that conservative management should not be prolonged.
• If conservative therapy fails to relieve the obstruction after 24 hours, most clinicians advocate lavage under sedation or general anaesthesia.
• The author's preference is to institute vigorous lavage (under general anaesthesia) by stirrup pump through a stomach tube. Obviously the patient's trachea should be intubated and the head is positioned over a supporting bag with the nose inclined downwards. In this way the impacted ingesta is progressively washed back out at the nostrils.
• Other clinicians prefer to attempt relief using a similar lavage technique with the patient standing but sedated.

Prognosis

The prognosis for a complete recovery after the relief of an oesophageal obstruction is good. The possibility of recurrence of the 'choke' or of long-term stricture development can be reduced by withholding dry fibrous foods for 72 hours at least, followed by the gradual re-introduction of a soft diet. Oesophageal motility is likely to remain weak for several days. The inhalational tracheitis or bronchitis is usually self-limiting but broad-spectrum antibiotic cover should be maintained for 7–10 days.

Further reading

Baker, G.J. (1985) Oral examination and diagnosis; management of oral diseases. In: *Veterinary Dentistry* (Ed. C.E. Harvey). W.B. Saunders, Philadelphia.

Dixon, P.M. (1993) Equine dental disease: a neglected field of study. *Equine Veterinary Education* **5**, 285–286.

Lane, J.G. (1993) *Proceedings of the 15th Bain-Fallon Memorial Lectures: Equine Head and Hind Limb Medicine and Surgery*. Australian Equine Veterinary Association, Artarmon.

Lane, J.G. (1994) A review of dental disorders of the horse, their treatment and possible fresh approaches to management. *Equine Veterinary Education* **6**, 13–21.

Richardson, J.D., Cripps, P.J. and Lane, J.G. (1995) An evaluation of the accuracy of ageing horses by their dentition. Parts 1, 2 and 3. *Veterinary Record* **137**, 88–90, 117–121 and 139–140.

2 *Gastroenterology 1. Colic*

2.1 *Introduction*

Acute abdominal pain (colic) in the horse is one of the most frequent emergency conditions encountered in practice. It is one which understandably causes owners considerable concern and apprehension, and about which few of them have any real understanding.

Colic is not a specific disease or even a diagnosis, it is only a symptom and represents a challenge of differential diagnosis. It simply indicates that the horse has pain, usually but not invariably in its abdomen and usually related to its gastrointestinal tract.

The horse with gastrointestinal pain can behave in a variety of ways:

- In response to mild pain it may occasionally paw the ground, turn its head to its flanks, stretch out or lie down for longer than normal.
- When moderate pain is present, the horse may show pawing, cramping with attempts to lie down, kicking at the abdomen, laying down and attempting to roll or rolling and turning its head to its flank. The horse also continues to move when not rolling.
- If the pain is severe, sweating, dropping to the ground, violent rolling and continuous movement or pawing are the signs usually displayed.

Such behaviour is not confined to horses with alimentary colic and many of the signs described may be shown by horses which have one of a number of painful conditions unrelated to the gastrointestinal tract (i.e. 'false colic').

False colics

- A mare with uterine torsion in the last trimester of pregnancy will exhibit signs of moderate colic due to tension on the uterine broad ligaments brought about by rotation of the uterus.
- A horse with acute exertional rhabdomyolysis may suddenly stop during exercise, drop to the ground, sweat and kick out.
- Severe impairment of blood supply to the hind limbs caused by aortoiliac thrombosis can similarly cause a horse to exhibit signs normally associated with severe colic due to intense muscle pain.
- Severe bladder distension due to urethral obstruction by a calculus, pleuritis, liver disease and laminitis can also simulate gastrointestinal colic.

An intelligent approach to the management of colic requires an understanding of the causes and mechanisms of gastrointestinal pain and the pathophysiological changes which occur as the result of intestinal obstruction.

Alimentary (true) colic

The majority of colic cases are associated with disruption of the normal gut motility brought about by a variety of factors such as diet, management and parasites. Certain anatomical features of the equine alimentary tract, particularly the large colon, also predispose to obstruction.

Several factors can contribute to the pain associated with alimentary (true) colic:

- An increase in intramural tension is probably the most common cause and may be brought about by distension associated with excessive fermentation or accumulations of fluid and/or gas oral to obstructions caused by impaction, displacements or strangulation obstructions.
- Spasm of intestine associated with hypermotility and disruption of the normal coordinated contractions of bowel is another frequent cause.
- Pain due to tension on mesentery may well accompany intestinal displacements, torsion, hernias and intussusceptions.
- Ischaemia of gut brought about by vascular occlusion due to a large variety of strangulation obstructions to which the horse's intestine is prone results in the rapid onset of severe pain due to hypoxia which later abates when the gut becomes necrotic.
- Mucosal inflammation and irritation present in conditions such as acute salmonellosis results in mild colic.

The pain associated with these factors is designated *visceral pain* and is manifested by the clinical signs described earlier. The pain which follows rupture of the stomach or intestine causing widespread peritonitis due to escape of ingesta is classed as *parietal pain*. In marked contrast to horses with visceral pain those with severe parietal pain show great reluctance to move and obvious boarding of the abdominal wall.

Depending on the cause of the problem one or more of these factors may be contributing to the pain in individual colic cases. For example, in horses with spasmodic colic, hypermotility and incoordinated contractions are the sole cause whereas in the early stages of a strangulation obstruction, ischaemia, hypermotility, distension and mesenteric tension may all be contributing to the pain exhibited.

Classification of colic

Although acute abdominal pain is a relatively frequent occurrence, the majority of cases are benign and respond readily to medical therapy. The remainder are potentially life threatening and require surgical interference if the life of the horse is to be saved.

Colic can be conveniently classified into seven types:

1. Spasmodic.
2. Impactive.

3. Flatulent.
4. Obstructive.
5. Non-strangulating infarction.
6. Enteritis.
7. Idiopathic.

Colic cases with a mild or uncomplicated disease process fall predominantly into the first three categories while those with serious life-threatening conditions usually have obstructive lesions.

The earlier these various disorders are recognized and specific therapy instituted, the better is the prognosis for recovery. In the early stages pain is the common factor and there may be little or nothing to differentiate the benign from the serious cases. A basic understanding of the pathophysiology of gastrointestinal obstruction is essential if their effects on the clinical parameters used to diagnose and evaluate colic cases are to be recognized and interpreted correctly.

2.2 *Pathophysiology of intestinal obstruction*

Any interference, mechanical or functional, with the progression of intestinal contents constitutes obstruction.

- The obstruction is said to be *simple* when the obstructive process is not complicated initially by vascular compromise of the bowel.
- In *strangulating obstruction* there is obstruction to both blood supply and the lumen of the intestine.
- Obstructions due to intravascular occlusion of the blood supply, thought to be due to thrombolic incidences by *Strongylus vulgaris* larvae in the cranial mesenteric artery or its branches are described as *non-strangulating infarction*.

Simple obstruction

Small intestine

1. Physical obstruction of the small intestine usually occurs by impacted food material, stricture, or foreign body (Table 1), thereby preventing the passage of the large volumes of fluid produced in the upper alimentary tract from reaching the absorptive surfaces of the lower intestine so that it becomes sequestered or may be lost by nasogastric reflux.

Table 1 Small intestinal obstructions

I. Mechanical obstructions

Simple obstruction
A. Intraluminal
  1. Impacted food
  2. Ascarid impaction
  3. Foreign bodies
B. Mural
  1. Ileal hypertrophy
  2. Neoplasia
  3. Proximal duodenal stricture (foals)
C. Extraluminal
  1. Congenital strictures
    (a) Non-strangulating mesodiverticular bands
    (b) Meckel's diverticulum
    (c) Atresias
  2. Acquired strictures
    (a) Inflammatory (adhesions, abscessation)
    (b) Trauma
  3. Compression
    (a) Intra-abdominal abscesses
    (b) Displaced large bowel

Strangulating obstruction
A. Internal hernias
  1. Epiploic foramen
  2. Diaphragmatic
  3. Mesentery of small intestine
  4. Gastrosplenic mesentery
  5. Broad ligament of uterus
  6. Mesodiverticular bands
B. External hernias
  1. Inguinal
  2. Umbilical
  3. Traumatic
C. Pedunculated lipomas
D. Intussusception
E. Volvulus
F. Fibrous bands and adhesions
G. Arterial thrombosis

II. Paralytic Ileus
A. Primary – grass sickness
B. Secondary
  Postoperative
  Peritonitis

2. During one day this volume almost equals the extracellular volume of the horse (approximately 125 litres).
3. Systemically the prime concern in simple obstruction is depletion of plasma volume and reduction in cardiac output together with acid base disturbances.
4. Gas production by bacterial action continues and is even enhanced by the static medium. With continued secretion of fluids and build-up of gas, the intraluminal hydrostatic

pressure (IHP) increases and distends the bowel.

5. As stretch receptors in the distended intestinal wall are activated, the pain increases and becomes continuous.
6. Peristaltic waves diminish and then cease altogether as the intestinal lumen is progressively filled, leaving an atonic rapidly distending tube.
7. Once IHP increases to above 15 cmH$_2$O, absorption of water by the mucosa stops and instead water begins to flow from the mucosa into the lumen.
8. The increasing pressure and expanding volume of fluid causes reflux into the stomach, how soon after the onset of the obstruction depending on where along the small intestine it is located.
9. Increased vascular hydrostatic pressure in the bowel promotes leakage of protein rich plasma into the peritoneal fluid. Few leucocytes and no erythrocytes appear in the peritoneal fluid within the first 12–24 hours but may become more numerous with the progression of degenerative changes and vascular compromise of the intestinal wall.
10. Damage may be sufficient to allow absorption of endotoxins and cause production of prostaglandins and leukotrienes which may further compromise cardiovascular function. However, endotoxic shock plays only a very limited part in the fatal outcome of unrelieved simple obstruction. Hypovolaemia and altered blood electrolytes are the usual causes of cardiovascular collapse.

The severity of clinical signs associated with a simple obstruction of the small intestine depends on the degree of obstruction (partial or complete) and the level of obstruction (proximal or distal).

● In general, proximal obstructions have a more acute onset, produce greater pain, generate a greater volume of gastric fluid sequestration and have a more rapidly fatal course than distal obstructions. In proximal obstructions, large quantities of chloride are lost particularly if gastric reflux is removed by a nasogastric tube, resulting in metabolic alkalosis.
● Later the metabolic disturbance becomes complicated by acidosis secondary to hypoperfusion.
● Clinical signs resulting from distal small intestine obstructions develop more slowly and are generally less severe due to the compliance of the intestine and the ability to continue some fluid absorption until IHP initiates secretion.

● Established distal small intestine obstructions are characterized by metabolic acidosis with low serum levels of HCO$_3$.

Large intestine

1. Simple obstruction of the large intestine (Table 2) is usually due to impaction with food material, enteroliths or other intraluminal masses, or a change in position of the colon, e.g. nephrosplenic entrapment, and may be partial or complete.
2. In general the clinical signs or rate of systemic degeneration are much less dramatic in simple obstruction of the large intestine than in simple obstruction of the small intestine.
3. Incomplete obstruction allows the passage of small amounts of ingesta and gas.
4. Dehydration is mild at first because water still passes into the caecum where it is readily absorbed.

Table 2   Large intestine obstruction

I.   Simple obstruction
   A. Congenital abnormalities
      Atresia of large or small colon
   B. Impaction
   C. Intraluminal concretions
      1. Enteroliths
      2. Trichobezoars
      3. Phytobezoars
   D. Foreign bodies
      1. Sand
      2. Nylon
   E. Displacement of large colon
      Nephrosplenic entrapment
      Right dorsal displacement
      Retroflexion
   F. Strictures
      1. Adhesions
      2. Fibrous bands
      3. Neoplasia

II. Strangulating obstruction
   A. Volvulus
      Large colon
      Caecum
   B Intussusception
      1. Caecocaecal
      2. Caecocolic
      3. Colonic
   C. Pedunculated lipoma (small colon)
   D. Vascular disease
      Thromboembolic infarction
      Rupture of mesocolon
      Submucosal haematoma (small colon)

5. The production of volatile fatty acid and gas by bacterial fermentation is reduced due to decreased amounts of ingesta.

6. If the obstruction becomes complete, ingesta, and particularly gas, accumulate much more rapidly. Distension becomes marked and may become so great as to exert pressure on the diaphragm and vena cava, resulting in impaired pulmonary function and venous return to the heart.

7. Prolonged and/or marked distension of the caecum and colon may cause interference with mucosal perfusion leading to devitalization and possibly fatal rupture.

Strangulating obstruction

Small intestine

1. Strangulating obstructions of the small intestine include incarcerations, intussusceptions and volvulus (Table 1), and represent a common cause of acute abdominal crisis.

2. The same fluid retention which occurs due to simple obstruction with eventual reflux into the stomach is present, but because vascular compromise of the intestine is present at the outset, the pathophysiological changes associated with strangulation obstruction are more acute and severe.

3. The mortality rate of surgical cases with strangulation obstruction can be high.

4. The vascular compromise may be venous, or venous and arterial, but typical lesions will cause venous occlusion before arterial occlusion with consequent venous congestion.

5. Within minutes of strangulation occurring the involved segment of bowel and its mesentery become deep red as veins and venules are distended with blood. If there is immediate concurrent arterial occlusion the intestine becomes cyanotic.

6. More often, thicker walled arteries and arterioles resist compression and continue to pump blood into the distended veins and venules. As the involved intestine is engorged with blood, vascular stasis quickly develops and the segment becomes red/black in colour. Almost immediately, the vascular endothelium becomes more permeable and plasma diffuses into the tissue.

7. Within a few hours degeneration of vascular epithelium becomes so extensive that blood pours out of the distended vessel into the tissue (venous infarction stage) and eventually into the lumen.

The mucosal villi are extremely sensitive to hypoxia and within minutes after oxygen deprivation, ultrastructural morphological changes are evident.

- The epithelial cells slough in sheets starting at the tip of the villus and working towards the crypts.
- Within 4–5 hours the mucosal epithelium is completely necrotic.
- By 6–7 hours the degenerative effects of hypoxia have extended through the external muscle layer.

As soon as the mucosal barrier is damaged Gram negative bacteria and endotoxins permeate the lamina propria and submucosa.

- Early in the development of the ischaemic lesions, the bacteria and endotoxins readily gain entry to the circulation via viable tissue adjacent to the lesion.
- By 6 hours or possibly earlier, as the muscularis degenerates, bacteria and toxins leak through the serosa into the peritoneal cavity from which they are readily absorbed.
- Release of endotoxins into the general circulation results in damage to endothelial cells and platelets. Platelets are immediately stimulated and release the potent vasoconstrictor substances, thromboxane and serotonin. Damage to the endothelium increases vascular permeability, prostacyclin is released and neutrophils are stimulated, especially in the lungs and site of intestinal injury.
- The endotoxic shock is dose-related and is more severe the greater the length of bowel involved.

The clinical picture is acute with severe pain which is continuous and shows no, or only temporary, response to analgesics.

- The heart rate increases progressively and pulse quality deteriorates.
- Mucous membranes become congested and the capillary refill time increases.
- The PCV and total protein also rise progressively and the respiratory rate increases in response to developing metabolic acidosis.
- At first the peritoneal fluid is slightly serosanguinous with a mild increase in protein and leucocytes. As the strangulation process continues, all these substances increase dramatically and the fluid becomes flocculent and turbid.

Toxic neutrophils indicate leakage of toxins and bacteria.

- The clinical course is rapid and most horses with an untreated strangulation obstruction of the small intestine will die within 24–30 hours of the onset of disease from irreversible septic shock and marked vascular collapse. However, the deterioration in the animal's condition is such that for surgical correction to be successful, it must be carried out within a few hours of the obstruction occurring. Eighty per cent or more of cases may recover if operated upon within 8 hours.

Large intestine

1. Strangulation obstructions of the large intestine (Table 2) include intussusception of the caecum, torsion and volvulus of the large colon and incarceration of the small colon.
2. The pathophysiology is similar to that previously described for the small intestine but there are points of variance.
3. The rate of systemic deterioration can vary markedly between caecocaecal intussusception in which it is slow, and 360° torsion of the large colon which is the most rapidly fatal of all the intestinal obstructions of the horse.
4. Such is the size of the submucosal space in the large colon that venous occlusion can result in the horse losing half its circulating blood volume into the wall of the gut within 4 hours of a 360° torsion occurring.
5. Hypovolaemia is rapidly profound and the mucous membranes become pale and cyanotic.
6. The degeneration of the large surface area of bowel wall allows massive leakage of endotoxin and bacteria into the peritoneal cavity and the effects of endotoxaemia are added to those of the hypovolaemia.
7. Because of the short clinical course prior to death, rupture is not normally seen.

2.3 *Pharmacological management of colic*

Aims of therapy

Types of drugs

A wide variety of therapeutic agents are used to treat equine colic. They include:

- analgesics to control visceral pain,
- agents to normalize intestinal contractions during adynamic ileus,
- anti-inflammatory drugs to reduce the adverse effects of endotoxin,
- agents to soften and facilitate the passage of ingesta,
- drugs to improve cardiovascular function during endotoxic and hypovolaemic shock.

The aims of therapy are:

- to relieve pain,
- to restore normal propulsive motility of gut without masking the clinical signs that must be monitored for proper assessment of the horse's condition and progress,
- correction and maintenance of hydration and electrolyte/acid–base balance,
- treatment of endotoxaemia.

Relief of pain

Relief of visceral pain in horses with severe colic is essential on humane grounds and to minimize injury to the horse and attending personnel during evaluation and therapy. Even in mild cases, owner distress over animal pain is a consideration.

- The most satisfactory method of pain relief is the correction of the cause of increased intramural tension resulting from distension or spasm. However, this may take time and it is frequently necessary to achieve temporary relief of severe pain chemotherapeutically to allow a thorough clinical examination without risk of injury to the horse and attending personnel.
- It is important to select a drug which will accomplish the desired effect without creating complications such as depressing gut activity, predisposing to hypovolaemia shock or, most important, masking the signs of developing endotoxaemia.

Non-steroidal anti-inflammatory drugs (NSAIDs)

Amongst the most useful analgesics for both surgical and non-surgical disease are the non-steroidal anti-inflammatory drugs. The therapeutic and adverse effects of these drugs result from inhibition of cyclooxygenase enzyme-mediated biosynthesis of prostaglandins.

The NSAIDs commonly employed – dipyrone, phenylbutazone, ketoprofen and flunixin meglumine – differ greatly in efficacy in the treatment of visceral pain in horses.

Dipyrone

Dipyrone is a very weak analgesic drug that provides only short-term relief in a few cases of very mild abdominal pain. Combined with hyoscine N-butylbromide it is effective in relieving intestinal spasm. Its failure to help reduce or stop pain in individual cases should signal that a condition exists which is more serious than a simple intestinal spasm or tympanic colic.

Phenylbutazone

Phenylbutazone provides no greater relief from visceral pain than does dipyrone. However, the toxic side effects of phenylbutazone are numerous and include gastrointestinal ulceration and nephrotoxicity. For this reason the dosage should not exceed 4.4 mg/kg every 12 hours.

Flunixin meglumine

- Flunixin meglumine is the most effective of the NSAIDs used to control visceral pain in horses and has been shown to block the production of prostaglandins, specifically thromboxane and prostacyclin, for 8–12 hours after a single dose.
- The duration of analgesia produced varies from 1 hour to more than 24 hours depending on the cause and severity of the pain.
- Although this drug has basic side effects similar to phenylbutazone, the greater risk associated with its use devolves from its ability to mask clinical signs of intestinal strangulation or obstruction by reducing heart rate, relieving pain and improving mucous membrane colour.
- If administered to horses in which the precise cause of colic has not been ascertained, it is essential to closely monitor rectal examination findings, nasogastric reflux, peritoneal fluid, heart rate and respiratory rate over the next few hours.
- It should be administered to control severe pain and diminish the effects of endotoxins in horses needing transport to a referral centre for surgery.

Sedatives

Xylazine

- Xylazine produces both sedation and visceral analgesia by stimulating alpha$_2$ adrenoceptors in the central nervous system (CNS), thereby decreasing neurotransmission. At a dose rate of 1.1 mg/kg IV, the visceral analgesia it provides is similar to that of flunixin and the narcotics.
- The duration of effect of xylazine is much shorter (usually 10–30 minutes) than that of flunixin making xylazine more useful for controlling pain during evaluation of the cause of colic and of the need for specific therapy.
- Potentially detrimental side effects of xylazine include bradycardia, decreased cardiac output, transient hypertension followed by hypotension, ileus and decreased intestinal blood flow, and may affect its use in horses in shock.
- In contrast to the bradycardia, hypertension and intestinal hypotension which last only a few minutes, the ileus and hypotension can be prolonged.
- A reduced dosage of 0.2–0.4 mg/kg IV can be administered in an attempt to reduce the severity and duration of the side effects. Alternatively it can be used at the lower dosage in combination with a narcotic agonist such as butorphanol.

Detomidine

- Detomidine, another alpha$_2$ adrenoceptor agonist, is a more potent sedative and analgesic than xylazine.
- The same complicating effects are likely to be present for detomidine as for xylazine.
- Detomidine will reduce intestinal motility similarly to xylazine and can mask many of the signs which assist the clinician to diagnose the cause of the colic.
- Since it is such a potent drug, any signs of colic observed within an hour of administration are an indication that a severe disease is present, one which may require surgery.
- Therefore it is a useful drug when used with caution and preferably at the low dosage of 10 μg/kg IV.

Romifidine

Romifidine has a similar action to xylazine and detomidine. At a dose rate of 40–80 μg/kg IV it provides potent analgesia lasting 1–3 hours.

Acepromazine

Phenothiazine tranquillizers have a peripheral vasodilatory effect which is contraindicated in horses with reduced circulatory volume because they block the life-saving vasoconstriction which maintains arterial blood pressure and assures, within limits, perfusion of vital organs.

Narcotic analgesics

The analgesic and sedative effects of these drugs result from interaction with central and/or peripheral opioid receptors.

Morphine

- Morphine and pethidine are opioid receptor agonists.
- They are potent analgesics but can cause excitement in horses unless used in combination with drugs like xylazine.
- Morphine is known to reduce progressive motility of the small intestine and colon while potentially increasing mixing movements and increasing sphincter tone.
- The disadvantages of morphine are sufficient to discourage its use in horses with abdominal disease.

Pethidine

Pethidine is a narcotic agonist with few side effects and provides slight to moderate analgesia of relatively short duration in horses with abdominal pain. Used repeatedly it can potentiate obstructions due to impactions by reducing colon activity.

Butorphanol

- Butorphanol is a partial agonist and antagonist which gives the best pain relief of the drugs in this group, with least side effects.
- It can be used in combination with xylazine in horses with moderate to severe abdominal pain.
- The dose can vary from 0.05 to 0.075 mg/kg. Doses exceeding 0.2 mg/kg can cause excitement.
- Butorphanol reduces small intestinal motility but has minimal effect on pelvic flexure activity.
- It is potent enough to stop colic for short periods of time when it is due to severe intestinal disease but the pain from large colon torsion or small intestinal strangulation may not be altered.

Pentazocine

Pentazocine is a partial agonist which is more effective than dipyrone but less effective than xylazine and flunixin in relieving visceral pain.

Spasmolytics

Increased frequency of intestinal contractions as in spasmodic colic, or spasms occurring oral to intraluminal obstructions such as impactions cause pain which can be relieved by spasmolytics. Spasmolytic drugs include cholinergic blockers such as atropine and hyoscine N-butylbromide.

Atropine

Atropine is not recommended for use in horses with colic because its effect in relaxing the intestinal wall and preventing contractions can last for several hours or even days creating tympany and complicating the initial problem with ileus.

Hyoscine

- Hyoscine has a shorter muscarinic cholinergic blocking effect compared to atropine and is effective in relaxing the bowel wall.
- It is available in Europe combined with dipyrone and is administered at a dosage of 20–30 ml IV.

Laxatives

Laxatives are commonly used on horses with colic to increase the water content and softness of ingesta thereby facilitating intestinal transit. The most common indication for their use is the treatment of large colon impactions.

Mineral oil

Mineral oil (liquid paraffin) is the most frequently used laxative in equine practice and is administered at a dose rate of 10 ml/kg by nasogastric tube. Its effects are considered mild and it is safe for prolonged use. Vegetable oils can be used in the same way.

Psyllium hydrophilic mucilloid

- Psyllium hydrophilic mucilloid is a bulk-forming laxative which causes the fluid and ion content of faeces to increase by absorbing water.
- It is particularly useful for treating impactions caused by ingested sand.

Osmotic laxatives

Magnesium sulphate and common salt can be used as an osmotic laxative in horses but because undiluted they will cause enteritis by osmotic damage to the mucosal cells, each dosage of 0.5–1.0 g/kg should be diluted in 4 litres of warm water and administered by nasogastric tube.

Dioctyl sodium succinate (DSS)

- DSS is an amonic, surface-active agent with wetting and emulsifying properties.
- It reduces surface tension and allows water and fat to penetrate the ingesta.
- DSS can cause damage to the mucosa and increases fluid permeability of colon cells.

Intravenous fluids

Balanced electrolyte solution administered intravenously will sometimes provide a stimulus for intestinal motility. This treatment works particularly well for colon impaction and appears to stimulate motility in cases of ileus of the caecum and large colon. 'Overhydration' with Hartmann's solution at 40–80 l every 24 h helps provide secretion of fluid to soften hardened impactions.

Drugs that alter intestinal motility

Postoperative ileus is the most common indication for pharmacological manipulation of intestinal contractile activity.

Neostigmine methyl sulphate

- Neostigmine directly stimulates intestinal contractions.
- The duration of effect is very short (15–30 minutes) and the drug may decrease propulsive motility of the jejunum and delay gastric emptying in horses. It can cause abdominal pain by stimulating spasmodic regional contractions.

The preferred method of correcting postoperative ileus is to specifically antagonize the inhibiting neurogenic or hormonal processes.

Metoclopramide

Metoclopramide appears to have a beneficial effect on stomach emptying and small intestinal motility when used as a constant drip infusion at 0.1 mg/kg/hour over several hours or constantly until some response is seen. Higher doses up to 0.5 mg/kg can cause untoward nervous signs.

Domperidone

Domperidone, a newer dopaminergic antagonist does not cross the blood–brain barrier and at a dose rate of 0.2 mg/kg IV has been shown to block dopaminergic receptors and prevent postoperative ileus induced experimentally. It has potential for use in clinical cases.

Cisapride

- Cisapride is a substituted benzamide with gastrointestinal prokinetic properties.
- The mode of action is believed to be enhancement of release of acetylcholine from intramural interneurons leading to increased calcium flux.
- 10 mg tablets available for the treatment of motility disorders in humans can be administered either orally or *per rectum* in horses.

Erythromycin

- Erythromycin stimulates enteric motilin receptors.
- Action is independent of antimicrobial activity.

Fluids

While universally employed to support horses with severe intestinal obstructions requiring surgery, the value of this simple medical therapy for colic in a field situation has not been fully appreciated. The type of fluid and rate of administration will change from the initial therapy which is designed to replace the deficits, to maintenance therapy which is designed to keep pace with ongoing requirements. A third category of fluid therapy is overhydration which is most commonly attempted in horses with large colon impaction.

2.4 *Common types of colic*

Spasmodic colic

Aetiology and pathogenesis

- Spasmodic colic is the most common form of colic in horses that accounts for some 40% of all cases.
- It is a functional intestinal disorder that is rarely associated with histological changes of the mucosa. It is attributed to an increase in vagal tone causing increased peristalsis and a propensity to spasm.
- Bouts of spasmodic colic can be precipitated by weather changes, overexertion, chilling and feeding errors, feeding technique, feed quality and quantity. An individual predisposition to this type of colic is not uncommon.

Clinical signs

- The disease is characterized by severe paroxysmal attacks of colic lasting from 5 to 10 minutes and separated by pain-free intervals during which the horse's appearance and behaviour are normal.
- Initially systemic effects are very mild.
- The respiratory and pulse rates increase little during bouts of pain and return to normal when the horse is quiet.
- Often the hyperperistaltic activity is audible at some distance from the horse and frequently has a metallic sound.
- Faeces may be passed frequently and in small amounts and may have a soft to semi-liquid consistency.
- Rectal findings are seldom remarkable but one or more spastically constricted loops of small intestine may be palpable which may then relax. In other cases small amounts of gas may be evident in the jejunum or caecum.
- Barring possible complications such as volvulus or intussusception, the colic symptoms will pass in 4 to 6 hours.

Treatment

- The administration of a spasmolytic/analgesic drug combination such as hyoscine/dipyrone will quickly abolish the spasm and thereby relieve the pain. It is therefore both diagnostic and therapeutic.
- The treatment may be repeated after several hours if necessary but most cases show no recurrence of colic when the effects of the initial injection wear off.

Differential diagnosis

- Attacks of colic associated with physical obstructions of intestine also commence with loud hyperperistalsis (resistance peristalsis) but do not respond promptly to spasmolytic therapy.
- Colic attributed to reduced blood flow due to thromboembolic lesions of the cranial mesenteric artery caused by migrating strongyle larvae may have a similar clinical presentation but recent experimental work has questioned the mechanism involved.

Impaction colics

Impactions are among the more common medical colics encountered by equine practitioners (Table 3). Diagnosis is seldom difficult and impaction colics, particularly those of the large colon, can usually be resolved with conventional therapy.

The primary objectives of therapy are:

- maintain hydration,
- provide gastrointestinal lubrication,
- stimulate gastrointestinal motility,
- control pain.

Although the majority of impactions are treated successfully without recourse to surgical interference, prolonged obduration and complete obstipation (e.g. due to enteroliths) must be recognized and dealt with before bowel necrosis and rupture occur.

In the majority of cases of impaction the obstructing material comprises ingesta of a drier than normal consistency, but extraneous materials such as sand or foreign objects, like nylon hay nets, may be the cause.

Table 3 Anatomical sites and common causes of impactions

Stomach
  Corn
  Shavings bedding in neonates
  Food – secondary impactions in horses with liver failure
Duodenum/proximal jejunum
  Coarse ingesta
Ileum
  Ingesta – primary impaction or secondary to ileal
    hypertrophy, tapeworm infestation, and grass
    sickness
Caecum
  Coarse roughage
  Often underlying motility problem
Large colon
  Sand
  Enteroliths
  Dehydration (e.g. ileal impaction secondary to anterior
    enteritis)
  Grass sickness
Pelvic flexure
  Coarse roughage
  Can be concurrent with right dorsal colon impaction
  Sand
  Grass sickness
Transverse colon
  Enteroliths
  Foreign bodies
  Sand
Small colon
  Enteroliths
  Foreign bodies
  Meconium in foals
  Faeces – may be associated with *Salmonella* infection
Rectum
  Cauda equina neuritis
  Perirectal abscesses

Prevention

Optimal management practices aimed at preventing impaction colic include:

- avoiding excessively fibrous feeds (especially horses which eat straw bedding),
- providing adequate water supply,
- maintaining adequate parasite control and dental care,
- removing foreign objects such as baling twine from food sources.

Clinical signs

- Rapid consumption of excessive amounts of corn can result in gastric and duodenal impactions.

- Pain is usually moderate and frequently intermittent.
- Signs include pawing, lying down and flank watching.
- Horses with an impacted pelvic flexure located within the pelvis adopt a stance for urination frequently and appear to find relief by lying in dorsal recumbency.
- The pulse may be slightly raised (40–50 per minute) with increases related to hypovolaemia and pain.
- The packed cell volume (PCV) and plasma protein are often normal but can be slightly increased if the impaction involves the small intestine or if it has been present for more than 24 hours in the large colon or caecum.
- Auscultation of the abdomen usually reveals a decrease in borborygmi but in horses with large colon impactions, bouts of pain are often concurrent with bowel activity.

Diagnosis

Rectal examination is the most important diagnostic procedure enabling firm masses which can be gently indented with the fingers to be identified within the bowel lumen.

- Impacted ileum may be recognized as a firm tubular structure the diameter of one's forearm to the left of the caecum early in the course of the condition before it is masked by numerous loops of distended jejunum.
- Primary impaction of the pelvic flexure is characterized by a firm evenly-filled viscus which is often located on the pelvic floor.
- The firmness and extent of the impaction should be noted so that the response to treatment can be evaluated at subsequent visits.
- The thickness of the wall of the colon should also be checked. Oedema indicates a degree of vascular occlusion usually due to torsion.
- Transverse colon impactions may be out of the examiner's reach and may be larger, thus requiring a more prolonged course of treatment with a guarded prognosis.
- Sand impactions may be suspected whenever faeces retrieved during rectal examination contain sand or grit. If water is added to faecal material in a rectal sleeve and massaged, the sand will settle into the fingers of the glove.

Secondary impaction of the colon is not uncommon in conditions causing dehydration such as ileal impaction, grass sickness and anterior enteritis.

This can be recognized by the fact that the colon is contracted down on the firm ingesta and the constrictions and sacculations of the ventral part are very distinct.

Caecal impactions are particularly difficult to assess since digesta may bypass the caecum while the impaction is present:

– Physical signs are similar to large colon impaction except that pain may be continuous and severe when distension is marked.
– The peritoneal fluid may demonstrate increased protein and cellular changes indicating compromised bowel.
– Impaction of the overhanging part of the base of the caecum can be palpated *per rectum* if the horse is not too large.

Small colon impactions present as a long tube evenly filled with faeces extending forward from the rectum. Generalized tympany of large colon and caecum is a feature of such impactions.

In neonates meconium retention can be felt *per rectum* with a finger at the pelvic inlet.

Treatment

Medical management of colonic impactions is relatively simple and involves the use of nasogastric intubation for lubrication and hydration, parenteral fluid therapy and the control of pain.

1. Lubrication of the intestinal tract is achieved using mineral or vegetable oil (4 to 8 litres) either on its own or mixed with electrolyte supplements.
   • This should be administered via a nasogastric tube by gravity or carefully using a stomach pump.
   • If necessary this is repeated at 12 and 24 hours.
2. While not necessary in horses with mild impactions of short duration, the intravenous administration of balanced electrolyte solution (10–15 litres) at least twice daily is of considerable benefit to those with severe impactions. The overhydration produced initiates fluid secretion into the intestine in order to directly hydrate and soften the mass of ingesta.
3. Since softening of the obstruction requires gut motility to mix the oil with the mass of ingesta, it is important to use an analgesic which does not depress colonic contractions. Flunixin meglumine 0.5–1.0 mg/kg at 8 to 12 hour intervals is the analgesic of choice. Hyoscine/dipyrone is a suitable alternative.
4. Due to the risk of rupture, horses with caecal impaction should always be considered candidates for surgery and may require an ileocolostomy to prevent recurrence of the problem.
5. Horses with impactions should be bedded on paper or shavings or muzzled if on straw. They should be allowed water ad libitum but all food should be withheld until the impaction has cleared.
6. Horses with impactions generally benefit from exercise.
7. The use of gastrointestinal stimulants such as neostigmine is not necessary and in severe cases bowel contraction, rather than propulsion, around the impaction causes pain.
8. Excessive tympany together with increasing episodes and intensity of pain requiring frequent administration of analgesics indicate the need for surgical intervention. It should be remembered that large colon impactions may be accompanied by torsion or displacements.
9. Surgical removal of impactions is indicated whenever a definitive diagnosis confirms that the obstruction cannot be cleared medically as with enteroliths or faecaliths or when sustained medical treatment has become unsuccessful and the horse becomes subject to bowel necrosis. This stage is reached much sooner in the case of caecal impaction than with large colon impaction. Early surgical intervention is also required in extensive small colon impactions due to the severe tympany and a rapid progression toward necrosis.
10. Meconium retention in neonates rarely requires surgical interference. Soapy enemas carefully administered via a soft rubber catheter together with intravenous fluid therapy and 8 oz of mineral oil orally are successful in clearing the impaction in the vast majority of cases.
11. Ileal impaction is the most common cause of simple obstruction of the small intestine.
    • It may be primary, or secondary to thickening of the wall of the distal ileum or the caecal mucosa at the ileocaecal orifice associated with a heavy tapeworm burden. It is also common in grass sickness cases.
    • Although impactions involving only a short length of ileum may clear spontaneously or in response to a spasmolytic

drug such as hyoscine, more extensive impactions require surgical intervention. Delay in carrying out surgery can result in postoperative ileus due to the great increase in intraluminal pressure brought about by sequestration of large volumes of fluid and gas in the jejunum.

Flatulent colic

Aetiology and pathogenesis

• Flatulent colic results from accumulation of excessive volumes of gas in the gastrointestinal tract. The overdistension of the viscera stimulates pain and pressure receptors causing mild to severe colic.
• The condition is usually due to increases in fermentation or ineffectual gastrointestinal motility or may be secondary to partial luminal obstruction.
• Distension inhibits vagal motility while fermentation continues.
• Since the release of gas is normally dependent on escape through the gastrointestinal tract, gas accumulates in the stomach, caecum and large colon.
• The source of the gas includes endogenous production of volatile fatty acids and other byproducts of fermentation of feedstuffs, and air in horses which are habitual crib biters and wind suckers.

The causes of flatulent colic include:

• interruptions in gastrointestinal motility from stress, excitement or pain,
• impactions,
• displacements,
• late pregnancy,
• ileus secondary to anaesthesia, surgical manipulation of intestines, vascular compromise (thromboembolic colic) and liver disease.

Contributory factors related to management include:

• feeding highly fermentable substrate (grain overload),
• feeding horses when exhausted or overheated,
• cold water engorgement and poor feed quality.

Behaviour-associated contributory factors include:

• aerophagia,
• inadequate mastication,
• rapid feed engorgement.

Clinical signs

• The clinical signs of flatulent colic depend on the rate of gas accumulation and the part of the gastrointestinal tract involved. They vary from merely being off feed to the acute distress which accompanies gastric distension.
• The temperature, pulse and respiratory rate will usually be elevated in proportion to the clinical signs.
• The mucous membranes are pale and the respirations become more rapid and shallow as the distended viscera occupy a greater proportion of the abdominal cavity and place pressure on the diaphragm.
• Because the stomach is situated immediately adjacent to the diaphragm, shallow respirations occur more consistently with gastric tympany.
• Rectal examination reveals gas-filled sections of intestine. Although the stomach itself is infrequently felt, the spleen may be felt extending more caudally than usual. The caecum is fixed at its base and therefore can be located in the upper right caudal quadrant of the abdomen. Distended large colon can readily be identified from its location, size and the presence of longitudinal bands except at the pelvic flexure.
• The shape of the abdomen changes in response to the intra-abdominal distension. Large colon tympany tends to result in bilateral abdominal distension, while caecal tympany often flattens and elevates the region of the right paralumbar fossa.
• Auscultation of the abdomen is valuable in determining the presence or absence of intestinal sounds.
• Percussion will aid in identifying more accurately the region of gaseous distension.
• The rate and location of gas accumulation tends to govern the intensity of pain. Gastric distension results in severe signs of pain while with distension of the caecum and colon the pain tends to be dull and intermittent.

Therapy

The primary objective of therapy is to evacuate the gases from the region of distension and prevent further formation.

1. Stomach tubing is always indicated as a diagnostic procedure in colic, and whenever gastric tympany is present, the elimination of gases through the tube will provide immediate, although possibly temporary, relief of clinical signs.
2. In very severe cases trocharization of the caecum can be employed to bring about a similar, rapid decompression. However, in the majority of cases the tympany is not immediately life threatening and these horses frequently benefit from 15 to 20 minutes trotting on a lunge rein.
3. Medical treatment should include supportive therapy to relieve pain, (α2 agonist $\pm$ butorphanol and intravenous fluids).
   • Mineral oil is often used to coat fermentable substrate and to lubricate the food material within the gastrointestinal tract for easier passage.
   • Metronidazole and/or neomycin by mouth, twice daily, can also be of value.
4. Decompression by trocharization should be used only when the sublumbar fossae are very distended, to prevent rupture. It should be taken into consideration that the character of the abdominal fluid will be changed shortly after trocharization so that the value of abdominal paracentesis for diagnosis is decreased. Trocharization of the caecum is carried out via the right sublumbar fossa. The site is clipped and surgically prepared. A local anaesthetic skin bleb and a small stab incision with a number 11 scalpel blade facilitates the insertion of a 10 cm 14 or 16 gauge needle through the abdominal wall into the caecum. A rush of gas from the needle will occur immediately and the needle should be left in place until the flow ceases. Ten to 20 ml of a broad spectrum antibiotic is injected through the needle as it is withdrawn as an aid to the prevention of local peritonitis. Systemic antibiotics may further suppress diffuse peritonitis.

Prognosis

The prognosis for uncomplicated cases of flatulent colic is usually good. However, prolonged or recurrent cases require further investigation for an underlying disorder affecting gastrointestinal motility or lumen patency.

2.5 *Grass sickness*

See Chapter 3.

2.6 *Anterior enteritis (proximal enteritis, gastroduodenal jejunitis)*

The term anterior enteritis is used to describe an acute clinical syndrome characterized by abdominal pain, ileus, gastric distension and hypovolaemic shock often complicated by endotoxic shock. This relatively new intestinal disease involving the duodenum and proximal jejunum was first recognized in Georgia, USA in 1977. It was subsequently seen with increasing frequency in the south eastern and south western United States and in Canada. The condition was reported in West Germany in 1981 and was first seen in the UK by the author in 1984.

Clinical signs and diagnosis

• The disease can be diagnosed for certain only at surgery or autopsy but in most cases the signs are said to be specific enough to allow a clinical diagnosis to be made.
• Horses present with moderate to severe colic frequently accompanied by marked sweating.
• Depression may replace the colic at 12–24 hours, although most horses continue to show intermittent pain.
• Ileus is a consistent physical finding.
• Gastric distension occurs secondary to the ileus, hypersecretion and decreased absorption of fluid within a few hours of the onset of the condition and in extreme cases may result in stomach contents being expelled via the nose.
• The volume of gastroenteric fluid obtained on nasogastric intubation varies from 5 to 30 litres. The fluid is usually foetid, alkaline and brown tinged. It may be positive for occult blood.
• Most horses have fever and an accompanying leucocytosis.
• Varying degrees of dehydration and endotoxic shock are seen. Heart rate (70–100) and respiratory rate (30–60) are elevated and capillary refill time is extended to 4 to 6 seconds. Mucous membranes are congested and injected and in cases presenting in severe shock, are cyanotic.

- Usually there are no intestinal borborygmi evident on abdominal auscultation.
- Rectal examination reveals a relatively empty intestinal tract except for a thickened or slightly distended segment of the distal duodenum as it courses over the base of the caecum. Distended loops of proximal jejunum may be palpated to the upper right quadrant. The large colon is reduced in size and contracted down onto the contents which are dry and firm secondary to the breakdown of intestinal fluid transport.

Laboratory data

- The packed cell volume and total plasma protein values reflect severe dehydration and are often in excess of 0.55 l/l and 85 g/l respectively.
- Serum electrolytes are usually normal. However, mild to moderate hypochloraemia is present in 50% of cases.
- There may be acidosis or alkalosis depending on the amount of gastric reflux and the severity of shock.
- Abdominocentesis findings tend to be unremarkable unless mural necrosis is advanced. The peritoneal fluid is usually straw coloured and either clear or slightly clouded. Microscopically some red blood cells are present with normal numbers of leucocytes. The total protein in the fluid is elevated to more than 30 g/l. The absence of blood staining of the fluid can be of value in differentiating this syndrome from strangulation obstruction of the small intestine.

Gross intestinal lesions

- At laparotomy or autopsy, varying lengths of the proximal small intestine are found to be slightly distended. Rarely is its diameter greater than 7 cm and the intraluminal pressure is usually less than 10 cmH$_2$O.
- The duodenum and proximal jejunum have red and yellow streaks. The serosal surface is mottled with petechial and ecchymotic haemorrhages.
- The wall of the affected gut is slightly thickened but is not as oedematous as infarcted or obstructed intestine.
- In some cases the lesions may progress to focal necrosis of the intestinal wall.
- Haemorrhages may also be seen in the meso-duodenum and mesojejunum together with sub-serosal oedema at the junction of the mesentery and intestine.
- The rest of the small intestine is contracted.
- No external signs are visible on the stomach.

Histopathology

- The histological lesions are confined to the duodenum and proximal jejunum in most cases but can extend from stomach to colon.
- There is submucosal and mucosal oedema, and hyperaemia with sloughing of the villous epithelium.
- In severe lesions there is neutrophilic infiltration and degeneration in the submucosa and haemorrhages in the muscularis and submucosa.
- The severity of the lesions varies between cases.
- The disease seen in Germany also has an associated haemorrhagic gastritis which is not commonly seen in cases in the UK or the USA.

Aetiology

- The aetiology of anterior enteritis is uncertain.
- *Clostridia* spp. and *Salmonella* spp. have been suggested as possible causes. The histological lesion is similar to clostridial enteritis seen in young pigs but is unlike the recognized clostridial enteritis in the horse which usually produce lesions in the caecum and colon. *Clostridium perfringens* have been found in over 60% examined by the author.

Treatment

In the absence of an identified cause for this condition, the management of anterior enteritis has been directed primarily at supportive therapy rather than at eliminating a specific aetiological agent. Various methods of treatment have been reported, both conservative and surgical.

The major *medical* therapeutic objectives are:

1. Maintaining adequate decompression of the stomach and intestine by nasogastric intubation as needed.
2. Controlling the effects of endotoxaemia.
3. Replenishing lost fluids and electrolytes.
4. Encouraging resumption of intestinal motility.

The use of antibiotics has been a matter of debate.

Maintenance of fluid and electrolyte balance in many cases of anterior enteritis requires a major effort and financial commitment; the need for infusion of up to 70–80 litres per day is not particularly unusual.

The paralytic ileus associated with this syndrome is the basis of the whole clinical problem and the most difficult thing to deal with therapeutically. Cisapride, which has prokinetic activity in relation to the intestines as well as the stomach, has not been as clinically effective as might have been expected from experimental studies.

Surgery is an option that some find unacceptable because the stress involved might make the prognosis worse. In the experience of some authors who favour medical therapy a high percentage of horses with anterior enteritis undergoing general anaesthesia and ventral midline laparotomy succumbed to circulatory shock and/or laminitis. However, if laparotomy and decompression of the intestine are completed rapidly and if adequate blood pressure is maintained under anaesthesia, there is no greater risk of postoperative shock or laminitis.

Following the isolation of *Clostridium perfringens* from one of the first horses referred to the author, the following treatment regimen was developed and employed for all subsequent cases:

• Horses suspected of having anterior enteritis are anaesthetized, and via a short midline laparotomy the characteristic serosal discoloration of the proximal small intestine is identified and other conditions eliminated by systematic examination of the alimentary tract.
• The intestine is decompressed by gently massaging its contents into the caecum.
• When large volumes of fluid contents are present, the caecum is evacuated via a small enterotomy incision near its apex.
• 2 g metronidazole is administered IV as soon as the diagnosis is confirmed.
• Hartmann's solution is administered throughout the operation.
• Every effort is made to keep the procedure as short as possible. The average operation time is 30–40 minutes.
• Nasogastric intubation is performed on recovery from anaesthesia and at 3 hourly intervals until no fluid is obtained on two successive occasions.
• Low dose flunixin (0.25 mg/kg three times daily) and metronidazole therapy is carried out for 2 to 3 days.
• Most cases show a steady fall in heart rate and packed cell volume which takes 24–72 hours to return to normal. Very few horses have any significant gastric reflux and this ceases 12 to 24 hours after surgery. Intravenous fluid therapy is continued during this period. Horses which have no postoperative gastric reflux and show a progressive return of normal gut activity are allowed small amounts of water to drink at hourly intervals until normal hydration is achieved and then slowly returned to normal rations.

The recovery rate with this treatment regimen has been extremely good (95%) with only one or two horses having postoperative complications.

The advantages of surgery in the treatment of this condition can be summarized as follows:

• It overcomes the difficulty in differentiating anterior enteritis from a physical obstruction and from grass sickness.
• By resorting to surgery without delay, complete decompression of the distended proximal small intestine can be achieved, thus encouraging the return of normal circulation and peristalsis.
• It also ensures that should the horse in fact have a physical obstruction, its correction is not delayed while conservative therapy of suspected anterior enteritis is instituted and its effects evaluated.
• As a result of the rapid return of normal gut activity and cardiovascular status, the horses require very little postoperative care and are discharged within 8 days of admission. This helps to keep down the cost to the client.
• The prolonged period of inactivity necessary after surgery is a disadvantage. However, when horses with anterior enteritis have been treated medically it is advisable to allow adequate time for them to recover fully because of the possibility of recurrence.

2.7 *Approach to diagnosis in colic cases*

The majority of cases of colic, probably in excess of 90%, respond to medical therapy.

The primary aim of the initial examination is to distinguish horses with a mild or uncomplicated disease process from those with a potentially life-threatening disorder requiring further monitoring, surgery or intensive care. The earlier these serious disorders are recognized and specific therapy instituted the better is the prognosis for recovery.

In cases of a serious nature, any attempt at a diagnosis is often made under stress and with less than favourable conditions, but in mild cases there will be adequate time to examine and initiate therapy without placing the patient at risk. However, even when a horse has mild colic, the veterinarian should complete a thorough examination and not be caught in a trap of letting the response to treatment guide the decision-making.

The ideal goal of the systematic examination is an aetiological diagnosis and it should include the following:

- Signalment
- Observation
- Clinical examinations
- Laboratory investigations

The cause of the colic and the length of time it has been in existence will largely determine whether a diagnosis can be made at the initial examination or requires the procedure to be repeated at 2 hourly intervals. It is important that the results are carefully documented. By comparing findings recorded at different times, the veterinarian is able to discern important trends in the course of the illness. This is particularly important if a subsequent examination is carried out by another veterinarian in the practice. A printed colic sheet listing the various procedures and providing spaces for recording the findings at each examination is of considerable value.

Signalment

1. The age of the horse should signal the veterinarian to consider specific conditions – for example meconium impaction in a foal 1 to 2 days old; ileal intussusception in yearlings or strangulating lipomas in horses older than 15 years.
2. Some conditions have a sex predisposition. Inguinal hernia affects stallions while large colon volvulus and uterine torsion typically affect mares.
3. The breed of horse may occasionally suggest certain disorders. Large bodied horses appear to have a high prevalence of nephrosplenic entrapment of the left colon and Standardbreds have a predisposition to inguinal hernia.

History

1. The most important factor of the history is the time which has elapsed since the onset of clinical signs. This may be known precisely but often can only be estimated, for example, in the case of horses which are found in colic at the owner's first inspection of the day, having been seen normal for the last time the previous evening. It is essential that a reasonably accurate assessment of the likely duration is made in order that the significance of the clinical findings can be evaluated.
2. The remainder of the history should include the general history relating to husbandry and management; the recent history and management and more specific details related to the present colic episode (Table 4).
3. The general history may not help to identify the specific cause of the colic episode under investigation but information such as a history of inadequate worming may be significant. Recent changes in housing, bedding materials, quantitative or qualitative changes in feed may be directly involved, e.g. horses which are brought in from pasture and bedded on straw eat the bedding in preference to hay and develop large colon impaction as a consequence.
4. In foals with heavy ascarid burdens, treatment with anthelmintics can lead to obstruction of the small intestine by dead worms. Caecocaecal intussusception following administration of an organophosphorus anthelmintic is another example where the recent worming history may be significant.

Table 4 History of the colic case

General history
1. Housed or at grass
2. Feed
3. Use
4. Daily routine
5. Parasite control
6. Past medical history

Recent history
1. When last fed
2. Consumption of feed and water
3. Any recent changes in feeding, bedding, housing or routine
4. Recent worming
5. Pregnancy
6. Recent exercise

Details relating to present colic episode
1. Degree and any changes in pain and how manifested
2. When last defecated
3. Sweating
4. Any treatment given and response
5. Previous episodes of colic or abdominal surgery

5. A history of previous illness may be important, e.g. in a horse with chronic colic an episode of strangles several weeks earlier may suggest a mesenteric abscess.

Questions relating to the present colic episode should specifically address the following:

- How severe has the pain been and has it altered during the time it has been observed?
- When did the horse last defecate and what was the character of the faeces?
- Has the horse shown specific behaviour such as playing with water or adopted any unusual postures?
- Could it have gained accidental access to too much highly fermentable feed?

Clinical examination

Observation

- Whilst the history is being taken, the horse may be inspected in its stall and its behaviour observed.
- The nature and the degree of colicky signs currently being shown are noted.
- Skin abrasions about the eyes and over the tuber coxae are indicative of rolling and other violent behaviour prompted by severe pain.
- Marks on the wall of the box caused by the horse's kicking and excessive disturbance of the bedding, or flattening of an area of grass in horses at pasture are further evidence of severe pain consistent with a severe intestinal obstruction.
- Horses in which a strangulating obstruction has occurred only within the past 3 or 4 hours or so may still be exhibiting signs of severe pain, whereas one in which the obstruction is of much longer duration and the segment of gut involved has undergone advanced necrosis will show no or very few signs of overt pain. However, although apparently calm it will be showing signs of intense depression, e.g. standing with its head low and taking no interest in its surrounding. This 'stage of indolence' is associated with severe endotoxaemia and is often mistaken by the owner of the horse as an indication it is improving.
- Such an evaluation of the circumstantial evidence and presenting signs at the time of examination allows a reasonably accurate assessment of the duration of the problem when the time of onset is unknown.
- Other signs to note are evidence of abdominal distension, sweating, or muscular tremors.

Table 5 Clinical examination

1. Cardiovascular system
   (a) Rate and quality of pulse
   (b) Appearance of mucous membranes
2. Examination of abdomen
   (a) Abdominal distension
   (b) Auscultation and palpation
   (c) Rectal examination
   (d) Paracentesis abdominis
   (e) Nasogastric intubation
3. State of peripheral perfusion and hydration
   (a) Capillary refill time
   (b) Packed cell volume
   (c) Total protein

- In stallions the scrotum should be observed for unilateral enlargement but palpation will probably be necessary later in the examination to confirm or eliminate inguinal hernia.

The veterinarian should now proceed to a systematic clinical examination of the horse to include the cardiovascular system, abdomen and state of peripheral perfusion and hydration (Table 5). If the colic is so severe that an orderly examination is impossible without risk to the horse or veterinarian, heavy sedation, preferably with xylazine, is necessary. In the majority of cases the pain is sufficiently mild to allow most of the examination to be performed without recourse to the use of drugs which might modify the heart rate or gut activity. However, on completion of examination of the cardiovascular system and auscultation of the abdomen, the administration of a sedative will greatly facilitate rectal examination which is such a vital part of evaluation of a colic case, and other procedures such as nasogastric intubation and paracentesis which may be performed.

Examination of cardiovascular system

Heart rate and pulse character
- The heart rate and character of the pulse are important criteria in assessing the colic patient.
- Pain, and the activity as a consequence of pain, have only a relatively minor effect on the heart rate which is influenced much more by haemoconcentration and diminished venous return, and by toxins absorbed from the intestine.
- There will be a close relationship between the pulse and the nature and duration of the colic.

• Infarctive disease is usually accompanied by a non-fluctuating elevation in heart rate which increases progressively as toxic shock develops.

• In contrast, the heart rate will be only slightly raised after 48 hours in horses with pelvic flexure impaction.

Mucous membranes

• The colour of the mucous membranes is of value in assessing the severity of the disturbance and the prognosis.

• The oral mucous membranes, provided they are not pigmented, provide the best surface because the conjunctivae are often congested due to trauma.

• Reddening of the membranes reflects developing haemoconcentration and at a later stage when the patient is in shock, vasodilatation adds to the reddening process.

• Patients with cyanotic mucous membranes invariably die.

Examination of the abdomen

Abdominal distension

• Observation of the degree of abdominal distension is helpful in making the distinction between involvement of the stomach and small intestine on the one hand and the caecum and large intestine on the other.

• The large intestines when distended are the only viscera large enough to cause noticeable enlargement of the abdomen in the adult horse (in the foal, small intestinal distension can cause abdominal enlargement).

• The pattern of distension will vary, e.g. distension of the right paralumbar fossa accompanies caecal dilatation, while general abdominal distension is seen in horses with small colon obstructions or as the result of flatulent colic.

Auscultation and palpation

• The abdomen should be thoroughly auscultated for several minutes.

• The best sites are along the caudal edge of the rib cage from paralumbar fossa to ventral abdomen on both right and left sides.

• The sounds normally heard are fluid gurgling mixed with gas.

• In almost all horses with abdominal pain, the propulsive sounds will be reduced.

• In cases of severe intestinal disease such as strangulation, all sounds will be absent within a very few hours of the obstruction occurring.

• Sounds will be reduced or even absent after the administration of drugs such as xylazine or detomidine.

• Increased sounds are heard in horses with spasmodic colic and during resolution of ileus in tympanic or simple cases of colic.

• The primary importance of auscultation is in monitoring the progress of the disease rather than arriving at a diagnosis.

• Palpation of the abdominal wall in the adult horse has little value other than in identifying 'boarding' in response to generalized peritonitis due to rupture of stomach or intestine.

Rectal examination

• Rectal examination is the single most important part of the clinical examination of the horse with colic and should be carried out in all cases whenever possible but must be approached with respect for both its value and the risk involved.

• It should be carried out after reviewing the pertinent aspects of the history and the remainder of the physical examination. In this way an attempt can be made to predict what should be felt and to compare the findings with those preconceived ideas.

• Adequate restraint is essential to prevent damage to the horse or examiner. Sedation with xylazine will aid a thorough and systematic examination of the caudal 40% of the abdominal cavity which is within reach.

• Several large intestinal obstructions can be diagnosed by this means including pelvic flexure impaction, nephrosplenic entrapment of the left colon, large colon torsion, caecal impaction and intussusception.

• Although rectal examination enables a specific diagnosis of very few obstructions of the small intestine such as inguinal hernia and ileal impaction, seldom does it provide no useful findings. Small intestine obstructions or adynamic ileus produce distended loops of bowel lying side by side. In the early stages of obstructions, careful, patient palpation over a period of several minutes may be necessary before a distended loop is recognized. Later multiple tightly distended loops pushing back into the pelvic inlet make examination difficult. The presence of distended small intestine almost always indicates a problem requiring surgical correction. Early identification greatly enhances the chances of recovery.

• The normal structures that are palpable include, in the left dorsal quadrant, the spleen, the caudal pole of the left kidney and, linking the two, the nephrosplenic ligament. Moving to the right and extending forward below the spine, the root of the mesentery can be palpated. In the right dorsal quadrant the base of the caecum is identified by the caudal and medial bands which normally are relaxed and run downwards, forwards and medially. Moving ventral to the pelvic brim the pelvic flexure of the large colon can usually be detected and, extending cranially from it, the large diameter left ventral colon with its clearly recognizable longitudinal bands and the narrow, smooth left dorsal colon. The space above this and to the left of the caecum is usually occupied by small intestine and small colon. The normal small intestine is usually not palpable unless it happens to contract when touched, but the small colon is easily recognized by the formed faecal balls it usually contains.

Paracentesis abdominis

• Analysis of the peritoneal fluid reflects the changes that occur in the tissues and organs within the abdominal cavity and on the peritoneal surface. In colic cases it assists in determining the type of disease and the severity of the lesion.
• The simplest method is to insert a 19 gauge 1.5 in needle through a prepared site on the ventral midline of the abdomen at its most dependent point. Entry of the needle into the peritoneal cavity is indicated by the flow of varying amounts of fluid which is collected in a tube with or without anticoagulant depending on the information required. In obese animals a longer needle may be required to penetrate the thick layer of retroperitoneal fat.
• The fluid obtained is evaluated by gross visual examination, total protein determination and, if necessary, microscopic evaluation.
• Normal fluid is pale yellow and clear.
• As the fluid changes with specific diseases, the fluid can become more turbid due to increases in protein, red blood cells (RBC) and white blood cells (WBC). Normal fluid will be present in horses with non-strangulating obstructions or strangulation obstructions within an hour or two of the obstruction occurring or when the infarcted bowel is not in direct contact with the peritoneal cavity as in diaphragmatic hernia.
• Paracentesis is particularly valuable in the early stages of severe colic, when serosanguineous fluid, which may require centrifugation to show the presence of red blood cells, helps to confirm the presence of infarcted bowel in advance of diagnostic rectal findings.
• Late in the course of strangulation obstruction, when distended loops of intestine on rectal and

positive gastric reflux have been confirmed, paracentesis may be difficult to perform without accidental penetration of bowel, and is not necessary for the decision to operate. However, if gastrointestinal rupture or very advanced gut necrosis are suspected, their confirmation by paracentesis indicates the need for immediate euthanasia.

Nasogastric intubation

• In addition to being of diagnostic value, decompression of the stomach via a nasogastric tube produces immediate alleviation of pain and reduces the risk of rupture.
• Gastric reflux of more than 2 litres is considered to be significant, and usually indicates a primary disorder located in the small intestine or stomach.
• However, in some large colon obstructions, e.g. nephrosplenic entrapment, the proximal small intestine is compressed preventing normal gastric emptying.
• Grass sickness and anterior enteritis are other possible causes of gastric distension.
• Normal gastric fluid has a pH of 3–6, but following intestinal obstruction, pH will be 6–8 due to the buffering effect of fluid from the small intestine.
• In horses with a history of recent access to excessive amounts of concentrated feed or those showing dyspnoea and spontaneous regurgitation of gastric contents down the nose, nasogastric intubation should be performed at the start of the examination to reduce pressure and prevent rupture.
• It is important in horses suspected of having gastric dilatation that continued efforts at decompression are made even though the initial attempt(s) at starting a siphon are not successful.

State of peripheral perfusion and hydration

Capillary refill time

• In conjunction with palpation of the extremities, this measure provides a direct means of assessing the state of peripheral tissue perfusion while providing indirect information on the degree of hydration and vascular tone.
• The application of digital pressure on the oral mucous membrane just above the incisor teeth is a simple way of assessing capillary refill time.
• Adequate peripheral perfusion, hydration and vascular tone are indicated by a normal refill of 1–2 seconds, and warm extremities.

An increase to 3 seconds or more and cool extremities indicate inadequate peripheral perfusion and excessive vascular tone or vasoconstriction.

Packed cell volume (PCV) and total protein

- Packed cell volume on its own is an unreliable indicator of the patient's intravascular hydration because of the wide range of normality.
- Progressively increasing PCV on repeated examinations, and values over 50% are considered significant.
- In the absence of a means of spinning down blood samples, they can be left to settle out.
- Since it is changes in PCV rather than a single percentage which are of assistance in evaluating colic cases, simple visual comparison of sequential samples is sufficient.
- When PCV is considered along with total protein (TP normal 65 to 75 g/l), it provides a very useful means of assessing intravascular hydration and acts as a guideline for fluid therapy. Raised levels of PCV and TP represent intravascular dehydration.

Imaging techniques

Although not routine clinical practice, there are indications for employing various imaging modalities in selected cases of equine colic.

1. *Radiology*: intestinal obstruction in foals, diaphragmatic hernia, enterolith and grass sickness.
2. *Endoscopy*: gastric ulcers.
3. *Ultrasonography*: intussusceptions, colonic displacements.
4. *Laparoscopy*: intra-abdominal mass.

Classification into categories

Although at first sight this may appear a formidable list of procedures, with experience the clinical examinations can be carried out in 15 to 20 minutes. At the initial examination it should be possible to classify the problem into one of the following three categories:

1. A benign problem requiring medical therapy, e.g. pelvic flexure impaction diagnosed by rectal palpation.
   Action: Administer the appropriate treatment and make arrangements to monitor progress.

2. A problem requiring surgical correction.
   Action: Arrange for immediate transfer to a surgical facility.
3. A problem which may require surgery but for which the evidence at that point is not conclusive.
   Action:
   - Administer an analgesic.
   - Ensure the horse is in a 'safe' environment.
   - Arrange to re-examine it in 2 hours' time.
   - Because of its ability to mask several of the clinical signs on which the decision to operate is based, flunixin should not be used at this stage.

At the second visit the same examination procedures are repeated and the results compared with those 2 hours earlier.

The horse may be found:

- to have improved,
- to have developed signs which indicate the need for surgery,
- to still be inconclusive.

If results are still inconclusive the arrangement may be made to re-examine the horse in 2 hours' time, but if there is the least cause for concern, consideration should be given to discussing the problem on the telephone with someone at a referral centre, when the decision may be taken to refer the horse for further investigation and, if necessary, surgery.

2.8 The decision for surgery

Surgical intervention is indicated:

1. When the exact cause of the colic can be diagnosed and the obstructing lesion requires surgery for its correction.
2. When there is no exact diagnosis but there is sufficient evidence to indicate that surgery is the only means of saving the animal's life.
3. When animals with recurrent colic over a period of days or weeks are suspected of having partial obstruction due to adhesions, neoplasia etc. (Table 6).

Most cases fall into the second category.

Despite tremendous advances in anaesthetic and surgical techniques and in postoperative management, the mortality rate in horses undergoing colic surgery remains quite high. Most horses which die as a direct result of colic

Table 6 Recurrent/chronic colic – possible causes

1. Partial occlusion of the gut lumen
   A. Small intestine
      Muscular hypertrophy of the ileum
      Hypertrophy of caecal mucosa at ileocaecal
      junction
      Intramural neoplasia
      Ileocaecal intussusception
      Adhesions
      Mesenteric abscess
   B. Large intestine
      Caecocaecal or caecocolic intussusception
      Recurrent displacements or mild torsions of the
      large colon
      Enteroliths
      Neoplasia

2. Gastroduodenal ulceration in foals and gastric
   ulceration in adults

3. Cranial mesenteric arteritis

4. Miscellaneous causes
   Oestrus
   Granulosa cell tumour of ovary
   Crib biting
   Renal calculi
   Chronic inflammatory bowel disease

succumb to acute circulatory failure (shock) secondary to intestinal ischaemia/infarction. Early recognition holds the key to improved survival rates so that surgical intervention occurs before the horse's condition begins to deteriorate.

In deciding the need for surgery, there is no single criterion that can be relied upon. All the information that the circumstances permit must be gathered and the facts must be weighed against each other so that a prognosis as well as a preliminary diagnosis can be rendered. The criteria most useful in identifying the acute surgical case are set out below in order of importance:

1. Degree of pain
● In some cases of strangulation obstruction, particularly 360° torsion of the large colon, the pain from the outset is so severe and unresponsive to analgesics that this alone is sufficient indication for resorting to surgery as soon as possible.
● Large colon displacements, ileal impaction and partial obstructions such as ileal intussusceptions are usually associated with moderately severe intermittent pain.

2. Rectal findings
● Positive rectal findings of obstructions such as large colon torsion or displacement, caecocaecal intussusception, enterolith obstruction of small colon, ileal impaction and ileocaecal intussusception are indications for immediate surgery regardless of the other clinical findings.
● In horses with other types of small intestinal obstruction, distended, taut loops of intestine are highly significant. It may be 8–10 hours before multiple loops are palpable in the caudal abdomen. Prior to this, careful, patient palpation over a period of several minutes may be necessary before a distended loop is recognized. Early identification greatly enhances the chances of recovery.

3. Heart rate and pulse quality
● Infarctive disease is usually accompanied by a non-fluctuating elevation in heart rate which increases progressively as toxic shock develops.
● A similar, but slower, increase will occur in horses with simple obstruction of the small intestine.
● In general, a pulse rate which has risen progressively to 60–70 per minute 6 hours after the onset of colic gives rise for concern, particularly if it remains high during quiet interludes and in the face of adequate analgesia.

4. Cardiovascular deterioration
● Progressive deterioration evidenced by a PCV of >55, mucous membranes injected, despite fluid therapy.

5. Absence of gut sounds

6. Nasogastric intubation
● Gastric reflux in excess of 2–3 litres is considered significant.
● If a primary gastric dilation can be ruled out, such reflux is indicative of small intestinal obstruction located anywhere between pylorus and ileocaecal junction, or ileus due to peritonitis, grass sickness or anterior enteritis. There is usually an accompanying progressive reduction in intestinal motility.

7. Paracentesis abdominis
● Positive changes in peritoneal fluid, viz an increase in RBC, WBC and protein, indicate morphological changes of the bowel.

• Sanguineous fluid is decisive evidence of infarction and an indicator for surgery.
• Reddish brown fluid containing a large number of WBC as well as RBC indicates more advanced changes and consequently a poorer prognosis.

Changes seen in the peritoneal fluid depend on a number of factors including the time which has elapsed since the obstruction occurred, the size and length of gut involved and whether or not it is in direct contact with the peritoneal cavity. From the point of view of the attending veterinary surgeon, referral of horses with colic of unknown cause should not be delayed until changes have occurred in the peritoneal fluid.

8. Abdominal distension
• Progressive abdominal distension which is becoming life threatening.

These criteria are only guidelines. Such is the great variety in the type of obstruction, the part and length of gut involved, the degree of obstruction etc., it is inevitable that some cases will present difficulties in diagnosis. Where evidence for and against surgery is evenly balanced, intuition based on clinical experience is often the deciding factor.

If the horse is to be referred to a surgical centre, it is preferable that this is done when the referring veterinary surgeon is less than certain of the need for surgery rather than wait until he has no doubt, under which circumstances the additional delay in arranging admission and transporting the animal may make the difference between success and failure. Practitioners are encouraged to contact staff at the centre to which they refer cases to discuss problem cases. The advice given may be to continue treatment at the premises or to refer the horse for further investigation and, if necessary, surgery, A significant number of these horses will recover without surgery and will be discharged within a day or two. Owners are appraised of the difficulties in identifying the cases requiring surgery and the advantages of hospitalization for further evaluation. Rarely if ever do they resent having transported the horse and are often delighted not to have to meet the considerable cost of surgery. It is important that horses in which the primary problem has progressed to severe irreversible cardiovascular compromise or gastric rupture are euthanased immediately and not subjected to transport.

2.9 *Preparation of the horse prior to transport to a surgical centre*

If a horse is to be referred to a university hospital or other centre and this involves a journey of any significant length, the following measures should be taken.

1. Decompress the stomach and, if necessary, leave the nasogastric tube in place and tape it to the head collar.
2. Administer an analgesic. If it is clear that surgery is necessary and a strangulation obstruction is suspected, flunixin is ideal because in addition to relieving the pain it will counter the effects of endotoxaemia.
3. If the horse is in shock plasma expanders may be given to improve the circulating blood volume. Crystalloids may be administered while awaiting the arrival of a horsebox but departure to the surgical centre should not be delayed for the purpose of administering the large volumes necessary to make any significant impression on the PCV. On arrival at the surgical centre a rapid improvement in the cardiovascular status of severely shocked horses can be achieved by the administration of 2 litres of hypertonic saline. This is not an option prior to referral because a large volume of isotonic solution such as Hartmann's solution is necessary within 2 hours of the hypertonic solution being given.
4. Rug the horse up and bandage its limbs.
5. Provide a detailed report of the treatment given to the horse prior to referral.
6. Provide the owner with accurate directions how to get to the hospital.
7. Owners should be strongly discouraged from travelling in the back of the horsebox or in the trailer with the horse.

2.10 *The surgical management of the equine colic case – general points*

Colic surgery is a team effort and the chances of success are greatest when the optimum number of people and back up facilities are available.

As stated previously, the patient in abdominal crisis is either in shock or predisposed to it and ideally should not undergo laparotomy until all its physiological parameters are within normal limits and the gastrointestinal tract has been decompressed. However, this is rarely a practical proposition. A balance between restoration of blood volume and complete rehydration must be found because if the whole of the calculated fluid deficit is given before anaesthesia, a substantial proportion will diffuse into the lumen of the intestine before the obstruction can be relieved. This will not only be lost from the circulation but it will also make the surgery more difficult. It is therefore advisable to administer as much balanced electrolyte solution as possible during preparation for surgery, and then to restore the remainder during the operation once the obstruction is relieved. This approach is satisfactory for horses with relatively mild deficiencies in circulating blood volume. However, acute restoration of the circulation in horses in severe shock is best achieved using hypertonic saline; 4 ml/kg of 7.5% saline given rapidly before induction of anaesthesia draws fluid into the circulation as well as increasing cardiac contractility and output. The effect can be dramatic and lasts well into the surgical period during which isotonic solutions are administered as usual.

It is generally agreed that the prognosis depends to a large extent on the duration of the operation which should be performed as expeditiously as possible without sacrificing good surgical technique. Whenever possible, the ventral abdomen should be clipped beforehand to reduce to a minimum the interval between induction and the first incision. This is particularly important in those horses with severe abdominal distension, where rapid decompression of the large intestine is essential if the patient is not to succumb to respiratory embarrassment caused by pressure on the diaphragm. The passage of a nasogastric tube and evacuation of fluid stomach contents prior to induction reduces the risk of gastric rupture, regurgitation and aspiration of fluid.

Premedication and anaesthesia

The anaesthetist frequently has to contend with the residual effects of a variety of drugs (e.g. sedatives, narcotics and spasmolytics) which have been administered between the onset of colic and referral for surgery. Colic patients are often quiet and depressed, but when sedation is required, the alpha-2 agents are the drugs of choice. Xylazine may be preferable to detomidine as it is shorter acting, but small doses of detomidine (5–10 μg/kg) may also be used.

Induction and maintenance

The objective should be to achieve:

- smooth induction so that the horse sinks quietly to the ground,
- a similarly smooth recovery a relatively short time after completion of surgery.

A variety of drugs and dose rates may be used depending on the preference and experience of the anaesthetist and the state of the patient. Whichever induction technique is chosen, it is important it is one with which the anaesthetist is fully familiar and it must be remembered that in toxic patients the doses required of any depressant drug will be considerably reduced.

The main requirements of anaesthetic maintenance are similar to any procedure except there is much greater emphasis on fluid replacement.

- Progress should be assessed by regular monitoring of PCV and plasma protein.
- Arterial blood pressure, mucous membrane colour and capillary refill time (CRT) provide valuable information as to the efficiency of the circulation.
- Cardiac support with the inotropes dopamine or dobutamine is widely accepted as effective therapy whenever hypotension is evident.

Respiratory depression may be a problem in the horse with colic, but the relative merits of positive pressure ventilation and spontaneous respiration must be balanced for each individual concerned.

Blood gas analysis, if available, will enable the existence and degree of acidosis or alkalosis present to be determined. In the absence of means of blood gas measurement, it is reassuring that once fluid therapy, kidney function and hepatic circulation are restored, the body rapidly adjusts its acid/base deficit.

Recovery from anaesthesia

If colic surgery has been successful in resolving the problem the horse is usually remarkably calm in the recovery period.

Laparotomy (celiotomy) technique

The ventral midline approach is used now almost universally for colic surgery.

- The incision allows easy, rapid access to the abdominal cavity with the minimum of haemorrhage.
- Great latitude of access and exposure of the viscera is possible, an important factor when we consider the frequency with which laparotomies are performed without the exact site of the obstruction being known.
- Adequate draping is necessary to protect the surgical field.
- The abdomen and legs of the patient are covered with a large cotton drape and the area adjacent to the incision is further protected with waterproof, plastic sheeting.

The initial incision is made accurately in the midline extending cranially from the umbilicus for 16 cm. This can be extended if necessary.

In order that a lesion does not go undetected in this, the largest and most complex of the body compartments, it is imperative that a routine, systematic exploration be employed.

- Much of the search is conducted virtually at arm's length; correlating palpable findings with the surgeon's knowledge of anatomical relationships. An accurate command of both normal and pathological anatomy is a considerable advantage.
- On incising the peritoneum the colour and character of any effusions, the distribution pattern of distended bowel and any discernible discoloration of visceral or peritoneal surfaces should be noted.
- If gas- or fluid-filled bowel is ballooning out of the abdomen, some decompression of the alimentary tract will be necessary before exploration can commence. In addition to facilitating exploration, decompression reduces intra-abdominal pressure, encourages peristalsis and simplifies closure of the abdomen.
- Decompression of the caecum, which can be partially exteriorized, can be quickly achieved using a 16 gauge needle attached to a suction line.
- Removal of gas from the large intestine is frequently necessary *in situ* by needle suction before any attempt can be made to exteriorize it.
- Lifting distended, sometimes friable, large colon must be done very carefully to avoid rupture.

- Evacuation of its contents is carried out by placing the pelvic flexure between the horse's hind legs, preferably on a colon tray, and performing an enterotomy in the terminal part of the left ventral colon. Dry contents are flushed from the lumen using a hose introduced up the left dorsal and ventral parts in turn via the enterotomy incision.
- Decompression of the small intestine can be achieved by stripping its contents into the caecum.
- When most of the small intestine is severely distended, decompression must be carried out in sections commencing distally. This means that the distal jejunum and ileum will be handled several times.

Gentle handling and ample lubrication with warm Hartmann's solution will minimize trauma and the risk of ileus. The caecum can be evacuated of the large volume of fluid it contains via an enterotomy incision at its apex.

- The initial gentle sweep of the abdominal cavity serves to check the sites of commonly occurring obstructions.
- Palpation is aimed at detecting firm masses, fluid distension and impaction or tympany of the large intestine. Abrupt changes in direction of intestine, tight mesenteric bands around or across intestine, or immobility of normally mobile portions of intestine indicate an area of involvement.
- If palpation fails to disclose the problem, the bowel must be exteriorized to facilitate visual examination.
- Normal small intestine can easily be exteriorized except for the proximal 1 metre and the terminal 15–20 cm.
- The apex and part of the body of the caecum can be lifted out, as can the left ventral and dorsal large colon, and parts of the right dorsal and ventral colon.
- The proximal 60–70 cm of the small colon and the rectum are inaccessible.
- Location of the obstruction can be achieved quickly and with less trauma to the intestine if the manipulation is commenced at the distal empty portion of the bowel and continues proximally. The terminal reference point of the segment of bowel which appears to be involved should be located, namely the ileum for the small intestine and the pelvic flexure or proximal small colon for the large intestine.

Examination of the small intestine

• The ileum can be located by exteriorizing the caecum and turning it backwards to reveal the dorsal band which bears the ileocaecal fold. If this fold is traced downwards to the lesser curvature of the caecum, it will lead to the ileum which is instantly recognized by the ileocaecal fold on its mesenteric border.

• If it cannot be exteriorized, the ileum must be involved in the obstruction.

• Compared to the remainder of the small intestine, the ileum is involved in a wide variety of obstructive conditions to a disproportionate degree, and in these patients the cause of the obstruction will be quickly identified.

• If the ileum is not involved, the empty flaccid intestine is traced proximally until the obstruction and distended bowel proximal to it are reached.

• Each length of bowel examined is returned to the abdomen as the adjacent bowel is lifted out, and a rough check is kept of the length examined.

• Eventually, in the absence of obstruction, the next part of the small intestine which cannot be exteriorized will be the duodenum.

Examination of the large colon

• Obstruction of the large intestine can usually be anticipated prior to laparotomy on the basis of the physical examination.

• Segments of large intestine are more easily differentiated on the basis of their appearance and position than are those of the small intestine.

• By taking note of the pattern and extent of the distension of the various parts, and taking into account the common causes and sites of obstruction, the location of the problem can be deduced without too much expenditure of time or energy.

• The caecum again serves as a landmark for the initial exploration. If its base and ventral longitudinal band cannot be palpated, a caecocaecal or caecocolic intussusception should be suspected.

• If the caecum can be exteriorized, the caecocolic fold is found and followed to the right ventral colon. This can then be traced cranially to the sternal flexure and then caudally to the pelvic flexure which is another easily recognizable part of the large colon. From there it can be followed back to the diaphragmatic flexure and on to the transverse colon cranial to the root of the mesentery. The transverse colon which is short in length

and fixed in position constitutes an abrupt constriction of the lumen and change in direction.

Evaluation of gut viability

The surgery necessary to relieve obstruction may vary from simply incising a constricting band of tissue to resecting several metres of intestine. The decision as to the necessity for resection and the length of bowel which needs to be removed often depends on a subjective assessment of bowel function.

• Any intestine of abnormal colour, decreased motility or thickened appearance must be considered suspect.

• After correction of obstructions causing secondary vascular embarrassment, observation of the bowel for 5–10 minutes for the return of colour, peristalsis and pulsation of vessels will aid in deciding for or against resection.

• The junction between viable and compromised bowel may be difficult to discern especially after displacement has been corrected and a significant improvement in the appearance of the bowel has taken place. Making a small incision in questionable bowel to determine how easily it bleeds and the appearance of the mucosa is fully justified.

Such clinical assessment of viability is not uniformly reliable, and its accuracy has been put as low as 36%. The use of these criteria become more beneficial with experience. It has been shown experimentally that following release of jejunal ligatures applied 50 minutes earlier, progressive degeneration continued even though there was gross evidence of perfusion and muscular activity soon after release. A number of alternative techniques have been investigated.

• The most popular clinically applicable methods of evaluating intestinal viability measure tissue perfusion by some direct or indirect method. Unfortunately, ischaemic damage can occur at the cellular level in spite of apparently adequate perfusion and can be impossible to discern intraoperatively.

• Intravenous fluorescein and Doppler ultrasound have been the most reported methods of detecting local perfusion of segments of bowel. Experience is needed to use either method.

• Fluorescein dye injected IV (6.6–11 mg/kg) is rapidly distributed to all perfused tissues. The serosal surfaces become yellow/green within 60 seconds and emit a yellow fluorescence when illuminated with long wave ultraviolet light. It is important to compare the segment being evaluated with unaffected small intestine or colon. When reduced fluorescence is generalized, little credence can be placed upon the procedure.

- The Doppler probe senses the passage of blood through vessels within the wall of the intestine. Signals from arterial flow in any form are considered to indicate viable bowel, with clinical and experimental evidence indicating a high degree of accuracy. One limitation is that the probe has to be placed in the exact area to be evaluated. When compared to sodium fluorescein fluorescence, the Doppler is generally no better in detecting non-viable segments.
- Surface oximetry measures the oxygen tension (mmHg) where the oxygen probe contacts the tissue surface. The PO_2 on the surface of the bowel (PsO_2) depends upon diffusion distance from the nearest vessel, local O_2 consumption, arterial (PaO_2) and local blood flow. Measurement of PsO_2 gives a qualitative estimate of tissue oxygenation beneath the 3 mm electrode. Applied to ischaemic bowel, values are compared to normal bowel and to PaO_2.

In summary, evaluation of bowel viability remains a perplexing surgical dilemma and at present there is no reliable method available. False interpretation of intestinal viability can result in continued shock, ileus, peritonitis and death or, less dramatically, but equally disappointing, in adhesion formation and secondary obstruction. Therefore, in equivocal cases, the surgeon should choose to resect suspect bowel rather than risk leaving compromised bowel *in situ*.

Resection of small intestine

A physiological limit of small intestine resection has been identified in the horse. Ponies in which 50% of the small intestine had been resected maintained their pre-surgical weight. These findings correlate well with clinical experience which suggests that in all but exceptional cases 8 metres is the maximum length which should be removed.

Resection and anastomosis

- Resection and anastomosis of the jejunum in the horse is simplified by the long mesentery, the

clearly visible blood vessels for ligation and the intestinal calibre which allows ample inversion.
- It is widely accepted that, when technically feasible, an end-to-end anastomosis is the simplest and most physiologically compatible method.
- Whenever possible the fluid-filled ischaemic bowel should be isolated with intestinal clamps before manipulation is begun. If not contained in this way, toxic fluids will reflux into normal intestine and be absorbed, resulting in rapid physiological deterioration of the patient. Failing that, the gut should be clamped as soon as it is freed.
- A suitable site for resection can subsequently be chosen proximal and distal to the strangulated bowel.
- The mesenteric vessels to the compromised bowel are double ligated, the ends of the proximal ligature being left long.
- The distal end of the gut is transected and the mesentery incised between the ligatures.
- As each vessel is cut, the long ends of the individual proximal ligatures are tied together. This greatly reduces the length of the gap in the mesentery to be closed when anastomosis has been completed. This is particularly helpful when a long length of intestine has been resected.
- With the infarcted gut now mobilized in this way, the distal end can be carefully lifted beyond the abdomen and drained into a suitable receptacle by removing the distal clamp.
- Removing the proximal clamp allows decompression of much of the distended bowel proximal to the ischaemic portion.

Open end-to-end anastomosis using one of a number of inversion suture patterns is still the most commonly employed method of intestinal anastomosis in the horse, but other methods have been evaluated experimentally and clinically. The author prefers a two layer closure comprising a simple continuous suture for the mucosa and a continuous Cushing seromuscular suture (Figure 1), or alternatively a single layer closure using interrupted Lembert sutures. Synthetic absorbable suture material (e.g. polyglactin or polyglycolic acid) is used in both types of anastomosis.

Closure of the mesentery

- After the anastomosis has been checked for patency and leakage, the remaining gap from

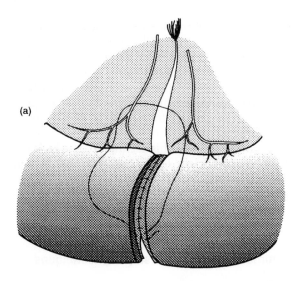

(a)

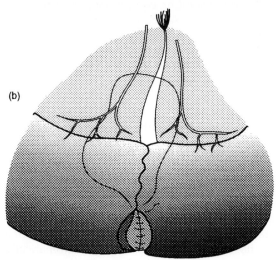

(b)

Figure 1 Two-layer end-to-end anastomosis. (a) Mucosa is closed with a simple continuous suture. (b) Anastomosis is completed with a continuous Cushing suture.

the stump of the mesentery to the mesenteric border of the intestine is closed with a continuous suture.

- In order to prevent adhesion formation to the extensive stump of the mesentery in which some ischaemic tissue remains distal to the ligature, after resection of a long length of bowel, it can be enveloped in two folds of adjacent mesentery, one drawn from each side.
- The intestinal segment and the mesentery are rinsed clean of blood using warm polyionic solution before being carefully replaced in the abdomen.

Anastomosis of intestinal segments of different diameters

- Dilatation of the proximal segment necessitates joining intestine of unequal diameters. While this can be overcome by cutting the smaller diameter segment obliquely, a side-to-side anastomosis is preferable, and is essential when chronic obstruction of small intestine due to progressive constriction of its lumen by neoplasia or ileoileal intussusception results in gross hypertrophy of the proximal bowel.
- Side-to-side anastomosis is used routinely by some for all jejunal anastomoses.
- It is also used for jejuno- and ileo-caecostomy, for bypassing obstructions and anastomosing adjoining segments of large colon.

Resection of the ileum

- The ileum is involved in obstruction disease almost as frequently as the remaining 21 metres or so of the small intestine. Many of these obstructions result in strangulation of bowel necessitating resection and anastomosis which, due to the inaccessibility of the terminal ileum via a ventral midline incision, can be technically difficult.
- Ileocaecal and jejunocaecal anastomoses whereby the natural ileocaecal junction is bypassed have proved very successful in overcoming the problems of restricted access and limited blood supply.
- A right-angled clamp is applied as low down the ileum as possible. After the contents have been stripped proximally for 20 cm an intestinal crushing clamp is applied and the ileum is transected just distal to this clamp.
- Oedema and friability frequently makes closure of the ileal stump difficult. A double row of inversion sutures is inserted.
- To avoid leaving potentially necrotic ileum *in situ*, it is necessary to progressively invaginate it into the caecum using a continuous Cushing suture. Alternatively, the ileum may be occluded using an automated stapler as close to the caecum as possible and then transected.
- The jejunum is clamped and transected at a suitable site proximal to the ischaemic bowel.
- After closure of the jejunal end with a double layer inversion suture, the jejunum is placed between the dorsal and medial bands of the caecum with its closed end pointing towards the base of the caecum.

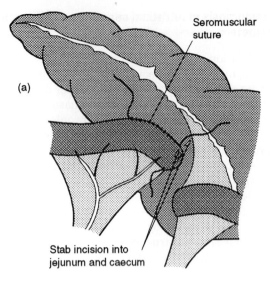

(a)

Seromuscular suture

Stab incision into jejunum and caecum

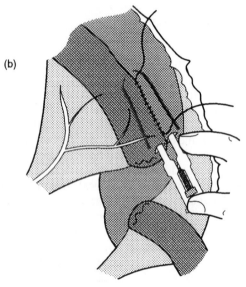

(b)

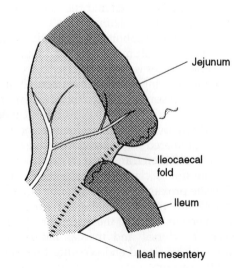

(c)

Jejunum

Ileocaecal fold

Ileum

Ileal mesentery

• A side-to-side anastomosis is now performed creating an opening 8–10 cm long using a conventional suture pattern or alternatively stapling equipment may be used (Figure 2).

• On completion of the anastomosis the mesenteric defect is closed by suturing the cut edge of the jejunal mesentery to that of the ileum and to the ileocaecal fold.

• A modification of this technique in which the ileum is anastomosed side-to-side to the caecum without resection can be used to bypass non-strangulating obstructions caused by hypertrophy or ileo-ileal intussusception.

Automated mechanical stapling techniques

• The use of stapling equipment in equine intestinal surgery is now becoming widespread. The various instruments have been developed for intestinal anastomosis in order to reduce surgery time and thereby increase the chances of survival of critically ill patients.

• The very fine stainless steel staples, which close to form a perfect B, preserve the blood supply to the tissues involved in the anastomosis and therefore avoid ischaemia.

• The linear staplers, which have 30 mm, 60 mm and 90 mm cartridges, insert staples in a double staggered row. The 4.8 mm size of staple is recommended for equine use. The application of these linear staplers include closure of intestine during resection of small or large intestine. As the instrument does not cut automatically, this must subsequently be performed with a scalpel.

• The gastrointestinal anastomosis instrument (GIA) inserts staples arranged in two double staggered rows 3.5 mm apart. A knife-blade cuts between them creating a side-to-side anastomosis. It is used for jejuno- and ileo-caecostomy, gastrojejunostomy and large colon anastomoses.

• Care should always be taken not to use stapling equipment if tissues are oedematous or thickened because of the risk of disruption and leakage.

Figure 2 Side-to-side jejunocaecal anastomosis using a Proximate Linear Cutter (Ethicon Ltd). (a) Jejunum is anchored to the caecum with a continuous seromuscular suture and a small stab incision is made into each. (b) The forks of the stapling instrument are inserted and locked together prior to pushing the firing knob. (c) The mesenteric defect is closed by suturing the cut edge of the jejunal mesentery to that of the ileum and to the ileocaecal fold.

Resection of large intestine

Generally resection of large intestine in the horse is performed very much less frequently than resection of the small intestine for two reasons.

- Firstly, many of the obstructions comprise displacement with no or only minimal interference with blood supply, or simple obstruction of the lumen, for example by enteroliths, which can be relieved by means of a simple enterotomy.
- Secondly when a strangulating obstruction is present, the length of bowel involved may be so great that resection and anastomosis is not considered feasible because of technical difficulties or because of likely postoperative nutritional or metabolic problems.

Caecum

Partial resection of the caecum is indicated when it shows infarctive changes due to intussusception or thromboembolism. A small amount of healthy caecum beyond the infarcted zone is included in the resection which is usually performed at the level of the attachment of the caecocolic fold. The medial and lateral caecal arteries and veins are double ligated in their course along the medial and lateral bands. The diseased portion is excised and closure carried out in the layers using a Cushing suture.

Total resection of the caecum together with an ileocolostomy requires an approach through a lateral right flank laparotomy in which the 17th and 18th ribs are resected.

Large colon

Clinical and experimental investigations have shown that horses tolerate resection of between 60 and 75 % of the large colon remarkably well.

Many of the technical difficulties can be overcome by the use of automated stapling equipment, but if the infarction due to torsion or thrombo-embolism is restricted to the left colon, resection can be carried out successfully using conventional techniques.

A side-to-side anastomosis is created between adjacent parts of the dorsal and ventral colons proximal to the infarcted portion. Delaying resection until after this procedure has been carried out helps to prevent the bowel retracting into the abdomen.

After ligation of the vessels and resection, the stumps are closed with a two layer continuous inverting Cushing suture.

Small colon

Following resection of infarcted small colon, continuity is restored by end-to-end anastomosis using simple interrupted Lembert sutures.

The large amount of fat in the mesocolon makes identification of the vessels more difficult than the jejunal mesenteric vessels. Particular care must also be taken when placing sutures at the mesenteric border to ensure a water-tight seal.

Closure of the midline incision (Figure 3)

Midline incisions heal more slowly than paramedian or flank incisions because of the relative lack of vasculature of the linea alba, but reconstruction can be accomplished quickly and easily with only minimal risk of herniation and evisceration. A wide variety of suture techniques and materials have been described.

- The peritoneum is thin and tears easily but providing adequate decompression of bowel has been carried out, it can be sutured using a continuous suture of polyglactin. However, experimental and clinical experience has shown that no detrimental effects result when the peritoneum is left unsutured.
- Closure of the linea alba with a continuous suture of 5 metric polyglactin doubled has proved reliable and effective in a large number of horses.
- However, in very large horses, or when performing colic surgery in heavily pregnant mares which may conceivably abort, 5 polyester fibre suture is preferred.
- The suture bites should be 1 cm from the margins of the incision and the edges approximated without undue tension.
- Thorough decompression of the intestine greatly facilitates closure.
- In extremely large or muscular horses, the far-and-near suture pattern has much to recommend it.
- The subcutaneous tissue is closed with a continuous suture of polyglactin, and the skin with a continuous mattress suture of nylon or stapled.
- Although the use of continuous suture patterns and absorbable materials would appear, theoretically at least, to be risky, it has proved to be a

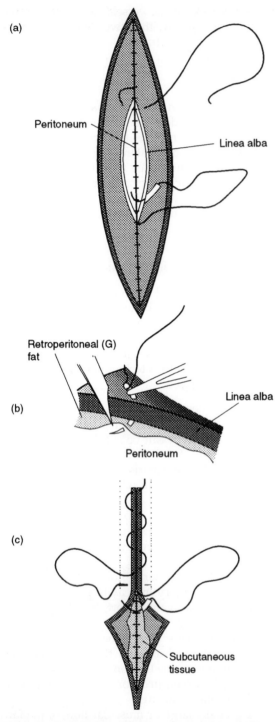

(a)

Peritoneum

Linea alba

Retroperitoneal (G) fat

(b)

Linea alba

Peritoneum

(c)

Subcutaneous tissue

Figure 3 Closure of the midline laparotomy incision. (a) The peritoneum is closed with a simple continuous suture of polyglactin and the linea alba with two continuous sutures of 5 metric polyglactin doubled. (b) Alternatively the peritoneum is included in the continuous suture used to close the linea alba. Care is taken to avoid including the retroperitoneal fat. (c) The subcutaneous tissue is closed with a continuous suture of 1 metric polyglactin, and the skin with a continuous horizontal mattress suture of monofilament non-absorbable material or with staples.

reliable method and has the advantage of significant saving in time and a reduction of sinus formation.

2.11 Postoperative management of the colic case

Adequate postoperative management of equine abdominal patients is just as important to patient survival as the most heroic corrective surgery. Its success will depend on adequate intensive care based on close monitoring of physiological parameters including acid–base, electrolyte and body fluid balance. Routine management of the uncomplicated surgical case is simple and places little strain on resources in terms of personnel or laboratory facilities, but patients with postoperative complications, particularly ileus, demand a great deal of supervision which may last several days.

• Limited oral intake is essential for all postoperative colics, especially following resection and anastomosis. Nothing should be allowed by mouth unless gut propulsive activity is present.
• When this function is assumed to have returned, small quantities (l litre) of water may be given at 2 hourly intervals.
• Small bran mashes or grass can be introduced during the third day and hay by the fourth postoperative day.
• Gentle walking exercise may aid recovery by decreasing wound oedema, reducing boredom and possibly encouraging defecation.

This management regimen will ensure prompt recovery of uncomplicated cases, but as the possible complications are many and potentially fatal, close postoperative monitoring is vital to ensure rapid diagnosis and correct treatment of problems as they develop. If this aspect of colic care is neglected, much of the previous efforts to save the animal may be wasted. This requires sequentially repeated examinations that will record signs giving early evidence of system dysfunction.

Monitoring protocol

The adoption of a protocol for monitoring postoperative colic cases, especially when carried out by a number of people over some time, should aid accurate assessment. A flow sheet is needed to systematically record all the required physical and laboratory data at each examination so that trends can be recognized and progress assessed.

The two major factors which affect cases adversely in the postoperative period are loss of gut propulsive activity (ileus) and cardiac insufficiency (shock).

The following parameters have proved valuable for early diagnosis of these and other complications:

- Heart rate and pulse quality
- Mucous membrane colour and capillary refill time
- Packed cell volume
- Pain
- Rectal temperature
- Wound integrity
- General demeanour
- Urination and defecation
- Gut sounds
- Nasogastric intubation
- Rectal examination
- Abdominal wall tension
- Willingness to move
- Digital pulses

Any treatment should be recorded including the volumes of fluid administered. The frequency of the flow sheet examination is determined by the clinician.

If constant vigilance is required because an acute change in condition is anticipated, the horse should be monitored every hour. This is particularly true in foals in which drastic changes in hydration and electrolyte status can occur very quickly.

Normally in a new case, the horse should be monitored every 3 hours until trends in the patient's condition can be determined.

Once heart rate, PCV and total protein levels have returned to normal or near normal, faeces have been passed and gastric reflux has been absent on two or three successive nasogastric intubations, the examinations can be carried out at intervals of 6–8 hours.

Catheter care

- Monitoring catheter patency and vein reaction to the catheter are important in proper fluid and drug administration as well as for prevention of thrombophlebitis, which in its most severe form can be life threatening.

- The catheter should be part of the daily monitoring, and the findings recorded on the flow chart.
- If there is any evidence of exudate at the site of catheter entry, or perivascular thickening, heat or pain, the catheter should be removed immediately.
- Horses suffering from severe endotoxaemia at the time of referral are often in a highly 'coagulable' state. Postoperative therapy in these cases may well continue for several days so vein patency is essential.
- If the jugular vein used shows signs of thrombophlebitis it is preferable to use the external thoracic vein rather than risk similar obstruction developing in the other jugular vein.

Fluid therapy

- Maintaining fluid balance in the postoperative horse or in the horse in shock is critical as it affects internal function and the normal body defence systems.
- In the case of small intestinal obstruction, 5–10 litres are necessary every 4 hours, whereas horses recovering from simple obstructions of caecum or colon require only 5 litres every 6–8 hours.
- Although over-hydration is useful in large colon impactions, it should be avoided in small intestinal ileus where excessive fluid in the vascular system appears to increase the volume secreted into the bowel.
- The fluid rate should therefore be adjusted to just maintain a level state of hydration.

Analgesia and anti-inflammatory therapy

- Treatment with NSAID analgesics in the critically ill horse is employed in all cases to reduce the effects of endotoxaemia, to maintain intestinal motility and to provide analgesia.
- When necessary low dose flunixin therapy (0.25 mg/kg three times daily) can be continued for 7–10 days without ill-effects, but if higher levels are used the risk of NSAID toxicity exists.
- Flunixin is also known to reduce development of strength in the abdominal incision.

Antibiotic therapy

- Antibiotics are commonly used in the prevention and treatment of infection and shock in the acute abdominal patient.

- The most effective and economic antibiotics are the aminoglycosides combined with penicillin.
- This combination is not totally effective against anaerobes, so metronidazole may also be used in some cases.

2.12 *Postoperative complications*

Shock

Shock is a constant hazard of colic cases and may be fatal, especially in the first few hours after surgery. It is hypovolaemic and/or endotoxic in origin. If intraoperative therapy has been sufficient, plasma volume may have been restored, but this may be a temporary improvement. Endotoxaemia is associated with altered haemostasis including disseminated intravascular coagulation.

- During the immediate postoperative period, while the horse is still recumbent, enriching the inspired air with oxygen to increase arterial oxygen tension is of benefit to the patient.
- A rising packed cell volume indicates the need for fluid, but plasma protein concentration should also be measured to avoid the overuse of crystalloid solutions which may produce a marked hypoproteinaemia.
- The possibility of postoperative ileus should be considered in such cases, and gastric fluid drained.
- Lactated Ringer's solution is the IV replacement fluid of choice but, if possible, the constituents of the replacement therapy should be related to laboratory results of plasma electrolyte and protein status.
- Acidosis is probable but not invariable.

Treatment of endotoxaemia and its related effects are more complex, although fluid and electrolytes are important.

The cyclo-oxygenase inhibitor flunixin is used routinely. It interferes with the metabolism of arachidonic acid to arrest the production of vasoactive metabolites mediating arterial hypoxia, platelet adhesion and lactic acidosis. The drug should be given during surgery (1.1 mg/kg body weight), if not administered previously, followed by 0.25 mg/kg at 8 hourly intervals.

It has recently been shown that endotoxin has a profound depressive effect on gut motility in horses. Evidence suggests that a considerable part of the mode of action is mediated by the prostaglandin cascade system. A comparative study of phenylbutazone and flunixin carried out on a postoperative ileus model suggested that phenylbutazone is superior to flunixin in inhibiting the effect of prostaglandin on gut activity.

Postoperative ileus

Postoperative ileus is a major problem which is often fatal. It is defined as a loss of coordinated bowel activity leading to physiological obstruction. Although many cases do have a silent abdomen, bowel activity does not always cease.

The critical feature is a loss of coordination between gastric and duodenal activity.

Frequently the animal makes a good anaesthetic recovery and may appear bright during the first part of the postoperative period. There is an absence of gut sounds after the first 3–5 hours. The packed cell volume and total protein rise steadily in the absence of effective transport of gut contents; any fluid therapy producing only temporary improvement. Deterioration in mucous membrane colour and capillary refill time accompanied by a corresponding rise in heart rate, are further evidence of circulatory collapse. Fluid accumulates in the stomach and small intestine and can be diagnosed by nasogastric intubation and rectal palpation.

Postoperative ileus falls into one of two categories.

- In some cases it is associated with a demonstrable cause such as mechanical obstruction, peritonitis or the continued presence of severely compromised gut.
- In other cases the ileus is idiopathic.

The problem is most common in the small intestine after distension from obstruction or strangulation.

Treatment of cases of known cause is specific, and requires relaparotomy to, for example, remove infarcted gut or break down an impaction.

Correct management of idiopathic cases is more controversial. Conventional management aims to maintain gastric decompression by nasogastric suction (10–15 litres may be removed at 3–4 hour intervals), hydration and electrolyte and acid–base balance by IV fluid therapy and attempts to restart gastric activity.

There is no generally accepted pharmacological treatment of postoperative ileus. Altering intestinal motility may not be possible if there has been severe ischaemia or distension. The bowel will not usually respond before 48 hours after this type of injury. Nevertheless any drug given for this purpose should be used as a prophylactic measure at the end of surgery when the gut has been decompressed.

The cholinergic drug cisapride which is now only available in tablet form can be administered orally at 0.1 mg/kg body weight, 2, 10 and 18 hours after surgery. Metoclopramide can be administered by constant drip over several hours at a dose rate of 0.1 mg/kg/hour.

The search for a drug which gives consistently beneficial results continues. Lignocaine administered as a constant intravenous drip at 0.05 mg/kg per minute over 24 hours has given promising results.

Myopathy

Postoperative myopathy is a possible complication of any extended surgical procedure requiring maintenance of a horse under general anaesthesia.

With animals in dorsal recumbency, the gluteal and longissimus dorsi muscles are most likely to be affected because of pressure combined with inadequate circulation in the hindlimbs caused by partial occlusion of abdominal blood vessels by distended viscera. An intraoperative fall in blood pressure is another contributory cause.

Prevention by positioning and padding and a short operating time is better than a cure. Affected animals are reluctant or unable to rise, or may show slight hind leg stiffness.

Euthanasia is necessary in isolated cases if no improvement is made and the animal becomes distressed.

Wound breakdown or infection

Wound dehiscence must be attended to promptly since failure of the incision leads to life-threatening evisceration.

However, the most common wound problem is superficial infection of the incision.

There is often no significant difference in the rate of incisional infection between horses undergoing enterotomy or resection and those in which the gut lumen is not invaded.

Affected animals show moderately severe oedema along the incision. One or more foci of exudate appear 5 to 7 days postoperatively. The oedema then subsides. Most of these infections will continue to discharge 1–4 weeks and then resolve.

A delayed complication of low grade infection is incisional hernia. Excessive exercise too soon after surgery may also contribute to such hernias. The hernia comprises skin, a thin layer of fibrous tissue and peritoneum.

The defect in the body wall is best repaired using polypropylene mesh (see Chapter 4).

Laminitis

Laminitis is an ever present threat to horses with an acute abdomen.

The cause and pathophysiology are still not fully understood and the ability to prevent the problem totally is still elusive. It appears to be associated with the systemic absorption of endotoxins. All horses with intestinal disease, particularly those with strangulation obstructions, are susceptible.

Low dose flunixin therapy postoperatively will help to minimize the likelihood of laminitis.

The feet of colic cases should be monitored frequently for increased digital pulsations and heat, and the animal's willingness to move freely noted. The onset of laminitis as determined by clinical signs is often the second, third or, occasionally, fourth day after surgery. Frog pads should be used to place weight on the horse's heels and frog.

Thrombophlebitis

See Chapter 7.

Peritonitis

Peritonitis results from leakage of protein, endotoxin or bacteria from the bowel. This may be due to necrosis of the entire bowel wall or leakage due to a mucosal injury only.

Recognition of peritonitis during the postoperative period is based on the presence of one or more signs including ileus, fever, colic, abdominal guarding and evidence of inflammation and sepsis in the peritoneal fluid.

The diagnosis is confirmed by analysis of peritoneal fluid.

Broad-spectrum antibiotics, NSAIDs and maintenance of hydration are the main elements of treatment.

Adhesions

Infection and the presence of ischaemic tissue predispose to adhesions which may occur within hours of surgery, but may not cause any ill effects for months or years. In some cases, the pain presumed to be caused by adhesions is mild and transient but if colic signs persist, a second laparotomy is indicated.

Postoperative diarrhoea

Diarrhoea may arise from damage to the colon as the result of displacement or torsion producing an inability to absorb fluid. This does not tend to persist but it is difficult to differentiate from more serious causes such as salmonellosis or clostridial overgrowth.

A precipitous drop in leucocyte count, pyrexia and depression may herald a *Salmonella* infection in advance of frank diarrhoea.

Further reading

Edwards, G.B., Gerring, E.L. and Arnold, A.F. (1992) Equine gastroenterology. *Equine Veterinary Journal* Supplement 13.

White, N.A. (1990) *The Equine Acute Abdomen*. Lea & Febiger, Philadelphia.

Gastroenterology 2. Hepatic and intestinal disorders

LIVER DISEASE

Liver disease is relatively common in the horse. However, liver failure is much rarer because the liver has a large reserve capacity and good capacity to regenerate. Liver failure will not occur until 70% or more of the organ has been damaged.

Chronic weight loss is the most common presenting sign of liver failure but other presentations include dullness, anorexia, behavioural abnormalities, skin lesions, pruritus, bleeding disorders, diarrhoea and colic.

Weight loss is a common, but non-specific, finding in chronic liver disease. It is related to failure of metabolic functions of the liver and reduced food intake.

Hyperammonaemia results when ammonia from portal circulation is not metabolized to urea within the liver and enters the systemic circulation. Raised plasma ammonia affects gluco-neogenesis causing utilization of branched-chain amino acids. The resultant decrease in ratio of branched-chain to aromatic amino acids affects neutrotransmission and may give rise to *hepatic encephalopathy* (see Chapter 11) or, very rarely, *peripheral neuropathy* which can lead to unusual complications such as gastric impaction (and colic) or laryngeal paralysis.

Accumulation of bilirubin in plasma may result in jaundice. There may be decreased hepatic metabolism of photodynamic phylloerythrin which, when exposed to ultraviolet light within superficial dermal circulation, results in necrotic skin lesions in white areas referred to as *photo-sensitization* (see Chapter 13). Pruritus occasionally occurs due to bile salt accumulation in the skin.

Altered faecal consistency is not uncommon in equine liver failure with diarrhoea in some cases, probably related to portal hypertension or thrombosis, and abnormally firm faeces occurring in others. Colic may arise due to hepatocellular swelling and obstruction of the biliary tract. A reduction in intestinal motility is a fairly frequent finding in cases of equine liver failure.

Failure of the liver to synthesize clotting factors may result in an increased *bleeding tendency*, especially after trauma. Spontaneous haemorrhage into the lungs or alimentary tract is rarely seen. Such haemorrhage usually occurs as a terminal event.

The underlying hepatic pathology is generally chronic but clinical signs are often relatively sudden in onset when the degree of organ failure exceeds the considerable functional reserve capacities of liver. Hepatic failure occurs in a wide variety of conditions which can be difficult to differentiate but clinical management of affected cases is often similar and directed at ameliorating hyperammonia and providing nutritional support.

The main differential diagnoses of equine liver failure are chronic enteropathies and chronic grass sickness.

3.1 *Diagnostic approach to liver disease*

History

● Age – in foals, liver failure associated with rare disorders such as Tyzzer's disease or porto-systemic shunt. Senile cirrhosis occurs in elderly animals.
● Multiple cases affected implies ingested hepatotoxin (e.g. pyrrolizidine alkaloid) or, very rarely, liver fluke infection. Also, hyperlipaemia with associated hepatic dysfunction may occur in groups of animals under the same management, and Theiler's disease is seen as a group disease in North Western US.
● Duration/procession of signs – insidious weight loss is common and non-specific for chronic hepatopathies. Neurological signs associated with hepatic encephalopathy can develop fairly suddenly in chronic advanced liver failure (e.g. pyrrolizidine toxicosis) or, more likely will be the presenting complaint in acute liver failure (e.g. Theiler's disease).

Physical examination

Few physical findings are diagnostic of equine liver disease. Generally the approach is to rule out other possible causes of weight loss, behavioural changes or skin lesions, e.g. signs of enteropathy, primary central nervous system (CNS) disease (Chapter 11) or primary skin disease (Chapter 13).

Jaundice occurs relatively infrequently in equine liver failure but is more likely in acute and/or cholestatic diseases. Horses commonly become mildly jaundiced from anorexia, even when the liver is not diseased.

Mucosal petechial/ecchymotic haemorrhages or bleeding due to clotting abnormalities occur uncommonly.

Peripheral oedema or ascites are rare in equine liver failure.

Photosensitization lesions occur in unpigmented skin especially of the head.

Laboratory investigation of liver disease

1. Plasma/serum liver enzymes
   - *Hepatocellular damage*:
     - glutamate dehydrogenase (GLDH) – liver specific
     - sorbitol dehydrogenase (SDH) – specific, unstable if stored (e.g. postal)
     - lactate dehydrogenase (LDH) – iso-enzyme 5 non-specific
     - aspartate transferase (AST) – non-specific
   - *Biliary tract damage or obstruction*:
     - gammaglutamyl transferase (γGT) – specific
     - alkaline phosphatase (AP) – non-specific
2. Bilirubin. Predominantly unconjugated regardless of disease type and can be elevated consequent upon prolonged anorexia without hepatic disease.
3. Liver function
   - *Bile acids* – particularly sensitive indicator of cholestasis.
   - *Ammonia* – plasma levels variably raised, and generally indicate severe liver failure; may be associated with decreased blood urea levels.
   - Bromosulphthalein (BSP) clearance – half-life of this dye is normally 2.0–3.7 minutes and may be extended in liver disease. Nowadays considered of doubtful usefulness.
4. Other analytes may be altered in hepatic disease e.g. hypoglycaemia, hypoalbuminaemia, decreased albumin:globulin ratio, raised levels of triglycerides and cholesterol.
5. Clotting function – prolonged prothrombin time.

Liver biopsy

In many cases biopsy can provide a definitive diagnosis (which laboratory tests cannot). Ideally, confirm normal clotting function prior to ultrasound-guided biopsy. Using a 14 cm needle, percutaneous biopsy can be performed 'blind' in the standing horse at the 12th, 13th or 14th right-sided intercostal spaces between the level of lines drawn from the tuber coxae to the point of the olecranon and the shoulder.

Diagnostic ultrasound in liver disease

By use of transabdominal ultrasonography it is possible to assess physical changes of the liver. Discrete lesions such as abscesses or choleliths can be visualized, and chronic fibrosis can be appreciated.

3.2 *Pyrrolizidine toxicity*

Ingestion of plants containing pyrrolizidine alkaloids is a common cause of equine liver failure. The plant species most frequently involved in the UK is *Senecio jacobea* (ragwort). In the USA, plants commonly incriminated include *Crotalaria* spp. (rattlebox), *Senecio* spp. (groundsel), and *Amsinckia* spp. (riddleneck). These plants are generally unpalatable to horses unless withered, e.g. following pasture-topping or within hay, or if grazing is severely restricted. Clinical signs of liver failure (see above) develop months to years after toxic ingestion and there may be multiple cases with variable severity of signs. Definitive diagnosis can be made by percutaneous biopsy. Treatment (see below) can be attempted; although the prognosis is poor, some cases survive.

3.3 *Theiler's disease*

The aetiology is unknown but historically the disease has been associated with serum administration. It commonly occurs as group outbreaks during autumn in north western USA but is only rarely recognized as an entity in Europe. Generally, affected cases develop peracute liver failure but individuals may have mild or subclinical signs with raised serum liver enzyme levels.

3.4 *Cirrhosis*

This is not well documented but is not uncommon. End-stage pathology is of other specific liver conditions or senile change. The most likely clinical presentation is chronic, progressive weight loss. Diagnosis is confirmed by biopsy. Supportive treatment may prolong life by weeks or months, but the prognosis is very poor.

3.5 *Liver fluke*

Fasciola hepatica infection is rare in the horse, but donkeys may be more susceptible. Clinical signs of liver failure can occur and it may be a group disease. Diagnosis is possibly confirmed by fluke eggs in faeces but immature, migrating parasites could cause signs prior to patency. Treatment is with triclabendazole, 15 mg/kg body weight *per os* (not licensed in the horse).

3.6 *Biliary calculi*

Biliary calculi (choleliths) occur rarely in the horse and may be asymptomatic or have a clinical presentation of recurrent colic in addition to other signs of liver failure (see above). Diagnosis is confirmed by ultrasonography, and prognosis is guarded, depending on the extent of hepatic fibrosis secondary to biliary obstruction. Treatment by surgery or cholelithotripsy is possible.

3.7 *Hydatid cysts*

Cysts of the horse-dog tapeworm *Echinococcus granulosus equinus* are common in equine livers in UK but they are virtually never associated with clinical disease.

3.8 *Other hepatic diseases*

Various other liver diseases have been documented in the horse but should be regarded as uncommon. Other diseases may affect liver function and some of these are described elsewhere in the text.

Portosystemic shunts (Chapter 20)
Chronic active hepatitis
Liver abscess
Equine herpesvirus (Chapter 19)
Biliary atresia
Mycotoxicosis
Hyperlipaemia (Chapter 9)
Hepatic carcinoma
Lymphoma (see 3.16)
Iron toxicity (haemochromatosis)
Tyzzer's disease (Chapter 20)
Cholangitis

3.9 *Treatment of liver failure*

Treatment of liver failure is basically supportive. Treatment is most likely to be successful in acute hepatic failure and is not indicated in horses with severely cirrhotic livers. The prognosis is poor for severe hepatoencephalopathy.

Sedation may be necessary in horses with signs of hepatoencephalopathy. Xylazine and detomidine administered in small doses are usually effective.

Intravenous glucose should be administered as a 10% solution if hypoglycaemia is present.

Attempts should be made to *decrease blood ammonia levels. Mineral oil* is administered by nasogastric tube. *Lactulose syrup* administered orally is digested by colonic bacteria into organic acids which create an osmotic diarrhoea. *Neomycin* or metronidazole administered orally decreases microbial production of toxins, but may predispose to salmonellosis.

A *low protein diet* should be fed.

Vitamin B₁, folic acid and *vitamin K₁* should be administered weekly.

Hydration, acid–base and electrolyte abnormalities should be corrected where necessary. Acidosis must be corrected slowly, since over-correction and alkalosis may exacerbate hepatoencephalopathy.

Antibiotics are indicated in cases of bacterial cholangitis.

Hyperlipaemia may be treated with insulin and heparin (see Chapter 9).

PANCREATIC DISEASES

Clinical disease due to pancreatic disorders is rare in the horse. Non-specific signs of weight loss, intermittent colic, jaundice and fever can arise from either chronic pancreatitis or pancreatic adenocarcinoma. Both disorders may give rise to increased levels of serum amylase and lipase as well as hypocalcaemia. Pancreatic diseases may also be associated with raised liver enzymes and hyperbilirubinaemia due to either biliary obstruction or pancreatic production of gamma glutamyl transferase (γGT) which is regarded as a 'liver-specific' enzyme. Confirmation of both chronic pancreatitis and pancreatic carcinoma is by either exploratory laparotomy or post-mortem examination. Acute pancreatitis is a very rare cause of severe abdominal pain with nasogastric reflux and circulatory failure such that it requires to be differentiated from strangulating intestinal obstruction and anterior enteritis.

3.10 *Grass sickness*

Grass sickness is a dysautonomia which is typically manifest by gastrointestinal signs. It is hypothesized but not yet proven that the aetiology of grass sickness (*equine dysautonomia*) is an environmental toxin. The disease is fairly common in regions of UK and parts of continental Europe. A virtually identical condition occurs in South America.

Epidemiology

Regional prevalence occurs with certain localities having higher risk for the condition and the incidence within regions varying from year to year.

Age prevalence peaks between 2 and 7 years old but the disease can occur at any age.

Seasonal prevalence exists with increased occurrence in April–July which probably relates to periods of dry, cool weather.

Grass sickness is more prevalent in animals introduced to premises within the last 2 months and/or which are outdoors all the time and/or which are not receiving supplementary feeding. Frequently more than one individual case is affected on same premises and the risk of grass sickness is much greater on grazing on which the disease has previously occurred.

Pathogenesis

Widespread and generally severe damage to neurons of the autonomic nervous system, enteric nervous system and certain somatic ganglia and nuclei of the central nervous system with resultant disruption of gastrointestinal motility.

Clinical signs

Acute (<4 days) or chronic (week to months) forms occur with some cases arbitrarily designated as 'sub-acute' (4–10 days).

Acute form
- Anorexia.
- Dysphagia.

- Colic (moderate to severe).
- Absence of gut sounds.
- Tachycardia (heart rate 70–80/min, or more).
- Congestion and dryness of mucous membranes.
- Dehydration.
- ±Patchy sweating.
- ±Muscle fasciculations/tremors.
- Nasogastric reflux – occasionally spontaneous appearance of green fluid at the nostrils or several gallons foetid yellow/green fluid obtained via stomach tube.
- Gastric rupture may occur.
- Crusty nasal discharge/rhinitis.
- *per rectum* – dry, tacky rectal mucosa; meagre rectal contents which are hard with mucosal casts on surface. Large intestine (especially large colon) is shrunken down onto hard, knobbly, impacted contents. Distended, fluid-filled loops of small intestine may be palpable, extending back towards the pelvic inlet.

Chronic form
From day to day marked variation in severity of signs.

- Dullness/hypoaesthetic/sleepy.
- Reduced intestinal motility.
- Marked weight loss/emaciation.
- Minimal faecal production – faeces hard and dry.
- Marked reduction of abdominal size – 'greyhound like'.
- Tachycardia.
- ±Abnormal stance – four feet placed closely together.
- ±Penile protrusion.
- ±Patchy sweating.
- ±Muscle fasciculation/tremor.
- ±Intermittent, mild colic.

Diagnosis

- Clinical signs.
- Contrast radiography: prolonged (>5 secs) oesophageal transit time of barium given into proximal oesophagus. Also may see barium pooling or retrograde movement.
- Oesophageal endoscopy – linear ulcerations.
- Definitive diagnosis requires histopathology: neuronal vacuolation and chromatolysis with variable inflammatory infiltrate. Usual material for histopathology is either coeliacomesenteric ganglion collected at post-mortem examination or ileal biopsy (at either exploratory laparotomy or post-mortem examination). Similar patho-

logical changes occur in other autonomic ganglia as well as in brain and spinal cord.

- Post-mortem examination.

Acute form

- Gastric distension with foetid fluid.
- Gastric/oesophageal mucosal ulceration.
- Large colon impacted with dark, dry, hard content.

Chronic form

- Emaciated carcass.
- Marked reduction of intestinal size.
- Dry, firm, large intestinal content.

Treatment

- Euthanasia.
- Selected chronic cases may survive given nursing/supportive therapy and use of the intestinal prokinetic agent, cisapride.

Prevention

It might help to keep equine animals indoors for at least part of every day, and/or feed supplementary roughage, during periods of peak incidence. This applies particularly to young or newly arrived animals, or when a case of grass sickness has already occurred on the premises.

GASTROINTESTINAL DISORDERS

The most common clinical disorders of the gastrointestinal tract are those giving rise to signs of acute abdominal pain or colic which are dealt with in Chapter 2. There are other clinical manifestations of intestinal dysfunction in the horse of which the most important are *acute diarrhoea or chronic weight loss and/or chronic diarrhoea*. The presence of diarrhoea almost invariably indicates large intestinal disease whereas weight loss may be associated with disorders affecting either the small intestine or the large intestine or both.

The principal pathological processes of intestinal disease are *protein losing enteropathy and/or carbohydrate malabsorption*. If only the latter is present, the clinical presentation will usually be of insidious weight loss, whereas with protein losing enteropathy (PLE) there will usually be fairly rapid weight loss and commonly peripheral

oedema will develop consequent upon hypoproteinaemia/hypoalbuminaemia. In acute disorders, fever, cardiovascular compromise and coagulopathy associated with endotoxaemia are common. Additional clinical signs which may be present in gastrointestinal disease include altered intestinal motility, anorexia, ptyalism, bruxism, dysphagia and, rarely, skin lesions.

A diverse group of gastrointestinal conditions may give rise to diarrhoea and/or weight loss but often these diseases cannot be readily differentiated on clinical findings. In practical circumstances the clinical management of such cases is often similar regardless of the diagnosis and is directed at symptomatic antidiarrhoeal medication and fluid/electrolyte/nutritional support. However, the prognosis for these conditions varies greatly, e.g. successful outcome following treatment of cases of larval cyathostomosis occurs in approximately 60% of cases whereas there is virtually 100% mortality in cases of intestinal lymphosarcoma. For this reason a specific diagnosis is preferable but unfortunately that can generally only be achieved by histopathological examination of intestinal biopsy specimens obtained at exploratory laparotomy. Animals with hypoproteinaemia secondary to protein losing enteropathy are high risk for wound dehiscence and this, together with the relatively high cost of equine abdominal surgery, means that a specific diagnosis is often only achieved at postmortem examination.

3.11 *Diagnostic approach to intestinal disease*

History

1. Age – foals and yearlings are more susceptible to gastrointestinal infections such as rotavirus (Chapter 20) and salmonellosis (Chapter 19). Larval cyathostomosis (Chapter 19) is more common in animals less than four years old, and grass sickness is also more prevalent in this age category. Chronic inflammatory bowel disease (CIBD) and intestinal neoplasia are more common in animals greater than ten years old.
2. Multiple cases are suggestive of an infectious cause, e.g. acute enterocolitis in salmonellosis (Chapter 19) or weight loss/diarrhoea of larval cyathostomosis (Chapter 19).

3. Duration/progression – peracute/acute systemic illness due to endotoxaemia occurs in various enterocolitides and also peritonitis. Cyathostomosis cases tend to have sudden onset, but rarely have marked systemic illness, and tend to have a timecourse of a few weeks. CIBD and intestinal neoplasia are generally insidious, with a duration of weeks to months.

Physical examination

There are virtually no characteristic physical findings for individual enteropathies, and the clinical approach is to rule out other disorders which may be associated with weight loss, e.g. liver disease with evidence of hepatic encephalopathy, then to undertake clinicopathological investigation relevant to intestinal dysfunction.

Colic, reduced borborygmi and cardiovascular compromise consequent upon endotoxaemia occur in acute enterocolitis and peritonitis which therefore necessitate differentiation from strangulating intestinal obstruction, non-strangulating infarction etc. (Chapter 2).

Various musculoskeletal signs which might be useful for differential diagnosis may be detectable in certain disorders primarily manifest as gastrointestinal in nature. In chronic grass sickness, cases often adopt a characteristic stance with all four feet placed close together under the trunk and such animals will often exhibit intermittent muscle fasciculations. Due to parietal abdominal pain, cases of peritonitis are often reluctant to move and do so with a rather 'wooden' gait. This feature should be differentiated from endotoxaemia-associated laminitis which can complicate both peritonitis and also enterocolitis.

Laboratory investigation

Blood biochemistry/haematology
There are no specific markers of gastrointestinal disease. The most relevant analyses to measure are total protein, albumin, globulin, alkaline phosphatase, fibrinogen and a complete blood count (CBC) and differential. In acute gastrointestinal disease, hydration status, acid–base balance and electrolyte (K, Na, Cl) disturbances should be assessed, together with renal function (creatinine, urea and phosphate). Serum protein electrophoresis is sometimes useful for differentiation of parasitic colitis (cyathostomosis) from other enteropathies. The level of abnormality of variables such as total protein, albumin, alkaline phosphatase and neutrophil levels relate to the severity of chronic enteropathies such that they may be helpful in assessing prognosis.

Peritoneal fluid cytology/biochemistry
Abdominocentesis is very useful in assessment of acute abdominal disorders (Chapter 2) but of limited value in chronic conditions. Peritonitis can be confirmed by detection of peritoneal fluid white cell count $> 5 \times 10^9/l$, total protein $> 10\,g/l$ and alkaline phosphatase of > 250 IU/l. Intestinal neoplasia and CIBD rarely exfoliate nucleated cells into peritoneal fluid in detectable numbers.

Intestinal function tests
Small intestinal absorptive dysfunction can be accurately detected by monosaccharide absorption tests, usually using glucose or, less commonly xylose. The protocol for the oral glucose tolerance test is:

- overnight fast and basal plasma glucose measurement time 0 min,
- glucose (20% solution) by stomach tube at dose of 1 g/kg body weight,
- plasma glucose measurement at times 30, 60, 90, 120, 180, 240, 360 min.

'Normal' small intestinal function is evidenced by a peak of plasma glucose at 120 min of 200% of basal level and return to basal levels by 360 min. A peak value of less than 120% basal value indicates total carbohydrate malabsorption and an increase of between 120 and 185% is classified as partial malabsorption.

Xylose absorption should give a similar shaped curve but interpretation is by comparison with established reference ranges.

Detection of carbohydrate malabsorption confirms the presence of small intestinal disease but the tests are not useful for differentiating the possible causes.

Histopathology
Chronic enteropathies can only be definitively diagnosed on the basis of histopathological features of biopsy material obtained by either laparotomy, rectal biopsy or post-mortem examination. The surgical risk and expense are high in animals with PLE and surgery is often not undertaken. Rectal biopsy is safe and simple from intrapelvic sites on the lateral rectum: diagnostic samples are obtained in about one third of chronic enteropathy cases.

Imaging modalities

Ultrasonography and laparoscopy are occasionally useful for investigation of animals presented with possible gastrointestinal disease, mainly to rule out rare conditions such as splenic neoplasia or urogenital disease.

3.12 *Chronic inflammatory bowel disease*

Chronic inflammatory bowel disease (CIBD) is a collective term for a group of chronic infiltrative enteropathies with very similar clinical presentations (usually of chronic weight loss) and clinical signs. These disorders are not as clearly defined in the horse as they may be in other animal species and humans. The major clinical differential diagnoses are intestinal neoplasia and chronic hepatopathies.

Epidemiology

Generally CIBD occurs spontaneously in individual, middle aged to old animals of any breed but it has been suggested that granulomatous enterocolitis is more common in Standardbreds less than 5 years of age.

Pathogenesis

The aetiopathogenesis of equine CIBD is uncertain but may represent immune-mediated phenomena. Various infectious agents may play a role in these enteropathies including strongyle parasites, *Mycobacterium paratuberculosis* (granulomatous enteritis), *Rhodococcus equi* (granulomatous enteritis) and *Histoplasmum capsulatum* (granulomatous colitis).

Clinical signs

- Weight loss
- ± Diarrhoea
- ± Intermittent colic
- ± Inappetence
- ± Peripheral oedema
- ± Pyrexia
- ± Skin lesions
- ± Mesenteric lymph node enlargement

Diagnosis

Clinical pathological findings are non-specific but may include:

- Hypoalbuminaemia.
- Hyperglobulinaemia.
- Neutrophilia.
- Anaemia.
- Hyperfibrinogenaemia.
- Raised serum alkaline phosphatase.
- Reduced glucose absorption (OGTT).

Definitive diagnosis is based upon histopathology of intestinal (or rectal) biopsies. The infiltrate may constitute a mixed cellular population or there may be a predominance of specific cell types such that CIBD may be classified as either granulomatous enteritis/colitis or eosinophilic gastroenteritis, eosinophilic granulomatous enteritis or lymphocytic plasmacytic enteritis. Similar pathological findings are commonly identified within mesenteric lymph nodes and also occasionally in skin lesions. The condition described as multisystemic eosinophilic epitheliotropic disease may have gastrointestinal involvement as well as cutaneous, hepatic and pancreatic lesions.

The major differential diagnoses for CIBD are alimentary lymphosarcoma, larval cyathostomosis, and chronic hepatopathies.

Treatment

Long term corticosteroid therapy (prednisolone) may result in clinical improvement during the course of treatment, but clinical relapses occur commonly, but not invariably, following cessation of medication. Other symptomatic treatments which may be useful include anti-diarrhoeal agents and/or anthelmintics and/or probiotics together with high protein nutritional supplementation.

Prognosis

Sustained clinical improvement is rarely achieved.

3.13 *Alimentary lymphoma*

Alimentary lymphoma is more common than either thoracic or cutaneous lymphoma (see Chapters 6 and 13) and most cases are presented with insidious weight loss, such that the major differential diagnoses are other chronic hepatopathies or chronic enteropathies.

Epidemiology

The disease may occur in young adults (2 to 6 years) but is apparently more common in animals more than 10 years old.

Pathogenesis

No infectious agent has been incriminated in equine lymphoma. The disease can result in both small intestinal carbohydrate malabsorption and/or protein losing enteropathy.

Clinical signs

- Weight loss
- ± Inappetence
- ± Intermittent/recurrent colic
- ± Peripheral oedema
- ± Diarrhoea
- ± Pyrexia

Diagnosis

Clinical pathological findings are non-specific but may include:

- Hypoalbuminaemia.
- Hyperglobulinaemia.
- Neutrophilia.
- Anaemia.
- Hyperfibrinogenaemia.
- Raised serum alkaline phosphatase.
- Reduced glucose absorption (OGTT).
- Peritoneal fluid cytology – rarely detect tumour cells.
- Decreased plasma levels of IgM.

Definitive diagnosis is based upon histopathology of intestinal (or rectal) biopsies.

Treatment

Temporary improvement can be achieved with palliative, symptomatic medication with either oral or systemic corticosteroids (prednisolone) and antidiarrhoeic agents, such as codeine phosphate. Cytotoxic therapy for treatment of equine alimentary lymphoma has not been reported.

Prognosis

The prognosis is extremely poor – most cases are euthanased on humane grounds within 6–12 months of onset of signs.

3.14 *Sand enteropathy*

Accumulation of sand in the gastrointestinal tract is a well-recognized but fairly uncommon cause of diarrhoea and/or colic.

Epidemiology

The equine animals at risk of developing sand enteropathy are those grazing areas of sandy soil with little pasture cover, and the risk is exacerbated if grain is fed from the ground to such animals. There is a relatively high prevalence in certain geographical regions, e.g. California, New Jersey.

Pathogenesis

Sand accumulates within the large colons and gives rise to either colonic irritation and/or physical obstruction which results in diarrhoea and/or colic.

Clinical signs

- ± Diarrhoea
- ± Colic
- ± (Rarely) weight loss

Diagnosis

- Per rectum detection of sand impaction.
- Visualization of sand sediment from faecal solution.
- 'Pouring sand' sounds on abdominal auscultation of ventral abdomen.
- Abdominal radiography.

Treatment

- Bulk laxatives (especially psyllium hydrophilia), initially via nasogastric tube and then in-feed.
- Mineral/vegetable oils via nasogastric tube.
- ± Parenteral fluid therapy.
- (Rarely) surgical removal of impacted sand.

Prognosis

The prognosis is generally good. Recurrence and/or cases in other animals under the same management can be prevented by avoiding over-grazing of pastures on sandy soil and feeding from fixed troughs.

3.15 *Idiopathic chronic diarrhoea*

In the horse, the cause of chronic diarrhoea often remains undiagnosed despite extensive investigative procedures.

Epidemiology

Some cases of idiopathic diarrhoea may be consequent upon earlier infectious enteropathies and/or fermentation disorders. Particularly in foals and yearlings diarrhoea may persist for several months before resolution which can be associated with a change to a pasture-based diet.

Pathogenesis

By definition the pathogenesis of these cases is not known.

Clinical signs

- Diarrhoea
- ± Weight loss

Diagnosis

Diagnosis is by exclusion of identifiable causes of diarrhoea.

Treatment

Symptomatic therapy can be utilized with variable clinical effect – recurrence of diarrhoea is not uncommon. Symptomatic antidiarrhoeals (e.g. codeine phosphate, iodochlorohydroxyquin) concurrently with either probiotics or natural yoghurt or transfaunated caecal contents are appropriate. Absorbents such as chalk, kaolin or activated charcoal are only useful in foals.

Prognosis

The prognosis is generally good for survival but recurrent, chronic diarrhoea may persist.

3.16 *Acute enterocolitis*

The term incorporates a variety of large intestinal disorders with very similar presenting and clinical signs of acute onset diarrhoea and colic. Causes of enterocolitis include salmonellosis (also see Chapter 19), Potomac horse fever (i.e. *Ehrlichia risticii* infection, Chapter 19), clostridiosis (also known as colitis X), antimicrobial therapy, non-steroidal anti-inflammatory drug (NSAID) therapy and toxicities such as either monensin/salinomycin or heavy metals. These disorders cannot be readily differentiated on the basis of clinical features and often there is rapid clinical progression with predisposition to sequelae of endotoxaemia including circulatory collapse, laminitis and thrombophlebitis.

Epidemiology

- Salmonellosis – increased risk in foals, stressed/hospitalized animals and those receiving antimicrobials: 'outbreaks' may occur.
- Potomac horse fever – regional occurrence – Eastern USA. Likely involves both an insect vector and an intermediate host.
- Colitis X – associated with *Clostridium perfringens* type A infection, but initiating factors unknown.
- Antimicrobial therapy – disruption of intestinal flora leading to diarrhoea has been associated with either lincomycin or tetracycline therapy, but other antibiotics can have a similar, possibly less severe, effect.
- NSAID toxicity – excessive or prolonged dosages and/or dehydrated animals.
- Monensin/salinomycin toxicity – ingestion of contaminated feedstuff.
- Heavy metal toxicity – rare.

Pathogenesis

- Salmonellosis – intestinal mucosal colonization results in inflammatory protein losing enteropathy (PLE) and endotoxaemia.
- Potomac horse fever – initial infection of peripheral monocytes and macrophages with later phase of infection within small intestinal and colonic mucosa. As a result there may be several days of fever and colic prior to onset of diarrhoea.
- Clostridiosis – marked colonic oedema and PLE.
- Antimicrobial therapy – per se altered fermentation by disruption of normal intestinal micro-

flora can give rise to diarrhoea. In addition, antibiotic therapy predisposes to both salmonellosis and also clostridiosis.
- Monensin/salinomycin – ionophores alter ionic transport across cell membranes: gastrointestinal, cardiovascular and neurological effects occur.

The pathophysiology of equine enterocolitis has not been defined in detail. The mechanisms which are likely to be involved include:

- Raised local levels of prostaglandins, prostacyclin and leukotrienes.
- Stimulation of fluid/electrolyte secretion and protein exudation into the bowel lumen.
- Increased permeability of intestinal microvasculature.
- Endotoxaemia.

Clinical signs

The clinical signs are somewhat variable, especially in Potomac horse fever, but generally cases of enterocolitis are extremely ill with rapid progression of:

- Markedly dull attitude.
- Fever.
- Decreased intestinal motility.
- Colic.
- Explosive watery diarrhoea.
- Endotoxaemia.
- ± Peripheral oedema.
- ± Laminitis.
- Rapid weight loss in survivors.

Diagnosis

The peracute nature of enterocolitis necessitates emergency treatment before a definitive, specific diagnosis is available. Successful intensive care of enterocolitis is ideally monitored by use of blood biochemical and haematological findings which are extremely dynamic in this condition. Typical clinical pathological features are:

- Dehydration/haemoconcentration – raised packed cell volume (PCV) and total protein (TP) but as the disease progresses there may be progressive decrease in TP due to intestinal protein loss; raised plasma creatinine and urea.
- Electrolyte imbalances – usually hyponatraemia and/or hypochloraemia and/or hypokalaemia.
- Metabolic acidosis.

- Leucopenia.
- ± Thrombocytopenia in Potomac horse fever.

Specific diagnosis may be obtained by:

- Salmonellosis – culture; may require multiple sequential faecal samples or post-mortem tissue/intestinal contents.
- Clostridiosis – culture of faeces/intestinal content with quantitative count of colony forming units.
- Potomac horse fever – serology; IFA or ELISA.

Gross post-mortem and/or histopathological findings vary depending on the time course of the disease. Necropsy findings usually include:

- Serosal discoloration; petechiae purple to black.
- Mucosal discoloration; haemorrhagic or necrotic black/brown.
- Mucosal oedema/thickening and sloughing of fibronecrotic debris.
- Watery, foul smelling intestinal contents.
- Mesenteric lymph node enlargement.
- Hyperaemia and/or petechial haemorrhages of lungs, liver and adrenal glands.

Treatment

- Intravenous fluid therapy with correction of specific electrolyte and acid–base disturbances and consider use of colloidals or plasma.
- Flunixin meglumine at anti-endotoxic dose of 0.25 mg/kg three times daily.
- Endotoxin antisera/purified immunoglobulin products.
- Frog supports.
- ? Antibiotics
  – generally contraindicated but appropriate in neonatal salmonellosis,
  – oxytetracycline is drug of choice in Potomac horse fever.
- Nutritional support.
- Critical care.

Prognosis

Mortality rate is high even after aggressive, expensive, intensive care and there is a high prevalence of complications. Cases which are diarrhoeic for more than 7 days are unlikely to survive. Acute enterocolitis does *not* usually result in chronic intestinal/digestive dysfunction in surviving cases.

3.17 *Non-steroidal anti-inflammatory drug toxicity*

Any non-steroidal anti-inflammatory drug (NSAID) can potentially lead to either gastro-intestinal and/or renal disease.

Epidemiology

Long-term treatment and/or overdosing with NSAIDs, which may arise from owner ignorance, often underlie NSAID toxicity. Animals with cardiovascular compromise and/or dehydration will be more prone to NSAID toxicity.

Pathogenesis

Inhibition of mucosal prostaglandins E_1 and E_2 which have a mucosal protective effect within the stomach, intestine and kidneys. Loss of mucosal protection can result in either protein losing enteropathy as a result of gastrointestinal ulceration or protein losing nephropathy.

Clinical signs

Variable severity of:

- Inappetence/anorexia.
- Peripheral oedema.
- Oral mucosal ulceration.
- Diarrhoea.
- Colic.
- Endotoxaemia.
- Laminitis.
- Decreased urine output and/or dilute urination.

Diagnosis

Usually a presumptive diagnosis is made from the history. Laboratory assessment of fluid/electrolyte and acid–base disturbances is useful to assist fluid therapy, and monitoring of renal function and plasma proteins levels is appropriate.

Endoscopy can allow visualization of oesophageal or gastric ulceration.

Treatment

- Discontinue NSAID therapy.
- Intravenous fluid/electrolyte therapy.
- Frog supports.

- Histamine receptor type – two antagonists (H_2 antagonists).
- Analgesia with butorphanol tartrate and/or alpha-2 agonists for colic (and laminitis).

Prognosis

Guarded in severe cases, e.g. diarrhoea, colic and laminitis, but slow recovery if signs are mild. Blood biochemical evidence of severe renal compromise generally indicates a poor prognosis.

3.18 *Other gastrointestinal disorders*

Many other conditions of the gastrointestinal tract occur with low prevalence in the horse. In addition, various disorders of other body systems may give rise to gastrointestinal signs and some of these are described elsewhere in the text.

Foal heat diarrhoea (Chapter 20)
Rotavirus (Chapter 20)
Coronavirus (Chapter 20)
Rhodococcus equi (Chapter 20)
Ehrlichia coli (Chapter 20)
Campylobacter spp.
Strongyloides westeri (Chapter 19)
Strongylosis (Chapter 19)
Cyathostomosis (Chapter 19)
Cryptosporidiosis
Coccidiosis
Giardiasis
Histoplasmosis
Cardiac failure (Chapter 7)
Cushing's disease (Chapter 9)
Hyperlipaemia (Chapter 22)
Peritonitis (Chapter 4)
Intestinal lymphangectasia
Gastric squamous cell carcinoma (Chapter 4)
Gastric ulceration (Chapter 20)
Cantharadin (blister beetle) toxicosis (Chapter 22)

Further reading

Brown, C.M. (1989) *Problems in Equine Medicine*. Lea & Febiger, Philadelphia.

Byars, T.D. (1983) Chronic liver failure in horses. *Compendium on Continuing Education for the Practising Veterinarian* **5**, S423.

Love, S., Mair. T.S. and Hillyer, M.H. (1992) Chronic diarrhoea in adult horses: A review of 51 referred cases. *Veterinary Record* **130**, 217.

Roberts, M.C. (1983) Protein-losing enteropathy in the horse. *Compendium on Continuing Education for the Practising Veterinarian* **5**, S550.

Whitlock, R.H. (1986) Colitis: Differential diagnosis and treatment. *Equine Veterinary Journal* **18**, 278.

Appendix. Differential diagnoses

1. Jaundice
Liver disease
Reduced food intake
Haemolysis
Biliary tract obstruction
Septicaemia
Leptospirosis

2. Acute diarrhoea in the adult horse
Larval cyathostomosis
Salmonellosis
Potomac horse fever
Clostridiosis
Antimicrobial therapy
NSAID toxicity
Other toxicities, e.g.
  heavy metals
  monensin/salinomycin
  plants
Endotoxaemia/septicaemia
Overfeeding or sudden dietary change
Anthrax
Purpura haemorrhagica
Anaphylaxis
Idiopathic

3. Chronic diarrhoea in the adult horse
Larval cyathostomosis
Mixed strongyle infections
Alimentary lymphoma
Inflammatory bowel diseases
Sand enteropathy
Peritonitis
Congestive heart failure
Liver failure
Hyperlipaemia
Idiopathic

4 *Abdominal cavity*

4.1 *Hernias*

Definitions

A hernia comprises the protrusion of an organ or part of an organ through the wall of the cavity normally containing it.

Hernias may be classified as direct or indirect, internal or external.

A *direct* hernia occurs through a rent or tear whereas an *indirect* hernia occurs through a natural passage such as the inguinal canal or umbilicus.

An *external hernia* occurs through the body wall producing a visible and palpable swelling covered by skin, whereas an *internal* hernia occurs within the abdominal cavity (Table 1).

Types of hernia

Hernias may be congenital or acquired. Most are reducible, but in some cases the contents of the hernias cannot be returned to their normal location due to incarceration, strangulation or adhesions.

An *incarcerated* hernia is one in which the passage of ingesta through the protruding loop of intestine is arrested. The blood flow in its wall, however, is maintained.

A *strangulated* hernia is one which is both irreducible and incarcerated, and in which the blood circulation is also arrested, resulting in gangrene unless speedy relief is afforded.

Hernias with intermediate sized rings are more prone to incarceration and strangulation because even moderate distension of the herniated intestine with gas or ingesta will result in compression of its lymphatic and venous drainage.

Umbilical hernias

Umbilical hernias are significantly more common in fillies than in colts, and may be hereditary.

The majority of small hernias close spontaneously as the foal gets older, and it has become customary to wait until the foal is 6–12 months old before attempting surgery. Large defects

Table 1 Types of hernia

External hernias
Umbilical
Inguinal/scrotal
Traumatic abdominal wall hernias
Ventral
Incisional hernias
Internal hernias
Epiploic foramen
Mesenteric
Diaphragm
Omentum
Mesocolon
Gastrosplenic ligament
Hepatogastric ligament
Hepatoduodenal ligament
Ductus deferens

show little tendency to spontaneous closure, and early attention to these cases is rewarded by the greater ease with which treatment can be carried out in the young foal.

Congenital hernias are present at birth and are due to failure of the abdominal wall to close. Acquired hernias are not present at birth, and develop at 3–4 weeks of age. Excessive straining to defecate or micturate, and infection of the umbilicus, may be causative factors. It has been suggested that many are the result of improper management/handling of the foal at birth including manual ligation of the cord.

The fibrous hernial ring is composed of the aponeurosis of the transverse muscle, the fused oblique muscles and the abdominal tunic.

Umbilical hernias may be oval in shape and vary in size from one to several centimetres in diameter.

The hernial sac comprises an inner peritoneal layer and an outer layer of skin linked by varying amounts of connective tissue. Intestine (small intestine or caecum), omentum or both may constitute the contents of the hernial sac.

Incarceration and strangulation of the herniated intestine are rare and most likely to occur when the hernial ring is intermediate in size and allows little room for distension of the loop of bowel without the risk of constriction.

A parietal or Richter's hernia is defined as incarceration of the bowel wall circumference within a hernial orifice. The bowel is not completely obstructed, and pain may be less severe or not evident until rupture is imminent. The ileum and less frequently the caecum may be involved.

Umbilical hernias complicated by infection of the remnants of the umbilical stalk are encountered only rarely in foals compared with calves. The umbilical structures should close within a week of birth and only fibrous remnants should remain at 6 weeks. In the event of infection one or more of these structures (one umbilical vein, two umbilical arteries and the urachus) will remain patent. Ultrasonography provides the best means of identifying which structure(s) is involved.

Examination of the hernia

In the vast majority of cases, gentle pressure on the protruding swelling will reduce the hernia, allowing identification of the hernial ring, which should be assessed for size, shape and rigidity.

Incarcerated hernias present as tense, painful swellings which are usually irreducible. Occa-sionally gas in the entrapped intestine may have been dispersed during transport to a surgical facility or by gentle pressure allowing reduction to be achieved. Although the immediate risk to the foal's life may have been removed, whenever possible repair of the hernia should be carried out as soon as possible.

Incision of the hernia sac and careful examination of the caecum and small intestine should be performed to rule out the possibility of ischaemic compromise which is particularly likely with a Richter hernia. Even if ischaemic damage is not considered likely, any delay in repair of the hernia should be kept to a minimum because of the possibility of a further episode of incarceration which on that occasion may progress to strangulation.

Closed reduction

A wide variety of methods of treatment have been used in the past, including blisters, transfixing skewers and wooden or metal clamps. Although clamps are still in use, the most commonly currently employed method of closed reduction is the application of elastrator rings at the base of the sac after ensuring that any contents have been returned to the abdomen. There may be some oedema between the rubber ring and the abdominal wall on the day after application, but any local inflammation usually resolves in 7–10 days.

Separation of the hernial sac vestige should be allowed to occur without assistance and takes approximately 3–4 weeks.

This technique depends on subcutaneous fibrous scar tissue to obliterate the defect, and is only applicable in treating small one finger defects.

With the availability of safe anaesthetic techniques and improved suture materials, there is little indication for employing a method which is less than certain to correct the hernia. Open reduction, whereby the defect in the abdominal wall is closed by apposing the edges of the ring or by the use of an inlay prosthesis, is therefore a much more satisfactory method of treatment.

Open reduction

The surgery is performed under general anaesthesia and strict aseptic conditions with the patient in dorsal recumbency.

An elliptical skin incision is made around the umbilical scar extending 2 cm beyond the margin of the hernial ring cranially and caudally. Care must be taken to avoid removing too much skin.

The peritoneal sac is carefully dissected away from the overlying skin and the abdominal wall until the margin of the ring can be identified.

Unless there is residual umbilical stalk present or ischaemic damage to the intestine is suspected, the hernial sac should not be incised but simply returned to the abdominal cavity.

The majority of hernial rings are oval in shape and their edges are sufficiently pliable to allow them to be closed by a series of overlapping mattress (Mayo) sutures of non-absorbable material.

The sutures are inserted 1–2 cm from the margin of the ring and are carried through the full thickness of the abdominal wall on both sides of the ring. A finger inserted into the inverted sac serves to guide the needle and prevent inadvertent damage to the intestine (Figure 1). The ends of each suture are held with haemostats until they are all in place. Simultaneous traction on the sutures overlap the edges of the ring and this is maintained while each individual suture is tied.

The subcutaneous tissue is apposed with a continuous suture of polyglactin, and the skin with a subcuticular suture of the same material. The application of an elastic bandage encircling the abdomen (or a stent bandage in the case of small hernias) will provide protection from contamination and eliminate dead space.

With large hernial rings, it may be necessary to bridge the defect with a prosthetic mesh or gauze. The mesh, which must be inert and non-reactive to the tissues, stimulates fibroplasia, resulting in it being enveloped in a thick fibrous bed that fills the defect and strengthens the abdominal wall.

The mesh is best placed in an extraperitoneal position between the internal rectus abdominal sheath and the peritoneum. The peritoneal sac is dissected down to the hernial ring and inverted into the abdominal cavity as described above. If the sac is sufficiently large, the mesh can be placed within it (Figure 2), but if it is not, the peritoneum is reflected peripherally from the deep fascial sheath of the rectus abdominis muscle for 1–3 cm to create a space for the mesh. The mesh is cut so that it overlaps the margin of the ring by the same amount. The sutures are pre-placed before tying. Sufficient tension is applied

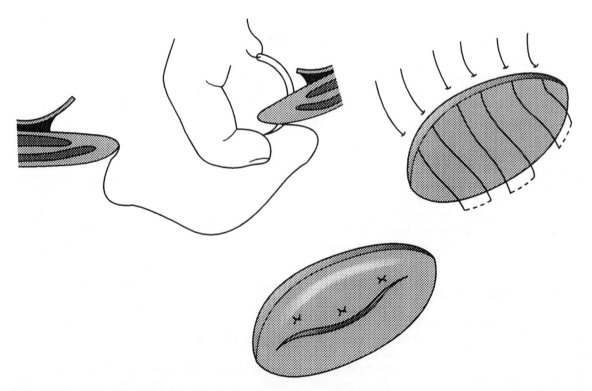

Figure 1 Repair of umbilical hernia by overlapping the margins using modified Mayo sutures.

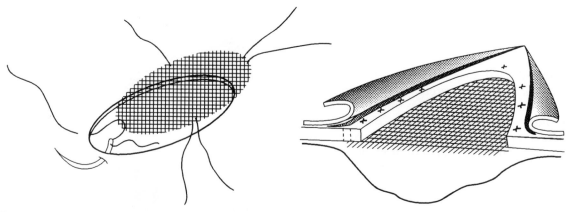

Figure 2   Repair of umbilical hernia using mesh prosthesis inserted within the inverted peritoneal sac.

so that the mesh is kept taut and flat. The subcutaneous tissues and skin are then carefully apposed over the mesh.

Ventral hernias

A ventral hernia is one that occurs through any part of the abdominal wall other than the umbilicus or inguinal canal.

They may be traumatic in origin or incisional. Kicks, collisions with blunt objects and straddling gates are common causes.

Common sites are low in the flank (just dorsal to the edge of the rectus muscle), along the costal arch and along the ventral abdomen.

The abdominal wall is weakest just dorsal to the rectus abdominis muscle, since the oblique abdominal muscles are aponeurotic here, and only the transverse abdominal muscle is present. Flank trauma usually causes the abdominal wall to split just above the rectus muscle. Usually the tear in each layer occurs along the direction of the fibres, and if damage to the external oblique is extensive, the inguinal ring may be involved. If the peritoneum too is torn, herniated intestine will come to lie beneath the skin and panniculus muscle.

A large tear will allow a large mass of viscera (e.g. large colon) to escape from the abdomen, but the size of the swelling is not necessarily an indication of the size of the defect because a considerable length of small intestine can escape through a small rent.

Inflammatory exudate accumulates in the surrounding tissues, but little change may occur in the herniated intestine during the first 2–3 weeks after injury. Nevertheless, the risk of strangula-tion of intestine necessitates early diagnosis and surgical treatment.

Diagnosis

Signs of depression, abdominal discomfort and cessation of defecation indicate intestinal obstruction requiring prompt intervention.

Diagnosis is not always straightforward, and a number of diagnostic procedures should be considered to differentiate a hernia from a haematoma or abscess:

- Palpation.
- Rectal examination.
- Auscultation.
- Ultrasonography.
- Exploratory surgery.

Palpation is complicated by the associated haemorrhage and oedema. Most defects are too ventral to be palpated *per rectum*. Aspiration, although helpful in identifying abscesses, is not advisable because of the risk of penetrating the bowel or introducing infection into a haematoma. Auscultation may reveal intestinal sounds which are more easily heard than over the remainder of the abdominal wall. *Ultrasonography* provides the most useful way of detecting herniated intestine.

Treatment

When intestinal obstruction necessitates immediate surgery, the tissues are very friable and have little suture holding power. It is not uncommon for disruption of the surgical repair to occur during recovery from anaesthesia. Therefore, when the hernia is not accompanied by signs of intestinal obstruction, it is advisable to delay surgery for 3–6 weeks until some swelling has subsided and deposition of collagen has increased the tensile strength of the damaged tissues.

Under general anaesthesia, the skin and sub-cutaneous muscle are carefully excised to reveal the herniated intestine. If examination of the intestine reveals no irreversible damage it is returned to the abdominal cavity. A midline laparotomy incision is helpful in identifying the precise site of the tear and allowing traction to be applied to the herniated gut.

The defect is closed by suturing each layer in turn.

When the defect is very large or its edges are too rigid to appose by suture, satisfactory repair may be achieved using mesh. Following closure of the peritoneum and transverse muscle by suture, a piece of polypropylene mesh is sutured to the deep face of the internal oblique aponeurosis.

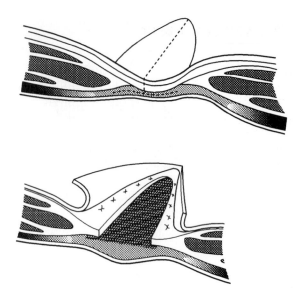

Figure 3 Repair of an incisional hernia using mesh prosthesis inserted into the space created by dissecting the peritoneum away from the margin of the abdominal wall defect.

Incisional hernias

Incisional or postoperative hernias are encountered relatively frequently following abdominal surgery.

Improper closure of the incision, sutures breaking or tearing through tissues and, of greatest importance, postoperative wound infection, are contributory factors.

The weakened abdominal wall undergoes loss of continuity and a hernia develops often after a delay of several weeks or months. The hernial rings vary considerably in size and can be very large.

Forceful approximation of the edges of a large fascial defect inevitably leads to failure and the use of a mesh prosthesis is required. Since the margin of the defect is less well defined than in umbilical hernias, it is necessary to dissect the peritoneum from the inner sheath of the rectus to create an adequate 'shelf' to support the mesh (Figure 3). Alternatively, a mesh inlay graft with the onlay apposition of supportive hernial sac fascia can be used (Figure 4).

Tissue healing is facilitated by obliterating dead space and preventing accumulation of serum. When the surgery is situated on the ventral abdomen, this can be achieved using elastic bandage or a belly bandage for 2 to 3 weeks after surgery. The horse should be given box rest with daily walking in hand for 2 months.

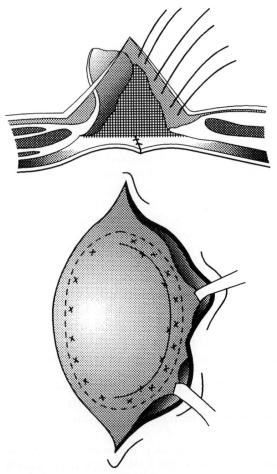

Figure 4 Repair of an incisional hernia using a mesh and fascial flap overlay technique

Prepubic tendon rupture

A tendinous rupture of the rectus abdominis muscles can occur in mares in late gestation or in early lactation. The prepubic tendon appears to degenerate separating its attachments to the pelvis and the onset is gradual.

A swelling appears cranial to the udder and may at first be mistaken for periparturient oedema.

The damage progresses (may be associated with further pregnancy) and eventually the contour of the ventral abdomen drops to the level of the hock accompanied by oedematous swelling of the subcutaneous connective tissue.

The large hernial ring runs transversely just anterior to the pelvis. Not all of the ring can be palpated *per rectum*. It can only be felt externally with the mare in dorsal recumbency.

It is not possible to repair the rupture.

Epiploic foramen incarceration

Incarceration of the small intestine through the epiploic foramen is the most common form of internal hernia in the horse and is especially common in older horses.

The epiploic foramen (the relatively narrow passage through which the greater and lesser peritoneal sacs communicate) is situated on the ventral surface of the liver dorsal to the portal fissure. It is bounded dorsally by the caudate lobe of the liver and the posterior vena cava, and ventrally by the right lobe of the pancreas, gastro-pancreatic fold and portal vein. The foramen is limited cranially by the hepatoduodenal ligament and caudally by the juncture of the pancreas and mesoduodenum.

In the adult horse, the passage is generally 10 cm long. In young horses, it is merely a potential space but in older horses, as the right lobe of the liver atrophies, the foramen enlarges making it easier for a loop of small intestine to enter.

Although the majority of horses in which this type of herniation occurs are at least 7 years of age, it can occur in considerably younger horses.

The intestine may enter the omental bursa from right to left, or it may slip through the foramen from left to right. The length of gut involved varies from a few centimetres to 17 metres.

Clinical signs

● The clinical signs are those of small intestinal obstruction (see Chapter 2), and vary with the nature and severity of the damage to the incarcerated bowel.
● Approximately 80% have irreversible vascular compromise of the herniated small intestine.

Diagnosis

● Diagnosis is usually made at exploratory laparotomy (see Chapter 2 for indications for exploratory laparotomy in acute abdominal pain).
● Sanguineous peritoneal fluid with a raised protein level is indicative of a strangulating lesion but when herniation occurs from right to left, the transudation enters the omental bursa and may not be collected by paracentesis.

Treatment

Conservative treatment is of no value and surgery should be performed at the earliest opportunity.

At laparotomy examination of the epiploic foramen is most easily performed from an operating position on the patient's left side using the right hand to explore the right hypochondral region. The hand is passed lateral and dorsal to the right dorsal colon and forward to the visceral surface of the liver. The only bowel that normally occupies the gutter between the right dorsal colon and the dorsal abdominal wall is the duodenum which is suspended by the short mesoduodenum permitting little lateral movement or mobility of this fixed part of the small intestine.

Distension of the herniated intestine with fluid and gas, and oedema of its wall, may make reduction difficult. *Attempts should not be made to enlarge the foramen, since this would result in fatal haemorrhage.* Traction applied to either the afferent or efferent intestine on the parietal side of the foramen should be gentle and along the plane of the foramen. At the same time, the surgeon's other hand is used to ease the incarcerated gut into the foramen. Strangulated bowel is resected and a suitable anastomosis performed. In cases where impaction of the loop with fibrous food material prevents reduction of ileal herniation, a further length of intestine can be pulled through the foramen to permit dispersion of the ingesta.

The prognosis for successful surgical correction of epiploic foramen incarceration is considered to be poor, particularly if a long segment of bowel is involved or if the severity of the lesion has gone unrecognized for a long period of time.

Diaphragmatic hernia

Diaphragmatic hernia is an uncommon occurrence in horses and is usually discovered at laparotomy or autopsy.

Diaphragmatic defects may be congenital or acquired but in most recorded cases there was convincing evidence that the diaphragm had ruptured either spontaneously or as a result of trauma. Most diaphragmatic hernias follow thoracic or abdominal trauma or strenuous exercise, parturition or extreme gastrointestinal distension.

The absence of haemorrhage at the margins of a defect found at autopsy identifies rupture which has resulted from post-mortem tympany.

Displacement into the thorax of large and small intestine, stomach, omentum, liver and spleen in one combination or another may occur.

Clinical signs

The clinical effects of diaphragmatic hernia are very variable.

- If only small intestine is displaced, signs of intestinal obstruction predominate, often with a rapidly fatal outcome.
- If large intestine moves into the chest, its greater bulk results in compression of the lungs and respiratory distress is more likely. In such cases respiratory and digestive signs may coexist, and the illness may be more protracted because large bowel obstruction is less rapidly fatal than incarceration of small intestine.

Diagnosis

- Absence of lung sounds or increased intestinal sounds in the chest.
- Dullness on percussion over the ventral thorax.
- Sanguineous fluid on thoracocentesis.
- A relative emptiness of the abdomen may be apparent on scrutiny or rectal examination (provided that the remaining segments of gut are not distended as a result of bowel obstruction).
- Thoracic radiography.
- Ultrasonography.

Treatment

- Surgical correction presents considerable problems and the prognosis in most cases of acquired diaphragmatic hernia is grave.
- The severe respiratory and cardiac embarrassment caused by the displaced viscera, and the large volume of fluid present in the chest, may result in death during anaesthetic induction.
- Adequate pulmonary ventilation during surgery is only possible using intermittent positive pressure ventilation.
- Bilateral pneumothorax can develop when the abdomen is opened or more frequently when the hernia is reduced.
- Large dorsal diaphragmatic rents are relatively inaccessible and retraction of herniated viscera is difficult. This is particularly so with congenital defects when the small opening may have to be enlarged before the herniated small intestine can be withdrawn from the chest.
- Once reduced, the infarcted bowel can be resected provided the length involved is not too great. However, it is not uncommon for all but the relatively fixed duodenum and ileum to pass into the chest.
- Any attempt at closure requires extending the abdominal incision cranially to the xiphisternum. Even then, access to the defect may be very restricted making closure by suture or the use of prosthetic mesh difficult.

4.2 *Peritonitis*

The peritoneum normally secretes a serous fluid which lubricates the abdominal cavity, minimizes adhesion formation, has minimal antibacterial properties and acts as a semipermeable barrier between the blood and the abdominal cavity. Inflammation of this mesothelial lining is termed peritonitis and is characterized by hyperaemia, peritoneal effusion and fibrin deposition, chemotactic phagocytosis and increased peritoneal permeability to toxins.

Although it may occur as a primary condition, it is more commonly seen as a secondary complication associated with infectious (bacterial, viral, fungal, parasitic) or non-infectious (traumatic, chemical, neoplastic) stimuli (Table 2). In primary peritonitis, the route of bacterial spread is not evident, but impaired defences may be involved. Bacteria enter the abdominal cavity in

Table 2 Causes of peritonitis

Infectious or septic	Non-septic	Parasitic	Traumatic	Iatrogenic
Surgical complications: • anastomosis failure • non-viable tissue • poor asepsis	Ruptured bladder, ureter or kidney	Verminous arteritis	Breeding or foaling accident	Rectal tear
	Chemical agents: • bile	Parasitic larval migration	Penetrating abdominal wound	Uterine perforation: • infusion • biopsy
Intestinal accidents with perforation	• gastric juice • pancreatic juice	Perforating lesions (ascarids, tapeworms)	Blunt abdominal trauma	• artificial insemination
Uterine rupture or perforation	Foreign body		Ruptured diaphragm	Enterocentesis
Metritis	Neoplasia: • ovarian • abdominal			Caecal trocharization
Urachal infection	Urolithiasis			Liver biopsy
Post-castration infection	Hepatitis			
Enteritis	Gastric rupture			
Septicaemia				
Cholangitis				

secondary peritonitis most commonly following disruption of the integrity of the gastrointestinal tract, or less frequently the genitourinary tract or abdominal wall.

Peritonitis may be further classified according to onset (peracute, acute, chronic) and the region affected (localized or diffuse). Its severity is related to a number of factors including the underlying problem, the nature of the infectious agent, the resistance of the host, speed of recognition and intervention, and response to initial therapy.

The inflammatory responses mobilize leucocytes and immunoglobulins, and cause a profound relocation of proteins, fluid and electrolytes from plasma. These fluid shifts can lead to cardiovascular collapse. Fibrinolytic activity is depressed and fibrin is rapidly precipitated either diffusely in septic peritonitis or following major gastrointestinal leakage, or focally around an intestinal perforation. Although initially of benefit by confining the contamination and infection, these processes may become deleterious, resulting in hypovolaemia, hypoproteinaemia, reflex ileus with bowel distension, ischaemia of bowel wall allowing absorption of bacteria and toxins, and adhesion formation.

Clinical signs

The clinical signs vary considerably depending on the cause and the extent of the disease.

1. Horses with peracute peritonitis (e.g. following gastric rupture) may be found dead or present with profound toxaemia, which rapidly leads to circulatory failure and death in 4–12 hours.
2. Acute diffuse peritonitis:
   • tachycardia
   • tachypnoea
   • congested to cyanotic mucous membranes
   • cold extremities
   • thready pulse
   • dehydration
   • depression
   Both visceral and parietal pain may be present but parietal pain characterized by immobility, splinting of the abdominal wall and sensitivity to extreme pressure is usually the major contributor.
3. Localized, subacute or chronic peritonitis:
   • dullness
   • decreased appetite
   • progressive weight loss
   • abdominal pain may be low-grade, intermittent or absent

- intermittent fever
- variable bowel sounds
- chronic diarrhoea in some cases.

Diagnosis

A definitive diagnosis can usually be made simply by examination of a peritoneal fluid sample for cytology and total protein. It may be turbid and off-white suggesting a high white blood cell count, homogeneously bloodstained suggesting haemoperitoneum or intestinal infarction, or turbid and brown/green in colour suggesting contamination with intestinal contents.

Early in the inflammatory process, the elevated white blood cell (WBC) count is due primarily to an increase in polymorphs while in chronic cases mononuclear cells and macrophages are increased.

Peritoneal fluid protein is significantly higher than normal.

Examination of Gram-stained smears may show free or phagocytosed bacteria.

Further evaluation of the degree of severity of peritonitis depends on laboratory estimation of fluid and electrolyte balance, blood gas analysis and haematology:

- In peracute and acute peritonitis, there is leucopenia with neutropenia and a degenerative left shift.
- Protein sequestration and fluid exudation into the peritoneal cavity leads to hypoproteinaemia and dehydration.
- In acute peritonitis of longer duration, and in localized or chronic peritonitis the changes in total WBC count are less dramatic.
- A decrease in albumin/globulin ratio is frequently present.

Rectal findings in cases of peritonitis are variable:

- Contamination of the abdominal cavity with gastrointestinal contents results in a gritty feeling to the serosal surface of bowel.
- In mares with uterine rupture, a fibrinous adhesion may be noted over the affected area.
- Distended bowel or secondary impaction may be evident while in other cases there may be no abnormalities palpable.

In foals, radiographs may show free fluid, ileus or free gas. Ultrasonography and laparoscopy can also be of diagnostic value.

Early exploratory laparotomy may be indicated for diagnostic, therapeutic and prognostic reasons, and is best performed while the horse is in reasonable condition.

Therapy

General therapy

- Early aggressive therapy is required if treatment is to be of benefit.
- The objective should be to correct the cause of the peritonitis if possible, and overcome the infection and the effects of inflammation.
- Pain relief, correction of fluid, electrolyte and acid–base disturbances, and treatment of cardiovascular and endotoxic shock will need to be addressed.
- Medical treatment is unlikely to be successful without surgical correction of the cause.
- Peritonitis may be associated with infection by any of the aerobic or anaerobic bacteria normally found in the intestinal tract. Alternatively, as in the case of abscesses, specific organisms such as *Streptococcus equi* or *Rhodococcus equi* may be involved. A positive culture is not always possible, and antibiotic therapy needs to be started as soon as possible. Penicillin is suitable as a first choice antibiotic because it is well tolerated and produces peritoneal fluid levels in excess of minimum inhibitory concentration and is bactericidal against most Gram positive aerobic organisms and most anaerobic organisms. For Gram negative aerobic organisms and *R. equi*, gentamicin is recommended. Metronidazole can also be used to treat anaerobic infections.
- Non-steroidal anti-inflammatory drugs are useful in combating toxaemia.
- Larvicidal anthelmintics such as ivermectin are indicated when parasitism is thought to be the cause.

Abdominal drainage and lavage

- Drainage of peritoneal fluid can be achieved using a cannula, Foley catheter or indwelling drain, but serious doubts exist about our ability to achieve mechanical removal of contaminants in the horse related to the size and limited access to many parts of the abdominal cavity.
- Premature obstruction of the drain with omentum or fibrin is often a problem, and local tissue irritation and cellulitis resulting from leakage of fluid into the subcutaneous tissues are other possible complications.
- Effective lavage of the peritoneal cavity requires large volumes (20–30 litres) of sterile Hartmann's solution.

• Failure to drain these large volumes effectively can increase morbidity and mortality.

Prognosis

If the causal lesion can be rapidly identified and corrected, the prognosis is fair to good. However, it is very poor if the peritonitis is the result of intestinal perforation. Few cases of localized adhesion formation or abscessation have a successful outcome; even if the immediate crisis is overcome, chronic ill-thrift and recurrent colic are frequent sequelae.

4.3 *Abdominal abscess*

The majority of internal abdominal abscesses involve the mesenteric lymph nodes and are believed to be the result of systemic spread of respiratory infections, but may be the sequel of foreign body penetration of the intestine or umbilical infection.

The causative organisms most frequently encountered are *Streptococcus equi, Streptococcus zooepidemicus, Escherichia coli, Salmonella* sp., and, in foals, *Rhodococcus equi.* Infrequently anaerobes may be involved.

Horses of any age may be affected, and those exposed to strangles are at greatest risk.

Heavily parasitized horses may be predisposed to abscesses as the result of migrating larvae invading mesenteric tissues allowing for secondary bacterial contamination. As the abscess enlarges and the associated adhesive peritonitis becomes more extensive, the adjacent small intestine may become compressed and/or constricted.

Clinical signs

The most common clinical signs are:

• Chronic weight loss.
• Intermittent low-grade colic.
• Inappetence.
• Low-grade fevers.
• Intermittent diarrhoea.

The colic may be the result of stretching of the mesentery, or adhesion or scarring of the intestine.

Occasionally, a large abdominal abscess may go unsuspected until the horse develops acute obstruction. Rectal examination may reveal a localized well-encapsulated mobile mass which may be painful to the touch. More frequently the abscess is very large, involves loops of bowel and is firmly adherent to the roof of the abdomen.

Peritoneal fluid may be normal, or reveal elevated white blood cells (predominantly neutrophils) and protein. If the abscess is mobile, it may be possible to obtain a needle aspirate percutaneously under ultrasound guidance. The purulent material should be submitted for both aerobic and anaerobic culture.

Treatment

• Long-term antibiotic treatment for a minimum of 30 days is recommended. Administration of antibiotics such as rifampicin, potentiated sulphonamides and metronidazole avoids the complications of long-term parenteral medication.
• Surgical intervention aimed at resecting the abscess is not recommended because of the serious risk of rupture and peritoneal contamination.
• In cases with small intestinal involvement, the obstructed intestine can be bypassed by side-to-side anastomosis of a proximal and distal segment, but horses in which numerous loops of bowel are found to be involved in extensive adhesions to the abscess should be euthanased.

4.4 *Abdominal neoplasia*

Neoplasms of the abdominal cavity are uncommon, and present a considerable diagnostic challenge. They include primary and metastatic tumours, and are generally seen in middle-aged to older animals. The majority of neoplasms involve the gastrointestinal system. Neoplasia of the urogenital system is much less common.

Gastrointestinal neoplasia

Neoplasia accounts for approximately 5% of horses presenting with signs of acute or chronic abdominal disease. Of the primary neoplasms encountered squamous cell carcinoma of the stomach, the alimentary form of lymphoma, and lipomas are the most common. Other types are seen rarely (Table 3). Metastatic spread occurs occasionally with malignant melanoma, transitional cell carcinoma, keratoma and others.

Table 3 Neoplasia of the gastrointestinal tract

Stomach
  Squamous cell carcinoma
  Adenocarcinoma
  Leiomyoma
  Fibrosarcoma

Intestine
  Lymphosarcoma
  Leiomyoma
  Leiomyosarcoma
  Adenocarcinoma
  Hamartoma
  Myosarcoma

Omentum and mesentery
  Lipoma
  Mesothelioma

Clinical signs

The presentation and clinical signs of abdominal neoplasia depend on the location and type of neoplasm. Since treatment is rarely possible or feasible, an early diagnosis is desirable to prevent unnecessary suffering. However, the signs are often vague, making early recognition and diagnosis difficult.

Clinical signs can include:

- Progressive weight loss.
- Depression.
- Reduced exercise tolerance.
- Pyrexia.
- Ventral oedema.
- Colic.
- Ascites.
- Abdominal distension.
- Diarrhoea.

Diagnosis

Cases suspected of having abdominal neoplasia should undergo a thorough clinical examination supported, where applicable, by haematology, serum biochemistry, peritoneal fluid evaluation, rectal palpation and abdominal ultrasonography.

Further diagnostic procedures that may be required include organ function tests, biopsy, laparoscopy and exploratory surgery.

Gastric squamous cell carcinoma

Squamous cell carcinoma is the most common gastric neoplasm in the horse. Middle-aged and older horses are most susceptible. There is a reported 4:1 male:female ratio.

The tumour usually originates in the oesophageal portion of the stomach, infiltrates the wall and projects like a cauliflower into the lumen. Metastatic nodules may occur in the liver, spleen, omentum, intestines, pleura and lungs, and there may be adhesions between the stomach and the liver or diaphragm.

Clinical features

- Chronic weight loss over 1–2 month period.
- Anorexia.
- Depression.
- Anaemia (PCV 12–28%) may develop as a result of haemorrhage into the stomach or depressed erythrogenesis.
- Pain is not usually present.

Diagnosis

- Passage of a nasogastric tube may meet resistance if the tumour involves the stomach adjacent to the cardia.
- Neoplastic cells may be found in fluid recovered by gastric lavage.
- A video- or fibreoptic endoscope 2 m in length will enable a definitive diagnosis by direct visualization and biopsy of the tumour.
- Ultrasonography from the left cranial abdomen may show thickening and abnormal echogenicity of the stomach wall.
- Ascites is commonly associated with the tumour, and secondary spread may be recognized as nodules in the liver, spleen, etc. Palpable masses or adhesions may be evident on rectal examination around the cranial mesentery.
- Exploratory laparotomy or laparoscopy allows more complete examination of the stomach region, and allows biopsy of the primary tumour mass or metastatic nodules.

Prognosis

By the time a diagnosis is made, the tumour has progressed beyond the point where any treatment is feasible. Euthanasia is the only option.

Lymphoma

Lymphoma is seen most commonly in horses more than 10 years of age, although it has been seen in animals as young as yearlings. It accounts for between 1.3 and 2.8% of all tumours seen in the horse.

Most lymphomas appear in lymph nodes or in tissues rich in lymphoid cells such as the spleen, bone marrow, pharynx and gastrointestinal tract. The alimentary form (see Chapter 3) occurs with slightly greater frequency than the mediastinal (thoracic) form (see Chapter 6). Alimentary lymphoma may occur as either a diffuse or a focal lesion.

Diffuse infiltration of either the small intestine and/or large intestine with involvement of local lymph nodes can result in both small intestinal carbohydrate malabsorption and/or protein losing enteropathy with a typical clinical presentation of progressive weight loss and/or diarrhoea.

Alimentary lymphoma may also result in single or multiple focal infiltration of the small intestine in focal lesions which are typically annular and progress in size to occlude the lumen. Enlargement of the mesenteric lymph nodes may sometimes accompany the focal intestinal lesion. The clinical course of focal intestinal lymphoma is chronic, extending over several weeks or months with intermittent, increasingly severe bouts of abdominal pain as the degree of obstruction increases.

Diagnosis

Clinical pathological findings are non-specific but may include:

- Hypoalbuminaemia.
- Hyperglobulinaemia.
- Neutrophilia.
- Anaemia.
- Hyperfibrinogenaemia.
- Raised serum alkaline phosphase.
- Reduced glucose absorption (OGTT).
- Peritoneal fluid cytology – rarely detect tumour cells.
- Decreased plasma levels IgM.

In addition, in focal lymphoma diagnosis may be suspected on the basis of:

- Marked muscular hypertrophy of several metres of intestine proximal to the lesion which occurs in response to the increased workload required to force ingesta through the narrowed intestine. This enlarged, thick-walled intestine may be palpable *per rectum* (the neoplastic mass itself is less likely to be palpable).

- Palpable enlargement of mesenteric lymph nodes.
- Demonstration of the bowel wall thickening by use of trans-rectal or trans-abdominal ultrasonography.

Prognosis

Horses with widespread lesions should be euthanased but others with a single primary lesion of small intestine sometimes make a long-term recovery following resection of the affected portion of bowel.

Lipomas

Pedunculated lipomas, benign fat aggregations attached to the mesentery, are common findings in horses and ponies in their mid teens or older, and have the potential to obstruct the small intestine, or, less frequently, the small colon. The risk of this disease is increased by obese body condition which is common in elderly ponies.

Clinical signs and treatment

Those whose pedicle is attached to the mesentery some distance from the mesenteric border of the intestine can cause strangulation of varying lengths of gut by wrapping tightly around a loop of intestine. This is accompanied by a sudden onset of severe, persistent colic and rapid degeneration of the obstructed intestine. Resection of the infarcted bowel is almost invariably necessary.

In a small proportion of cases, the pedicle is attached at the mesenteric attachment of the intestine. When the lipoma reaches a large size, its weight can cause partial simple obstruction of the intestine, resulting in moderately severe, sometimes intermittent, colic. At laparotomy, the lipoma can be removed but resection of bowel is rarely necessary.

Urogenital tract neoplasia

Ovarian neoplasia

See Chapter 14.

Testicular neoplasia

See Chapter 14.

Renal neoplasia

See Chapter 8.

Bladder neoplasia

Neoplasia of the bladder is rare. Cystoscopy using a video or fibreoptic endoscope is the preferred means of obtaining a tissue sample from an intraluminal mass. Ultrasonography is also useful, particularly in distinguishing a cystic calculus from a tumour.

Further reading

Auer, J.A. (1992) *Equine Surgery*. W.B. Saunders Co., Philadelphia.

Bristol, D.G. (1986) Diaphragmatic hernias in horses and cattle. *Compendium on Continuing Education for the Practicing Veterinarian* **8**, S407.

Holt, P.E. (1986) Hernias and ruptures in the horse. *Equine Practice* **8**, 13.

Scott, E.A. (1979) Repair of incisional hernias in the horse. *Journal of the American Veterinary Medicine Association* **175**, 1203.

5 *Disorders of the ear, nose and throat*

CONTENTS

Conchal necrosis and metaplasia
Facial and sinus trauma
Intranasal foreign bodies
Subcutaneous emphysema

5.17 *Idiopathic headshaking (IHS) in horses*

5.18 *Diagnostic approach to conditions causing airway obstructions in horses*

5.19 *Common upper respiratory tract obstructive disorders of horses*

5.20 *Recurrent laryngeal neuropathy (RLN)*

5.21 *Dorsal displacement of the soft palate (DDSP)*

5.22 *Epiglottal entrapment (EE)*

5.23 *Sub-epiglottal cysts*

5.24 *Arytenoid chondropathy*

5.25 *Fourth branchial arch defects (4-BAD)*

5.26 *Causes of dynamic airway collapse*

Mechanisms of dynamic collapse during exercise

Pharyngeal collapse
Dynamic DDSP
Intermittent epiglottal entrapment
Ary-epiglottic fold collapse
Dynamic RDPA
Dynamic laryngeal collapse

5.27 *Other causes of airway obstruction in the exercising horse*

Choanal stenosis
Pharyngeal lymphoid hyperplasia (PLH)
Palatal cysts
Palatal defects
Pharyngeal cysts
Pharyngeal paralysis
Pharyngeal and laryngeal neoplasia
Congenital tracheal collapse
Acquired tracheal obstructions
Tracheotomy intubation

5.28 *Miscellaneous throat conditions of horses*

Wind-sucking and crib-biting
Salivary gland disorders
Thyroid neoplasia
Parotid melanomas
Facial palsy
Horner's syndrome
Jugular phlebitis
Nuchal fractures
Cervical injection abscessation

5.1 *Diseases of the external ear*

Anatomical considerations

The external ear consists of a semi-rigid open-ended tube supported by the auricular and annular cartilages, and lined by modified integument. The canal comprises a vertical segment covered by pigmented skin and rich in wax-producing cells, and a very narrow horizontal section which is non-pigmented and leads to the pretympanic region. The auricular muscles are innervated by the auriculo-palpebral branch of the facial nerve and loss of ear motility indicates an injury close to the emergence of the nerve trunk from the facial canal.

Clinical signs of otitis externa

- Abnormal ear carriage may indicate aural pain or malfunction of the auricular muscles.
- Discharge at the natural opening of the meati or staining of the skin of the parotid region may be present with or without an unpleasant smell.
- Soft tissue swellings.
- Resentment of handling around the ears.

Investigation of ear disorders

- A distant inspection may reveal abnormal carriage of the ear or of the head as a whole.
- Swellings or overt otorrhoea voided over the parotid area or a discharging sinus tract at the rostral margin of the pinna may be seen. The

discharge may be malodorous if secondary infection is present.

● Digital palpation may reveal soft tissue swellings in the canal. It is normal for the lining of the vertical ear canal to be covered with dark waxy secretions.

● Smears may be taken to identify parasitic mites by microscopy.

● Detailed otoscopy can only be performed under general anaesthesia. Appropriate equipment must be on hand to inspect the very narrow horizontal canals in this species. A 4 mm rigid arthroscope makes an effective otoscope.

Temporal teratoma

● Teratomatous lesions may develop adjacent to the external ear in horses. While the majority of teratomas at this site contain identifiable dental tissues some are of dermal origin.

● The characteristic presenting sign of temporal teratoma consists of a persistent discharging sinus tract which opens at the rostral margin of the pinna 2–3 cm from the natural opening of the ear.

● Young horses are invariably involved, i.e. under 1 year of age when signs first appear.

● There may or may not be a visible or palpable swelling.

● Radiographs are useful to differentiate dermal from dental teratomas, to locate the sac where the teratoma lies and to establish the size of the lesion which is to be resected.

Treatment consists of resection following dissection along the discharging tract. Where deep lesions are involved care is required to avoid damage to the facial nerve and the ear canal.

Parasitic otitis

● Otodectic mites may cause aural irritation but are easily identified either with a hand lens or by examination of smears. The acaricidal preparations used to treat parasitic otitis in small animals are effective in horses.

● The ears appear to be attractive to small biting flies during the summer months and behaviour typical of local irritation will be exhibited. Insect repellents applied to the skin at the base of the ears provide effective protection.

Chronic keratinization plaques

A form of papillomatosis with the formation of discrete white plaques on the underside of the pinnae is common. The aetiology is not known but some clinicians believe that they are the result of repeated insect harassment (see 13.7).

Foreign bodies

Foreign bodies rarely become trapped in the external auditory meati of horses. *Acute onset* of aural discomfort, holding the affected side of the head down, rubbing, otorrhoea and headshaking are the likely presenting signs.

Neoplasia: sarcoids

● The pinnae and surrounding tissues are common sites for the development of equine sarcoids.

● The full range of lesions including occult, verrucose, nodular and fibroblastic may be found at this location.

● The diagnosis is most often based on physical appearance but differentiation from other rarer integumental tumours requires biopsy sampling.

● Surgical excision at this site can be difficult and is likely to be followed by recurrence. The pinna is not a good site for cryotherapy as distortion of the auricular cartilage leaves a poor cosmetic result.

● Topical application of heavy metal cytotoxic cream has been advocated for this condition, or solitary sarcoids may be treated by intralesional BCG (bacillus Calmette–Guérin) injections.

Neoplasia: other ear tumours

Other tumours which may occur in and around the external ear include squamous cell carcinoma, adenoma, adenocarcinoma and, in grey horses, melanoma.

5.2 Diseases of the middle ear

Anatomy and function of the middle ear

The middle ear comprises the space within the tympanic bulla and includes the ear drum, auditory ossicles and the tensor tympani and stapedius muscles. The internal auditory tube runs from the rostral wall of the middle ear to the nasopharynx and provides the means for pressure equilibration across the tympanic membrane and mucus clearance from an enclosed space. The middle portion of this tube passes through a diverticulum, the guttural pouch (see 5.3).

Otitis media

Infections may become established in the middle ear after rupture of the ear drum, by microbial passage from the guttural pouch and by haematogenous spread. Otitis media is rarely identified as an isolated entity in the horse, but more frequently it is recognized after infection has extended to involve adjacent structures.

- Horses with otitis media are likely to present with aural discomfort and a tendency to hold the head rotated with the afflicted ear down.
- Purulent otorrhoea may arise when the ear drum has ruptured from the middle ear outwards.
- The middle ear is a difficult structure to investigate in the living horse. Otoscopy and palpation of the ear drum are unreliable techniques to confirm defects.
- Endoscopy of the auditory tube diverticulum (ATD) (see 5.3) permits inspection of the ventral aspect of the tympanic bulla and of the internal os of the eustachian tube.
- The tympanic bulla is not a good subject for diagnostic radiographs because of superimposition of the petrous temporal bones.

Osteitis of petrous temporal bone

Suppurative otitis media may extend to involve the surrounding structures of the petrous temporal and stylohyoid bones. Ankylosis of the tympano-hyoid articulation is the usual sequel leading to pathological fracture of the great cornu of the hyoid. The clinical signs of the osteitis are variable but include facial palsy and dysphagia with limited motility by the tongue. There may be signs of peripheral vestibular disease if the infection has extended to involve the inner ear.

Otitis interna/peripheral vestibular disease

The inner ear constitutes the end organs of hearing and proprioception, i.e. the cochlea, semicircular canals, utricle and saccule.

- Deafness is practically unrecorded in horses but whether this reflects an absolute rarity or a lack of observation by attendants is unclear.
- The term otitis media should *not* be used to describe the state of neurological disturbance where there is head tilt, ataxia, circling and nystagmus; this is indicative of disturbance of the vestibular system, particularly the peripheral vestibular apparatus of the inner ear.
- Otitis interna may arise as an extension of suppurative otitis media and be concurrent with osteitis of the petrous temporal bone.
- The diagnosis is based upon the presenting signs, the exclusion of other neuropathies such as cervical spondylopathy ('wobbler syndrome'), endoscopy of the ATDs and radiography in both lateral and ventrodorsal projections.

5.3 *Diseases of the auditory tube diverticulum (ATD) (guttural pouches)*

Anatomy of ATDs

The ATDs are balloon-like structures lying between the base of the cranium dorsally and the pharynx and oesophagus ventrally. The volume of each pouch is approximately 300 ml, and medially the two ATDs are in contact with one another, divided only by a thin layer of areolar tissue. The stylohyoid bone divides each pouch into lateral and medial compartments.

- Each pouch is in contact with the base of the skull so that those structures which enter and leave the cranium through the foramen lacerum must cross the pouch: internal carotid artery, cervical sympathetic nerve and cranial nerves IX (glossopharyngeal), X (vagus) and XI (accessory).
- The facial nerve (VII) lies in the submucosa of the lateral compartment dorsally.
- The internal maxillary artery and vein cross the wall of the lateral compartment and here the pouch lies beneath Viborg's triangle.
- The walls of the ATDs are composed of ciliated columnar mucous membrane and a dynamic

clearance system removes mucus and particulate debris.

The drainage ostia are slit-like openings under cartilaginous flaps which lie on the dorsolateral wall of the pharynx and they are quite close together, separated by the pharyngeal recess. Thus, although slight discharges from one pouch may produce a predominantly unilateral nasal discharge, the more copious the discharge, the more likely it is to be bilateral.

Signs of ATD diseases

The signs of disorders of the guttural pouches reflect either compression of adjacent organs when they become distended or damage to the structures which cross them.

- Swellings of the ATDs may be visible externally at the parotid region or will partially obstruct the pharynx leading to dyspnoea or dysphagia.
- Erosion of the internal carotid artery can cause spontaneous haemorrhage to the nares which on occasion is so severe that the horse exsanguinates.
- ATD disorders provide the potential for a very wide range of neuropathies to such an extent that the possibility of guttural pouch disease should be considered practically whenever a horse is presented with a cranial nerve deficit.

Physical examination of ATDs

External palpation in the parotid area is helpful to detect swellings produced by tympany, empyema, abscessation of adjacent lymph glands or neoplastic foci particularly in the parotid lymph glands.

On occasions guttural pouch mycosis may produce painful foci deep to the base of the ear when the head of the stylohyoid bone or the tympanohyoid articulation have become involved. However, this condition rarely produces an external swelling.

Endoscopy of ATDs

The simplest way to pass an endoscope into each pouch is by using a wire leader passed through the biopsy channel of the endoscope. This channel is invariably eccentric and thus, the wire can be used to raise the cartilage flap before advancing into the duct beyond.

Apart from abnormalities inside the ATDs, endoscopy should check for laryngeal and pharyngeal extension of ATD disease.

Depression at the pharyngeal recess and partial obscuring of the larynx may result from distension within the ATD.

Pharyngeal and laryngeal hemiplegia can result from mycotic infections.

Radiographic examination of ATDs

The ATDs are normally filled by air and the contrast thus provided makes for good diagnostic radiographs.

The erect lateral projection is used and may reveal free gas/fluid interfaces, loss of air contrast through replacement by inspissated pus or soft tissue substitution, e.g. indentations from lymph node swelling in the caudal wall.

Complete occlusion of an ATD can occur in cases of chronic empyema or chondroid formation.

Topical treatment of ATDs

A 35 cm long 30 ml Foley balloon catheter offers a suitable indwelling device for repeated topical infusion of medication. The catheter is passed up the ventral nasal meatus using a metal stiffener slightly bent at the leading end. This is rotated under the cartilage flap of the ostium which lies on the lateral pharyngeal wall at the same level as the eye.

Long-term catheterization may lead to weakening of the ostium and erosion of the cartilage flap.

Surgical approaches to ATD

1. *Hyovertebrotomy.* An incision is made parallel and immediately cranial to the wing of the atlas. The parotid salivary gland is reflected forwards. An endoscope introduced into the ATD *per nasum* serves to illuminate the membranous lining deep in the surgical site once the loose connective tissue has been bluntly separated.
2. *Viborg's triangle.* Access to the ATDs by this approach is very restricted except in conditions where there has been stretching of the tissues through distension of the pouch which in turn increases the overall size of Viborg's triangle.

3. *Paralaryngeal (Whitehouse) approach.* With the horse in dorsal recumbency, a ventral midline incision is made over the larynx. The dissection passes lateral to the larynx, trachea and cricopharynx to reach the pouches ventromedially. Entry to the ATD is made medial to the stylohyoid bone. The depth of incision limits the value of this approach.
4. *Modified Whitehouse approach.* Although the surgery is again performed with the patient in dorsal recumbency, the site of the incision corresponds to that used for prosthetic laryngoplasty, i.e. it lies ventral to the linguofacial vein and then follows the same route to enter the pouch. The Whitehouse approaches are advocated because they allow access to the roof of the ATD, the possibility to explore the lateral compartment digitally and access to both ATDs through the same incision.

5.4 *Guttural pouch tympany*

Aetiology

In this condition the ATD ostium acts as a non-return valve so that air can enter the pouch but cannot escape.

Clinical signs and diagnosis

• This is a condition of foals which usually manifests itself within a few days of birth and it is thought to arise from a congenital malfunction of pharyngeal opening of the pouch.
• The disorder appears to be more common in fillies than colts and is almost invariably unilateral.
• Air accumulates and produces a tympanitic swelling in the parotid region which is initially non-painful and non-inflammatory.
• Established cases invariably show evidence of opportunistic infection because a mucopurulent nasal discharge is generally present by the time afflicted foals are submitted for corrective surgery.
• The laxity of the medial septum between the ATDs may lead to swelling on the normal side, and hence false diagnoses of bilateral tympany may be made.
• Dysphagia and dyspnoea may be exhibited by virtue of the size of the distension.
• Occasionally ATD tympany is an acquired disorder of the adult horse.

Treatment

Three principles have been applied for the relief of ATD tympany:

1. Dilation of the pharyngeal ostium on the affected side.
2. The creation of a fistula between the normal and distended pouches by the removal of a section of the medial septum.
3. Blunt fistulation between the ATD and the pharyngeal recess.

A simple conservative technique to remedy the disorder has been suggested consisting of the long-term implantation of an indwelling Foley catheter placed through the defective pharyngeal ostium *per nasum* and left in place for up to 8 weeks.

The purpose of the medial wall fistulation technique is to facilitate the egress of air from the abnormal ATD through the pharyngeal ostium of the normal side. Transendoscopic laser surgery provides an option for non-invasive fistulation through the medial septum when this facility is available.

Prognosis

The prognosis for ATD tympany is usually favourable regardless of whether the catheterization or fistulation technique is used.

5.5 *Diverticulitis of the guttural pouch*

Aetiopathogenesis

There are poorly defined and poorly understood conditions in which inflammation of the mucous membrane lining of the ATDs occurs and which can loosely be termed 'diverticulitis'. They include strangles abscessation in the lymphoid tissue of the walls of the pouches, empyema, chondroid formation and chronic diverticulitis.

A catarrhal inflammation of the ATD mucosae probably accompanies most upper respiratory tract bacterial and viral infections and the tympany described above is also likely to be accompanied by inflammatory changes, hence the term tympanitis.

'Strangles'

See Chapter 19.

• This is an infectious condition of horses caused by *Streptococcus equi* which consists of a suppurative lymphadenitis particularly of the lymph glands associated with the upper respiratory tract including the ATDs.

• Occasionally the free movement of air through the drainage ostia of the ATDs is obstructed by the physical presence of the lymphadenopathy and a variable degree of tympany may be exhibited.

• Temporary tracheotomy is indicated for those horses which show life-threatening airway obstruction.

Chronic ATD empyema and chondroids

• Empyema of the ATDs occurs when mucus and/or pus accumulates within the pouches because it is failing to drain satisfactorily.

• The primary aetiological factor in ATD empyema is a dysfunction of mucociliary clearance followed by stagnation of mucus, opportunist bacterial infection and finally purulent exudation. There is a possible aetiological association with tympany.

Regardless of the precise aetiology of empyema, pus which is stagnant within the pouch eventually becomes inspissated and progressively leads to the formation of solid concretions – *chondroids*.

• The clinical signs of empyema include a bilateral purulent nasal discharge and swelling of the parotid region.

• The distension of the affected pouch into the pharynx may produce obstructive dyspnoea.

• The nasal discharge is sometimes malodorous.

• Lateral radiographs confirm the loss of air contrast from within the ATD, and if the pus is still fluid, an air/fluid interface will be demonstrable.

• An indwelling self-retaining Foley balloon catheter may be used for drainage of the ATD and for long-term irrigation in the management of chronic cases.

• The removal of inspissated caseous pus is not possible by conservative means and thus surgery is required to extirpate chondroids.

• Empyema is often bilateral and, if so, a ventral Whitehouse approach is preferred so that both pouches can be entered through the same incision.

Chronic diverticulitis

• Chronic catarrhal inflammation of the ATDs may be encountered with no history to suggest previous strangles infection.

• Chronic diverticulitis without the presence of empyema may present with a syndrome of neuropathies where any combination of deficits of the glossopharyngeal, vagus, facial, spinal accessory and sympathetic nerves may be present. It is assumed that the nervous pathways are damaged as an extension of the inflammatory process in the ATD walls.

• The diagnosis is established by a functional assessment of the cranial nerves mentioned, combined with the endoscopic identification of a roughened thickening of the ATD lining.

• The nervous form of diverticulitis carries a poor prognosis.

5.6 *Guttural pouch mycosis (GPM)*

Aetiopathogenesis

The fungal plaques of guttural pouch mycosis (GPM) are usually found in one of two characteristic sites:

• The majority on the roof of the medial compartment.

• Others on the lateral wall of the lateral compartment.

There is a close association between the predilection sites and the underlying internal carotid (ICA) and external carotid (ECA) arteries respectively.

Clinical signs

The development of an invasive fungal plaque on the mucosal wall of the ATD of a horse will produce consequences ranging from nil to fatal.

• Spontaneous epistaxis at rest is the most frequent sign noted by owners and usually consists of a small quantity of fresh blood at one nostril in the first instance.

• A number of further minor haemorrhages may follow but, if untreated, exsanguination is a probable final outcome.

• It is unusual for the first episode of epistaxis to be fatal, but the course of the disease from first to final haemorrhage rarely spans more than 3 weeks and is more likely to be a matter of days.

• Pharyngeal paralysis is the most frequent neuropathy which accompanies GPM and the inclusion of ingesta in a nasal discharge from any horse is an indication to inspect both ATDs by endoscopy as well as to assess pharyngeal function.

• Endoscopic evidence of pharyngeal paralysis includes persistent dorsal displacement of the palatal arch, the presence of saliva and ingesta in the nasopharynx, weak pharyngeal contractions and a failure of one or both of the pharyngeal ostia of the ATDs to dilate during deglutition.

• Laryngeal hemiplegia is the next most frequent cranial nerve deficit encountered in horses with GPM but it is rarely responsible for the only signs observed by the owner.

• GPM may produce a wide range of other signs referable to the head and upper neck. These include facial palsy and Horner's syndrome; reluctance to lower the head to the ground and stiffness in the upper neck; parotid pain; otorrhoea; epiphora and photophobia.

• Abnormal head posture may be associated with pain in the atlanto-occipital joint when the mycosis has extended into this joint.

Diagnosis

The clinical signs are not specific but whenever a horse is presented with spontaneous epistaxis the possibility of GPM should be explored because delayed treatment may result in a fatal outcome.

• A definitive endoscopic diagnosis of a mycotic plaque in the ATD is not always straightforward; two caveats should be heeded.
  – First, the stress of handling the horse may precipitate a fatal epistaxis.
  – Second, endoscopic visibility within the affected pouch may be poor after a recent haemorrhage and accurate location of the lesion will not be possible.

• If the epistaxis has been recent, it is sufficient to identify the stream of blood flowing from the pharyngeal drainage ostium.

• In all cases of mycosis, the contralateral pouch should be checked for extension of the disease through the medial septum and for concurrent bilateral mycosis.

• A full endoscopic assessment of laryngeal and pharyngeal function is required for an accurate prognosis.

Treatment

• Medical treatment of GPM, be it by the use of topical or systemic antimycotic drugs or by a combination of both, is frequently unsuccessful.

• Surgical occlusion of the branches of the carotid artery is recommended.

• The internal carotid is not an end-artery and therefore the placement of a simple ligature on the cardiac side of the lesion will not always be successful because retrograde haemorrhage may occur.

• Occlusion of the distal segment with a balloon-tipped catheter combined with proximal ligation of the ICA is superior.

• Topical antimycotic medication as an adjunct to arterial occlusion is probably not necessary.

Prognosis

• Those cases of GPM not showing neurological complications can usually be brought to a successful conclusion by arterial occlusion surgery.

• Although a small proportion of horses showing pharyngeal paralysis recover normal swallowing function, destruction on humane grounds is a more likely outcome and is indicated as soon as the patient shows signs of dehydration or aspiration pneumonia.

• Laryngeal hemiplegia resulting from GPM can be managed as for the idiopathic form of recurrent laryngeal neuropathy (see 5.20, 'Treatment').

5.7 *Other ATD disorders*

Trauma

• The rectus capitis ventralis muscles insert onto the basisphenoid bones which form a narrow bridge between the foramina lacera in the dorsomedial aspect of the ATDs.

• Fractures at the junction of the basisphenoid and occipital bones may occur in horses that have sustained violent head trauma by rearing over backwards.

• Some patients with this injury are unable to stand but show collapse and epistaxis.

- Endoscopy can be used to confirm that the origin of the epistaxis lies in the ATDs and radiography can also make a valuable contribution to diagnosis.
- Apart from blood showing as free fluid in the floor of the ATDs, a step in the base of the skull will be visible on radiographs.
- The condition is irreparable even for those horses able to stand after the immediate injury – most are rendered partly quadriplegic.
- Foreign body penetration into the retropharyngeal tissues by wire can occur in horses.
- The clinical signs include epistaxis, nasal discharge, dyspnoea, dysphagia and pain in the upper neck with restricted movement.
- The radiographic identification of metallic material in the caudal wall of the ATD is straightforward but projections in two planes are required for an accurate stereotactic location of the object.

Neoplasia

- All regions of the horse richly endowed with lymphoreticular tissue are potential sites for lymphoma development and this tumour can arise in the tissues abutting onto the ATDs.
- Ectopic melanosis is a common feature of the mucosa of the ATD of grey horses. Primary melanomas can arise here.

5.8 Disorders of the external nares

Anatomical features

The nostrils contribute more than 50% to the total resistance to flow of the entire upper respiratory tract during quiet breathing. This can be reduced considerably by active dilation during exertion. The C-shaped alar cartilages, back-to-back at the midline, provide rigidity for the otherwise soft structures of the external nares. Dilation of the nostril margins is achieved through the action of the nasolabialis muscles which receive their motor supply through the dorsal buccal branches of the facial nerves. The alar folds which attach to the ventral conchus mark the dorsal margin of the airway through the nasal vestibule, although the blind pocket of the false nostril lies above this.

'Wry nose'

- A congenital deformity of the nose resulting from gross foreshortening of the premaxilla on one side.
- The deformity is not thought to be genetically transmitted but may be due to abnormal positioning in utero.
- The deformity is externally obvious.
- Even radical surgery is unlikely to render the horse suitable for exercise.

Hypertrophy of alar folds

- It is normal for the alar folds which form the floor of the false nostril sometimes to vibrate during exhalation. This is the origin of the vibrant expiratory noise known as 'high blowing'.
- Occasional horses exhibit a comparable vibrant sound during inspiration.
- Confirmation that the origin of the noise lies at the alar folds is achieved by placing full thickness mattress sutures from the skin at the dorsal aspect of the nose across the openings of the false nostrils. The technique is performed under local anaesthesia so that the noise can be compared before and after suture placement. A positive result is an indication for resection of the alar folds.

'Atheroma' of false nostril

- Sebaceous cysts occasionally develop in the lining of the false nostril.
- These are painless and can be seen at the dorsal aspect of the nose rostral to the naso-maxillary notch.
- Although the swellings can be sizeable they do not obstruct respiration and are of cosmetic significance only.
- Removal by careful dissection from the dorsal skin surface is straightforward and recurrence is improbable.

Facial paralysis

See Chapter 11.

Flaccidity of a nostril margin through dysfunction of the nasolabialis muscle represents an aerodynamic disaster to an athletic horse. Many cases of facial palsy are of iatrogenic origin and during facial surgery, i.e. dental extractions, the branches of the facial nerve should be respected.

Trauma

• Wounds to the nostrils are typically sustained when a horse pulls backwards having caught the margin of its nose on a hook.
• These injuries demand meticulous management in the acute stage with layer-by-layer anatomical restoration.
• Inadequately managed nostril tears will lead to stricture of the nostril aperture and a major reduction in athletic capacity.

Alar cartilage necrosis

Neglected penetration injuries of the alar cartilages may be followed by the extension of suppuration into the cartilage matrix. Careful resection of the diseased tissue is required because loss of mechanical stability at this location represents a serious complication.

5.9 *Diagnostic approach to nasal and paranasal sinus disease*

Anatomical considerations

The paranasal sinuses are extensive air-filled spaces lined by mucoperiosteum. The normal removal of mucus is a dynamic process depending on mucociliary flow to the drainage ostia which do not lie at the lowest points in the sinuses. Once the nasal meati are reached mucus is lost by a combination of evaporation and further mucociliary flow towards the nasopharynx.

The five paired paranasal sinuses of the horse are:

1. Frontal/conchofrontal
2. Caudal maxillary
3. Rostral maxillary
4. Ethmoidal
5. Sphenopalatine

• The frontal sinus is divided into conchofrontal (CFS) and frontal (FS) portions. Drainage takes place through the frontomaxillary foramen into the caudal maxillary sinus (CMS).

• The ethmoidal and sphenopalatine sinuses also drain via the CMS into the middle nasal meatus.
• The rostral maxillary sinus (RMS) has an independent drainage ostium, again into the middle nasal meatus.
• The RMS is divided into a lateral bony and a medial turbinate portion within the ventral conchus (ventral conchal sinus, VCS). They are separated by the infraorbital canal and a sheet of bone joining it ventrally to the roots of the cheek teeth. In the young horse the lateral bony compartment is largely occupied by the roots of the cheek teeth and regardless of age, the VCS is not easily accessible for surgery other than via the floor of the CFS.
• The roots of the 4th, 5th and 6th cheek teeth lie within the maxillary sinuses: they are most prominent in young horses and recede towards the floor of the sinuses with age.
• The roots of the 3rd cheek tooth form the rostral wall of the RMS.
• When dental periapical suppuration is the cause of sinusitis, the tooth roots are approached with a trephine site located as directly over the roots as vital structures such as the nasolacrimal canal, infraorbital canal, vein and artery of the angle of the eye will permit.

Common presenting signs

• The clinical signs of paranasal sinus diseases almost invariably include a nasal discharge, which may be mucoid, purulent, haemorrhagic or a combination of these.
• There may also be facial swelling and obstructive dyspnoea.
• Some expansive lesions in this area will displace orbital tissues resulting in exophthalmos but it is exceptional for a sinus disorder to extend caudally into the cranium to provoke central nervous signs.
• The intranasal structures are richly vascular and it is not surprising that trauma and destructive conditions frequently lead to epistaxis.

History

• Note should be made of possible contact with infectious respiratory disease and of the duration and nature of any nasal discharge.
• It is unusual for sinusitis to be bilateral and it is logical that the discharge will be largely unilateral

when its origin lies proximal to the caudal limit of the midline septum.

● When a horse is presented with unilateral epistaxis, enquiries should be made regarding associations with exercise to eliminate a diagnosis of exertion-induced pulmonary haemorrhage (see 6.8).

● Epistaxis due to guttural pouch mycosis may be acute and, even if episodic, the course of the history is unlikely to exceed 3 weeks (see 5.6).

● A diagnosis of progressive ethmoidal haematoma (PEH) is more likely to be correct when episodes of epistaxis span a longer period, especially if the blood is not fresh.

● A foetid nasal discharge points to suppuration but this could arise from a wide range of chronic sinus lesions.

Physical examination

● The facial area should be inspected for evidence of deformity of the supporting bones through swelling or trauma.

● Subcutaneous emphysema may be detected after trauma in some cases where the sinus walls have been disrupted.

● Percussion of the walls of the paranasal sinuses is an unreliable technique but increased resonance may be perceived when the walls become thin or dullness may develop when the sinuses are completely filled by fluid or soft tissue.

● The airflow at each nostril should be checked to assess obstruction of the nasal meati.

● The clinical crowns of the cheek teeth are examined for the presence of fracture, displacement or impaction of degenerate ingesta.

● The patency of the nasolacrimal duct can be checked by catheterization and infusion of saline solution from either end.

Endoscopy

Endoscopy of the nasal area is performed in two ways:

● First, by conventional passage of the instrument into the nasal meati.

● Second, by direct inspection of the sinus contents through small trephine holes.

This latter technique is most commonly performed in the CMS. All endoscopy of this region is best performed on the standing horse because orientation is straightforward and the nasal

tissues of the recumbent animal become discoloured and engorged.

Nasal endoscopic checklist:

1. Nasal meati – are they narrowed?
   Compare with contralateral side
2. Is narrowing of the meati the result of conchal distension?
   Dorsal conchus – CFS   Ventral conchus – VCS
3. Is narrowing due to a soft tissue mass?
   Does the colour of the mass indicate a PEH, cyst or tumour?
   Can a mass be seen extending caudal to the midline septum when the endoscope is passed via the opposite nostril?
4. Sinu-nasal drainage ostium in caudal middle meatus:
   Is there discharge/blood present?
   Is the ostium dilated or compressed?
5. Ethmoidal labyrinth:
   Is there any sign of blood/PEH?
6. Conchal mucosa – check for:
   Mycosis
   Ulceration/haemorrhage
   Necrosis
7. After surgery – check for:
   Evidence of persistent infection including mycosis
   Satisfactory sinu-nasal fistulation
8. Direct sinus endoscopy – check for:
   Empyema
   Dental periapical reactions
   Mycosis
   PEH

Radiography

The good contrast provided between bone and air renders the nasal chambers and paranasal sinuses excellent candidates for radiographic diagnosis.

Erect lateral, lateral oblique, lesion-oriented oblique and ventrodorsal views may be required for a comprehensive investigation.

The radiographic signs of sinu-nasal disease include:

● free fluid interfaces in the sinuses;

● loss of normal air contrast through substitution by fluid or soft tissue;

● depression or elevation of the supporting bones of the face;

● distortion of normal structures such as the tooth roots, sinus walls, midline septum and infraorbital canals.

Biopsy

Even after full endoscopic and radiographic investigations, surgical exploration may be performed before a specific diagnosis has been made. Suspect tissues should be biopsied to differentiate neoplastic disorders from other disease processes.

5.10 *Treatment of sinu-nasal disorders*

Treatment objectives

- Accurate diagnosis of the primary sinu-nasal disorder and removal of diseased tissue.
- Restoration of the normal drainage mechanisms or the creation of alternative drainage through a sinu-nasal fistula.
- Adequate visibility within the sinuses and nasal meati for accurate diagnosis and surgery.
- Means to control haemorrhage during both surgery and in the recovery period.
- A safe airway during surgery and recovery.
- Facilities for topical postoperative treatments and for monitoring progress.
- An early return to exercise.
- A pleasing cosmetic result.

Medical management

Non-surgical treatments for sinusitis include antibiotics, mucolytics, steam inhalations, volatile inhalations and continued controlled exercise. The objective is the return of normal mucociliary clearance. Most cases of simple primary sinusitis will be resolved either naturally or with minimal veterinary assistance provided that the necessary supportive management is instituted promptly.

Trephination

- Simple trephination also aims to restore normal sinus drainage but with the addition of irrigations and topical antibiotic infusions to clear stagnant mucus and eliminate secondary infection.
- Trephination is performed using local anaesthetic infiltration with the horse standing.
- The preferred site for trephination is into the CMS in the angle formed between the margin of the bony orbit and the facial crest.

- Indwelling balloon catheters provide a good means for regular irrigation over a number of days until the discharge to the nostril ceases.
- The RMS is less available for simple trephination especially in young horses where the lateral compartment is largely occupied by the roots and reserve crowns of the third and fourth cheek teeth.

Facial flap surgery

- In the face of chronic sinusitis, sinus cyst and PEH, the natural drainage system may be physically obstructed. Fistulas can be made by removal of the floor of the CFS and medial wall of the VCS so that there is free communication between the sinus cavities and the nasal meati.
- Extensive frontonasal flap surgery is required for this, and additional drainage from the CMS is achieved by removal of the septum dividing it from the RMS.
- The bulla of the RMS may bulge caudally into the CMS when it is inflated by pus and this is easily punctured and partly excised.
- In older horses a secondary fistula through the bone plate ventral to the infra-orbital canal provides communication between the lateral bony compartment and the VCS.
- In surgical practice the fistulas described provide convenient routes by which to lead sock-and-bandage pressure packs to the nostrils (see below).
- Frontonasal or maxillary flap surgery is required for extensive excisional procedures such as the removal of sinus cysts, PEHs and selected tumours as well as for the relief of chronic sinusitis and fistulation techniques.
- Radical exposure of the nasal chambers, paranasal sinuses and their contents can be achieved through the bony walls of the supporting bones.
- The surgical options are:
  - between fronto-nasal and lateral (maxillary) approaches;
  - whether to reject or preserve the bone flap.
- Lesser decisions relate to the shape of the bone flap and the direction in which the skin/periosteal flap is raised.
- The lateral approach into the maxillary sinuses provides limited access and it should be reserved for those instances where the disease process is restricted to the maxillary compartments.

• Incisions are made through skin and periosteum in the same plane before the periosteum is peeled away from the underlying bone.

• The bone flap is best fashioned with an oscillating saw but in practice hand saws or a series of overlapping trephine holes are alternatives.

• Once the sinus contents are exposed, the disease focus is identified and removed.

• Closure of the incision can be achieved with a single layer of mattress sutures but accurate alignment is required for the best cosmetic result in horses with natural facial markings.

• Temporary bilateral carotid occlusion can reduce haemorrhage and improve visibility during the intraluminal stages of sinus flap surgery.

• This technique comprises the prior placement of a snare around each common carotid artery which can be drawn tight for the 15–20 minutes required to complete the intranasal stages of the operation.

• The advantages in terms of haemorrhage control must be weighed against the disadvantages of prolonging the surgery.

• Pressure packing within the sinus cavities and nasal chambers is essential to control haemorrhage on completion of the surgery and during the initial recovery period, i.e. 48–72 hours. Sock-and-bandage packing consisting of lengths of cotton bandage packed into tubular stockinet socks is suitable. The open end of the stockinet is led to the nostril.

• A cuffed endotracheal tube is essential to protect the lower airways from the inhalation of blood, pus, surgical debris and irrigation fluids during surgery.

• Vigorous lavage, possibly from a hosepipe, is frequently used to displace inspissated pus from the recesses of the sinuses.

• For this inflation of the cuff should be checked and the head lowered.

• During anaesthetic recovery, until the horse regains its feet, a nasopharyngeal tube should be placed through the contralateral nasal chamber and secured at the nostril.

• Tracheotomy intubation is not necessary.

• Blood clots and devitalized tissue are inevitably left after facial flap surgery and opportunist infections, frequently mycoses, are likely.

• A Foley balloon catheter implanted into the CMS (see above) offers a convenient route for post-surgical irrigation and medication.

• The topical medication should include an anti-mycotic agent.

• Inspection of the sinus contents to monitor progress after sinus flap surgery can be achieved by endoscopy *per nasum* through the iatrogenic fistulas or laterally through the trephine hole into the CMS.

• In spite of the radical nature of some sinus surgical procedures, an early return to exercise is recommended as an integral part of treatment.

• Forced nasal ventilation increases the evaporation of residual discharges when stagnation might otherwise encourage postoperative infections to become established.

5.11 *Primary and secondary empyema*

Aetiopathogenesis

• Primary sinus empyema results from the stagnation of mucus through damage to the dynamic mucociliary clearance system, generally by infection with upper respiratory tract viral agents.

• Initially the dependent portions of the sinuses fill with mucus which passively spills through the drainage ostia into the nasal meati.

• Bacterial opportunism follows exacerbating the mucosal inflammation and leading to purulent exudation.

• Hyperplasia of the sinus lining is a feature of sinusitis which narrows the drainage ostia.

• Inspissation of pus develops in the later stages and also occludes the ostia.

• The conchal walls of the sinuses are not rigid and in the face of obstructed drainage there is a tendency to inflation and thereby to obstruction of the nasal airways.

• Secondary (dental) sinusitis is a sequel to dental periapical suppuration.

• The roots of the third to sixth maxillary cheek teeth lie within the maxillary sinuses and are covered by a thin layer of alveolar bone and mucosa. Whenever these teeth are devitalized by fracture or infundibular necrosis there is the possibility of secondary sinusitis.

Clinical signs

• In the acute stages primary sinus empyema produces a mucus-based unilateral nasal discharge.

• As the condition becomes more chronic so the discharge becomes more purulent and malodorous.

• The discharge of secondary (dental) sinusitis is invariably purulent and often malodorous. It is generally less profuse than with primary empyema.

• Primary and secondary sinusitis are rarely bilateral conditions.

• The discharge is occasionally blood flecked.

• Facial swelling, over the maxillary sinuses, and nasal obstruction are later features of primary empyema.

Diagnosis

• Based on the history and clinical signs.

• Physical examination takes note of the nasal discharge and any facial deformity.

• The airflow at the external nares is compared.

• Percussion may show loss of resonance if the sinus spaces are filled by pus but is unreliable when filling is incomplete.

• An oral inspection is used to check the cheek teeth for fractures, displacement or infundibular necrosis.

• Endoscopic features have been outlined above (5.9, 'Endoscopy') but at the least this will show a flow of discharge from the caudal region of the middle nasal meatus where the sinus drainage ostium is located.

• Radiographs either show free horizontal gas/fluid interfaces or, when the sinuses are full, total loss of air contrast. It is important to assess the possibility of dental suppuration as the cause of the sinusitis.

Treatment

• Early cases can be treated non-surgically using systemic antibiotics, volatile or steam inhalations and continued light exercise (Figure 1).

• Those which do not respond to conservative measures should be managed by the implantation of a catheter into the appropriate sinus compartment(s) but this usually means the CMS which communicates with all of the sinuses except for the RMS.

• The catheter is used for topical antibiotic infusion in addition to physical irrigation. A free flow of lavage to the nostrils implies that the drainage ostia are clear and this is an optimistic sign.

• Refractory cases, typically where there is poor drainage during irrigation and a putrid nasal

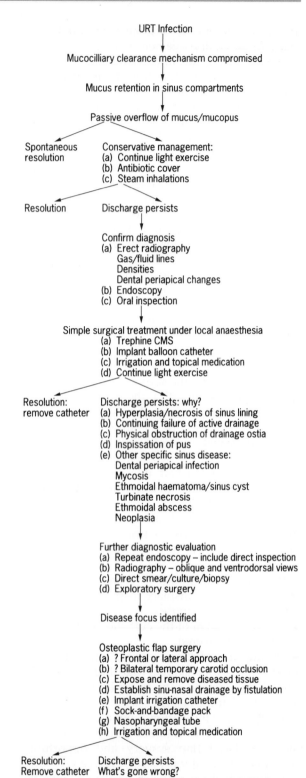

Figure 1 Management of primary sinusitis in the horse. URT, upper respiratory tract; CMS, caudal maxillary sinus. Reproduced with permission from Lane, J. G. (1993) The management of sinus disorders of horses – Part 1. *Equine Veterinary Education* **5**, 5–9.

discharge, should be considered potential candidates for facial flap surgery.

- Endoscopic and radiological re-assessment is used to confirm the exact location of the empyema and to decide which technique to use.
- The objectives of this radical surgery in the management of chronic sinusitis are to break down the intercompartmental barriers thus converting the sinuses into a common air space and to create generous fistulae into the nasal meati.

Prognosis

A minority of cases of sinus empyema require any form of surgical intervention and of those which do, the overwhelming majority are resolved by simple trephination and catheterization.

5.12 *Progressive ethmoidal haematoma*

Aetiopathogenesis

- The aetiology of PEH is not known.
- There is no evidence that any form of neoplastic process is responsible for the repeated submucosal haemorrhages which cause these relentlessly expanding lesions to develop on the surface of the ethmoidal turbinate labyrinth.
- Lesions may arise on the nasal or sinus aspects of the ethmoidal 'onion'.
- The mucosal capsule splits intermittently to release a bloody discharge but the overall trend is towards expansion.
- This in turn may compromise sinus drainage with a secondary retention of mucus, or the nasal airways may become obstructed causing dyspnoea.
- In extreme cases the dyspnoea may cause distress even at rest and the mass may be extruded at the nares.

Clinical signs

- Afflicted horses are 4 years of age or older, the incidence increasing with age.
- Repeated low-grade haemorrhage from one nostril is the most common presenting sign.
- The blood is not fresh and epistaxis is not related to exercise.
- Between haemorrhages a dirty nasal discharge is often present.

- Varying degrees of nasal obstruction will be present and in competition horse's noisy breathing may be the first symptom noted by the rider.
- A facial swelling is a late feature of PEH.
- Rare cases cause pressure on, or infiltrate through, the cribriform plate, typically ventrally so that central nervous signs including blindness are occasionally reported.

Diagnosis

- Diagnosis is based on the clinical history, physical examination, endoscopy and radiography.
- Percussion of the sinuses may show increased resonance if the walls are becoming thin.
- Endoscopy *per nasum* will reveal those PEHs based on the nasal surfaces of the ethmoid. The lesions appear as smooth-walled masses pushing forward from the caudal nasal region. The colour of the lesions is very variable ranging from yellow/orange to grey/green.
- Some PEHs arise on the sinus aspect of the ethmoids and are not visible *per nasum* although a stream of blood may be seen emerging from the sinus drainage ostium.
- Direct sinus endoscopy through the CMS is required for a definitive diagnosis of these PEHs.
- Radiography in the standing position should reveal a soft tissue mass extending rostral or dorsal to the ethmoidal 'onion' into the CFS or FS respectively.

Treatment

- Ablation via a frontal facial flap is the treatment of choice.
- Lesions within the sinuses are easily accessible but nasal aspect PEHs require removal of the floor of the CFS.
- The lesions are rarely withdrawn without rupture of the mucosal sac but the basal area should be subjected to thorough curettage.
- Neodymium (Nd) YAG laser destruction is a suitable technique for small lesions.

Prognosis

The prognosis for successful ablation by facial flap surgery is good but recurrence may occur in up to 25% of cases within 18 months.

5.13 *Sinus cysts*

Aetiopathogenesis

• The aetiology of sinus cysts is not known but there appear to be features common with PEHs inasmuch as the two conditions may occur concurrently and both show evidence of repeated haemorrhage.
• Cysts typically contain vivid yellow fluid indicative of blood pigment degradation.
• Sinus cysts typically arise in the region of the drainage ostium so that expansion either occurs into the sinus or into the nasal meati.

Presenting signs

Nasal obstruction and facial swelling are the typical presentation signs of sinus cysts. The facial swelling is generally over the conchofrontal or maxillary sinuses but a small number of cases show a midline frontal distension. Rarely proptosis may be seen.

Diagnosis

• Sinus cysts tend to occur either in the first year of life or in horses over 4 years old.
• The presenting signs, physical examination, endoscopy and radiography provide the necessary diagnostic information.
• Sinus cysts are large space occupying lesions and can easily be confused with a neoplastic disease. However, cysts are very much more frequent in horses than nasal tumours.
• The physical examination may reveal a considerable swelling over the facial region with or without obstruction to nasal air flow.
• Increased resonance on percussion can be expected if there is thinning of the nasal bones.
• Cysts which have expanded in a nasal direction can be seen at endoscopy as discrete rounded masses typically in the middle meatus.
• Those which are confined to the sinuses cause a more diffuse narrowing of the nasal airways to the point where passage of the endoscope to the nasopharynx is obstructed.
• Radiographs will reveal a homogeneous soft tissue density with at least some of its margins well demarcated.
• On lateral standing views free gas/fluid lines may be seen indicative of impeded sinus drainage.

• Ventrodorsal views are helpful to demonstrate the limits of the lesion in a rostrocaudal dimension as well as the extent of any septal deviation.
• If there is a safe available site, aspiration into the cyst provides definitive confirmation of the diagnosis by the release of characteristic vivid yellow fluid.

Treatment

Frontonasal flap surgery is effective and the cyst wall can be peeled away from the inside of the sinuses. In the event of incomplete ablation small areas of residual cyst tissue do not appear to cause complications.

Prognosis

The prognosis for successful surgical ablation is excellent and recurrence is not likely.

5.14 *Mycotic rhinitis and sinusitis*

Aetiopathogenesis

Although mycotic opportunism is common after surgery or secondary to other suppurative conditions such as dental periapical abscessation, horses are encountered where these infections arise on the sinu-nasal tissues without obvious underlying disease. The aetiology is not known but the infection consists of a destructive rhinitis/sinusitis, occasionally producing sinu-nasal fistulas.

Clinical signs

Horses with mycotic infections in the nasal region usually show a low-grade unilateral purulent discharge which may be malodorous. On the rare occasions when erosion of a significant blood vessel has occurred, there may be epistaxis.

Diagnosis

• The external physical examination is unlikely to be helpful.
• Similarly radiographic findings may appear to be relatively normal with no more than small gas/fluid lines and such a finding in a horse with a notable nasal discharge is highly suggestive of a mycotic infection.

- The presence of mycotic plaques can be confirmed by endoscopy either *per nasum* or directly into the CMS.

Treatment

- Topical medication with the benzimidazole agent enilconazole provides an effective and simple remedy.
- A Foley balloon catheter is placed into the CMS and the sinus cavity acts as a reservoir for the medication which is infused twice daily.
- Resolution may require prolonged treatment, i.e. 4–6 weeks.

Prognosis

Primary sinu-nasal mycosis carries an excellent prognosis provided that the course of treatment is sufficiently long.

5.15 *Sinus and nasal neoplasia and polyps*

Aetiopathogenesis

True tumours of the sinus and nasal regions are rare in the horse.

- Squamous cell carcinoma, adenocarcinoma, osteomas and osteosarcomas have all been reported.
- Odontogenic tumours, i.e. tumours derived from the tooth-forming tissues, are rarely encountered, usually in young horses.
- Polyps, i.e. pedunculated inflammatory proliferations enclosed in mucous membrane, are likely to represent a complication of dental periapical disease.

Clinical signs

The clinical signs are likely to be confused with those of a severe primary sinus empyema, cyst or progressive ethmoidal haematoma, i.e. a putrid nasal discharge possibly mixed with blood; nasal obstruction and facial swelling. In addition there may be proptosis when the tumour has infiltrated the bony orbit and displaced the globe outwards. Some nasal polyps protrude to the nostrils.

Diagnosis

The usual physical, endoscopic and radiographic procedures which might be applicable to a case of empyema, cyst or PEH are indicated.

- In horses with proptosis, trans-ocular ultrasonography should be used to assess the integrity of the bony orbit.
- Attempts to aspirate fluid from the lesion will fail to produce pus or fluid but needle aspiration could be a means to obtain biopsy material, for example after exploratory trephination.
- Radiographs may show a lesion with an outline less well demarcated than with a cyst or empyema. Identifiable mineralized dental tissue may be evident in cases of well-differentiated odontogenic tumour. In cases of suspected polyp the dental features on radiographs should be reviewed as well as checking the clinical dental crowns by oral inspection.

Treatment

Frontonasal flap surgery may be used on an exploratory basis and this may or may not lead on to extirpation depending on the feasibility of total removal.

Prognosis

The prognosis for sinu-nasal tumours in horses is highly variable and each case must be treated on its merits. Well-circumscribed benign lesions often lend themselves to successful removal by frontonasal flap surgery and the size of the lesion need not be a deterrent.

5.16 *Other sinu-nasal disorders*

Nasal septal deviation

Congenital deviation of the nasal septum is invariably present in cases of wry nose but may also occur as an independent entity. It may not come to light until the patient commences training and investigations into the cause of abnormal respiratory noise take place.

While a diagnosis of septal deviation may be suggested by endoscopy, the diagnosis can only be confirmed by radiography in the ventrodorsal plane showing that the septum does not adhere to a midline position.

Septal resection is a feasible treatment for septal disorders in horses.

Other nasal septal disorders

Infections of the nasal septum are rare in the United Kingdom but in other countries this is a site where granulomatous thickening may occur in response to infections such as cryptococcosis. In addition to specific antifungal medication, septal resection may be indicated to relieve the obstructive effect.

Conchal necrosis and metaplasia

Metaplastic calcification of the conchal cartilages may occur as an end-stage of dental suppuration which has extended into the nasal tissues. Horses afflicted with this condition will be presented with a foetid nasal discharge but signs directly referable to dental disease may not have been noted. Endoscopy will show necrotic debris on the surfaces of the conchal scrolls but radiographs provide the definitive diagnosis in the form of turbinate 'coral' formation.

Facial and sinus trauma

Horses involved in all forms of athletic sport are vulnerable to facial trauma in falls, stick-and-ball injuries as well as kicks.

The guiding principles which relate to the management of cases of facial trauma are no different from those which apply to other wounds:

- control of haemorrhage and preservation of vital functions such as respiration in the acute phase;
- anatomical restoration where desirable for functional or cosmetic reasons; removal of devitalized tissue;
- control of secondary infection.

Intranasal foreign bodies

Intranasal foreign bodies are uncommon in horses. The sudden onset of acute nasal discomfort with intense sneezing and facial rubbing are the likely signs, particularly if there has been recent epistaxis. Some foreign bodies are visible as soon as the alar margins are raised but others are only identified at endoscopy.

Subcutaneous emphysema

The presence of air in the subcutaneous tissues suggests one of three events: (1) leakage of air from within the respiratory tract; (2) repeated entrapment of air in an external wound; (3) the presence of gas-forming organisms.

1. Trauma and surgery of the upper respiratory tract, including the paranasal sinuses, larynx and trachea, may lead to air being forced between the skin and the underlying layers. Emphysema typically arises when the air cannot move freely to the nares during expiration and is therefore forced through a defect in the wall of the tract into the subcutaneous tissues. Oedema and spasm after laryngeal surgery, or nasal packing after frontonasal surgery are examples of iatrogenic causes of emphysema.
2. Wounds in the axillary region frequently cause progressive entrapment of air with each movement of the forelimb.
3. Clostridial (gas gangrene) infections typically stem from the deep inoculation of the infective agent and unless identified promptly they are rapidly fatal.

The objectives in treatment of subcutaneous emphysema are straightforward: either prevent further air entering the subcutaneous space by closure of the defect, or allow the air to escape more easily by an alternative route. Facilities for emergency tracheotomy or laryngotomy should always be on hand in establishments where airway surgery is performed. Neglected subcutaneous emphysema can lead to pneumothorax and fatal pulmonary collapse after air has entered by way of the mediastinum.

5.17 *Idiopathic headshaking (IHS) in horses*

Clinical signs

The term 'headshaking' is used to describe the abnormal condition when a horse shakes its head in the absence of obvious external stimuli and with such frequency and violence that it becomes difficult or dangerous to ride or appears to be distressed.

The typical presenting features of a headshaker include:

- The headshaking consists of rapid vertical head flicking and rarely are the movements horizontal.
- The behaviour occurs during ridden exercise once the horse has warmed up.
- The horse is inclined to sneeze/snort at the walk and trot.
- There is an obvious seasonal tendency for the condition and in the northern hemisphere most cases begin between March and June. The condition generally is at its worst in late spring but can last until the early winter. During the first few seasons the winter resolution and spring relapses are obvious but many horses eventually become afflicted throughout the year.
- The horse was purchased during the winter months.
- There is almost invariably evidence of irritation at the nostrils. This may consist of sneezing, snorting, rubbing the nose or even striking at it with the forefeet.
- When being walked the horse will rub its nose along the ground or constantly nudge its handler in the back.
- The headshaking is particularly likely to occur on warm humid days when the horse is exercised under trees.
- There is sometimes engorgement of the superficial veins on the face together with excess lacrimation.

Horses of all breeds and over a wide age range may be afflicted by headshaking. It is unusual to encounter IHS in horses racing on the flat or over jumps. Most appear to be involved in restrained exercise such as dressage, eventing, showing or general purpose riding.

Horses do not often exhibit IHS when at rest in the stable or at grass but signs generally begin once the animal has warmed up at exercise. Owners will often describe the headshaking behaviour as resembling a horse with a bee sitting on the end of the nose.

Proposed aetiology

On the basis of convincing circumstantial evidence, it is proposed that IHS is an expression of allergic rhinitis. However, this hypothesis has not yet been supported by specific immunological tests.

Clinical investigation

A review of the presentation and history is of paramount importance. The major diagnostic challenge is to eliminate demonstrable disorders of the ears, eyes, cervical spine, auditory tube diverticula, upper respiratory tract, central nervous system (CNS), cranial nerves, teeth and oral cavity.

Thus clinical examination includes a general health assessment; a neurological examination; external inspection of the head; flexion tests of the neck in both horizontal and vertical plains; endoscopy of the upper respiratory tract, including a tracheal wash; and an ophthalmoscopic examination. A demonstration of the behaviour is staged within the limits of safety to the rider and the effect of a bilateral infra-orbital nerve block assessed. At a later stage intradermal monospecific antigen testing is applied. Under a general anaesthetic a detailed otoscopic inspection of both ear canals and smear examinations for mites should be performed (see 5.1, 'Investigation'). The oral cavity and teeth are checked carefully for potential sources of discomfort, particularly those which could interfere with the bit, and, when indicated, radiographs of the dental arcades are made. In typical cases of IHS most of the investigations above are unhelpful.

Recently a photic form of headshaking has been described in which a pattern of behaviour very similar to that described above has been attributed to exposure to bright sunlight. Obviously, photic headshaking could be expected in the summer months also and care is required to differentiate the condition from IHS. The use of a visor with tinted lenses or testing the horse at dusk as well as in the middle of the day will produce a dramatic improvement of photic headshaking.

Treatment

- The use of aids such as nose fringes/muslin masks can be helpful in the short term.
- A number of medical regimens have tried to control IHS and these have included systemic corticosteroids, inhaled corticosteroid (beclomethasone), inhaled sodium chromoglycate, systemic antihistamines and flunixin meglumine. None is at all effective, either because the treatment has no effect or because of impracticalities of administration.
- Complete and sustained resolution can be achieved by bilateral infra-orbital neurectomy in

approximately 40% of cases. Presumably this has its effect by complete desensitization of the end of the muzzle where some of the 'itch' of the rhinitis occurs. Only in those horses which give a positive response to such a diagnostic nerve block should surgical neurectomy be considered.

• Cyproheptadine may be useful for management of photic headshaking.

5.18 *Diagnostic approach to conditions causing airway obstructions in horses*

Functional concepts of conducting airways

Olfaction is relatively unimportant to the horse and the conchal scrolls of the nasal chambers are anatomically simple, and the nasal meati are streamlined for a species which is an obligatory nasal breather.

The movement of air through the respiratory tract is achieved by the creation of pressure gradients during inspiration and expiration.

• During the inspiratory phase the pressure within the lumen of the airways is lower than that within the tissues of the walls of the tract as well as in the external environment.
• During expiration the gradients are reversed.
• The greater the work of breathing, the greater are the collapsing forces applied to the walls of the upper respiratory tract, so that during inspiration at exercise they are very considerable, as much as 40 cmH$_2$O.
• During quiet breathing, the upper respiratory tract, principally the nostrils and larynx, provides 70–85% of total resistance, but when required this can be reduced to under 50% by strategies such as the active dilation of the nares and larynx and by straightening the airway.
• Airflow through the conducting airways increases from 4 litres/second at rest to 70 litres/second at the gallop and video-endoscopy of horses exercising on a high speed treadmill confirms that although the airways dilate in response to increased demand, the same inward and outward movements of the pharyngeal walls and soft palate can be seen on inspiration and expiration.
• An essential component of the overall airway dilation is the maximal abduction of the rima glottidis achieved by the action of the intrinsic laryngeal musculature. Treadmill endoscopy confirms that the full abduction is sustained through all phases of the respiratory cycle and continues during the immediate post-exercise recovery period. Failure of this function, for example in laryngeal hemiplegia or arytenoid chondropathy, leads to dynamic collapse of the flaccid structures into the airway during inspiration causing restriction of airflow with associated noise.

• Dynamic dysfunction at the level of the pharynx and larynx accounts for the majority of cases of obstructive dyspnoea in athletic horses.
• The structural rigidity provided by the conchal cartilages and the tracheal rings provides stability through much of the upper respiratory tract but in three key areas of the airway, the nostrils, pharynx and larynx, resistance to collapse is provided by active muscular dilation. These are coincidentally the sites at which much of the resting airway resistance occurs and it is suggested that relatively minor lesions or dysfunctions at these sites of high resistance may significantly increase total impedance to airflow.

Respiration and locomotion

At the walk, trot and when pacing there is no relationship between locomotion and the respiratory cycle. However, at the canter and gallop a 1:1 relationship exists, i.e. one respiratory cycle is completed in the time taken for one stride. At the canter and gallop inspiration occurs during the extension phase of the forelimbs. Conversely, expiration occurs during the weight bearing phase of the forelimbs and for ridden exercise this coincides with the rider moving forwards in the saddle.

Horses may require to swallow during exercise and respiration cannot continue through deglutition; it is suspended after the inspiratory phase and resumes with expiration on completion of swallowing. For horses at the canter and gallop deglutition must be completed exactly in the time taken for a whole number of strides, usually one.

Intranarial larynx

The horse is designed to be an obligatory nose-breathing animal and never to breathe through its mouth. It is equipped with an intranarial larynx whereby the cartilages of the larynx are locked into the caudal wall of the nasopharynx by the palatopharyngeal arch which acts as an airtight seal. The palatal arch requires to be able to disengage momentarily for deglutition, but at all other times the larynx remains in its intranarial position.

Clinical signs of obstructive dyspnoea

The signs of airway obstruction include increased respiratory effort, increased respiratory noise and compromised athletic performance. The increased work of breathing exaggerates the collapsing forces so that some horses which appear to be normal at rest show signs only during exercise. Dynamic collapse of the soft structures abutting onto the walls of the airway may exacerbate the obstruction and audible respiratory sounds are produced. Occasionally the airways are so severely obstructed that breathing at rest is embarrassed, for example in the face of an intranasal mass or arytenoid chondropathy.

Respiratory noises at exercise

When horses are exercised the process of inspiration should be silent to the unaided human ear. In contrast, vibrant sounds generated by the alar folds frequently make expiration a noisy process – 'high blowing'.

Respiratory obstructions may arise through structural distortion of the walls of the airways or through abnormal function. When there is structural change or when the malfunction is consistent the inspiratory sounds which are heard will be reliably present at a given speed, provided that ambient conditions of temperature and humidity remain unchanged. However, in some circumstances the dysfunction is momentary and therefore the sound which is heard has an abrupt onset and often an equally abrupt conclusion.

History

Horses are presented for respiratory assessments at pre-purchase examinations and because of nasal discharge, untoward respiratory noises, acute and chronic coughing, prolonged post-exercise tachypnoea, fatigue at exercise and disappointing performances. In the context of poor performance, it is important to discover whether the performance is unproven and may result from an inherent lack of ability, or whether the patient has been an effective athlete but is no longer successful.

Before commencing an examination of the upper respiratory tract the bodily condition of the patient should be noted, as overweight, unfit horses are inclined to produce 'stuffy' respiratory noises resulting from pharyngeal flaccidity. The temperature should be taken and any nasal discharge noted; the lymph glands should also be palpated looking for evidence of current upper respiratory tract infections.

Palpation tests

During the examination at rest palpation of the larynx should check for:

- the cartilage structure of the larynx (see 5.25);
- the presence of atrophy of the intrinsic musculature, typically the dorsal crico-arytenoideus muscle and resultant prominence of the muscular process of the arytenoid cartilage;
- evidence of previous surgery, i.e. ventral laryngotomy cicatrix or scar from laryngoplasty surgery;
- responses to the 'slap' test; these are better assessed by palpation than by endoscopy;
- the arytenoid depression test whereby the right muscular process is depressed in order to close the right side of the larynx. In cases of severe recurrent laryngeal neuropathy the left side of the larynx will already be closed. Thus, closure of the right side will markedly restrict the airway and provoke stridorous sounds.

Palpation of the trachea should seek evidence of disruption of the normal ring architecture by previous trauma or surgery. Congenitally flattened rings may also be detected.

Endoscopy at rest

An endoscopic inspection of the conducting airways during quiet breathing forms the basis for most diagnosis of airway obstructions in practice. A full endoscopic examination should include both nasal chambers, the nasopharynx, epiglottis, soft palate, larynx and trachea. Apart from the overall conformation of the lumen of the airway, the relationships between structures such as the soft palate and epiglottis may be noted and the resting movements of the larynx observed. Note is also made of the presence and origin of any discharge, including blood.

During the examination the patient should be stimulated to swallow on multiple occasions in order to give the best opportunity to identify those anomalies such as epiglottal entrapment and small sub-epiglottic cysts which may not be consistently visible.

Radiography of the throat

Radiographs can be used to provide an additional dimension to respiratory investigations, particularly to reveal structures obscured from endoscopic view, for example the tissues ventral to a soft palate which is permanently displaced dorsal to the epiglottis.

Conduct of exercise tests

Although an exercise test is an important part of the overall examination, and no pre-purchase assessment is complete without one, the consent of the owner of the horse, the suitability of the location, the fitness of the horse and the competence of the rider/handler should all be established before the test begins.

All ridden and lunged exercise tests to detect respiratory sounds should include a canter in both directions in a confined area. A ridden test is preferred because in a collected canter the poll is flexed and the resultant curvature of the airway exaggerates any untoward noises produced. The adventitious noises can be timed with respect to the phase of the respiratory cycle, i.e. inspiratory versus expiratory.

Endoscopy after exercise

Although it is standard procedure to include an examination as soon as possible after completion of the exercise test, this is probably the least informative time to perform endoscopy. No dynamic collapse is likely to be seen and some of the subtler anomalies apparent during quiet breathing will have been abolished, especially by the full sustained abduction of the larynx.

Radio-stethoscope

The sounds generated in the upper respiratory tract can be analysed by recording through a telemetric link to a microphone attached to the throat of horses at exercise. The duration of the inspiratory and expiratory phases can be measured accurately and the frequencies and amplitude of the sounds can be used as the basis for diagnosis of the location and nature of disease.

Treadmill testing of horses during exercise

The advent of improved endoscopic equipment and treadmills upon which horses can exercise at speeds up to 14 m/second has provided the means by which to study the dynamic changes which occur in the conducting airways at exercise. Comparison of the results of resting endoscopy and findings during exercise suggests that diagnosis at rest yields a significantly inaccurate result in as much as 50% of cases.

The advantages of treadmill testing include improved specificity of diagnosis and an increased repertoire of diagnosis. It also gives the opportunity for simultaneous physiological tests, not only to assess whether the anomalies observed endoscopically are compromising respiratory function but as the means to test the efficacy of surgical methods of correction.

5.19 Common upper respiratory tract obstructive disorders of horses

Obstructions of the conducting airways are diagnosed in two circumstances:

1. Horses which produce audible respiratory noises, typically during inspiration.
2. During routine pre-purchase examinations.

In order of frequency in Thoroughbred horses, the causes of structural and/or functional airway collapse are:

- recurrent laryngeal neuropathy (RLN),
- dorsal displacement of the palato-pharyngeal arch (DDSP),
- epiglottal entrapment (EE),
- fourth branchial arch defects (4-BAD),
- arytenoid chondropathy (AC).

The absolute prevalence of each of these entities is not known.

5.20 Recurrent laryngeal neuropathy (RLN)

Aetiopathogenesis

RLN causes a permanent dysfunction of the intrinsic muscles of the larynx which receive their motor innervation through the recurrent laryngeal branch of the vagus nerve. The result is partial obstruction of the airway evident during exercise and compromised athletic performance through hypoxia. The condition almost invariably involves the left side of the larynx and very rarely right-sided or bilateral cases are encountered. The disease manifests itself as a failure to achieve or to maintain full symmetrical arytenoid abduction under conditions of greatest respiratory demand. The resistance to normal airflow causes turbulence in the airstream which is the source of the characteristic abnormal inspiratory sounds – 'whistling' or 'roaring'.

RLN consists of a distal axonopathy whereby the larger myelinated nerve fibres degenerate from the motor end-plate proximally towards the cell body of the neuron. The effect is one of atrophy of those muscles predominantly supplied by the large myelinated fibres, and for this reason the major adductor, the crico-arytenoideus lateralis (CAL), is afflicted before the major dilator of the rima glottidis, the crico-arytenoideus dorsalis (CAD). However, defects of adduction are rarely noted by owners although they form the basis of some clinical tests such as the 'slap' reflex. It has been suggested that the structural changes in the nerves arise through an underlying defect of axonal transport so that the condition may be related to the absolute length of the recurrent nerve fibres. The recurrent laryngeal nerves include by far the longest lower motor neurons in the horse and the left nerve is significantly longer than the right. Clinical signs of RLN, with exercise intolerance and stridor at exercise, become apparent with involvement of the principal abductor, the CAD muscle, and the degree of neurogenic myopathy correlates with the severity of the nerve lesion.

Less common causes of RLN include:

- trauma to the recurrent nerve by perivascular injection of irritant medicaments,
- damage to the vagal trunk by guttural pouch mycosis or strangles abscessation,
- toxicity by heavy metals such as lead and organophosphate poisoning,
- nutritional deficiencies such as thiamine.

Distal axonopathies often show an inherited basis and there is evidence to support this contention in the horse.

During exercise the arytenoid cartilages are normally held in full symmetrical abduction which is sustained throughout all stages of the respiratory cycle and this abduction will be present for a period after completion of the exercise. Failure of the neuromuscular unit results in partial obstruction of the airway. As the cross-sectional area of the rima glottidis is reduced, the pressure differentials within the larynx increase to maintain the airflow necessary to sustain exercise. The collapsing forces rise and the paralysed cord is drawn even further across the airway (Venturi effect). When the demands for inspiratory flow reach their peak, afflicted horses show flow limitation, increased inspiratory resistance and depression of arterial oxygen tension.

Prevalence

Horses of any age from birth onwards may be afflicted with RLN, although it is not clear:

- whether the disorder is invariably present from birth but simply not recognized by the owner
- whether the clinical signs only manifest themselves when the horses reach an age when they are subjected to the necessary level of exertion
- whether the disorder is progressive.

Horses over 16 hands tall are most susceptible and RLN becomes increasingly rare below 15.2 hands.

The prevalence of RLN in the Thoroughbred is not known and there are widely varying estimates (0.96–95%) in the literature. The frequency of true hemiplegia, i.e. where there are no active abductory or adductory movements whatever by the left arytenoid cartilage and vocal folds, is in the order of 2%.

The clinical signs of RLN usually appear before the horse is 6 years of age.

Clinical signs

- Horses afflicted with RLN usually produce consistent inspiratory sounds which can be heard throughout the period of exertion at the canter and gallop.
- The sounds themselves may range from a low-grade musical 'whistle' similar to the noise produced by blowing over the top of an empty bottle, to a harsh 'roaring' noise like sawing wood.
- Disappearance of the sounds can be expected within a short period of pulling up; horses with RLN recover a resting respiratory rate in a normal period.
- Occasionally horses with RLN produce adventitious respiratory noises only under extreme exertion and, unless examined by endoscopy during high-speed treadmill exercise, it is not possible to determine whether the noise stems

from abrupt dynamic collapse of the paralysed arytenoid cartilage or from secondary DDSP.
• The athletic potential of horses that exercise aerobically is likely to be compromised by RLN. However, the impact on the performance of horses that are involved in anaerobic sports, such as sprint racing, will be less marked.

Diagnosis

1. Palpation.
   • Palpation of the larynx should seek evidence of atrophy of the intrinsic laryngeal musculature especially on the left side.
   • An assessment of the strength of the 'slap' response is more accurately judged by palpation than by endoscopy.
   • The arytenoid depression test, whereby the right side of the larynx is forced to adduct by pressure on the right arytenoid muscular process, is more likely to provide a convincing increase in stridor at the conclusion of exercise than at rest.
   • Palpation should also seek evidence of a cicatrix from previous surgery.
   • During palpation of the larynx note should be taken of the spacing between the cricoid and thyroid cartilages. Deformities of the thyroid laminae are frequently present as part of the fourth branchial arch defect syndrome (see 5.25) and particular attention should be paid in cases of apparent right-sided RLN.
2. The 'Grunt-to-the-Stick' test depends upon startling the horse by threatening with a cudgel. Laryngeal fixation in an incompletely closed position together with a rapid rise in pressure within the airway produces a low-pitched grunt. This is a test of the competence of laryngeal adduction but the results are inconsistent.
3. Endoscopy.
   • The asymmetry of the rima glottidis in cases of true left laryngeal hemiplegia is usually obvious (Figure 2).
   • During equine laryngoscopy, the perspective distortion which arises from the eccentric position of the endoscope in the nasopharynx must be taken into account. Thus, when the endoscope is introduced through the right nostril, false negative diagnoses are possible, but from the left side the left arytenoid cartilage may give the false impression of inadequate abduction. Whenever doubt exists, the

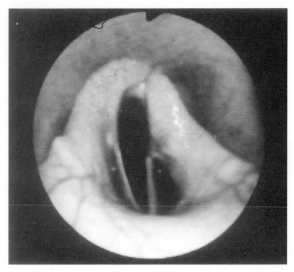

Figure 2   Marked laryngeal asymmetry.

endoscopy should be performed through each nostril in turn.
• A grading system with reproducible parameters is necessary if the subjectivity of endoscopy of the larynx is to be eliminated, particularly when left laryngeal dysfunction is incomplete. A suggested grading system is provided below:

Grade 1.   All movements, both adductory and abductory, are synchronized at rest and after exercise. Any appearance of asymmetry arises as an artefact of the position of the endoscope and when the right and left nostrils are used in turn the perspective distortion is cancelled. This being the case a 'mirror' effect operates such that when the endoscopy is performed through the right nasal chamber, the right arytenoid may appear less abducted and vice versa.

Grade 2.   All major movements are symmetrical with a full range of abduction and adduction. Transient asynchrony, flutter or delayed or biphasic abduction may be seen especially by the left arytenoid.

Grade 3.   Although the left arytenoid is still capable of full abduction, activity is generally reduced on the left compared with the right with periods of prolonged asymmetry, particularly during quiet movements. Full bilateral abduction can be stimulated transiently by partial asphyxiation using nostril closure but it is not sustained.

Grade 4. The left arytenoid is no longer capable of full abduction and during adduction compensation by the right arytenoid crossing the midline may be evident. Asymmetry is marked but some residual movements are present.

Grade 5. True hemiplegia, i.e. a complete absence of active movement on the affected side; no response to the 'slap' test will be provoked.

Grades 1 and 2 are considered to be within the acceptable limits of clinical normality; Grades 4 and 5 are considered abnormal and horses showing arytenoid motility in these grades would be expected to produce abnormal inspiratory noises during the exercise test. Grade 3 comprises equivocal dysfunction where some horses show no untoward inspiratory sounds at exercise, while others produce a characteristic 'whistle'.

High-speed treadmill endoscopy is necessary to provide a complete assessment of laryngeal function because the interpretation at rest may be misleading. Treadmill testing is particularly helpful to clarify the significance of Grade 3 motility.

4. Exercise test.
5. Other diagnostic tests which are not widely used but which may be of future interest include the radio-stethoscope with sound frequency analysis, electromyographic recording of laryngeal muscle activity and measurement of conduction time in the 'slap' reflex.

Treatment

A number of procedures have been proposed to relieve the obstructive effects of RLN. The most notable of these are:

- the various ventriculectomy and cordectomy procedures,
- prosthetic laryngoplasty,
- temporary and permanent tracheostomy,
- subtotal arytenoidectomy,
- nerve/muscle pedicle grafting.

1. Ventriculectomy (Hobday or Williams procedure) depends upon the removal of the mucous membrane lining from the laryngeal ventricle and excision of the vocal fold. The benefits of the Hobday procedure are at best slight, and the technique should be reserved for horses with less marked RLN and those horses that, on the treadmill, are shown to be obstructed by the dynamic collapse of the vocal fold rather than by the arytenoid cartilage.

2. Abductor prosthesis operation (prosthetic laryngoplasty, 'tie-back') is considered to be the treatment of choice for RLN in most countries.
   - The procedure and its variants aim to implant a ligature between the caudal border of the cricoid cartilage and the muscular process of the arytenoid to mimic the action of the CAD muscle as if it were in a semi-contracted state.
   - However, the procedure should be regarded as a gross physiological disturbance because when the rima glottidis is fixed in an abducted position, the ability of the larynx to protect the lower airways during deglutition is compromised and a degree of dysphagia is inevitable.
   - Nevertheless, most horses show relief of laryngeal obstruction and are only subclinically dysphagic.
   - Physiological studies have confirmed that prosthetic laryngoplasty is effective in the restoration of normal respiratory function and in the prevention of dynamic collapse of the paralysed arytenoid in cases of RLN.

3. Temporary tracheotomy tubing (see 5.27)
   - The purpose of these tubes is to provide an alternative airway and to bypass the site of airway obstruction.
   - They may be used when other surgical techniques for RLN have failed but their major virtue is that intubation is performed under local analgesia and disruption of the training programme is minimal.
   - Tracheotomy tubing provides a short-term expedient to race horses that would otherwise be side-lined by alternative surgery.
   - When the tracheotomy tube is eventually removed the defect heals quickly by second intention and the option to perform a ventriculectomy or laryngoplasty operation will not have been compromised.

4. Permanent tracheostomy, the creation of a fistula between the tracheal lumen and the skin surface of the ventral neck, has been used for horses and ponies but the results are generally not aesthetically acceptable. There is a regular requirement for nursing to remove exudation from the skin adjacent to the stoma and to maintain local hygiene.

5. Total, partial and subtotal arytenoidectomy aim to remove the intralaryngeal structures

which are causing obstruction. Thus, the usual indications for arytenoidectomy are the removal of infected cartilage in cases of chronic chondropathy (see 5.24) and the removal of the left arytenoid cartilage when other techniques to treat RLN have failed.

6. Nerve/muscle pedicle grafting aims to transplant cubes of muscle taken from the omohyoideus together with their motor supply through the first and second cervical nerves into the atrophied CAD muscle to restore abductory function to the larynx. Following surgery the grafts grow in response to mechanical stimulation so that at least a year must be allowed to achieve optimum results. Abduction of the arytenoid cartilage only occurs during exertion because the omohyoid is an accessory muscle of respiration and the technique has the advantage over prosthetic laryngoplasty that no complications can arise from aspiration through a permanently abducted rima glottidis.

Prognosis

• Prosthetic laryngoplasty is far from ideal as a treatment for RLN but it remains the best practicable option currently available. Although it is recognized that this surgery can produce complications in the forms of coughing, nasal reflux of ingesta or recurrence of dyspnoea, the risks are justifiable in horses that cannot otherwise be effective athletes.

• Nerve/muscle pedicle grafting is a promising alternative which is most likely to be applicable to horses where RLN is confirmed at an early stage and when the prolonged convalescent period is likely to be less restrictive.

5.21 *Dorsal displacement of the soft palate (DDSP)*

Aetiopathogenesis

The function of the arcus palato-pharyngeus is to provide an airtight seal that locks the larynx into the caudal wall of the nasopharynx. This mechanism renders the horse at exercise an obligatory nose-breather where the intranarial siting of the larynx provides streamlining of the airway.

Rostrally the palatal arch passes ventral to the epiglottis; laterally, lateral to the aryepiglottic folds; and posteriorly, caudal to the corniculate processes of the arytenoid cartilages. Thus, the free border of the palate is not visible by endoscopy when the larynx occupies its normal intranarial position.

DDSP arises as an acute respiratory obstruction which occurs while a horse is at fast exercise and when the free border of the palatal arch becomes dislodged from its normal sub-epiglottic position and the unsupported soft tissue is inhaled into the rima glottidis.

Treadmill endoscopy has clarified the sequence of events leading to dynamic DDSP. Jerking movements are generated at the junction of the hard and soft palates leading to billowing waves in the soft palate which pass caudally towards the free border. This is followed by retraction of the larynx and irregularities of respiratory rhythm. Finally the palatal slips from beneath the epiglottis to obstruct the laryngeal airway. Deglutition rarely if ever precedes DDSP but afflicted horses swallow afterwards to restore the larynx to its intranarial site.

DDSP is frequently a symptom rather than a disease in its own right. Amongst the underlying causes which have been proposed are:

• Conditions causing fatigue, e.g. unfitness; primary cardiovascular disorders; primary pulmonary diseases, particularly small airway inflammation; and other concurrent obstructions of the conducting airways such as RLN.

• Disorders of the palate itself or which compromise its function, e.g. congenital and iatrogenic defects; ulceration of the free border; intrapalatal cysts; and pharyngeal paralysis.

• Disorders of the epiglottis, e.g. hypoplasia; deformity; entrapment; sub-epiglottic cysts; and epiglottitis.

• Conditions causing mouth breathing, e.g. neglected enamel points; retained temporary premolar caps; bits that are too harsh for the patient's mouth; and excessive flexion of the neck when being ridden, typically seen in dressage and show horses.

• Conditions provoking pharyngeal discomfort, e.g. pharyngeal lymphoid hyperplasia; pharyngitis; pharyngeal cysts; current upper respiratory tract infections; the presence of excessive discharges such as mucopus in chronic obstructive pulmonary disease (COPD) or blood in exercise-induced pulmonary haemorrhage (EIPH); and neoplasia.

Clinical signs

- The abrupt respiratory obstruction which accompanies DDSP not only causes a loud vibrant noise but precipitates a serious interference with the progress of the horse.
- In most cases, the horse completely loses its stride rhythm as it makes gulping attempts to restore the larynx into the intranarial position.
- Occasionally a horse will continue running noisily but with the severe handicap produced by partial asphyxiation.
- As soon as the normal anatomical configuration is restored, the horse is able to resume galloping and will not appear distressed thereafter.
- DDSP generally occurs when a horse reaches the point of maximum exertion, typically in the later stages of a race or during a competitive gallop in training. Racehorses, including trotters and pacers, are mostly involved but the dysfunction can occur in other occupations such as eventing.

Diagnosis

The diagnostic challenge in cases of DDSP is to identify the predisposing factor(s) by a diligent physical examination.

- Although a ridden exercise test should be included for cases of suspected DDSP it is unusual for a choking up episode to occur without the exertion of a race or competitive gallop.
- Nevertheless, even when a physical evaluation is combined with endoscopy, broncho-alveolar lavage and detailed clinical pathology, there are frequent cases where a specific cause is not found, and then by a process of elimination DDSP is deemed to be idiopathic.
- Intermittent DDSP during resting endoscopy is frequently observed in normal horses and should not be regarded as an indication of potential dynamic dysfunction during exercise.
- However, persistent DDSP should be regarded as significant, and is an indication for further investigation such as radiography or endoscopy *per os*.

Treatment

Conservative measures
- Every attempt should be made to eliminate the predisposing factors, including unfitness, or,

alternatively, to provide additional time or medication for recovery from respiratory tract infections.
- Routine dental attention should be directed to the removal of enamel points from the cheek teeth and to displace loose temporary premolar caps.
- Aids to prevent mouth-breathing such as a dropped or crossed noseband should be tried, and a change of bit to a simple rubber snaffle or, if applicable, a bitless bridle may be recommended.
- The position of the bit in the mouth may be modified by an Australian noseband.
- Tongue straps or tongue-ties are used to discourage caudal retraction of the tongue and in turn to inhibit deglutition.

Surgical treatments
The results of surgical procedures performed to inhibit DDSP are varied and will depend on how rigorous the methods of diagnosis and selection have been at the outset.

1. Although interferences to the free border of the palatal arch include chemical and physical cautery, the most frequent technique comprises resection of the edge of the palate, staphylectomy.
   - This technique appears to be illogical inasmuch as the effect of the surgery is to increase the size of the intrapharyngeal ostium so that the intranarial configuration of the larynx would be expected to be less stable. However, there is agreement that a proportion of horses are improved by staphylectomy – 59% in one survey – and it has been suggested that the improvement arises through a reduction in the bulk of the tissues available to obstruct the rima glottidis.
   - Staphylectomy is performed under general anaesthesia and through a conventional laryngotomy incision at the cricothyroid membrane.
   - The major detractions of staphylectomy are the need for general anaesthesia and the possibility that excessive removal of palatal tissue, or damage to the pharyngeal wall, will precipitate a permanent dysphagia.
2. Inhibition of the laryngeal retraction which precedes DDSP may be achieved by section of the strap muscles – sterno-thyro-hyoideus myectomy – a procedure which can be performed on the standing horse under local analgesia, but which is more safely and more accurately carried out under general anaesthesia. The overall success rate of 60% which has

been recorded after myectomy is not significantly different from that achieved by staphylectomy.

3. On the basis that myectomy and staphylectomy performed independently produce approximately 60% success, some surgeons hold that the two techniques performed together increase the possibility of inhibiting DDSP.

4. The intra-oral technique – oral palato-pharyngoplasty (Ahern procedure) – to resect a partial thickness bi-elliptical section of the soft palate from its junction with the hard palate caudally has the merit that it reduces flaccidity at the point where the prodromal billowing arises.

Prognosis

A cautious prognosis must be given for all horses in which DDSP is diagnosed. The results of the surgical treatments outlined above are, at best, unpredictable.

5.22 *Epiglottal entrapment (EE)*

Aetiopathogenesis

• In this condition the cartilage of the epiglottis becomes enveloped by a fold of glosso-epiglottic mucosa arising between the epiglottis itself and the base of the tongue and extending laterally as the aryepiglottic folds.
• The aetiology of EE is usually not known as the condition can be reproduced on most equine laryngeal post-mortem specimens but it is not clear why some horses develop the condition in life and others do not.
• The aetiology of EE is no mystery when the epiglottis is congenitally hypoplastic or where it is associated with a sub-epiglottic cyst. These possibilities should be checked by endoscopy and/or radiography before surgical correction is attempted.

Clinical signs

The signs associated with EE are highly variable and include:

• exercise intolerance with inspiratory and/or expiratory noises at exercise,
• intermittent gurgling from secondary DDSP,
• coughing after eating.

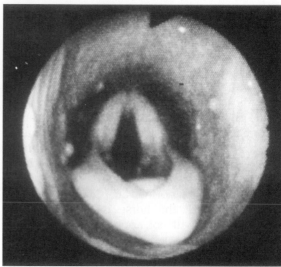

Figure 3   Epiglottal entrapment.

Reports of the prevalence of EE in endoscopic surveys of athletic horses at rest suggest an incidence in the range of 0.75% to 3.3%.

Diagnosis

• Definitive diagnosis of EE is achieved by endoscopy which shows that the epiglottis has lost its wrinkled cartilage border and that the superficial blood vessels are obscured by the entrapping mucosa (Figure 3).
• Occasionally the mucosa overlying the epiglottis is ulcerated.
• When persistent DDSP is present, the epiglottis cannot be seen at all, in which case a lateral radiograph of the pharynx is indicated to determine whether or not entrapment is present. On this projection the epiglottis should measure at least 7.0 cm from tip to hyoid articulation; an epiglottis with a length less than 5.5 cm is indicative of hypoplasia and surgery is contraindicated.
• EE may be intermittent and it is important, as a routine part of the endoscopic procedure, to stimulate a series of deglutition sequences in an attempt to provoke the condition. However, EE may be present only during vigorous exercise so that high speed treadmill endoscopy provides the best opportunity to establish a diagnosis of intermittent entrapment (see 5.26).

Treatment

The treatment options for epiglottal entrapment are:

1. resection via ventral laryngofissure,
2. axial division *per os*,
3. axial division *per nasum*,
4. trans-endoscopic Nd:YAG laser resection.

Methods 1 and 2 require general anaesthesia but both 3 and 4 can be performed on the standing horse with the obvious advantage of minimal disruption of training and racing schedules.

Methods 2 and 3 utilize a hooked bistoury to make a longitudinal cut in the loose mucous membrane overlying the epiglottal cartilage. The procedure of axial section of the EE is performed under endoscopic surveillance – the endoscope is passed through one nostril while the bistoury is introduced through the other. The ary-epiglottic mucosa is quite tough and care is required to prevent a palatal injury when the hook suddenly cuts free from the entrapment. Method 2 is safer and represents the technique of choice albeit with the risk of anaesthesia.

Prognosis

All of the methods of treatment mentioned above yield a high rate of uncomplicated resolution of EE. The possibility of recurrence of entrapment is greatest with the axial section techniques but even this is uncommon. Iatrogenic trauma to the epiglottal cartilage can provoke granulomas and other distortions which may compromise the relationship between the epiglottis and the soft palate. Chronic coughing associated with low-grade dysphagia is a rare but recognized complication of resection of the glosso-epiglottal mucosa.

5.23 *Sub-epiglottal cysts*

Aetiopathogenesis

Developmental cysts are occasionally recognized in the pharynx of horses and represent causes of dyspnoea and/or dysphagia.

- The most frequently encountered of these lesions is the sub-epiglottic cyst which is thought to be derived from the embryological remnants of the thyroglossal duct, a structure which runs from the level of the epiglottis to the anterior mediastinum.
- It is believed that sub-epiglottic cysts are present from birth although they may not be discovered until the horse is mature and commences training.
- The cysts consist of smooth-walled, sometimes multilobular, structures filled with straw-coloured slightly tenacious fluid.
- They arise from within the loose glosso-epiglottic mucosa lying between the base of the tongue and the epiglottis. It is very rare for a sub-epiglottic cyst to be found which is not located within an epiglottal entrapment.

Clinical signs

The age and manner by which the cysts cause clinical signs is dependent on their size.

- Large cysts can be a cause of dysphagia and respiratory obstruction in foals. Such foals may present within a few days of birth with reflux of milk from the nares and will require an endoscopic examination for differentiation from foals with palatal clefts.
- Older animals with cysts may present with a variety of respiratory signs including nasal discharge from dysphagia and abnormal respiratory sounds at exercise.
- Horses with small sub-epiglottic cysts may present with a history of choking up under exertion and will require differentiation from DDSP.

Diagnosis

- The diagnosis is easily established by endoscopy provided that the cystic lesions are available to be seen.
- In some horses with this condition persistent DDSP is present, in which case it will be necessary to resort to other diagnostic procedures such as plain and contrast radiography.

Treatment

- The objective of treatment is to ablate the cyst by sharp excision which can be achieved *per os* using an ecraseur.
- Resection by conventional ventral laryngofissure is generally simpler and safer. The technique is similar to that used for the treatment of epiglottal entrapment.
- Nd:YAG laser destruction can also be used.

Prognosis

The cystic lesions can often be excised intact and a favourable prognosis can be given. Recurrence is unlikely.

5.24 *Arytenoid chondropathy*

Aetiopathogenesis

Arytenoid chondritis (chondropathy) consists of the development of suppuration within the matrix of one or both arytenoid cartilages. The mechanism of development of micro-abscessation with discharging tracts is not clear but young male Thoroughbreds are usually affected. The condition appears to be more prevalent in the USA than Europe.

Clinical signs

The signs associated with arytenoid chondritis arise through a combination of airway obstruction and compromised glottic protection. Thus, stridorous noises are heard when the horse is exerted and if there is bilateral involvement there may be airway obstruction at rest. Coughing may be evident at any stage.

Diagnosis

- The diagnosis of arytenoid chondritis is primarily made by endoscopy showing distortion of the affected cartilage. As the micro-abscesses develop the cartilage thickens and shows axial displacement towards the midline and reduced motility.
- In the early stages, particularly when the left side is involved, casual endoscopy may suggest a diagnosis of RLN. As the condition advances, so the distortion of the cartilage becomes more obvious and granulomatous eruptions appear on the medial face of the corniculate process.
- Contact lesions may develop on the contralateral arytenoid cartilage.
- Lateral radiographs of the larynx usually show focal mineralization even in early cases.

Treatment

The progress of arytenoid chondritis may be arrested in the early stages by the prolonged (i.e. 6 weeks) use of potentiated sulphonamide medi-cation but once the chronic stage has been reached, the only treatment option is arytenoid-ectomy.

- Total arytenoidectomy implies that the entire arytenoid cartilage together with the corniculate process is removed.
- In partial arytenoidectomy the muscular process and articular facet are left *in situ* and in sub-total arytenoidectomy part or all of the corniculate process is also left in place.
- The greater the extent of cartilage resection the greater is the possibility that the ability of the larynx to protect the lower airways during deglutition will be compromised and that marked dysphagia with aspiration pneumonia will ensue.

Prognosis

Partial arytenoidectomy offers the best compromise to salvage a horse afflicted with laryngeal chondritis for breeding or for quiet exercise, but full athletic capacity cannot be restored by any surgery.

5.25 *Fourth branchial arch defects (4-BAD)*

Aetiopathogenesis

This is a syndrome of irreparable congenital defects resulting from a failure of development of some or all of the derivatives of the fourth branchial arch.

- The structures which may be defective are the wings of the thyroid cartilage, the cricothyroid articulation, the cricothyroideus muscles and the cricopharyngeal sphincter muscles. Any permutation of aplasia or hypoplasia of these structures may arise uni- or bilaterally.
- The absence of a firm bond between the wing of the thyroid and the cricoid cartilages deprives the larynx of a stable skeleton to facilitate the function of its intrinsic musculature. For example, in the face of such defects, the action of the crico-arytenoideus dorsalis muscle will be ineffective and the extent of arytenoid abduction is reduced. Clearly, this may convey a false impression of RLN on the affected side or sides.
- The absence of the cricopharyngeus muscles has two obvious effects: firstly the inability to close the upper oesophageal sphincter which

results in involuntary aerophagia; secondly, there is no means to anchor the palatal pillars into a position caudal to the apices of the corniculate cartilages resulting in rostral displacement of the palatal arch (RDPA).

Prevalence

The prevalence of 4-BAD in Thoroughbred horses is not less than 0.3% and the condition has been identified in other breeds such as the Hanoverian, warmbloods and the Haflinger. There is no current evidence that the syndrome is genetically transmitted.

Clinical signs

The presenting signs of horses with 4-BAD are very variable and reflect the severity of the absence of the structures involved. However, in order of frequency, the signs are:

- abnormal respiratory sounds at exercise,
- belching,
- nasal discharge,
- coughing,
- recurrent colic.

The involuntary aerophagia and eructation sometimes observed by owners may be confused with the noises produced by 'wind-suckers' (see 5.28).

Diagnosis

- A complete evaluation of the extent of 4-BAD can only be made at exploratory surgery or post mortem, but the combined findings of palpation, endoscopy and radiography are generally sufficient to justify a diagnosis.
- When the cartilage components are defective, an unusually wide gap can be palpated between the caudal margin of the thyroid and the rostral edge of the cricoid whereas in the normal larynx the two structures overlap.
- The two endoscopic features to alert the clinician to the possibility of 4-BAD are RDPA (see above) where the caudal pillars of the soft palate form a cowl which partly obscures the corniculate processes dorsally and may even leave the upper oesophagus open, and defective arytenoid motility.
- A small number of cases of 4-BAD can only be detected as dynamic RDPA during treadmill exercise (see 5.26).
- When the upper oesophageal sphincter is absent lateral radiographs will reveal a continu-

ous column of air extending from the pharynx into the oesophagus. The RDPA is seen as a 'dew drop' intruding into this air column from the dorsal wall.

Treatment

There are no effective means to reconstruct the absent structures.

Prognosis

Horses afflicted with 4-BAD are generally ineffective athletes but may be useful in less arduous occupations as pleasure horses. Repeated aerophagia leaves those animals without an upper oesophageal sphincter susceptible to episodes of colic which may be life threatening.

5.26 *Causes of dynamic airway collapse*

Mechanisms of dynamic collapse during exercise

Throughout the respiratory cycle of the exercising horse there are large intraluminal pressure swings, up to 40 cmH$_2$O, within the airway so that during inspiration in particular, the tissues abutting onto the extrathoracic airway must resist marked forces of collapse. In this regard the soft structures of the external nares and the pharynx and larynx are most vulnerable.

It is most unlikely that dynamic collapse can be seen by endoscopy during quiet breathing, unless by partial asphyxiation by forced nostril closure. It has only been since the advent of high-speed treadmills and of equipment to perform endoscopy during peak exertion that the dynamic causes of airway collapse have been confirmed.

Pharyngeal collapse

It is quite normal for the walls of the pharynx to collapse slightly during exercise and for the soft palate which makes up the floor of the nasopharynx to billow slightly upwards, but weakness of the muscular structures surrounding the airway at this level will produce a marked obstruction to air flow and reduced performance associated with abnormal inspiratory noises.

Dynamic DDSP

DDSP is a dynamic event which occurs only under the conditions of extreme exertion, and treadmill endoscopy offers the best means by which to observe the events which lead to the spontaneous displacement of the palatal arch above the epiglottis (see 5.21) and to differentiate idiopathic DDSP from other forms.

Intermittent epiglottal entrapment

Frequently EE is not a stable anatomical arrangement but may consist of the intermittent gathering of the glosso-epiglottic mucosa over the apex of the epiglottis. Although most cases of intermittent EE can be provoked by the repeated stimulation of deglutition sequences, a small number are not confirmed by endoscopy until treadmill exercise is used.

Ary-epiglottic fold collapse

The ary-epiglottal mucosal folds extend from the lateral margins of the epiglottis to the arytenoid cartilages. Dynamic collapse of one or both of these folds towards the midline is a relatively common observation during treadmill endoscopy of horses with a history of consistent harsh inspiratory noises at exercise. The inversion of the soft tissues causes a major obstruction of the rima glottidis but the aetiology is unknown and no treatments have been devised to relieve the condition.

Dynamic RDPA

The 4-BAD syndrome has been explained above (5.25), but even with diligent palpation, radiography and endoscopy, a definitive diagnosis may not be achieved at rest, particularly when the defects are minor. The only evidence of this lesser expression of 4-BAD may be dynamic rostral displacement of the palatal arch observed during treadmill endoscopy.

Dynamic laryngeal collapse

During quiet breathing the reliability of endoscopy as a means to interpret laryngeal function is far from satisfactory (see 5.20, 'Diagnosis'). In the absence of the collapsing forces at inspiration, resting horses with RLN may recruit sufficient motility to appear relatively normal. However, exercise may lead to fatigue of the residual abductor musculature so that treadmill endoscopy reveals dynamic collapse of the affected arytenoid cartilage and vocal fold.

5.27 Other causes of airway obstruction in the exercising horse

Choanal stenosis

Congenital narrowing of the airways at the level where the nasal meati meet the nasopharynx can be a highly subjective diagnosis. This site corresponds with the location of the bucconasal membrane in the developing foetus but this should perforate and retract well before term in order that the foal can commence nose breathing immediately after birth. Persistence of the bucconasal membrane can occur as a membranous or bony septum uni- or bilaterally to cause severe obstructions to nose-breathing with no air movement through the diseased side. Bilateral cases are likely to asphyxiate rapidly. There is no effective remedy for choanal stenosis and afflicted horses show limited athletic capacity.

Pharyngeal lymphoid hyperplasia (PLH)

PLH consists of extensive follicles of lymphoid hyperplasia on the walls of the nasopharynx and pharyngeal recess. PLH, also known as 'follicular pharyngitis', has a 100% prevalence in young horses and the significance which should be attached to the finding is doubtful. There is little interference with the performance of those adolescent animals which have marked PLH, but some clinicians believe that the disturbance of laminar airflow over the protuberances causes adventitious noise and the discomfort of engorged follicles provokes episodic gurgling through secondary DDSP.

Palatal cysts

Cysts, possibly of salivary origin, occasionally arise within the tissues of the soft palate and have been incriminated as a cause of abnormal respiratory noise in horses. They may not be easily identified by endoscopy and contrast radiography of the oropharynx is helpful to outline them. Access for surgical dissection is difficult but ventral laryngotomy offers the best option. Iatrogenic fenestration of the soft palate is a likely surgical complication when excision is attempted and the prognosis for horses with these cysts becoming useful athletes is not good.

Palatal defects

Defects of the hard and soft palate may be congenital or iatrogenic (see 1.3). Although the overwhelming majority of animals with palatal defects are presented with a history of dysphagia, the more subtle signs of longstanding clefts include a cough not invariably related to feeding and respiratory noise associated with palatal instability. Epiglottal entrapment is a frequent concurrent finding with longstanding congenital defects.

Iatrogenic palatal defects arise through over-enthusiastic resection surgery for DDSP (see 5.21, 'Treatment') and the most common sequel is chronic palatal instability leading to more severe signs of DDSP.

Pharyngeal cysts

Congenital cysts arising from the pharyngeal walls arise occasionally and the stage at which clinical signs are noted probably depends on their size. Diagnosis by endoscopy is invariably straightforward. The origin of these cysts is not known but they are generally amenable to surgical excision.

Pharyngeal paralysis

Although guttural pouch mycosis is the most common cause of pharyngeal paralysis (hemiplegia) (see 5.6) this neuropathy can arise following heavy metal poisoning and in botulism. Although dynamic collapse of the pharyngeal walls and intractable DDSP would lead to partial asphyxiation during exercise, this is most unlikely to be a major presenting sign (see 1.4).

Pharyngeal and laryngeal neoplasia

All tissues that are rich in lymphoreticular elements are intermittently susceptible to lymphoma

development and the nasopharynx and larynx are no exceptions. Other tumours at these locations are very rare. However, it should be noted that arytenoid chondropathies (5.24) frequently resemble tumours.

Congenital tracheal collapse

Congenital narrowing of the trachea through flattening of the cartilage rings is uncommon in horses. However, it is occasionally encountered in miniature Shetland ponies. Afflicted horses are presented with persistent coughing and adventitious respiratory sounds at exercise. There is no effective means to correct this deformity.

Acquired tracheal obstructions

The tracheal cartilage rings are vulnerable to fracture by kicks from other horses or by running against paddock rails. Inept tracheotomy intubation (see below) may also produce transection of tracheal rings comparable to fractures. The likely result of these injuries is narrowing of the airway in the form of a stricture or stenosis. Such lesions are usually palpable from the exterior and the luminal distortion can be confirmed by a combination of endoscopy and radiography.

Only narrow stricture bands may be treated by tracheal resection and anastomosis but even so the tension in the repaired incision is such that recurrence of the cicatrix is common. Longer segments of tracheal distortion may be treated by the application of an external prosthesis against which the collapsed cartilage rings are conformed. The prognosis for the successful repair of acquired tracheal stenoses is guarded.

Tracheotomy intubation

Tracheotomy intubation comprises the implantation of a tube directly into the trachea to provide an alternative airway when the upper respiratory tract is completely or partly obstructed or when it may become obstructed, for example after surgery. It can be used as the primary means to manage pharyngeal or laryngeal obstructions or when other methods to treat RLN have failed (see 5.20, 'Treatment').

● The surgery is performed through a ventral midline incision on the standing, possibly sedated, horse under local anaesthesia.

- After clearing the overlying muscle and fascia, an incision is made into the lumen without transection of a complete tracheal cartilage ring. Thus, semi-circles of cartilage are removed from adjacent tracheal rings leaving a narrow bridge of cartilage on either side of the hole by which to maintain the structural stability of the trachea.
- A self-retaining metallic tube is placed for racing purposes. A similar technique may be used for anaesthetic maintenance when the presence of an endotracheal tube passed *per os* is an encumbrance to the surgeon.

5.28 *Miscellaneous throat conditions of horses*

Wind-sucking and crib-biting

Wind-sucking and crib-biting are well-recognized examples of equine stereotypic behaviour whereby horses grasp fixed objects between their incisor teeth, arch the neck and emit a characteristic noise.

- Deglutition and the passage of air through the oesophagus to the stomach do not occur.
- The behaviour involves the contraction of the strap muscles of the neck in order to create a pressure gradient across the oesophageal wall so that air suddenly rushes from the pharynx into the upper oesophagus. As the muscles relax, the air returns to the pharynx.
- The role of the crib-biting component of the activity is that the grasping of fixed objects in the stable environment facilitates the arching of the neck and contraction of the strap muscles.
- The characteristic grunting sound associated with wind-sucking derives from the rush of air from pharynx to oesophagus.

The surgical methods used to treat wind-sucking all aim to inhibit the effectiveness of contraction of the ventral muscles of the neck, and Forssell's operation and its variants excise or denervate the sternohyoideus, sternothyroideus, omo-hyoideus and sternomandibularis muscles.

Salivary gland disorders

Salivary gland disorders are uncommon in horses.

- The relatively superficial position of the parotid gland and its duct renders them vulnerable to laceration wounds. Saliva is saturated with calcium salts and any leakage of saliva to the skin surface can be differentiated from serum, for example, by the chalky deposits on the surrounding area.
- Fresh wounds to the parotid duct should be closed by simple anastomosis around a pre-placed catheter which is passed from the exterior into the buccal cleft through a stab wound before entering the duct via the parotid papilla.
- Wounds to the glandular tissues themselves are generally self-limiting but can produce considerable leakages of saliva for 2–3 weeks while the defects resolve.
- Chronic salivary fistulation is rare but complete excision of the injured gland would be required to achieve resolution.
- Strictures of the duct may follow trauma and this will produce a distended painless fluid-filled structure corresponding to the course of the duct. The glandular tissue distal to the stricture will atrophy but the cord-like distension remains.
- Salivary calculi invariably involve the parotid system and generally come to obstruct the major duct close to the parotid papilla. The resultant swelling is similar to that which follows a stricture but the calculus is palpable.
- Sometimes the sialolith can be delivered through the papilla using forceps, otherwise a direct surgical incision onto the calculus is made.
- Seasonal sialadenitis is an idiopathic, usually bilateral, swelling of the paestid glands which is typically seen in grazing animals in spring/summer. This condition has no clinical significance other than owner concern regarding the physical appearance of the swollen glands.

Thyroid neoplasia

- Benign adenomas and C-cell tumours of the thyroid glands produce discrete mobile swellings on one or other side of the larynx.
- The lesions should not be confused with normal thyroid glands which are the size of a small hen's egg and are frequently suspended by a loose pedicle on either side of the cricoid cartilage.
- Thyroid tumours are not usually functional and therefore their significance simply relates to the physical presence of the swelling which is likely to cause concern to the owners long before

there is compression of the upper respiratory tract.

• These tumours are easily removed by surgery provided that care is taken with their vascular supply and a ventral midline approach is recommended.

• Malignant tumours of the thyroid glands are rare.

Parotid melanomas

Melanomas are common tumours of grey horses from middle age onwards. They are most commonly located in the perineum but the parotid region is the site next most frequently involved. The parotid swellings themselves are not primary tumours but secondary deposits in the lymphoid tissue which permeates the parotid salivary gland. The primary melanomas are derived from ectopic melanosis in the lateral compartment of the adjacent auditory tube diverticulum.

• There are no effective treatments for parotid melanomas.

• Medical management using cimetidine has been reported as helpful but is often ineffective.

• Any attempt to excise the secondary parotid lesions should be avoided.

• Thus, the significance of these tumours should be clarified with the potential purchaser of a grey horse with parotid swellings. Expansion of the untreated lesions will initially limit mobility at the upper neck and spread to adjacent sites may cause dyspnoea or dysphagia.

Facial palsy

See Chapter 11.

In many instances facial paralysis is of iatrogenic origin and in most cases this insult is avoidable. The buccal branches are vulnerable during dental extractions but the nerve tracts can be identified and retracted or bypassed. During general anaesthesia and recovery from it, the nerve trunk is particularly vulnerable to insult by unprotected head collars as it passes over the caudal border of the vertical ramus of the mandible.

Fortunately facial nerve palsies often show spontaneous complete or partial recovery in the months following injury but the time taken for the improvement to occur depends on the distance between the site of trauma and the denervated muscle.

Horner's syndrome

See Chapter 11.

The two most likely causes of Horner's syndrome are injury to the cervical preganglionic pathway, for example by perivascular reaction to the vagosympathetic trunk, and guttural pouch mycosis where the mycotic plaque infiltrates the nerve pathway in the region of the cranial cervical ganglion. The level at which the hemifacial sweating commences provides a firm guide to the level of the injury. In cases of perivascular reaction the skin over much of the side of the neck may be persistently damp.

Jugular phlebitis

See Chapter 7.

Nuchal fractures

Avulsion fractures of the nuccal crest of the occipital bone arise from direct trauma to the poll region. Afflicted horses show acute onset inability to raise the head from the ground but their coordination is otherwise normal. Radiographs confirm the diagnosis. Avulsion fractures should be managed conservatively as a fibrous union will form within weeks and a full range of mobility will return. In the early stages food and water should be offered from ground level.

Cervical injection abscessation

Suppuration may develop in the segmental muscles on either side of the nuccal ligament through contaminated injections. The development of a hot painful swelling at the side of the neck in the days following an intramuscular injection makes the diagnosis straightforward. Afflicted animals may be febrile and are likely to show restricted neck movement. Treatment based on first principles dictates that the abscessation should be encouraged to drain and ultrasonography can be helpful to establish the extent of free pus in the lesion and the optimal site for lancing. Chronic abscesses at this site are inclined to infiltrate between the fascial planes and may require aggressive surgery to expose and drain all of the infected tissue.

Further reading

Beech, J. (ed.) (1991) *Equine respiratory disorders.* Lea and Febiger, Philadelphia and London.

Lane, J.G. (1993) *Proceedings of the Fifteenth Bain-Fallon Memorial Lectures: Equine Head and Hind Limb Medicine and Surgery.* Australian Equine Veterinary Association, Artarmon, NSW.

APPENDICES

Appendix 1. Differential diagnostic list of causes of respiratory obstruction and/or abnormal respiratory noise in the horse

The following list itemizes the potential causes of obstructive dyspnoea on the basis of location in the upper respiratory tract.

Nostrils
Wry nose
Post-traumatic stenosis
Collapse resulting from facial palsy
Alar fold hypertrophy

Nasal chambers
Deviation and deformity of midline nasal septum
Sinus empyema
Sinus cyst
Progressive ethmoidal haematoma (PEH)
Polyp formation
Neoplasia

Nasopharynx
Choanal atresia/stenosis
Palatal defects: congenital, iatrogenic
Lymphoid hyperplasia (PLH)
Dynamic collapse of pharyngeal walls
Dorsal displacement of soft palate (DDSP)
Intrapalatal cysts
Pharyngeal cysts
Pharyngeal paralysis
Neoplasia
Extramural distortion by: strangles abscessation, ATD distension, neoplasia

Larynx
Epiglottal hypoplasia
Epiglottal entrapment (EE)
Sub-epiglottic cyst
Epiglottitis, including foreign body-induced
Dynamic epiglottal instability
Fourth branchial arch defects (4-BAD syndrome)
Dynamic ary-epiglottic fold collapse
Recurrent laryngeal neuropathy (RLN) idiopathic, iatrogenic and other acquired
Dynamic vocal cord instability
Laryngeal granuloma
Arytenoid chondropathy
Neoplasia

Trachea
Congenital collapse
Traumatic ring fracture
Post-traumatic, including iatrogenic, stenosis/stricture

Appendix 2. Differential diagnosis of non-infectious nasal discharge in the horse

See table opposite.

1. History (● = typical sign, x = occasional finding)
2. Diagnostic procedures (a) (● = often positive, x = occasionally helpful)
3. Diagnostic procedures (b) (● = often positive, x = occasionally helpful)

Column groups: **SINU-NASAL CONDITIONS** (Acute sinus empyema, Chronic sinus empyema, 2° dental sinus empyema, Ethmoidal haematoma, Sinus cyst, Conchal necrosis, Sinu-nasal neoplasia) · **ATD CONDITIONS** (ATD mycosis, ATD empyema, ATD diverticulitis) · **DYSPHAGIA** (Palatal defects, Pharyngeal paralysis, Laryngeal disorders, Oesophageal obstruction, Grass sickness) · **1° PULMONARY CONDITIONS** (EIPH, COPD/small airway inflammation, Pleuro-pneumonia)

	Ac. sinus emp.	Chr. sinus emp.	2° dental sinus emp.	Ethmoidal haematoma	Sinus cyst	Conchal necrosis	Sinu-nasal neoplasia	ATD mycosis	ATD empyema	ATD diverticulitis	Palatal defects	Pharyngeal paralysis	Laryngeal disorders	Oesophageal obstruction	Grass sickness	EIPH	COPD/small airway inflam.	Pleuro-pneumonia
Discharge																		
Acute epistaxis				x			x	●								x	x	
Recurrent epistaxis				●			●									x	x	
Exercise induced epistaxis																●	x	
Mucopurulent	●	x		x			x		x				x	x			●	●
Purulent	●	●	x	x	●	●	x	x	x	●			x	x			●	●
Malodorous		●	●			●			●	x								●
Ingesta								x			x	●		●				
Unilateral	●	●	●	●	●	●	●	x	●	●			●	●			●	●
Bilateral						●			x	x	x	x	●	●	●		●	●
External swelling	●	●	x	●			●		x									
Coughing				x					x	x		x	●	●	●	x	●	●
Respiratory obstruction	x			x		●	●	x	x		●	x	●					
External observation																		
Exaggerated expiratory effort																	●	
Unequal airflow at nares		x		x														
Trial allergen-free management																	●	
Facial distortion	x			x			●	x										
Palpation						●	●	x	●				●					
Auscultation														●		●	●	●
Percussion	x	x		x														
Oral examination			●			●					x							
Oesophageal manometry (Ventigraph)															●			
Exercise test													●			●	●	
Attempt pass stomach tube														●	●			
Endoscopy																		
Nasal meati	●	●	x	●	●	●	●	x										
Direct sinus endoscopy	x	●	x	●	●	x	●											
Pharynx/larynx/ATDs								●	●	●	●	●	●	●	●			
Trachea including aspiration																●	●	●
Radiography/ultrasonography																		
Erect lateral sinu-nasal area	●	●	x	●	●	●	●											
30° oblique maxilla	x	x	●	x	x	x												
Ventrodorsal Pharynx/larynx	●	●	●	●			●	●	●	●								
ATD/oesophagus								x					x	x	x			
Carotid angiography								x										
Chest													x	x	x	x	x	● +U
Exploratory surgery and biopsy	x			●		x	●								●			

6 *Lower respiratory tract*

CONTENTS

6.1 *Diagnostic approach to lower respiratory tract diseases*

The clinical signs associated with respiratory diseases include *coughing, nasal discharge, dyspnoea* and *exercise intolerance*.

History

History and signalment are important in aiding diagnosis of horses with respiratory diseases. Important points include:

• Age – many contagious diseases, including strangles and *Rhodococcus equi* infection, are most frequently seen in young horses, whereas allergic diseases such as chronic obstructive pulmonary disease (COPD) are usually seen in mature horses.
• Health of in-contact horses – similar clinical signs among in-contact horses suggests contagious disease.
• Environment – COPD is most likely in stabled horses or horses exposed to hay and/or straw. *Dictyocaulus arnfieldi* infection is most likely in horses grazing pasture contaminated by donkeys.
• Seasonality – seasonal disease in horses at grass is suggestive of summer pasture-associated obstructive pulmonary disease (SPAOPD).
• Stress – severe respiratory disease occurring in a recently stressed horse (such as after long distance travel or surgery) should arouse suspicion of pleuropneumonia.

Physical examination

The physical examination should be performed in a quiet environment with the horse relaxed and rested. Examination during and after exercise may be required subsequently.

Systemic signs

• Pyrexia
• Weight loss
• Elevated heart rate
• Weak pulse
• Dehydration
• Signs of pain

Respiratory rate, pattern and character

• *Normal respiration* in the resting horse is *slow* (8–16 breaths/min) with minimal chest or abdominal wall movement. Increased depth of breathing (with or without an increased rate) is abnormal, and its character should be noted.
• *Expiratory dyspnoea* with incorporation of the abdominal muscles producing a biphasic or double expiratory lift is typical of small airway obstruction.
• *Inspiratory dyspnoea* (sometimes associated with a stertorous or stridorous adventitious noise) is indicative of upper airway obstruction. Occasionally, inspiratory dyspnoea may occur with severe restrictive lung diseases (e.g. pneumonia, interstitial disease).
• *Combined inspiratory and expiratory dyspnoea*, usually with tachypnoea, is suggestive of severe upper or lower airway obstruction, diffuse pulmonary disease or pleural disease.

Nasal discharge

• *Unilateral* nasal discharges usually originate from the nasal chamber, paranasal sinuses or guttural pouches.
• *Bilateral* discharges can arise from the upper or lower respiratory tracts.
• *Serous* nasal discharges are commonly seen in viral infections, although they frequently change to *mucopurulent* or *purulent* with secondary bacterial infection.
• The presence or absence of *odour* or *food material* in the discharge is also helpful in determining the cause.

Cough

• Coughs arising from upper airway infections are usually *harsh, dry, hacking* and *non-productive*.
• Lower airway coughs are usually *deep, soft* and *productive*. The intra-narial position of the equine larynx usually precludes the coughing up of sputum directly into the mouth, but the observation of *swallowing after a cough* indicates that the cough is productive.
• *Short, painful coughs*, associated with reluctance to move or to lie down, suggest pleural pain.

Palpation

• The cervical trachea is palpated for abnormalities of structure.

• The bases of the jugular grooves are palpated for the presence of a mass which may indicate a mediastinal tumour that has extended rostrally through the thoracic inlet; these cases often have subcutaneous oedema as well, due to venous obstruction.

• Distension of the jugular veins or the presence of an abnormal jugular pulse indicates primary cardiac disease or compression of the heart/vessels by a mass or fluid.

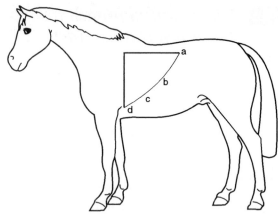

Figure 2 Normal area of auscultation of the lungs. a: tuber coxae at the 18th rib; b: mid thorax at the 13th rib; c: level with the shoulder at the 11th rib; d: elbow.

Auscultation

Auscultation is performed on both sides of the chest and over the cervical trachea. Lung sounds will vary depending on the body condition and depth of breathing. In fat horses, airflow sounds may be difficult to appreciate; these sounds can be accentuated by using a *re-breathing bag* (place a large plastic bag over the nose and let the horse breathe into and out of the bag until the arterial carbon dioxide tension increases, thereby increasing the depth of respiration) (Figure 1) or by temporarily *occluding the nostrils*. The normal margins of the lung fields are level with the tuber coxae at the 18th rib, mid thorax at the 13th rib, shoulder at the 11th rib, and then curving down to the level of the elbow (Figure 2).

• Normal airflow sounds are most readily appreciated at the area around the carina, and may be difficult to perceive at the lung periphery.

• Normal airflow sounds are slightly louder on the right side than the left, and louder during inspiration than during expiration.

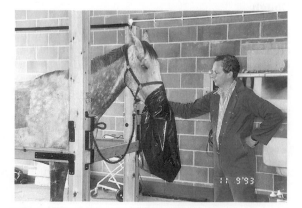

Figure 1 Use of a re-breathing bag. The horse is forced to breathe into and out of a large bag secured over the nose. This results in increased depth of respiration, which accentuates normal and abnormal lung sounds.

• A generalized increase in the intensity of airflow sounds is suggestive of lower airway disease such as COPD.

• A localized absence of sounds may indicate a pulmonary or pleural abscess/tumour.

• Absence of sounds in the ventral thorax (often bilateral) suggests a pleural effusion.

• Absence of sounds in the dorsal thorax suggests a pneumothorax.

Adventitious sounds (i.e. abnormal sounds) include *crackles (rales), wheezes (rhonchi)* and *pleural friction sounds.*

• Crackles are detected in COPD and acute obstructive pulmonary disease, and pulmonary oedema.

• Wheezes are musical notes that occur in obstructive lower airway diseases including COPD and bronchopneumonia.

• Pleural friction sounds are crunching/creaking sounds that may be detected in early pleuritis.

Percussion

A plexor and pleximeter may be used, or, alternatively, the fingers can be employed to sharply tap over the intercostal spaces (Figure 3).

• Normal lung tissue sounds resonant and hollow.

• Fluid or soft tissue sounds dull and flat.

• Pain on percussion is observed in early pleuritis.

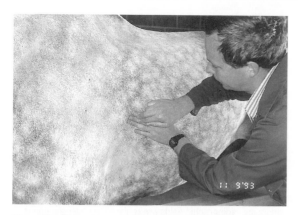

Figure 3 Thoracic percussion. The fingers of one hand are sharply tapped onto those of the other hand, which is placed over the intercostal spaces.

Endoscopy

In most horses, an endoscope can be introduced from the nasopharynx into the larynx without inducing significant coughing. However, in horses affected by lower airway diseases, this manoeuvre may induce a severe cough response. Coughing may be abolished by spraying a dilute lignocaine solution over the larynx (via a catheter passed down the biopsy channel of the endoscope). Sedation with xylazine, detomidine or romifidine may also diminish the cough response.

The trachea is assessed for strictures/collapse and for the presence of discharge; the latter often pools at the distal cervical trachea, where its nature and volume can be assessed, and samples aspirated for cytology or bacteriology if required.

There is normally a sharp angle between the two mainstem bronchi (the carina), but this angle may appear blunt due to mucosal inflammation/oedema in chronic lower airway diseases.

The source of any observable lower airway discharge should be determined with regard to whether it originates from both bronchial trees (i.e. bilateral) or only one bronchial tree (i.e. unilateral). If unilateral, the discharge may be followed down the bronchial tree towards its source. Passage of the endoscope into the bronchi frequently provokes coughing, which may be reduced by sequential infusion of lignocaine solution at each bronchial division.

The bronchi themselves are assessed for inflammation and collapse. Lungworms (*Dictyocaulus arnfieldi*), foreign bodies and endobronchial tumours may be identified.

Tracheal aspiration

Samples of lower airway secretions may be obtained for cytology or culture.

Tracheal aspirates can be collected by endoscopy or by a transtracheal technique. In the former, the endoscope is positioned in the distal cervical trachea, and 30 ml of sterile saline infused through a catheter passed down the biopsy channel. The fluid usually forms a pool at the thoracic inlet from where a sample can be aspirated. Aspirates obtained in this way are suitable for cytological examination. Aspirates from normal horses contain mainly ciliated epithelial cells and macrophages. Approximately 10% of the cells are neutrophils, although some stabled horses may have up to 40% neutrophils.

- An increase in numbers of neutrophils indicates inflammatory lower airway disease, such as COPD, bronchopneumonia, etc.
- Large numbers of eosinophils are seen in lungworm infections.

Tracheal aspirates obtained through the endoscope can be used for bacterial culture, but they may be contaminated by upper airway bacterial flora (unless a guarded catheter is used).

Samples obtained by transtracheal aspiration are collected aseptically and are suitable for both cytology and culture. An area over the lower third of the cervical trachea is clipped and prepared aseptically, and an over-the-needle cannula inserted between two tracheal rings into the tracheal lumen. A catheter is then threaded through the cannula and passed to the level of the thoracic inlet where lavage with 30–100 ml of sterile saline is performed (Figure 4). In cases of lower airway or pulmonary infection, a Gram-stained smear of a sample obtained in this way may give an early indication of the types of bacteria involved before culture results are available. Both aerobic and anaerobic cultures should be performed in cases of pneumonia/lung abscess.

Bronchoalveolar lavage (BAL)

BAL is used to obtain samples of lower airway secretions, primarily for cytology, from the small airways and alveoli. The technique may be performed through an endoscope (which is lodged in a bronchus prior to lavage) or blindly using a catheter passed *per nasum* into the bronchial tree.

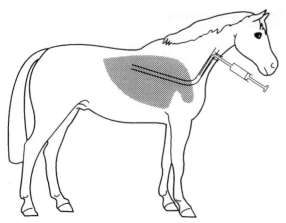

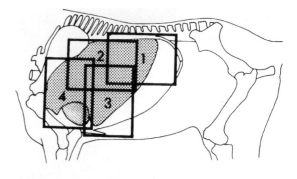

Figure 6 Thoracic radiography in the adult horse. A series of overlapping radiographic fields are required to cover the entire thorax.

Figure 4 Transtracheal aspiration. A catheter is passed into the tracheal lumen through a cannula placed between two tracheal rings in the cervical trachea. Saline is infused and aspirated at the level of the distal cervical trachea.

The catheter is advanced into the bronchi until it becomes lodged (usually at a 4th or 5th generation segmental bronchus). Sterile saline (300 to 500 ml) is infused and then aspirated (Figure 5). The predominant cell types in BAL of normal horses are macrophages and lymphocytes. COPD is characterized by an increase in neutrophils. BAL cytology provides a more realistic picture of the cell types in the small airways, but it samples only a very small lung segment. BAL is, therefore, only helpful in diffuse lung diseases such as COPD. In focal diseases (including exercise-induced pulmonary haemorrhage (EIPH), pneumonia, lung abscess) BAL cytology may appear normal.

Thoracic radiography

In adult horses, only lateral views are possible. Four overlapping fields are often required to cover the entire thorax in adult horses (Figure 6). An air gap is used between the patient and the film to avoid the use of a grid. Lesions that can be detected include pulmonary consolidation/pneumonia, lung abscesses, advanced EIPH lesions, lung infiltrates such as neoplasia, granulomas and fibrosis, and pleural effusions.

Diagnostic ultrasound

Diagnostic ultrasound is well suited to the investigation of pleural diseases. The volume and character of pleural effusion can be assessed, as can fluid loculations, fibrin tags, adhesions and pleural thickening. Consolidated areas of lung and other pulmonary soft tissue lesions may be visualized only if they extend to the pleural surface. Needle biopsy of such lesions may be possible under ultrasound guidance.

Thoracocentesis

Thoracocentesis allows the collection of samples of pleural fluid for analysis (including cytology and bacteriology); it can also be used in the treatment of pleuritis by allowing the drainage of large amounts of fluid. The precise site at which the chest is entered will vary depending on the amount of effusion; ultrasound guidance can be helpful. The usual site is either the right side at the 7th intercostal space, or the left side at the 7th or 8th spaces in the ventral third of the chest. Care must be taken to avoid the lateral thoracic vein

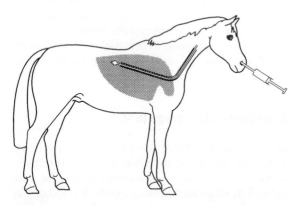

Figure 5 Bronchoalveolar lavage. A catheter is passed into the distal bronchial tree, where saline is infused and aspirated.

and the heart. The area is clipped and local anaesthetic infiltrated under the skin and into the intercostal muscles down to the pleura. A stab incision in the skin allows the introduction of a cannula (such as IV cannula, teat cannula or metal bitch urinary catheter) which is pushed into the pleural cavity along the cranial border of the rib. Fluid will normally drain by gravity, but care must be taken to avoid introduction of air into the cavity. Normal horses have a small quantity of clear, watery and pale straw-coloured fluid. The nucleated cell count of the fluid is low ($<4 \times 10^9$/l) with approximately 70% neutrophils, 20% large mononuclear cells, and small numbers of lymphocytes and eosinophils. The total protein content is normally less than 30 g/l. Effusions are classified as transudates, modified transudates, exudates or chylous.

- Transudates have normal characteristics and may be found in some early neoplastic diseases, congestive heart failure, hypoproteinaemia, etc.
- Modified transudates are similar but with added cells (e.g. mesothelial cells, neutrophils or neoplastic cells) or protein. They are usually associated with neoplasia.
- Exudates have high cell counts ($>10 \times 10^9$/l) and high protein concentrations (>30 g/l). The majority of the cells are neutrophils. Exudates are usually thick and cloudy, and are seen in pleuritis/pleuropneumonia, and sometimes with neoplasia.
- Chylous effusions are rare; they are milky white in appearance, and contain large numbers of lymphocytes.

Haematology

Haematological alterations in lower respiratory tract diseases are often minimal or non-specific. Hyperfibrinogenaemia, hyperglobulinaemia, hypoalbuminaemia and mild anaemia may be observed in infectious, inflammatory and neoplastic diseases.

Other diagnostic tests

Other diagnostic techniques that may be usefully employed in some situations include lung biopsy and pleuroscopy. Pulmonary function tests (such as intrapleural pressure measurement) and arterial blood gas analysis are occasionally required.

6.2 *Diagnostic features of the common lower respiratory tract diseases of the adult horse*

See Table 1.

6.3 *Chronic obstructive pulmonary disease (COPD)*

COPD is also known as chronic small airway disease (SAD), chronic pulmonary disease (CPD), broken wind, heaves, chronic alveolar emphysema.

This is a common condition that results from obstruction of small airways (bronchioles); some cases may have bronchitis; in late stages, some horses develop emphysema, and rarely cor pulmonale.

COPD occurs in all breeds of horses, ponies and donkeys. The incidence tends to increase with age – usually horses older than 4 years. In performance horses, low grade COPD may cause few overt clinical signs other than *exercise intolerance* and *poor performance*. There is also a possible association with exercise-induced pulmonary haemorrhage (EIPH).

Aetiology

In most cases, *pulmonary hypersensitivity* associated with inhalation of organic dusts, primarily *hay and straw dusts*, occurs. Hypersensitivity to fungal and thermophilic actinomycete spores (major component of hay and straw dust, especially from 'heated' bales) is involved in most cases. Spores of *Faenia rectivirgula* (formerly known as *Micropolyspora faeni*), *Aspergillus fumigatus*, etc., have been implicated. COPD is primarily a disease of the stabled horse. Some cases appear to be sensitive to pollens (see also summer pasture-associated obstructive pulmonary disease). In the UK, oilseed rape pollen has been associated with signs of COPD in some cases.

Pathogenesis (Figure 7)

Inhaled fungal and actinomycete spores (and other possible allergens) deposit in the bronchioles where hypersensitivity reactions are initiated. These include:

Table 1 Diagnostic features of lower respiratory tract disease

Disease	Diagnostic features
COPD/SPAOPD/chronic lower airway inflammation	Endoscopy – lower airway exudate/bronchial inflammation Tracheal aspirate – neutrophilia BAL – neutrophilia
EIPH	Endoscopy – blood in airways Tracheal aspirate/BAL – red blood cells and haemosiderophages Radiography – opacity in dorsocaudal lung (advanced cases)
Lungworm	Endoscopy – larvae in bronchial tree Tracheal aspirate – eosinophilia/larvae BAL – eosinophilia
Neoplasia	Endoscopy – usually normal; rarely endobronchial mass Tracheal aspirate/BAL – usually normal; rarely neoplastic cells Radiography – pulmonary mass/pleural effusion Ultrasound – pleural effusion/mass Thoracocentesis – cytology may show neoplastic cells Biopsy – diagnostic Pleuroscopy – may show pleural mass
Pleuritis/pleuropneumonia	Endoscopy – lower airway exudate Tracheal aspirate – neutrophilia; Gram stain/culture BAL – may be normal or neutrophilia Radiography – pulmonary consolidation/pleural effusion Ultrasound – pleural effusion Thoracocentesis – exudate; culture
Focal pneumonia/lung abscess	Endoscopy – lower airway exudate Tracheal aspirate – neutrophilia; Gram stain/culture BAL – may be normal Radiography – pulmonary consolidation Haematology – anaemia, hypoalbuminaemia, hyperfibrinogenaemia
Tracheal stenosis	Endoscopy – tracheal narrowing Radiography – tracheal narrowing
Tracheobronchial foreign body	Endoscopy – foreign body Tracheal aspirate – neutrophilia Radiography – may be focal pulmonary consolidation
Chronic interstitial lung disease	Endoscopy – normal Tracheal aspirate/BAL – neutrophilia/lymphocytosis Radiography – miliary pulmonary infiltrate Lung biopsy – diagnostic

- Type 1 (immediate) response – mast cell degranulation.
- Type 3 (immune-complex) response.
- Type 4 (delayed) response.

Spores and other particles also have a non-specific irritant effect.

The net results of these reactions are:

- Spasm of small airways (smooth muscle contraction)
- Mucus hypersecretion
- Inflammatory bronchiolitis.

These reactions result in *small airway obstruction*; airflow is impeded, especially during expiration. Most of these reactions are totally reversible if exposure to the offending allergens is eliminated. In longstanding cases, some structural changes to the bronchioles may occur, e.g. metaplasia of the epithelium, hyperplasia of mucus-secreting goblet cells. In severe cases, chronic airflow obstruction results in alveolar overinflation and eventually areas of emphysema. In a minority of cases, secondary infection by opportunist bacteria may occur.

Clinical signs

The onset of disease is frequently insidious. Alternatively, the disease may follow an acute respiratory infection.

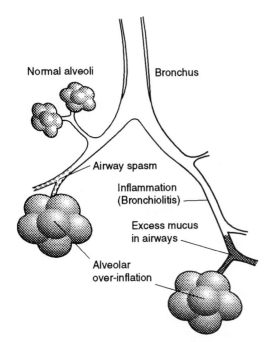

Normal alveoli

Bronchus

Airway spasm

Inflammation
(Bronchiolitis)

Excess mucus
in airways

Alveolar
over-inflation

Figure 7 Diagram demonstrating the pathological features of COPD.

The severity of the disease is extremely variable, ranging from subclinical to mild to severe. If left untreated, severity tends to worsen. The clinical signs may be continuous or intermittent.

Subclinical disease
This is most likely to be recognized in performance horses demonstrating *exercise intolerance* with no other overt clinical signs.

Mild clinical disease
- There is usually a *chronic cough* that is occasional and sporadic; it is frequently noticed at the start of exercise or whilst feeding.
- Normal respiratory rate and normal respiratory character.
- There may be a slight serous/mucoid bilateral *nasal discharge* (especially after exercise)
- *Exercise intolerance* (performance horses).

Severe clinical disease
- *Chronic cough* that may occur at any time, but is most marked if the horse is exerted and during feeding.
- *Increased respiratory effort* with *expiratory dyspnoea*. Expiration becomes more markedly biphasic, with use of the abdominal muscles; an 'abdominal lift' occurs at the end of expiration resulting in a *double expiratory effort*. In longstand-

ing cases, hypertrophy of the external oblique abdominal muscles leads to the development of a *heave line*. Expiratory airflow at the nostrils becomes biphasic.
- Resting respiratory rate may be normal or mildly elevated (16–20/min).
- There is usually a *bilateral nasal discharge*, but this is not invariably present and may be worse after exercise or when the head is lowered. In some horses, the discharge may appear to be predominantly unilateral. The nature of the discharge varies from serous to mucoid to mucopurulent.
- Exercise intolerance is marked in performance horses, and the recovery period after exercise is prolonged.

Diagnosis

1. History and clinical signs.
2. Increased sensitivity of laryngeal cough reflex.
3. Auscultation:
   - fluid sounds over distal cervical trachea
   - bronchial sounds audible over larger than normal area
   - crackles
   - wheezing
   - crackling sounds audible to naked ear at nostrils.
   Subtle changes in lung sounds may be enhanced by the use of a re-breathing bag.
4. *Endoscopy:*
   - accumulation of variable quantities of mucopurulent discharge in the trachea (especially at the thoracic inlet) and bronchi
   - congestion and thickening of the airway mucosa of the distal trachea, carina and mainstem bronchi
   - 'blunting' of the carina due to swelling/oedema of the mucosa
   - in severe cases, there may be observable collapse of the trachea and bronchi during expiration and coughing.
5. Tracheal aspirate: neutrophilia.
6. Bronchoalveolar lavage: variable cytological change – usually increase in neutrophils.
7. Thoracic radiography: normal or mild interstitial reticular pattern.
8. Intradermal allergen tests/serum precipitins (mould species): non-specific reactions are common, and these tests are unreliable.
9. Inhalation challenge test: expose horse to mouldy hay/straw and observe for worsen-

ing of clinical signs, or changes in tracheal aspirate/BAL cytology.

10. Pulmonary function tests, e.g. intrapleural pressure measurement, arterial blood gas analysis: non-specific changes in severe clinical disease, but may be no changes in milder disease.
    - Intrapleural pressure: maximum ΔPpl – normal < 6 mmHg
    - Arterial oxygen: PaO_2 – normal 90–110 mmHg.
11. Test management: manage from pasture with no access to hay or straw.
12. Test therapy: bronchodilators.

Treatment

To relieve clinical signs
1. 'Dust-free' management
   - Manage from pasture with no access to hay or straw.
   - Minimize dust levels in stable:
     - Bedding: shavings/shredded paper/peat/synthetic bedding/rubber mats/sand, etc.
     - Maintain clean, dry bed (avoid deep litter).
     - Ventilation: ensure adequate ventilation rates.
     - Ensure horse is in a separate airspace (or else all horses in the same airspace must be managed under similar dust-free conditions).
     - Avoid overhead lofts.
     - Keep muck heap as far away from the stable as possible.
     - Horse should be out of the stable when it is mucked out (and for 30 minutes afterwards).
     - Feeding: If possible, feed an alternative to hay, e.g. 'complete diet' nuts, silage, vacuum-packed hays.
     - If hay is to be fed, it should be good quality, and thoroughly soaked prior to feeding (up to 12 hours).
     - Consider use of dust extractor in the box.
2. Bronchodilators
   - Most effective is clenbuterol (not available in the USA); may be administered orally, intravenously or by nebulization
   - Methylxanthines, e.g. theophylline.
3. Mucolytics and expectorants, e.g. dembrexine.
4. Corticosteroids. Usually for short-term use only. In horses requiring long-term therapy,

maintain horse on minimal dose to alleviate signs, every other day.

To prevent recurrence of disease
1. Maintain strict 'dust-free' conditions
2. Sodium cromoglycate. Administered by nebulization. The horse should be free from signs when the drug is given.

Prognosis

Lung changes of COPD are mostly reversible until structural damage (emphysema) occurs. Most cases have a favourable prognosis provided that exposure to allergens can be kept to a minimum.

Prevention

Maintain good stable hygiene, especially during the course of any infectious respiratory disease.

6.4 *Acute obstructive pulmonary disease*

Acute airway obstruction may occur as an acute exacerbation of COPD or SPAOPD of similar aetiology and pathogenesis.

Clinical signs

Usually seen within 20 to 30 minutes of stabling:

- Marked dyspnoea – mainly expiratory with forced abdominal efforts
- Tachypnoea – up to 40/min
- Sweating
- Anxious facial expression
- Dilated nostrils
- Protrusion of the anus with each expiratory effort
- Paroxysmal coughing
- Congestion of the mucous membranes
- Tachycardia – up to 80–90/min
- Normal to mildly elevated rectal temperature

Diagnosis

1. Clinical signs.
2. Auscultation:
   - harsh lung sounds with widespread crackles and wheezing

- crackles audible at the nostril to the naked ear.

Treatment

- Turn out into fresh air immediately.
- Bronchodilators, e.g. clenbuterol (preferably administered IV).
- Corticosteroids, e.g. dexamethasone or betamethasone (preferably administered IV).
- Consider prophylactic antibiotic cover (especially if corticosteroids are used).
- In extreme cases, atropine (up to 5 mg IV) will provide effective and fast bronchodilation. (NB. the use of atropine in horses can result in ileus and abdominal pain)

6.5 *Summer pasture-associated obstructive pulmonary disease (SPAOPD)*

The clinical signs and pathophysiology of SPAOD are similar to COPD, but occurring in grazing horses at grass in the summer. It occurs sporadically thoughout the UK and USA, but is especially common in south eastern USA.

Aetiology

The aetiology is uncertain, but probably involves a pulmonary hypersensitivity to environmental allergens including pollens. Anectdotal reports in the UK suggest an association with oilseed rape pollen, but this has not been confirmed by immunological methods or challenge tests.

Clinical signs

Signs are similar to COPD: expiratory dyspnoea and exercise intolerance. Coughing is not usually as marked as with COPD. Sometimes anorexia and weight loss.

Treatment

Drug therapy is as for COPD. In addition, the horse should be stabled and fed a diet of hay and nuts.

6.6 *Chronic lower airway inflammation*

Lower airway inflammation associated with mild clinical signs, but often causing exercise intolerance and poor performance in athletic horses (especially racehorses). Some cases follow an initial viral infection ('chronic post-viral coughing'). Initial viral infection may be subclinical (especially equine herpesvirus (EHV) 1 and 4 infections).

Aetiology and pathogenesis

The aetiology may vary from case to case, but probably includes one or more of the following:

- Chronic bacterial bronchitis/bronchiolitis, e.g. *Streptococcus zooepidemicus, S. pneumoniae, Pasteurella* species, *Bordetella bronchiseptica.*
- Mycoplasma infections.
- Airway hyperreactivity.
- Mucus cell hyperplasia of the lower airways.
- Hypersensitivity similar to COPD.

Clinical signs

- Pyrexia.
- Chronic cough (especially during exercise).
- Mucopurulent nasal discharge (variable).
- Exercise intolerance in performance horses.

Diagnosis

- Clinical signs.
- Endoscopy: tracheal discharge.
- Tracheal aspiration/BAL:
  - cytology usually shows increased numbers of neutrophils,
  - culture to identify potential pathogens.

Treatment

- 'Dust-free' management as for COPD.
- Bronchodilators.
- Mucolytics.
- Antibiotics in cases where infection is suspected or confirmed.
- Immune modulator drugs, e.g. mycobacterial cell wall fractions (uncertain efficacy).

6.7 *Lower airway infections*

Bacterial and mycoplasmal lower airway infections have been identified as causes of pyrexia and mild respiratory disease in young thoroughbred racehorses. The clinical signs are similar to chronic lower airway inflammation (see above), but may arise as an outbreak among susceptible horses. A variety of bacterial species have been implicated as for chronic lower airway inflammation. Treatment is similar (see above).

6.8 *Exercise-induced pulmonary haemorrhage (EIPH)*

Haemorrhage into the lungs, usually in the dorso-caudal area of the diaphragmatic lobe, occurring during fast exercise.

Epistaxis (i.e. the presence of blood at the nostrils) occurs in up to 5% of racehorses after galloping. This blood usually originates from the lungs. Endoscopic evidence of blood in the trachea is seen in up to 60% of horses examined after racing. Tracheal aspirates of horses in training show haemosiderin-laden macrophages in nearly 100% of horses undergoing fast work. In other words, some degree of lung haemorrhage is probably universal among racehorses undergoing fast work.

Aetiology

A number of different theories have been proposed:

- Stress failure of pulmonary capillaries. Pulmonary capillaries have extremely thin walls to allow rapid exchange of respiratory gases across them. Mechanical failure of the walls of the capillaries may occur when the pressure inside them rises to high levels during exercise.
- Haemorrhage occurs from areas of lung neovascularization, where there has been proliferation of the bronchial arterial system as a response to low-grade lower airway disease, e.g. COPD.
- Haemorrhage occurs in areas of lung subjected to high pressure swings and stress.
- Haemorrhage occurs in the lung secondary to partial asphyxia due to an upper airway obstruction such as laryngeal hemiplegia.

Clinical signs

Most horses are affected by EIPH with no obvious overt clinical signs. In a small number of cases, there may be epistaxis after racing. Occasionally, a massive fatal pulmonary haemorrhage may occur.

The effect of EIPH on racing performance is variable, and in most it is probably minimal. In some cases, there may be reduced exercise tolerance, sometimes to the point where the horse pulls up during a race. In these cases, the affected horse may show respiratory distress, with an anxious facial expression and some coughing. Repeated swallowing may be observed as the blood is cleared from the trachea into the pharynx.

Some horses may continue to bleed into the lung for several days or even weeks after racing. These horses tend to be dull and lethargic but non-pyrexic. Haematology may show a progressive anaemia.

Diagnosis

- Endoscopic examination of the trachea after strenuous exercise.
- Tracheal aspirate/BAL cytology: stain for haemosiderin (Pearl's Prussian Blue).
- Radiography: opacity in dorsocaudal lung field (must be performed within 7 to 10 days of galloping to identify a recent haemorrhage).

Treatment

Treatment of EIPH is mainly empirical. A large number of prophylactic treatments have been proposed, but their efficacies are largely unproven.

1. Any underlying small airway disease (COPD, viral infections, etc.) should be treated.
2. A dust-free environment should be available.
3. Horses that have suffered haemorrhage that is believed to have affected performance should be rested to allow healing of damaged capillaries and lung tissue.
4. Antibiotic cover may be indicated to prevent secondary infection of affected areas.

The following prophylactic treatments have been employed (use of these will be dictated by the relevant racing authorities):

- Frusemide (furosemide)
- Oestrogens

- Disodium cromoglycate
- Clenbuterol

6.9 *Lungworm (Dictyocaulus arnfieldi) infection*

See also Chapter 19.

Donkeys are the natural host of *D. arnfieldi*, and commonly carry asymptomatic infections. Horses usually become infected by grazing pasture contaminated by donkeys. Eggs passed out in donkey faeces can develop rapidly into infective larvae which can survive 6–7 weeks on pasture under suitable conditions (damp/shade). The larvae cannot overwinter.

Horses become infected by ingesting larvae, which migrate to the lungs. In most horses, larval development becomes arrested and egg-laying adults do not arise. The disease is usually recognized in late summer/autumn.

Clinical signs

Chronic coughing (often paroxysmal in nature). Signs may be indistinguishable from COPD.

Diagnosis

- History and clinical signs.
- Faecal examination for presence of larvae (Baerman technique). This is usually negative since most infections are non-patent.
- Endoscopy may reveal larvae in the trachea or mainstem bronchi.
- Tracheal aspirate/BAL: pronounced eosinophilia. In some cases, larvae may be recovered by tracheal aspirates or BAL.
- Response to treatment.

Treatment

Ivermectin (0.2 mg/kg) by mouth. There may be a temporary worsening of clinical signs for a few days after treatment, followed by a rapid improvement.

6.10 Parascaris equorum *infection*

See also Chapter 19.

This is an unusual cause of coughing in foals, weanlings and yearlings, and is associated with the migration of larvae through the lungs, resulting in mild eosinophilic pneumonia.

Clinical signs

Signs are cough, serous nasal discharge, inappetence and weight loss.

Diagnosis

- Clinical signs and history. Absence of fever may help to distinguish *P. equorum* infection from bacterial infections.
- Tracheal aspirate/BAL: eosinophilia.

Treatment

Ivermectin or fenbendazole by mouth.

6.11 *Inhaled foreign bodies*

This is an uncommon cause of chronic coughing. The foreign body may lodge in the pharynx/larynx or in the tracheobronchial tree.

Various types of foreign bodies may be involved. In the lower airways they usually involve twigs or brambles (thorns act as barbs which prevent the bramble from being coughed up).

Bronchial foreign bodies often enter the right mainstem bronchus, and may cause secondary pneumonia or lung abscess, or may penetrate the pleura leading to pleuritis.

Clinical signs

- Sudden onset of coughing – often paroxysmal.
- Pharyngeal foreign bodies may cause dysphagia and painful swallowing (differentiate from oesophageal obstruction).
- Tracheobronchial foreign bodies result in halitosis (malodorous breath) and purulent nasal discharge.

Diagnosis

- Endoscopy.
- Radiography.

Treatment

Surgical removal under general anaesthesia, or standing (under sedation) using an endoscopic biopsy instrument.

6.12 *Pulmonary/pleural/ mediastinal neoplasia*

Neoplasia is uncommon. Diagnosis depends on radiography, biopsy, pleural fluid cytology, etc.

Primary lung tumours

These are rare, e.g. myoblastoma (granular cell tumour), bronchial and alveolar carcinomas, haemangiosarcoma.

Lung metastases

Metastases are uncommon, e.g. lymphosarcoma, various carcinomas (e.g. renal), melanosarcoma.

Clinical features of lung tumours

Lung tumours usually present as chronic progressive dyspnoea with weight loss. There may be a chronic cough and intermittent/persistent pyrexia. There may be an associated pleural effusion (with worsening dyspnoea). Clinical signs associated with lung metastases often relate more to the primary site of tumour formation than to thoracic involvement.

Primary pleural tumours

These are generally mesotheliomas.

Pleural metastases

Examples are gastric squamous cell carcinoma, other carcinomas.

Pleural tumours usually present as dyspnoea (may have apparent sudden onset) with pleural effusion and weight loss.

Pleural fluid cytology may be diagnostic in pleural neoplasia and pulmonary neoplasia with pleural effusion (neoplastic cells).

Mediastinal tumours

Lymphosarcoma can affect horses of all ages. Usually multicentric, and commonly involves the mediastinal lymph nodes. These may become large enough to act as a space occupying lesion compressing the lungs, trachea, oesophagus and major blood vessels, resulting in dyspnoea, dysphagia and distension of the jugular veins.

A mass may be palpable at the base of the jugular groove (extension of neoplastic lymphoid tissue through the thoracic inlet and involvement of the deep caudal cervical lymph nodes) – this may be accessible to biopsy.

Many cases also produce pleural effusion and ventral thoracic oedema. Pleural fluid cytology may be diagnostic – large numbers of lymphoid cells and lymphoblasts showing variation in size and shape. (NB: normal pleural fluid cytology does not exclude lymphosarcoma or other neoplasia.)

6.13 *Pleuropneumonia*

This is commoner in the USA than the UK.

- Pneumonia
- Pulmonary abscess } alone or in combination
- Pleuritis (pleurisy)

Aetiology and pathogenesis

1. Stress, e.g. long-distance travel ('transit fever'), surgery.
2. Secondary bacterial infection after viral respiratory disease.
3. Bacteraemia, e.g. strangles.
4. Inhalation pneumonia secondary to dysphagia:
   - oesophageal obstruction (choke)
   - pharyngeal paralysis
   - structural abnormalities
   - grass sickness
   - iatrogenic
   also inhaled foreign bodies.
5. Direct thoracic trauma and chest penetrations.
6. Pulmonary emboli and infarction, e.g. secondary to jugular phlebitis and thrombosis.

Pathology

The pathology is variable. Usually there are discrete areas of pneumonia/abscessation. Occasionally generalized pneumonia involves the whole lung. Pleuritis with pleural effusion is usually bilateral. In chronic cases, there may be extensive fibrin formation within the pleural cavity, with adhesion formation and pleural abscessation. Abscess/granulation tissue may localize cranial to the heart forming a *cranial thoracic mass*.

Organisms

A variety of organisms may be involved: *Streptococcus* spp., *Staphylococcus* spp., *Klebsiella* spp., *Pasteurella* spp., *E. coli*, *Bordetella bronchiseptica*, *Nocardia* spp., *Mycoplasma felis*.

Anaerobic bacteria are common, e.g. *Bacteroides* spp.

Clinical signs

- Initially fever and pain (reluctance to move; abduction of the elbows) must be differentiated from more common causes of acute pain, e.g. colic, laminitis, rhabdomyolysis.
- Later, recurrent/persistent fever, inappetence, tachypnoea and dyspnoea (inspiratory and expiratory), cough, weight loss, pectoral and sternal oedema – must be differentiated from thoracic neoplasia, interstitial lung diseases (tuberculosis, granulomatous pneumonia, etc.).
- Nasal discharge is variable – occasionally blood-tinged. May be malodorous breath with anaerobic infections.
- In cases with a cranial thoracic mass, there may be pointing of a foreleg, distension of jugular veins and tachycardia.

Diagnosis

May be difficult in the early stages.

1. Clinical signs.
2. Thoracic auscultation – may be normal in the early stages:
   - pleural friction sounds
   - ventral dulling of lung sounds with heart sounds audible over a larger than normal area, indicative of pleural effusion
   - localized areas of reduced lung sounds, indicative of pulmonary consolidation/pneumonia/abscessation
   - adventitious lung sounds (crackling/wheezing/pleural friction rubs)
3. Thoracic percussion:
   - pain response by horse (especially in early stages of pleuritis)
   - reduced resonance ventrally, indicative of pleural effusion
4. Radiography:
   - consolidated lung
   - pleural effusion
5. Haematology – variable:
   - leucocytosis, neutrophilia and hyperfibrinogenaemia may occur, but haematology may be normal initially; in the acute stages there may be leucopenia
6. Thoracocentesis – cytology and bacterial culture (including anaerobic culture)
7. Tracheal aspiration/BAL – cytology and culture
8. Ultrasonography:
   - consolidated lung and abscesses (adjacent to the pleural surface only)
   - assess presence, quantity and nature of pleural effusion
   - fibrin, adhesions, loculated fluid, cranial thoracic mass

Treatment

- Appropriate systemic antibiotics (preferably identified by bacteriological cultures) for prolonged periods.
- Analgesics – non-steroidal anti-inflammatories.
- Supportive nursing care.
- Drainage of pleural fluid – continuous drainage via indwelling thoracic drain with one-way valve, or repeated drainage by thoracocentesis.
- Intrapleural antibiotics, e.g. metronidazole.
- Drainage of localized pleural/cranial thoracic abscess (using ultrasound guidance).

6.14 Rhodococcus equi *pneumonia*

Rhodococcus equi is responsible for pneumonia of foals, especially in the 1–6 month age group. The pathogenicity of this bacterium may be dependent upon the presence of a certain plasmid. The organism survives in the soil, and the disease tends to become endemic on certain farms. Infection may occur by inhalation or ingestion, and the prevalence of disease increases with dusty environments and dry weather.

Two clinical forms of *R. equi* pneumonia are recognized. The subacute form is characterized by a diffuse miliary pyogranulomatous pneumonia with a short clinical course usually resulting in death. The chronic form is characterized by solitary or multifocal pyogranuloma, and has a prolonged clinical disease of weeks to months.

Clinical signs

- *Subacute form.* Acute onset of fever, tachypnoea and dyspnoea. Coughing and nasal discharge are variable. Often die within a few days of onset of clinical signs. Post-mortem examination reveals lung abscesses and diffuse pneumonia.
- *Chronic form.* Fever, depression, dyspnoea and tachypnoea, weight loss and unthriftiness. Coughing and nasal discharge are variable.
- *Intestinal form* is sometimes recognized in older foals. Weight loss, diarrhoea and recurrent colic. Abscessation of the mesenteric lymph nodes may occur.

Diagnosis

- Clinical signs. History of disease on the premises.
- Haematology: neutrophilia, hyperfibrinogenaemia.
- Transtracheal aspirate culture (negative in 30–60% of cases). Cytology shows many degenerate neutrophils and Gram positive coccobacilli.
- Thoracic radiography: nodular lung lesions (may be cavitary) and lymphadenopathy. Some cases have pleural effusion.
- Agar gel immunodiffusion test (AGID) serology for antibody against 'equi factor'.

Treatment

- Erythromycin (25 mg/kg by mouth, three times daily) and rifampicin (5 mg/kg by mouth, twice daily). Erythromycin alone may be effective if economics do not justify or permit the use of both drugs. Treatment must be continued 4–12 weeks until radiology and plasma fibrinogen are normal.
- Plasma therapy. Hyperimmune plasma used within the first week of life is an effective preventive treatment.
- General nursing care/provision of adequate ventilation.

Prognosis

The prognosis is fair. Approximately 80% recover with erythromycin and rifampicin treatment, with good prognosis for athletic soundness.

6.15 *Interstitial pneumonia/ chronic interstitial inflammation*

Chronic interstitial disease involving mycobacterial infections (especially Mycobacteria of the *avium-intracellulare* group) are occasionally recognized. Other chronic interstitial pneumonias and inflammatory/fibrotic diseases of unknown aetiology also occur. Non-mycobacterial granulomatous interstitial pneumonia may occur as part of a generalized granulomatous disease of unknown aetiology. Eosinophilic interstitial pneumonitis is also occasionally identified. These interstitial diseases can eventually result in *fibrosing alveolitis*. Environmental exposure to coal dust/silica, etc., can result in *pneumoconiosis*.

Clinical signs

- Chronic, progressive dyspnoea, with or without coughing.
- Weight loss.
- Persistent or recurrent pyrexia.

Diagnosis

- History and clinical signs. Lack of response to usual treatments for lower airway diseases.
- Auscultation – harsh lung sounds with variable wheezing and crackling.
- Thoracic radiography – interstitial infiltrate (may appear nodular or miliary).
- Bronchoalveolar lavage – variable cytology. Smear and culture for Mycobacteria. Particulate material within macrophages may be seen in cases of pneumoconiosis.
- Lung biopsy.

Treatment

There is no treatment. Mycobacterial infections are potential public health risks. Long-term anti-inflammatory drugs or corticosteroids may be beneficial in chronic interstitial inflammatory diseases, especially if given early in the course of the disease before fibrosis occurs.

6.16 *Fungal pneumonia*

Pathogenic fungi include *Coccidioides immitis*, *Histoplasma capsulatum* and *Cryptococcus neoformans*. Pulmonary infections by these fungi are usually only recognized in specific geographical locations.

Opportunist pulmonary infections by other fungi may occur in immunocompromised horses. These include *Aspergillus* species, *Candida* species, *Mucor* species and *Rhizopus* species.

Diagnosis

- Tracheal aspirate – fungal elements identified by cytology. NB: fungal hyphae and spores are commonly found in tracheal aspirates from normal horses; to be significant, these elements must be present in very large numbers.
- Lung biopsy.

Treatment

Antifungal drugs – amphotericin B, ketoconazole, miconazole, etc.

6.17 *Pulmonary oedema*

Pulmonary oedema is rarely recognized as a primary problem. It may be seen as a secondary feature or in association with a number of other diseases:

- Upper airway obstruction
- Septicaemia/septic shock
- Congestive heart failure
- Pneumonia
- Overhydration
- Smoke inhalation
- Acute alveolitis

Anaphylaxis sometimes occurs following injection or oral administration of drugs. A similar reaction may arise following the ingestion of certain foods (especially proteins – soya and wheat origin) or inhalation of organic dusts. Immediate immune reactions usually result in subcutaneous oedema and skin plaques, but may cause pulmonary oedema.

Clinical signs

The clinical signs will reflect the primary disease as well as the lung disease. Affected horses are often cold and clammy, weak and ataxic, with a subnormal temperature. The pulse is weak and rapid. Respirations are rapid and shallow. Fluid (may be frothy and blood-tinged) discharges from the nose, and may drool from the mouth. In severe cases, there is marked dyspnoea, collapse and death.

Diagnosis

- Clinical signs and evidence of predisposing disease.
- Auscultation – fine crackles and sometimes wheezing.
- Thoracic radiographs.

Treatment

Treatment should be aimed at eliminating the underlying cause as well as treating the pulmonary oedema.

- Diuretics (frusemide IV or IM).
- Corticosteroids if allergic mechanism is involved.
- Broad-spectrum antibiotic cover, especially if corticosteroids are used.
- Non-steroidal anti-inflammatory drugs.
- Nasal oxygen.

6.18 *Drowning/near drowning*

Rare, but can occur in horses undertaking swimming exercise. Fresh water inhalation leads to atelectasis and hypoxaemia. Salt water inhalation may lead to severe pulmonary oedema and dehydration. Aspiration pneumonia may follow.

Treatment is as for pulmonary oedema. In addition, bronchodilators may be beneficial.

6.19 *Pulmonary congestion*

Commonly occurs in recumbent horses (e.g. during general anaesthesia, or neuromuscular diseases – tetanus, botulism, etc.). This is rarely severe enough to compromise pulmonary function, but if prolonged may predispose to secondary infection.

Occasionally, severe pulmonary congestion may arise during strenuous exercise, especially in unfit horses. This may also involve a degree of EIPH and pulmonary oedema. The horse shows rapid, heaving respirations, with the head held down; haemorrhagic froth may appear at the mouth and nostrils.

Treatment

- Rest in quiet environment.
- Antibiotic cover.
- Diuretics.

6.20 *Haemothorax*

Uncommon. May occur when there is damage to either visceral or parietal pleural vessels:

- Trauma to chest wall and fractured ribs.
- Erosion of vessels by pulmonary abscess/ neoplasm.
- Haemangiosarcoma involving pleura.
- Severe EIPH.
- Bleeding disorders.

The clinical signs resemble those of pleural effusion. Diagnosis is based on thoracocentesis. Treatment is aimed at treating the underlying cause. Free blood should be drained from the thorax to prevent severe adhesion formation.

6.21 *Pneumothorax*

This is uncommon and is usually related to trauma.

- Penetrating wounds to the thorax.
- Puncture or rupture of the trachea.
- Rupture of the oesophagus.
- Broncho-pleural fistula secondary to pleuropneumonia.

Open pneumothorax results when a wound allows air to enter and leave the pleural cavity. *Closed pneumothorax* involves trapping air within the chest. *Tension pneumothorax* occurs when a flap of tissue acts as a valve allowing air to enter but not leave the thorax.

Clinical signs

- Tachypnoea and dyspnoea.
- Sometimes cyanosis.

Diagnosis

- Clinical signs and evidence of cause.
- Auscultation – absence of normal lung sounds dorsally.
- Percussion – increased resonance dorsally.
- Thoracic radiography.
- Ultrasonography.

Treatment

The underlying cause should be treated where possible. Any open wound should be cleaned and sealed.·

A chest drain with a one-way valve (e.g. Heimlich valve) should be introduced into the dorsal thorax to drain off the free air.

6.22 *Ruptured diaphragm*

This is rare. Acquired diaphragmatic defects are commoner than congenital defects. They are usually associated with chest trauma, parturition or strenuous exercise.

Clinical signs

Variable (depending on the extent of the defect; which viscera enter the chest; and how much compromise to lung function occurs). Intestine passing through the defect may obstruct and/or strangulate, causing colic.

- Acute to chronic colic.
- Dyspnoea.
- In longstanding cases, a pleural effusion may form.

Diagnosis

- Auscultation:
  - muffling of heart/lung sounds

– borborygmi in chest (NB: some referred intestinal sounds are normally heard within the chest).
- Radiography (possibly with barium contrast)
- Rectal examination – 'empty' abdomen

Treatment

Treatment is by surgical repair via laparotomy.

6.23 *Pleural transudates*

Transudative pleural effusions are rare and arise as a consequence of a disease process that does not affect the pleural cavity directly. They are sometimes detected in early thoracic neoplasia.

- Hypoproteinaemia, e.g. malabsorption, protein-losing enteropathy, protein-losing nephropathy. These more commonly result in ventral subcutaneous oedema, but may result in pleural and/or peritoneal effusions.
- Increased capillary hydrostatic pressure – congestive heart failure, space-occupying lesion in the thorax.

Clinical signs

The clinical signs relate simply to the presence of a pleural effusion. Other signs referable to the primary disease problem are likely to be more obvious.

- Laboured breathing (inspiratory and expiratory dyspnoea) with flared nostrils.
- Reluctance to move or to lie down.

Diagnosis

- Auscultation – absence of lung sounds ventrally.
- Percussion – dullness in ventral chest.
- Radiography.
- Ultrasonography.
- Thoracocentesis – transudates are typically straw-coloured fluids with low total nucleated cell count ($<10 \times 10^9/l$), low total protein ($<30\,g/l$) and low specific gravity (<1.017).

Treatment

Treat the primary disease.

NB: Transudative effusions may occur in early neoplastic chest diseases and ruptured diaphragm. It is important to ascertain the cause of the effusion in cases where a pleural transudate is identified.

6.24 *Smoke inhalation*

Damage to the respiratory tract occurs because of the effects of heat as well as the chemical effects of smoke. Most damage arises within the upper respiratory tract, involving inflammation and oedema of the mucosa. Pulmonary damage and oedema may occur in severe cases. Small airways may become obstructed by inflammatory cells, necrotic epithelial cells and carbonaceous material. Secondary infection and pneumonia may occur.

Clinical signs

The clinical signs depend on the amount and type of smoke inhalation.

- Depression/ataxia/coma.
- Fever (102–104°F) for up to 7 days.
- Dyspnoea.
- Cough.

Treatment

- Provide ventilatory support as necessary (humidified oxygen by nasal tube).
- Treat shock/toxaemia as necessary.
- Tracheostomy may be necessary if there is upper airway obstruction.
- Antibiotics (broad spectrum).
- Non-steroidal anti-inflammatory drugs or corticosteroids.
- Provide 'dust-free' environment.
- Mucolytics and/or bronchodilators as necessary.

Further reading

Beech, J. (1991) *Equine Respiratory Disorders*. Lea & Febiger, Philadelphia.

Brown, C.M. (1989) Coughing and laboured breathing. In *Problems in Equine Medicine* (Ed. C.M. Brown), Chapter 7. Lea & Febiger, Philadelphia.

Mair, T.S. (1994) Differential diagnosis and treatment of acute onset coughing in the horse. *Veterinary Record suppl. In Practice* **16**, 154–162.

McGorum, B. (1994) Differential diagnosis of chronic coughing in the horse. *Veterinary Record suppl In Practice* **16**, 55–60

Robertson, J.T. and Reed, S.M. (1991) Respiratory disease. Medicine and surgery. *Veterinary Clinics of North America: Equine Practice* **7**(1). W.B. Saunders & Co, Philadelphia.

Sweeney, C.R. & Smith, J.A. (1990). Diseases of the respiratory system. In *Large Animal Internal Medicine* (Ed. B.P. Smith), Chapter 29. C.V. Mosby Co, St Louis.

Appendix. Differential diagnoses of conditions presenting with respiratory signs

1. Acute/sudden onset coughing
Viral, bacterial and parasitic infections
1. Contagious diseases, e.g.
   EHV-1 and -4
   Equine influenza
   Equine viral arteritis
   Streptococcus equi (strangles)
   Streptococcus zooepidemicus
   Dictyocaulus arnfieldi
2. Non-contagious e.g. bacterial pneumonia/ pleuropneumonia
   Acute obstructive pulmonary disease
   Foreign body
   Acute dysphagia and food aspiration
   Oesophageal obstruction
   Smoke inhalation
   Trauma to larynx, trachea or chest
   Pulmonary haemorrhage
   Pulmonary oedema

2. Chronic coughing
COPD
Chronic lower airway inflammation
SPAOPD
Chronic bacterial pneumonia/pleuropneumonia
Pulmonary abscess
Dictyocaulus arnfieldi infection
Parascaris equorum larval migration
Chronic dysphagia and food aspiration
Chronic lesions of pharynx, larynx and trachea, e.g.
   retropharyngeal abscess
   arytenoid chondritis
   epiglottic entrapment
   subepiglottic cyst
   pharyngeal paralysis
   tracheal stenosis/collapse
Fungal pneumonias
Congestive heart failure
Tumours/polyps in airway

Thoracic neoplasia
Chronic interstitial lung diseases

3. Bilateral purulent nasal discharge
Secondary bacterial infections (in viral infections)
Streptococcus equi (strangles)
Streptococcus zooepidemicus
Bacterial pneumonia/pleuropneumonia/pulmonary abscess
COPD
Guttural pouch empyema/chondroids/mycosis
Pharyngeal/retropharyngeal abscess
Foreign body (nasopharyngeal/tracheobronchial)
Conidiobolomycosis (in endemic areas)

4. Unilateral purulent nasal discharge
Paranasal sinusitis/dental infection/sinus cyst/ neoplasia
Mycotic rhinitis
Nasal foreign body
Nasal tumour/polyp/cyst
Guttural pouch empyema/chondroids/mycosis

5. Nasal return of food
Oesophageal obstruction (choke)
Cleft palate
Streptococcus equi (strangles)
Guttural pouch mycosis/diverticulitis/empyema
Retropharyngeal abscess
Grass sickness
Gastric dilation
Small intestinal obstruction
Proximal enteritis (duodenitis/proximal jejunitis)
Myopathies
Botulism
Lead poisoning
Gastroduodenal ulceration
Megaoesophagus

6. Epistaxis
EIPH
Guttural pouch mycosis
Progressive ethmoidal haematoma
Trauma
Nasal/paranasal sinus tumour
Foreign bodies
Clotting/bleeding disorders, e.g.
   thrombocytopenia
   purpura haemorrhagica
   disseminated intravascular coagulation
   warfarin toxicity
Conidiobolomycosis

7. Dyspnoea in adult horse
COPD/acute obstructive pulmonary disease
Pneumonia/pleuropneumonia/pulmonary abscess
Retropharyngeal abscess
Streptococcus equi (strangles)
Paranasal sinus disease
Nasal/nasopharyngeal tumour/cyst
Pneumothorax
Diaphragmatic hernia
Thoracic neoplasia
Interstitial pulmonary disease
Cardiac disease
Shock
Anaemia
Pain
Tracheal collapse
Acute laryngeal conditions

8. Malodorous nasal discharge
Sinusitis (usually secondary to dental disease)/sinus neoplasia
Foreign body
Ethmoidal haematoma
Nasal tumour
Pneumonia/pulmonary abscess
Mycotic rhinitis
Guttural pouch mycosis

7 Cardiovascular system

CONTENTS

7.1 Physical examination

A careful examination of the cardiovascular system should be included as a part of every clinical examination:

- The arteries, veins and mucous membranes are inspected visually and palpated.
- The heart is auscultated and palpated for the presence of precordial thrills.
- The other body systems should be evaluated for extracardiac signs of cardiac dysfunction and failure.
- Many equine cardiac problems are apparent only at exercise. The history should include careful evaluation of previous performance and, if necessary, the horse should be examined during and after exercise.

Arterial pulses

- The transverse facial, the facial, the digital, brachial and femoral arteries are readily palpable. Most clinicians routinely palpate the facial and digital arteries.
- The abdominal aorta can be palpated *per rectum* if necessary.
- The rate and rhythm of the arterial pulse are recorded.

- Normal adult horses have a pulse rate of 30 to 50 beats per minute (bpm) at rest while newborn foals generally have a faster pulse rate (60–80 bpm).
- The quality of the pulse should also be assessed. The normal pulse is strong with a symmetrical profile.
- Abnormalities of the pulse include weakness (low pulse pressure), a bounding quality (strong systolic pulse with a rapid run-off to a weak diastolic pressure) and variable pulses (pressure varies from beat to beat).

Veins

- The jugular veins should be distended to check their patency and palpated for the presence of swelling or thrombi.
- The normal jugular pulse extends only one third up the neck when the horse's head is in a normal position.
- If venous occlusion is suspected, the vessels proximal to the lesion should be checked for distension.
- The jugular venous fill serves as a guide to circulating volume and will be reduced in a hypovolaemic animal.

Mucous membranes

- The oral and ocular mucous membranes are usually examined.
- Their colour and moistness serve as a guide to circulation and perfusion. Normal mucous membranes are pink and moist with a capillary refill time of less than 2 seconds.
- In the shocked animal, the mucous membranes are pale, or if there is endotoxaemia, they are often congested with a purplish ring around the gum margins (toxic ring).
- Petecheae and injection of the vessels should also be noted.

Auscultation and palpation of the heart

The cardiac silhouette is located in the third to fifth intercostal spaces and therefore, the majority of it is auscultated underneath the muscles of the forearm.

- There are four heart sounds and all of these can be audible in the normal horse.

- The first heart sound coincides with the onset of systole and is associated with closure of the atrioventricular valves and opening of the semilunar (aortic and pulmonic) valves.
- The second sound coincides with the onset of diastole and is associated with the closure of the semilunar valves and opening of the atrioventricular valves. The second heart sound can be split in normal horses if the semilunar valves close asynchronously.
- The third heart sound occurs early in diastole. It arises as blood decelerates rapidly at the end of the rapid ventricular filling phase. This sound is only audible in about one in three horses.
- The fourth heart sound is associated with atrial contraction and occurs late in diastole, immediately before the first heart sound. This sound is audible in the majority of horses.
- Cardiac murmurs are a common finding in horses. They should be characterized according to the:
  - Timing in the cardiac cycle.
  - Location.
  - Radiation.
  - Quality.
  - Intensity.
  - Presence or absence of a precordial thrill.

Timing
It is helpful to palpate the arterial pulse while auscultating the heart to determine the phase of the cardiac cycle in which a murmur is occurring. Murmurs can be either systolic, diastolic or continuous (throughout systole and diastole) and this is further divided into:

- Pansystolic/pandiastolic – obscuring the heart sounds before and after that phase of the cardiac cycle.
- Holosystolic/holodiastolic – beginning immediately after one heart sound and lasting until immediately before the next heart sound.
- Early, mid or late systolic/diastolic – occupying only one part of that phase of the cardiac cycle.

Location
Murmurs are usually loudest over one part of the heart and identification of this site aids the clinician in determining the origin and significance of the murmur. The heart valves are located as follows:

- Left atrioventricular valve – in the left fifth intercostal space, midway between the level of

the point of the shoulder and the point of the elbow.
- Aortic valve – in the left fourth intercostal space, at the level of the point of the shoulder.
- Pulmonic valve – in the left third intercostal space mid way between the level of the point of the shoulder and the point of the elbow.
- Right atrioventricular valve – in the right fourth intercostal space mid way between the level of the point of the shoulder and the point of the elbow.

Radiation

The radiation of a murmur refers to the direction in which it fades out. The direction of radiation is influenced by the direction in which the turbulent jet of blood that is causing it is travelling. This is described in anatomical terms, for example caudodorsally, and caudoventrally. Murmurs that do not radiate are referred to as localized.

Quality

A variety of terms are used to describe the quality of murmurs, for example coarse, harsh, soft, blowing, and musical. The changes in volume of the murmur are also considered. Murmurs may be crescendo–decrescendo, decrescendo and plateau or band-shaped if they do not vary in volume.

Intensity

The intensity or loudness of a murmur is used in combination with the presence or absence of a precordial thrill to assign a grade as follows:

- Grade one – a very quiet murmur which is only audible after several seconds of listening.
- Grade two – a soft murmur that is audible after a few seconds of listening.
- Grade three – a loud murmur that is audible immediately the stethoscope is placed over it.
- Grade four – a very loud murmur without a precordial thrill.
- Grade five – a very loud murmur with a precordial thrill.
- Grade six – a murmur that can still be heard when the stethoscope is removed from the chest wall slightly.

7.2 Clinical signs of heart failure

- Left-sided heart failure produces pulmonary oedema and respiratory signs. The respiratory system should be auscultated carefully for evidence of pulmonary oedema (increased respiratory rate, coughing, nasal discharge, wheezes or crackles on auscultation).
- Right-sided heart failure leads to ventral oedema and accumulation of fluid in the pleural and peritoneal cavities. Occasionally, bowel oedema causes diarrhoea.
- Biventricular congestive failure is associated with both right- and left-sided signs.
- Low cardiac output associated with conditions such as certain arrhythmias, myocardial failure and pericardial disease can lead to weakness, collapse and renal dysfunction.

7.3 Ancillary diagnostic aids in cardiology

Echocardiography

Echocardiography is the technique of choice for evaluating horses with cardiac murmurs and allows the cause and significance of the majority of cardiac murmurs to be determined definitively. It is also indicated for horses with myocardial or pericardial disease. Echocardiography encompasses two-dimensional, M mode and Doppler echocardiography and usually all three techniques are used in combination.

Two-dimensional echocardiography provides a slice-type of image of the internal structures of the heart and allows the structure of the valves, the interventricular septum, the ventricular and atrial walls and the great vessels to be visually inspected (Figure 1). Specific lesions, such as

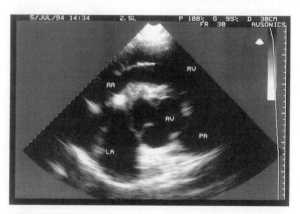

Figure 1 Two-dimensional echocardiogram of the structures at the heart base. The internal anatomy of the right atrium (RA), right ventricle (RV), pulmonary artery (PA), left atrium (LA) and aortic valve (AV) are visible.

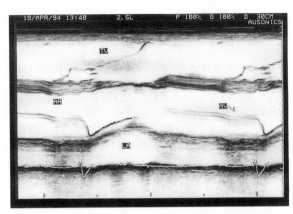

Figure 2 An M mode echocardiogram of the structures at the heart base. The right atrioventricular valve (TV), aortic root (AR), aortic valve (AV) and a portion of the left atrium (LA) are visible. An ECG is superimposed to time cardiac events.

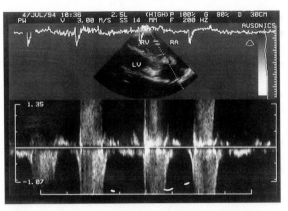

Figure 3 A pulsed-wave Doppler echocardiogram with a corresponding two-dimensional image illustrates the position of the sampling volume (the area between the parallel lines). It has been placed within the right atrium (RA). On the spectral tracing, high velocity blood flow is present in systole indicating that this horse has right atrioventricular regurgitation. An ECG is superimposed to time cardiac events. Notice that this horse has atrial fibrillation (RV = right ventricle, LV = left ventricle).

focal or generalized thickening of a valve or ventricular septal defects, can be demonstrated and, in addition, the effects of cardiac lesions, such as ventricular dilatation or hypertrophy can be identified.

M mode echocardiography refers to a one-dimensional image that is displayed in a graph form of location against time (Figure 2). It is used to make precise measurements of cardiac structures throughout the cardiac cycle and to measure various functional parameters.

Doppler echocardiography identifies both the speed and direction of blood flow. This can be depicted either in a spectral form (Figure 3), a graph of blood flow against time or, using colour flow Doppler, information on blood flow is displayed superimposed on two-dimensional or M mode echocardiogram to provide a map of intracardiac blood flow. Using Doppler echocardiography, abnormal blood flow associated with valvular regurgitation or intra- and extracardiac shunts can be demonstrated. The degree of valvular regurgitation can be semi-quantitated by determining the area occupied by the regurgitant jet.

Electrocardiography

Electrocardiography refers to the recording of electrical potentials generated by depolarization and repolarization of the myocardial cells. In routine clinical practice this is recorded from the body surface. In the normal heart, the wave of depolarization is initiated by the pacemaker cells at the sinoatrial node which is located within the right atrium. From here it spreads across the atria by moving from cell to cell and through specialized interatrial conduction tissue. Having travelled through the atria, the wave of depolarization arrives at the atrioventricular node where it is delayed slightly, and then travels through the bundle of Hiss and Purkinje network to the ventricles. Once the myocardial cells are depolarized, there is a refractory period before they repolarize. On the electrocardiogram (ECG) each of these phases can be documented (Figure 4):

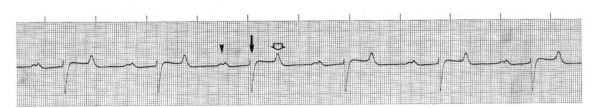

Figure 4 A base–apex ECG from a normal horse illustrating the normal p (arrowhead), qrs (arrow) and t (open arrow). The p wave is bifid and qrs is negative in this lead (0.5 cm/mV, 25 mm/s).

- The p wave represents atrial depolarization.
- The p–r interval represents the normal delay at the atrioventricular node.
- The qrs complex represents ventricular depolarization.
- The t wave represents ventricular repolarization.

In horses, the p wave is usually bifid, but the shape of the t wave is very variable. In some species, for example man and dog, the size of the qrs complex is related to ventricular mass. In horses, and other ungulates, this is not the case because these species have a very extensive Purkinje network and conduction is independent of myocardial cell number or mass. Thus, in horses the ECG can only document conduction and electrical activity and cannot be used to identify hypertrophy. Therefore, the use of electrocardiography in horses is primarily indicated to characterize arrhythmias.

Various leads systems can be used to record the equine ECG. The unipolar and bipolar limb leads, which were developed for use in man, can also be applied to the horse. The base–apex lead is obtained by attaching a positive electrode to the left thorax, over the heart base, and a negative electrode over the right jugular furrow or higher in the neck at the top of the scapula. This is often used to monitor rhythm because large, easily identifiable complexes are produced. Other workers prefer a semi-orthogonal system where leads are applied to both sides of the chest, the ventrum and dorsum and cranial and caudal to the heart. No one lead system has a clear advantage over any other.

ECGs recorded for a short time at rest are sometimes insufficient. Many arrhythmias occur only at exercise or in the immediate post-exercise period. Others vary in their frequency at rest. Radiotelemetric electrocardiography is performed using a small transmitter that is attached to the horse and a receiver that displays the ECG at a distant point. This system is extremely valuable for investigating exercise-induced arrhythmias. Ambulatory ECG recorders allow an ECG to be recorded for a 24 hour period on magnetic tape that is subsequently analysed by computer. This allows the frequency of arrhythmias to be documented more accurately than in the standard ECG and, because the horse can be left alone in a loose box, environmental influences can be removed.

A systematic approach to the interpretation of ECGs allows dysrhythmias to be identified easily:

- Measure the heart rate.
- Are all the p–p intervals equal? If not, consider sinus arrhythmia, sinoatrial block, sinoatrial arrest or supraventricular premature depolarizations.
- Are all the r–r intervals equal? If not, consider atrioventricular block, ventricular premature depolarizations, ventricular tachycardia, atrial fibrillation or ventricular fibrillation.
- Is there a p for every qrs–t? If not, consider atrial fibrillation, ventricular premature depolarizations or ventricular tachycardia.
- Is there a qrs for every p? If not, consider atrioventricular blocks or unconducted atrial premature depolarizations.
- Are there any pauses? If so, consider sinoatrial block, sinoatrial arrest, or atrioventricular blocks (including unconducted supraventricular premature depolarizations).
- Are there any premature complexes? If so, consider supraventricular or ventricular premature depolarizations.
- Are all the complexes the same configurations? If not, consider ventricular premature depolarizations, ventricular tachycardia or ventricular fibrillation.

Cardiac catheterization

Catheters placed in various chambers of the heart can be used to document pressures within specific chambers or vessels and to withdraw blood for blood gas analysis. This can be used to demonstrate intra- or extracardiac shunts associated with congenital defects and is sometimes used to assess the severity of valvular regurgitation.

Radiography

Thoracic radiography is rather limited in its usefulness in the adult horse. Dorsoventral radiographs cannot be obtained successfully but lateral radiographs can be used to document pulmonary oedema and gross cardiac enlargement. In the foal, radiography is more useful and angiography can be used to demonstrate congenital defects. However, echocardiography has largely replaced these techniques.

Cardiac isoenzyme analysis

Serum concentrations of isoenzymes of creatine kinase (CKMB) and lactate dehydrogenase (LDH 1 and 2) that are derived primarily from the heart can be increased in horses with acute myocardial disease. However, these isoenzymes are located in other organs as well as the heart and increases are also observed in horses with other conditions such as gastrointestinal disease.

7.4 *Cardiac murmurs*

Cardiac murmurs are extremely common in horses. Determining the clinical significance of equine cardiac murmurs can cause some consternation amongst clinicians. However, following a careful clinical evaluation and, if necessary echocardiography, it is usually possible to place each murmur into one of three categories:

- Physiological.
- Pathological but not clinically significant.
- Pathological and clinically significant.

Physiological murmurs are associated with normal cardiac function. The specific forms of cardiac pathology in which cardiac murmurs are present include:

- Valvular insufficiency.
- Ventricular septal defect.
- Atrial septal defect.
- Patent ductus arteriosus.
- Complex congenital defects.

Unlike small animals, valvular stenosis in horses is extremely uncommon and usually only occurs in combination with other congenital defects. In the simple congenital defects (e.g. ventricular septal defect) the clinical significance of the defect depends primarily on the size of the defect and the associated shunt.

In valvular insufficiency, the factors that determine its clinical significance are:

- The specific valve involved.
- The type of pathology.
- The degree of regurgitation.
- The rate of progression.

Pathological but not clinically significant murmurs include:

- Most cases of aortic insufficiency.
- Most cases of right atrioventricular insufficiency.
- Some cases of left atrioventricular insufficiency.
- Small ventricular septal defects.

Pathological and clinically significant murmurs include:

- Rapid onset aortic, pulmonic or right atrioventricular insufficiency.
- Many cases of left atrioventricular insufficiency.
- Large ventricular septal defects.
- Other congenital defects.

Physiological murmurs

- Blood flow out the great vessels can generate physiological murmurs that are characteristically grade 1–3/6, holo- or mid-systolic, loudest in the left fourth intercostal space at the level of the point of the shoulder, crescendo–decrescendo and blowing.
- The origin of physiological murmurs during diastole is less clear but they are readily recognized as grade 1–3/6, early or late, decrescendo sounds that are usually loudest over the left or right heart base and are often squeaky in nature.

7.5 *Aortic insufficiency*

Pathology

- The aortic valve is the commonest site for degenerative lesions, which are nodular or generalized fibrous thickenings of the valve cusps.
- Doppler echocardiographic studies have shown that mild aortic insufficiency is common in horses with no cardiac pathology and no cardiac murmurs.
- Valvular prolapse (floppy valve) is a common finding on echocardiography but it is rarely associated with significant aortic regurgitation. Severe aortic valvular prolapse may accompany ventricular septal defect.
- Inflammatory lesions (valvulitis) of the aortic valve can occur, and in fact, may be more common than was previously recognized.
- Bacterial endocarditis results in large vegetative lesions of the valves.
- One cusp may tear (flail cusp) leading to acute, severe aortic insufficiency. This occurs spontaneously or sometimes secondary to ventricular septal defect.

Haemodynamic effects

• Aortic regurgitation produces left ventricular volume overload. In response to increased end-diastolic pressure and ventricular wall tension, ventricular contractility is increased which increases the arterial pulse pressure in systole.
• The regurgitation of blood reduces the diastolic arterial pressure.
• Severe left ventricular dilatation can dilate the left atrioventricular valve annulus causing left atrioventricular valvular regurgitation. The horse then becomes more likely to develop congestive heart failure.

Signalment

• Degenerative lesions of the aortic valve are commonest in middle-aged or older horses and ponies.
• Horses of any age or breed can be affected with the other forms of aortic insufficiency.

Clinical signs

• The characteristic murmur of aortic insufficiency is grade 2–6/6, loudest in the left fourth intercostal space, at the level of the point of the shoulder, radiating caudoventrally, and is sometimes also audible in the right fourth intercostal space. It is pan-, holo- or early diastolic, and is decrescendo and coarse. In some horses it has a bizarre creaking or groaning quality.
• In most horses, the murmur of aortic insufficiency is detected as an incidental finding during routine physical examinations.
• Aortic insufficiency alone rarely causes poor performance.
• Horses with bacterial endocarditis usually present with fever.
• The pulses become hyperkinetic (bounding, strong systolic pressure with rapid run-off to reduced diastolic pressure) as left ventricular volume overload increases and this is the best clinical guide to the severity of the lesion.
• Affected horses should be evaluated carefully for the presence of an accompanying murmur of left atrioventricular valvular insufficiency.

Assessment

• Echocardiography is used to demonstrate valvular lesions, semi-quantitate the size of the regurgitant jet, assess the degree of left ventricular volume overload and to eliminate the presence of left atrioventricular valvular insufficiency.
• Electrocardiography is used to investigate any concurrent arrhythmias.
• A complete blood count, serum fibrinogen and blood culture should be performed in any horse suspected of having bacterial endocarditis.

Prognosis

• The prognosis is very good for horses with degenerative lesions of the aortic valve. Affected horses should be re-examined echocardiographically every 12 to 24 months so that the rate of progression can be determined.
• Lesions with an acute onset such as flail cusp and bacterial endocarditis carry a guarded prognosis.
• In bacterial endocarditis it may be possible to obtain a bacteriological cure with appropriate antibiotics. However, there is usually irreparable structural damage to the valve.

7.6 *Pulmonic insufficiency*

Pathology

• The pulmonic valve is an uncommon site for valvular pathology.
• Rupture of the pulmonic valve (flail cusp) and bacterial endocarditis have been described.
• In horses with congestive heart failure, the pulmonic valve can begin to leak secondary to pulmonary hypertension.

Haemodynamic effects

• Acute onset, severe pulmonic insufficiency leads to right ventricular volume overload and right-sided heart failure.

Signalment

• Horses of any age, breed or sex can be affected.
• Bacterial endocarditis of the pulmonic valve can be a sequel to septic jugular thrombosis.

Clinical signs

• The characteristic murmur of pulmonic insufficiency is grade 2–6/6, loudest in the left third intercostal space, at the level of the point of the

elbow, radiating ventrally. It is pan-, holo- or early diastolic, and is decrescendo and coarse.
- Mild and moderate degrees of pulmonic insufficiency can be present with no murmurs.
- Horses with severe pulmonic insufficiency show signs of right-sided heart failure, such as jugular distension and pulsation, ventral oedema, pleural effusion (on percussion and auscultation the ventral thorax is dull), and ascites (rarely clinically apparent in horses).
- Horses with bacterial endocarditis usually present with fever.

Assessment

- Echocardiography is used to demonstrate valvular lesions, semi-quantitate the size of the regurgitant jet, and assess the degree of right ventricular dilatation.
- A complete blood count, serum fibrinogen and blood culture should be performed in any horse suspected of having bacterial endocarditis.
- Thoracic radiography and tracheal aspirates or bronchoalveolar lavage are indicated if concurrent embolic pneumonia is suspected.

Prognosis

- The prognosis for horses with severe pulmonic insufficiency and right-sided heart failure is poor.

7.7 Right atrioventricular insufficiency

Pathology

- Degenerative and inflammatory lesions can affect the right atrioventricular valve but this is an uncommon site for valvular pathology.
- Right atrioventricular insufficiency is common in all types of horses, particularly Steeplechasers and Standardbred racehorses. These horses usually have no evidence of right atrioventricular valvular pathology or have valvular prolapse (floppy valve).
- Right atrioventricular valvular insufficiency can develop secondary to pulmonary hypertension in horses with congestive heart failure.
- Bacterial endocarditis can affect the right atrioventricular valve, and this is usually secondary to septic jugular thrombosis.

- Rupture of a chorda tendinea of the right atrioventricular valve leads to acute, severe valvular insufficiency.

Haemodynamic effects

- Severe right atrioventricular valvular insufficiency leads to right atrial dilatation and right ventricular volume overload. However, it is unusual to see signs of right-sided heart failure with right atrioventricular insufficiency alone.
- Mild and moderate right atrioventricular valvular insufficiency is generally very well tolerated.
- Right atrial dilatation can predispose the horse to the development of atrial fibrillation.

Signalment

- Horses of any age, sex or breed can be affected.
- Right atrioventricular valvular insufficiency has been documented most frequently in Steeplechasers and Standardbred racehorses.

Clinical signs

- The characteristic murmur of right atrioventricular valvular insufficiency is grade 2–6/6, loudest in the right fourth intercostal space, mid way between the point of the shoulder and the point of the elbow, radiating cranially. It is pan-, holo- or mid-systolic and can be either coarse or blowing and crescendo–decrescendo or band-shaped.
- Right atrioventricular valvular insufficiency is often detected as an incidental finding.
- If it is severe, it can lead to poor performance or exercise intolerance.
- Abnormal jugular pulsation is present in severe right atrioventricular insufficiency.
- Horses with bacterial endocarditis usually present with fever.

Assessment

- Echocardiography is used to demonstrate valvular lesions, semi-quantitate the size of the regurgitant jet, and demonstrate the degree of right ventricular volume overload and right atrial dilatation.
- Electrocardiography is indicated if there are concurrent arrhythmias.
- A complete blood count, serum fibrinogen and blood culture should be performed in any horse suspected of having bacterial endocarditis.

Prognosis

• The majority of horses with right atrioventricular valvular insufficiency and either no echocardiographic evidence of valvular lesions, or mild valvular prolapse, or focal valvular thickenings, have an excellent prognosis.
• These horses should be examined approximately every 24 months to determine the rate of progression of the insufficiency.
• Horses with acute onset severe lesions such as rupture of a chorda tendinea or bacterial endocarditis have a poor prognosis.

7.8 *Left atrioventricular insufficiency*

Pathology

• The left atrioventricular valve is the second most common site for degenerative lesions. These are focal or generalized thickening of the valve cusps.
• Inflammatory lesions (valvulitis) may occur more commonly than was previously recognized.
• Prolapse of the left atrioventricular valve (floppy valve) can cause a murmur but is not usually associated with significant regurgitation.
• Rupture of a chorda tendinea can occur spontaneously or secondary to inflammatory or degenerative lesions.
• Left atrioventricular valvular insufficiency can arise secondary to dilatation of the valve annulus following left ventricular dilatation (aortic insufficiency, cardiomyopathy).
• Bacterial endocarditis can affect the left atrioventricular valve.

Haemodynamic effects

• Left atrioventricular valvular insufficiency leads to increased left atrial pressure and dilatation.
• This in turn leads to pulmonary hypertension and pulmonary oedema.
• The left ventricular end-diastolic volume is increased.
• Pulmonary oedema leads to respiratory dysfunction.
• Left atrial enlargement can lead to atrial fibrillation.
• Pulmonary hypertension can lead to pulmonary artery dilatation and rupture.

• Right-sided heart failure can follow left-sided heart failure.

Signalment

• Any breed, age and sex of horse can be affected.

Clinical signs

• The characteristic murmur of left atrioventricular valvular insufficiency is grade 2–6/6, loudest in the left fifth intercostal space, midway between the point of the shoulder and the point of the elbow, radiating caudodorsally. It is pan-, holo- or mid-systolic, band-shaped, and can be either coarse or blowing.
• In severe left atrioventricular valvular insufficiency, the third heart sound is increased (because of increased ventricular filling).
• Left atrioventricular valvular insufficiency is often, but not always, associated with poor performance.
• Severe left atrioventricular insufficiency leads to respiratory signs: exercise intolerance, increased respiratory rate and effort at rest or after exercise, nasal discharge, and wheezes on auscultation.
• Atrial fibrillation can accompany left atrioventricular valvular insufficiency.
• Horses with left-sided heart failure also often have signs of right-sided heart failure such as jugular distension and pulsation.
• Pulmonary artery rupture can lead to collapse or sudden death.
• Horses with bacterial endocarditis usually present with fever.

Assessment

• Echocardiography is used to identify valvular lesions, such as focal or generalized thickening, ruptured chorda tendinea, or vegetative lesions, to assess the degree of left ventricular volume overload and left atrial dilatation, and to semi-quantitate the degree of regurgitation. The diameter of the pulmonary artery should be measured to determine the degree of pulmonary artery dilatation.
• Electrocardiography is used to assess any concurrent arrhythmias.
• Thoracic radiography is indicated if pulmonary oedema is suspected.
• A complete blood count, serum fibrinogen and blood culture should be performed in any horse suspected of having bacterial endocarditis.

Prognosis

• Left atrioventricular insufficiency is the form of valvular heart disease which is most likely to lead to poor performance or cardiac failure.
• Horses with valvular prolapse or mild left atrioventricular insufficiency can often perform to their owners' expectations.
• If left atrioventricular valvular insufficiency is confirmed, the horse should be examined every 6–12 months to assess the rate of progression.
• Horses with pulmonary artery dilatation are at risk for collapse or sudden death.
• Acute severe lesions, such as rupture of a chorda tendinea or bacterial endocarditis, carry a grave prognosis.

7.9 *Ventricular septal defect*

Pathology

• The commonest site for ventricular septal defect (VSD) is in the membranous portion of the septum, immediately below the aortic root.
• Less commonly, the defect is in the muscular portion of the septum, and here it can be a series of channels rather than a single defect.
• When located in the membranous portion of the septum, the defect can affect the support of the aortic valve causing concurrent aortic insufficiency.

Haemodynamic effects

• Blood flow through the VSD travels from the left ventricle to the right ventricle in uncomplicated cases.
• The volume of blood leaving the right ventricle is increased causing a relative pulmonic stenosis.
• If the shunt is large, right ventricular pressure overload occurs.
• The pulmonary circulation is increased and the volume of blood returning to the left ventricle from the lungs is increased, leading to left ventricular volume overload.
• Concurrent aortic insufficiency exacerbates left ventricular volume overload.

Signalment

• Any breed of horse can be affected, but congenital cardiac defects are thought to be more common in the Arabian and Standardbred breeds.
• The defect is present at birth, but most horses are 2 or 3 years old before clinical signs become apparent.

Clinical signs

• Horses with VSDs have at least two murmurs (three if aortic insufficiency is present).
• Blood flow through the VSD produces a characteristic murmur that is grade 4–6/6, pansystolic, loudest in the right fourth intercostal space at the costochondral junction, and is band-shaped and coarse.
• Relative pulmonic stenosis produces a characteristic murmur that is grade 3–6/6 (usually one grade less than the VSD murmur in any individual), holosystolic, loudest in the left third intercostal space midway between the point of the elbow and point of the shoulder, and is crescendo–decrescendo.
• If the defect is small, the VSD may be an incidental finding and the horse can be performing up to its owners' expectations.
• With larger defects, the signs can range from poor performance and exercise intolerance to stunting and failure to thrive. Left-sided or congestive heart failure may eventually develop.

Assessment

• Two-dimensional echocardiography is used to visualize and measure the size of the VSD and to assess the degree of left ventricular volume overload.
• Doppler echocardiography is used to estimate the pressure gradient between the left and right ventricles, to document right ventricular hypertension and to demonstrate any concurrent aortic insufficiency.
• Cardiac catheterization can be used to confirm the presence of a left to right shunt and to document right ventricular hypertension.
• Electrocardiography is used to assess any concurrent arrhythmias.

Prognosis

• The prognosis for horses with VSD is dependent on the size of the defect.
• Thoroughbreds and Standardbreds with a membranous defect of less than 2.5 cm in two mutually perpendicular planes have an excellent

prognosis for survival and can have a useful athletic career.

- Horses with larger defects and severe aortic insufficiency have a guarded to poor prognosis.

7.10 Other congenital cardiac defects

- A wide variety of congenital cardiac defects have been reported in the horse.
- In the simple defects, such as atrial septal defect and ductus arteriosus, the severity of the clinical signs and the prognosis is probably dependent on the size of the defect.
- In complex congenital defects, such as tetralogy of Fallot, right ventricular atresia and malformations of the great vessels, the clinical signs are usually severe and congestive heart failure is apparent early in life.
- Echocardiography is the technique of choice for diagnosing specific congenital defects.
- The prognosis is usually very guarded.

7.11 Treatment of congestive heart failure

In congestive heart failure, the goals of therapy are:

1. To reduce congestion and oedema.
2. To improve tissue perfusion.
3. To allow the heart to function more effectively.

- Frusemide (0.5 – 2 mg/kg, IV, IM or by mouth) is used as a diuretic to reduce congestion and oedema.
- Nitroglycerine ointment is a venedilator and is used to reduce pulmonary oedema.
- Arterial dilators improve tissue perfusion and reduce afterload, allowing the heart to function more effectively, but their use has not been investigated extensively in the horse. The pharmacokinetics of hydralazine have been established but protocols for its use in horses with heart failure have not been published.
- Digoxin is indicated if there is atrial fibrillation and a ventricular rate of greater than 60/minute. The aim is to slow the ventricular response and allow the heart to fill and contract more effectively. Digoxin is administered orally at 0.01 mg/

kg twice daily. Serum concentrations should be monitored to ensure that therapeutic, and not toxic, concentrations are maintained. Side effects of digoxin include gastrointestinal signs such as colic and diarrhoea, and digoxin can induce ventricular dysrhythmias.

7.12 Dysrhythmias and myocardial disease

Horses are frequently affected by dysrhythmias. In the majority of cases, these are physiological in nature but, in some horses they are indicative of underlying myocardial disease. Myocardial disease can be either focal or generalized. Focal myocardial disease is usually associated with dysrhythmias, whereas generalized myocardial disease (cardiomyopathy) can lead to ventricular dysfunction with or without dysrhythmias. There are many causes of myocardial dysfunction in horses, including hypoxia, endotoxaemia, electrolyte disturbances, toxins such as the ionophore antibiotics (monensin, salinomycin), and drugs such as anaesthetic agents. Active or recent viral infections can lead to dysrhythmias. Many workers believe that immune-mediated myocarditis can occur as a sequel to respiratory virus infection. Dysrhythmias may occur only during or after exercise. In some cases, these dysrhythmias are pathological, while in others, they can be attributed to 'autonomic imbalance', because the vagus is slowing the heart while there are high circulating levels of catecholamines and other vasoactive substances released during exercise.

Dysrhythmias can be classified as bradydysrhythmias or tachydysrhythmias, depending on whether they slow down or speed up the heart rate, and they can also be defined on the basis of their site of origin in the heart.

7.13 Physiological dysrhythmias

Second degree atrioventricular block

- Atrioventricular block refers to slowing or blocking of conduction at the atrioventricular node, and three types are recognized. In first degree atrioventricular block, conduction is delayed for greater than 0.5 seconds but not blocked completely. In second degree atrioventricular block, conduction through the atrioventricular node is blocked intermittently, and in third degree atrioventricular block, there is no conduction and the atria and ventricles operate independently.

- Second degree atrioventricular block is the commonest physiological dysrhythmia in the horse. It is mediated by the vagus (parasympathetic system).
- On auscultation, there is a regular underlying rhythm with intermittent pauses during which only the fourth heart sound is audible.
- On ECG, there is a regular underlying rhythm with intermittent p waves that are not followed by a qrs complex.
- Up to one in three beats may be blocked in normal horses. Occasionally, two or more beats are blocked in succession.
- In normal horses, the second degree atrioventricular block is abolished by removing vagal tone (such as excitement, exercise, and vagolytic drugs including atropine and glycopyrrolate).
- One or two blocked beats are occasionally seen in horses immediately after strenuous exercise.

Sinus arrhythmia

- This is a less common physiological dysrhythmia in the resting horse, but it is often seen immediately after exercise.
- On auscultation, there is a gradual slowing and speeding of the heart rate.
- On ECG, the p–p interval and the r–r interval gradually increase and decrease.
- Wandering atrial pacemaker often accompanies sinus arrhythmia. This means that conduction is initiated in different cells within the sinoatrial node and is recognized as slight variations in the configuration of the p wave.
- In normal horses, sinus arrhythmia is abolished by removing vagal tone (such as excitement, exercise, and vagolytic drugs including atropine and glycopyrrolate).

Sinoatrial block and arrest

- These are uncommon physiological dysrhythmias in the horse in which conduction is delayed at the sinoatrial node. They are mediated by the vagus (parasympathetic system).
- On auscultation, a regular underlying rhythm with intermittent pauses is heard.

- On ECG, there is a pause of less than two normal p–p intervals (sinoatrial block) or two or greater p–p intervals (sinoatrial arrest).
- In normal horses, these dysrhythmias are abolished by removing vagal tone (such as excitement, exercise and vagolytic drugs including atropine and glycopyrrolate).

7.14 *Pathological dysrhythmias*

Atrial premature depolarizations and tachycardia

- Atrial premature depolarizations (APDs) can occur in association with any form of myocardial disease.
- Four or more APDs occurring in sequence is defined as atrial tachycardia.
- Infrequent APDs (less than 5 in 24 hours) are occasionally seen in normal horses.
- Isolated APDs are sometimes seen immediately after exercise as the heart slows and these are considered insignificant provided that they are isolated, infrequent and do not occur during exercise.
- APDs are frequently detected in horses after treatment for atrial fibrillation.
- On auscultation, a premature beat is heard.
- On ECG, a premature p wave with an abnormal configuration is present. This may or may not be followed by a qrs–t complex, depending on whether it is conducted or not. The qrs–t complex is of normal configuration.
- Specific anti-dysrhythmic treatment should not be undertaken until any underlying cause is identified and treated.
- In horses in which post-viral or immune-mediated myocarditis is suspected, corticosteroids and rest may be successful.
- Digoxin to slow the ventricular response rate is indicated for rapid atrial tachycardia.

Atrial fibrillation

- Atrial fibrillation is the most common clinically significant dysrhythmia in the horse.
- The horse is predisposed to the development of atrial fibrillation because of its high vagal tone which promotes electrical heterogeneity in the atrial myocardium, and because it has a large heart which has sufficient mass to sustain atrial fibrillation.

• It can occur in isolation as a primary disorder or secondary to a variety of cardiac diseases in which atrial enlargement is present, e.g. left atrioventricular insufficiency, right atrioventricular insufficiency, atrial septal defect, and complex congenital cardiac defects.

• In horses with uncomplicated atrial fibrillation, the clinical signs depend on the horse's occupation: horses in light work often show no signs, whereas competition horses and racehorses present with poor performance or exercise intolerance.

• Atrial fibrillation can be a consequence of conditions causing congestive heart failure, but is rarely a cause of clinical signs of congestive heart failure.

• In some horses, atrial fibrillation is paroxysmal and reverts to normal sinus rhythm without treatment within 24 hours. This has been documented most often in horses with gastrointestinal disease and during exercise. Potassium deficiency may predispose horses to developing paroxysmal atrial fibrillation.

• On auscultation, an irregularly irregular heart rate with no fourth heart sound, and variable intensity heart sounds are heard.

• The pulses vary in their strength.

• On ECG, there is no regular rhythm, the r–r intervals are variable and the p waves are replaced by f waves, irregular undulations of the base line (Figure 5).

• Horses with atrial fibrillation should be assessed with the aim of identifying any underlying cardiac disease: auscultation is used to identify cardiac murmurs; echocardiography is used to identify atrial enlargement and characterize any underlying cardiac disease; cardiac isoenzyme assay is used to identify active myocardial pathology.

• Horses with uncomplicated atrial fibrillation can be treated with quinidine sulphate. Quinidine is effective because it prolongs the myocardial refractory period. It is administered by nasogastric tube at 22 mg/kg every 2 hours for four or five treatments and thereafter every 6 hours until the atrial fibrillation resolves or toxic side effects develop. The duration of the qrs complex is measured before each treatment and, if it is greater than 25% longer than its pretreatment value, treatment is abandoned because it is likely that toxic concentrations are present.

• Cardiac side effects of quinidine include rapid supraventricular tachycardia due to its vagolytic action, and ventricular tachycardia due to its proarrhythmic action. It is also an alpha-adrenergic antagonist and produces hypotension. These cardiac dysrhythmias can be detected most easily if the ECG is monitored continuously during treatment. Rapid supraventricular tachycardia is treated with intravenous digoxin (0.002 mg/kg IV) to slow the ventricular response rate, sodium bicarbonate (1 mEq/kg IV) to reduce the circulating concentrations of quinidine, and polyionic fluids intravenously to increase the blood pressure. Quinidine-induced ventricular tachycardias have responded to treatment with magnesium sulphate (2 g IV boluses up to a total dose of 25 g) or propanolol (0.05-0.16 mg/kg IV).

• Extracardiac side effects of quinidine include tympanitic colic, diarrhoea, upper airway oedema and stridor, ataxia and laminitis. The gastrointestinal side effects are most common and these tend to be dose-dependent. If they are severe, quinidine administration must be abandoned.

• After successful conversion to sinus rhythm, a 24 hour ECG should be obtained to determine if there is a significant number of APDs present. If the 24 ECG is normal the horse can return to exercise immediately. If APDs are present, the horse should be rested until the 24 hour ECG is normal (usually 4 to 8 weeks).

• The prognosis for successful treatment of atrial fibrillation depends on the presence of underlying heart disease and also on the duration of the condition prior to treatment. In horses with long-

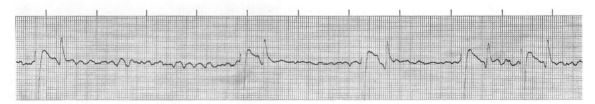

Figure 5 An ECG from a 4-year-old Thoroughbred gelding with atrial fibrillation. The r–r intervals are completely variable. There are no p waves and these have been replaced with f waves, identified as irregular undulations of the baseline (base–apex lead, 0.5 cm/mV, 25 mm/s).

standing atrial fibrillation, recurrence is more likely.

● Quinidine is contraindicated in horses with congestive heart failure. In these horses, treatment with digoxin and furosemide is indicated (see above).

Ventricular premature depolarizations and tachycardia

● Ventricular premature depolarizations (VPDs) can occur in association with any form of myocardial disease.
● Four or more VPDs occurring in sequence is defined as ventricular tachycardia.
● Ventricular tachycardia is the commonest dysrhythmia seen in horses with gastrointestinal disease.
● Infrequent VPDs (less than 5 in 24 hours) are occasionally seen in normal horses.
● Isolated VPDs are sometimes seen immediately after exercise as the heart slows and these are considered insignificant, provided that they are isolated, infrequent and do not occur during exercise.
● Frequent VPDs and sustained or paroxysmal ventricular tachycardia during exercise are clinically significant and can lead to collapse or even sudden death.
● On auscultation, a premature beat is heard.
● On ECG, a premature qrs–t complex with an abnormal configuration is present (Figure 6). If all the premature complexes have the same configuration, they are termed monomorphic, and if they have more than one configuration, they are termed polymorphic.
● Specific antidysrhythmic treatment should not be undertaken until any underlying cause is identified and treated.
● In horses in which post-viral or immune-mediated myocarditis is suspected, corticosteroids and rest can be successful.

● Antidysrhythmic therapy is indicated in horses with ventricular tachycardia, if the dysrhythmia itself is life threatening. The following criteria are used to identify these cases:
  – The ventricular rate is greater than 100 per minute.
  – The ventricular tachycardia is polymorphic.
  – Signs of low cardiac output are present (weakness, collapse, weak peripheral pulses, pale mucous membranes).
  – The r on t phenomenon is present (the qrs complex is superimposed on the preceding t wave).
● Specific antidysrhythmic therapy for ventricular tachycardia includes quinidine gluconate (0.7–3 mg/kg/hour as an IV infusion; side effect – hypotension), lignocaine (0.5 mg/kg IV boluses up to 2 mg/kg: side effect – convulsions and seizures), procainamide (1 mg/kg/min IV), and magnesium sulphate (2 g IV boluses up to 25 g). Propranolol (0.05–0.16 mg/kg IV) has been used with limited success.

Ventricular fibrillation

● Ventricular fibrillation describes the state in which there is no organized electrical activity in the heart.
● It is a terminal event that is most easily recognized under general anaesthesia and in foals in intensive care.
● On auscultation, no heart sounds are audible and there is no peripheral pulse.
● On ECG, there are no recognizable complexes, and these are replaced by chaotic undulations of the baseline.
● Ventricular fibrillation is an emergency and requires immediate resuscitation. The principles of cardiopulmonary resuscitation in horses are the same as those recommended for other species:
  – A, airway: ensure there is an effective airway – endotracheal intubation.

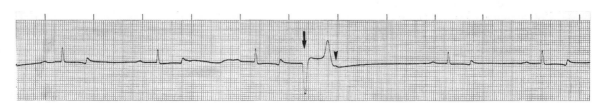

Figure 6 An ECG from a 13-year-old Thoroughbred gelding illustrating a ventricular premature depolarization (arrow). It is premature, large and negative, and is not preceded by a p wave, whereas the sinus complexes are smaller, positive and all have p waves before them. Immediately after the ectopic t wave, a small, unconducted sinus p wave (arrowhead) is visible.

– B, breathing: in foals an Ambu bag is effective, in adults a demand valve can be used.
– C, circulation: initiate external cardiac massage immediately – apply pressure to the chest; consider the use of adrenaline (1–5 mg/kg IV or via a tracheal catheter) to increase vascular tone; internal cardiac massage should be considered if external methods are ineffective.

• The treatment of choice for ventricular fibrillation is electrical defibrillation. However, this is only feasible in foals, weanlings and small ponies. Lignocaine (0.5 mg/kg IV boluses up to 2 mg/kg) and bretyllium may be effective but the prognosis is extremely poor. Bretyllium is used at 5–10 mg/kg in humans; dosage recommendations for horses are not available.

Advanced atrioventricular block

• Second and third degree atrioventricular block can arise secondary to inflammation or fibrosis at the atrioventricular node and in association with certain drugs, notably halothane. This is also the commonest form of dysrhythmia seen in foals with hyperkalaemia associated with uroperitoneum.
• In advanced atrioventricular block that develops under anaesthesia, treatment with atropine (0.01–0.2 mg/kg IV) or glycopyrrolate (0.005 mg/kg), and/or dopamine (1–5 µg/kg/min) or dobutamine (1–5 mg/kg/min) is recommended.
• If myocardial inflammation is suspected, corticosteroids may be effective.
• Permanent transvenous pacemakers have been used successfully in horses with third degree atrioventricular block.

Asystole

• Asystole describes complete absence of cardiac electrical and mechanical activity.
• It is a terminal event which is most easily recognized under general anaesthesia and in foals in intensive care.
• On auscultation, no heart sounds are audible, and there is no peripheral pulse.
• On ECG, there is a straight line with no electrical activity.
• Asystole is an emergency and requires immediate resuscitation. The principles of cardiopulmonary resuscitation in horses are summarized above.

• Adrenaline (1–5 µg/kg IV) should be administered for asystole.

7.15 *Pericarditis*

• The pericardium is a thin, highly vascular membrane that encloses the heart and proximal portions of the great vessels.
• Inflammation of the pericardial sac is fairly uncommon in horses, but potential causes include bacterial and viral infections, blunt or penetrating trauma and neoplasia. It can be secondary to septic endocarditis or pleuropneumonia. However, the majority of cases are idiopathic.
• Pericarditis can be either effusive or constrictive, and both types can coexist.
• In effusive pericarditis, there are large volumes of free fluid within the pericardium which compress the heart and lead to cardiac tamponade as pressure within the pericardial space increases. The right-sided structures are most susceptible because they have lower pressures, but as the volume of fluid increases, the left side of the heart is also compressed.
• Pericardial effusions often contain large amounts of fibrin and variable quantities of protein and inflammatory cells.
• In constrictive pericarditis, the pericardium becomes thickened, impeding diastolic filling.
• The clinical signs of pericarditis vary depending on the amount of pericardial effusion and the rate of fluid accumulation. Presenting signs can include fever, depression, anorexia and weight loss. Specific cardiovascular signs reflect right-sided and low output cardiac failure. These include tachycardia, jugular vein distension, marked ventral oedema and pleural effusion, and decreased renal output.
• On auscultation, the heart sounds are muffled.
• On ECG, the heart rate is fast and usually regular, but the amplitude of the complexes is decreased.
• Echocardiography confirms the presence of effusion, fibrin tags and thickening of the pericardium, and demonstrates impaired cardiac filling.
• Horses with effusive pericarditis have been successfully treated with broad spectrum antibiotics and pericardial lavage. An indwelling drain is inserted into the pericardium from the left fifth

intercostal space. Echocardiography is used to select the optimum site. Lavage and instillation of antibiotics can be repeated twice a day. The prognosis for these horses is good, provided aggressive therapy is initiated early.

• Constrictive pericarditis carries a more guarded prognosis. Pericardectomy to surgically remove thickened pericardium has been attempted with limited success.

7.16 *Vascular disease*

Jugular thrombophlebitis

• Jugular thrombophlebitis frequently arises as a complication of venepuncture and vascular catheterization and can be either septic or non-septic.

• Sepsis is associated with needle or catheter contamination during insertion, migration of bacteria along a catheter from the skin, contaminated intravenous solutions or haematogenous spread.

• On clinical examination, the affected vein is enlarged. A cylindrical intraluminal mass can be palpated or the vein may feel corded. The patency of the vessel is reduced or absent. If sepsis is present, the vein is usually hot and painful. Venous occlusion leads to distension of the superficial vessels proximal to the thrombus, and, if the condition is bilateral, there is oedema of the muzzle, supraorbital areas and upper airway.

• Ultrasonography can be used to differentiate perivenous swelling from thrombophlebitis, to assess the degree of patency of the vessel, and to demonstrate cavitation of the thrombus which is consistent with sepsis.

• In septic thrombophlebitis, the thrombus should be aspirated to obtain a sample for bacteriological culture and antimicrobial sensitivity. If associated with a catheter, the catheter itself can be cultured.

• Treatment of thrombophlebitis includes topical and systemic anti-inflammatory drugs such as dimethyl sulphoxide ointments, and phenylbutazone or flunixin. Hot compresses can be applied over the area three or four times a day. The head should be tied in a raised position if there is extensive oedema. Occasionally emergency tracheostomy is necessary. Horses with septic thrombophlebitis should be treated with broad

spectrum antibiotics until specific sensitivity patterns are obtained.

• The prognosis in non-septic jugular thrombophlebitis is good: the vessel will often recanalize with time. Occasionally, upper airway oedema secondary to jugular thrombophlebitis causes poor performance.

• The prognosis in septic thrombophlebitis is guarded: potential sequelae include bacterial endocarditis, pulmonary thromboembolism and septicaemia.

Aortoiliac thrombosis

See Chapter 15.

Vascular rupture

• Vascular rupture is the commonest cause of sudden death of horses during exercise.

• Pulmonary artery rupture can be spontaneous or a sequel to cardiac diseases that produce pulmonary hypertension.

• Rupture of the middle uterine artery occurs in middle-aged or older broodmares in the periparturient period. These mares are found dead or present with abdominal pain. Some survive with supportive therapy.

• Aortic rupture has been described most frequently in aged breeding stallions. However, it can occur in any age or type of horse. It can be the sequel to aortic aneurysm or degenerative changes in the arterial wall. In some horses, a sinus of Valsalva aneurysm has been diagnosed echocardiographically prior to rupture, and abdominal aortic aneurysms are occasionally detected on rectal examination. However, aneurysms of the aorta are often undetected prior to rupture.

Further reading

Bernard, W, Reef, V.B. Sweeney R.W. *et al* (1990). Pericarditis in horses: six cases 1982–1986. *Journal of the American Veterinary Medical Association* **196**: 468.

Brown, C.M. Kaneene, J.B. and Taylor, R.F. (1988) Sudden and unexpected death in horses and ponies: an analysis of 200 cases. *Equine Veterinary Journal* **20**, 99.

Else, R.W. and Holmes, J.R. (1972) Cardiac pathology in the horse: 1. Gross pathology. *Equine Veterinary Journal* **4**, 1.

Else, R.W. and Holmes J.R. (1972) Cardiac pathology in the horse: 2. Microscopic pathology. *Equine Veterinary Journal* **4**, 57.

Marr, C.M. and Reef, V.B. (1995) Pathophysiology and diagnosis of cardiovascular disease. In *The Horse. Diseases and Clinical Management* (Eds C.N. Kobluk, T.R. Ames and R.J. Geor). W.B. Saunders, Philadelphia. p. 113.

Marr, C.M. and Reef, V.B. (1995) Cardiac arrhythmias. In *The Horse. Diseases and Clinical Management* (Eds C.N. Kobluk, T.R. Ames and R.J. Geor). W.B. Saunders, Philadelphia. p. 137.

Marr, C.M. and Reef, V.B. (1995) Disturbances of blood flow. In *The Horse. Diseases and Clinical Management* (Eds C.N. Kobluk, T.R. Ames and R.J. Geor). W.B. Saunders, Philadelphia. p. 157.

Muir, W.W. and McGuirk, S.M. (1985) Pharmacology and pharmacokinetics of drugs used to treat cardiac disease in horses. *Veterinary Clinics of North America* [Equine Practice] **1**, 335.

Patteson, M.W. and Cripps, P.J. (1993) A survey of cardiac auscultatory findings in horses. *Equine Veterinary Journal* **25**, 409.

Reef, V.B. (1990) Pericardial and myocardial diseases. In *The Horse. Diseases and Clinical Management* (Eds C.N. Kobluk, T.R. Ames and R.J. Geor). W.B. Saunders, Philadelphia. p. 185.

Reef, V.B., Levitan, C.W. and Spencer, P.A. (1988) Factors affecting prognosis and conversion in equine atrial fibrillation. *Journal of Veterinary Internal Medicine* **2**, 1.

Reef, V. B. (1990) Echocardiographic examination in the horse: the basics. *Compendium of Continuing Education for the Practising Veterinarian* **12**, 1312.

Reimer, J.M. (1992) Cardiac arrhythmias. In *Current Therapy in Equine Medicine* (Ed. N.E. Robinson), 3rd Edn. W.B. Saunders, Philadelphia, p. 383.

Appendix. Differential diagnosis of conditions presenting with cardiovascular signs

1. Systolic murmur loudest over the left hemithorax
Physiological murmur associated with aortic ejection
Left atrioventricular valvular insufficiency
Left atrioventricular valvular prolapse
Tetralogy of Fallot
Other complex congenital cardiac defects

2. Systolic murmur loudest over the right hemithorax
Right atrioventricular valvular insufficiency
Ventricular septal defect
Right atrioventricular atresia
Other complex congenital cardiac defects

3. Diastolic murmur
Physiological murmur associated with ventricular filling
Aortic valvular insufficiency
Pulmonic valvular insufficiency

4. Dysrhythmia
Second degree atrioventricular block
Sinus arrhythmia
Sinus pause or arrest
Atrial premature depolarizations or tachycardia
Atrial fibrillation
Ventricular premature depolarizations or tachycardia
Ventricular fibrillation

5. Ventral oedema
Protein losing enteropathy
Lymphadenopathy
Vasculitis
Congestive cardiac failure
Right-sided cardiac failure
Pericarditis
Pleuropneumonia
Cranial thoracic mass
Hepatic fibrosis and portal hypertension
Advanced pregnancy

6. Pleural effusion
Pleuropneumonia
Cranial mediastinal lymphosarcoma
Other thoracic neoplasia
Pericarditis
Right-sided cardiac failure

7. Jugular distension
Cranial mediastinal lymphosarcoma or mass
Jugular thrombosis
Congestive cardiac failure
Pericarditis

8. Poor performance
(Note only cardiovascular conditions are listed here; other causes such as respiratory and musculoskeletal conditions should also be considered)
Left atrioventricular valvular insufficiency
Atrial fibrillation
Exercise-induced dysrhythmias (atrial or ventricular premature depolarizations)
Ventricular septal defect
Jugular thrombosis
Cardiomyopathy

9. Collapse

Narcolepsy/cataplexy
Epilepsy
Vascular rupture
Supraventricular or ventricular premature depolarizations or tachycardia
Advanced second degree or third degree atrio-ventricular block
Complex congenital cardiac defects
Dehydration
Anhydrosis
Rhabdomyolyis
Vasovagal syndrome
Neurological conditions

8 Diseases of the urogenital system

CONTENTS

8.1 Evaluation of the urinary system

Renal function and water balance in the normal horse

- Water intake: varies greatly depending upon diet, ambient temperature, exercise, lactation and psychogenic factors. Range: 20–90 litres/day.
- Urination frequency: 7–11 times daily (foals urinate hourly).
- Urine volume: 2–16 litres daily.
- Urine character: pale yellow to brown (may darken upon standing). *Viscid* due to mucus secreting cells in the renal pelvis. Often *opaque* due to suspension of calcium carbonate crystals. Horses fed legume hay form large amounts of calcium carbonate crystals and thus tend to have more opaque urine than horses fed grass hay.

Physical examination

Only the caudal pole of the left kidney can be palpated *per rectum*. Evaluation is *highly subjective*, but:

- Enlargement and pain response may be noted if the horse is in acute renal failure.
- Shrinkage, firmness and irregular surface may be noted if the horse is in chronic renal failure.

Ultrasonic examination

- Equipment – 3.0–3.5 MHz transducer for percutaneous examination (5.0 MHz for foals); 5.0–7.5 MHz transducer for examination *per rectum*.
- Location – level of tuber coxae and 15th to 16th intercostal space for right kidney and paralumbar fossa for left kidney.

- Indications:
  - Distinguishing acute and chronic renal disease. Acute – swollen kidney with decreased echogenicity. Chronic – small, irregular kidney with increased echogenicity.
  - Diagnosis of renal cysts, urinary calculi, urinary neoplasia, uroperitoneum, etc.

Endoscopic examination

Endoscopic examination is useful in diagnosis of cystitis, urinary calculi, pyelonephritis, sources of haematuria, etc.

Percutaneous renal biopsy

Usually Vim–Silverman type or Tru-Cut (Travenol) needles are used.

- Ultrasonically guided.
- Assistant guided – the left kidney is grasped *per rectum*; needle puncture of the kidney can then be felt. Serious haemorrhage can result. Perform only if information gained is necessary to determine treatment. Of most value for assessment of suspected chronic renal failure.

Laboratory assessment of urinary tract disease

1. Serum urea nitrogen (SUN) – concentration rises when glomerular filtration rate (GFR) decreases. Not a reliable indicator of GFR because it is affected by non-renal factors. Anorexia and liver disease decrease concentration of SUN; increased protein intake increases concentration of SUN.
2. Serum creatinine – concentration rises when GFR decreases. Production (from muscle) is fairly constant. Not significantly absorbed or secreted by renal tubules. Therefore, creatinine approximates GFR. Azotaemia (elevated

concentration of SUN and/or creatinine) is not necessarily indicative of renal disease or the severity of renal disease.

3. Creatinine clearance – a reliable index of GFR in horses. Determined by comparing creatinine concentrations in serum (Scr) and urine (Ucr) and the rate of urine production. Reference range is 1.39 to 1.87 ml/min/kg. Concentrations below the reference range indicate decreased GFR. Clearance cr = Ucr/Scr × ml/min/kg body weight.

4. Serum electrolytes
   • Tendency toward hyponatraemia, hypochloraemia, and hyperkalaemia in renal failure. Degree of abnormality, if any, depends upon diet, appetite and duration of renal failure.
   • Hypo-, normo-, or hypercalcaemia can occur in renal failure. Depends upon diet, appetite, duration of failure, and age of the horse. Hypercalcaemia in renal failure is unique to the horse and is poorly understood.
   • Hypo-, normo-, or hyperphosphataemia can be seen in equine renal failure.

5. Fractional excretion (clearance) of electrolytes – in renal tubular disease, electrolytes may be inappropriately excreted in urine. Because the clearance of creatinine is constant over time, the excretion of electrolytes can be compared to the excretion of creatinine. The formula for determining fractional excretion of an electrolyte (FE$_e$) is derived in the following manner:

$$FE_e = \frac{Clearance\ e}{Clearance\ Cr} \times 100$$

$$FE_e = \frac{Ue/Se \times urine\ vol/time/kg\ body\ wt}{Ucr/Scr \times urine\ vol/time/kg\ body\ wt} \times 100$$

$$FE_e = \frac{Scr}{Ucr} \times \frac{Ue}{Se} \times 100$$

Values > reference range indicate increased loss of electrolyte in urine, and may reflect inability of renal tubular cells to reabsorb these electrolytes (sodium Na, inorganic phosphorus P)

FE$_{Na}$ – normally ≤1%; useful for differentiating prerenal and renal azotaemia. See Prerenal azotaemia, clinicopathologic signs (p. 159).

FE$_p$ – normally ≤1%; increases occur not only in renal disease but also in primary or pseudohyperparathyroidism and secondary nutritional hyperparathyroidism.

6. Urine to plasma or serum ratios for urea nitrogen (un), creatinine (cr) and osmality (osm). Useful in distinguishing between renal and prerenal azotaemia, but measurements for renal and prerenal azotaemia may overlap. Based on a small number of azotaemic horses, reported measurements are:
   • Uun/Pun – 15.2–43.7 (prerenal); 2.1–14.3 (renal)
   • Ucr/Pcr – 51.2–241.5 (prerenal); 2.6–37 (renal)
   • Uosm/Posm – 1.7–3.4 (prerenal); 0.8–1.7 (renal)

7. Urinary enzymology – when renal tubular cells die, enzymes contained within these cells are released into the urine. Abnormally high concentrations of *gamma glutamyl-transferase* (GGT) indicate renal tubular damage. Comparison of UGGT concentration to Ucr concentration corrects for the effect of urine concentration on enzyme concentration.

$$\frac{UGGT}{Ucr} \times 100 = < 50\ in\ normal\ horses$$

Elevation indicates that tubular necrosis is occurring. Urinary concentrations of GGT are unaffected by serum concentrations of GGT. Concentration of UGGT is useful in monitoring for aminoglycoside-induced renal tubular necrosis.

8. Urinary specific gravity (USG) – tends to be between 1.030 and 1.060, but fluctuates widely. Random urine samples may indicate hyposthenuria, isosthenuria (USG 1.008–1.019) or hypersthenuria. Foals tend to be hyposthenuric because they have a large fluid intake. Possible explanations for dilute urine in the adult horse include:
   • Excessive water intake from psychogenic causes
   • Renal failure
   • Fluid therapy
   • Diabetes insipidus, central or renal
   A water deprivation test may distinguish between these causes if the cause is not obvious. For the water deprivation test, the horse is weighed and held off water until changes in USG make the cause obvious, or until the horse has a 5% weight loss. USG in the isosthenuric range in a dehydrated horse suggests renal disease.
   • USG < 1.020 in horses with clinical dehydration and/or azotaemia is highly suggestive of renal failure due to renal disease.

- Azotaemia associated with USG >1.030 indicates prerenal azotaemia.
9. Urinary pH. Normally *alkaline* (pH is usually between 7.5 and 8.5). Urine may be acidic in cases of:
   - Prolonged anorexia.
   - High grain diets.
   Urine of foals tends to be acidic.
10. Urinary sediment
   - Casts – presence of granular or cellular casts usually indicates renal disease; casts dissolve quickly in alkaline urine. Leucocyte casts are indicative of bacterial nephritis.
   - Bacteria – the presence of small numbers do not necessarily indicate urinary infection.
   - White blood cells – the presence of small numbers (≤8/high power field) are not abnormal.
   - Crystals – normal urine may contain crystals of calcium carbonate, triple phosphate, and oxalate.
11. Urinary protein – commercial dipsticks may falsely indicate the presence of protein in alkaline urine. The sodium sulphosalicyclic acid test should be performed to determine if the horse has proteinuria. Proteinuria without presence of blood or cellular debris is likely of renal origin, and may indicate glomerulonephritis.
12. Assessment of discolored urine – myoglobin, red blood cells or haemoglobin can cause reddish brown discoloration of urine. To differentiate:
   - If CPK is high – probably myoglobinuria.
   - If serum is clear – probably myoglobinuria; if coloured – probably haemoglobinuria.
   - Examine urine after centrifugation. If supernate is clear, then haematuria is the likely cause of discoloration.
   - Urine electrophoresis.

Renal disease vs. renal failure

Renal disease tends to be inapparent until *renal failure* occurs, and renal failure can occur without the presence of renal disease. Renal failure is the inability of the kidneys to excrete nitrogenous wastes and is characterized by *azotaemia* (elevated concentration of serum urea nitrogen and/or creatinine). Renal failure occurs when 75% of nephrons become temporarily or permanently non-functional. Azotaemia can occur in the absence of renal disease merely from decreased renal blood flow (*prerenal azotaemia*), or from disease of the urinary tract distal to the kidneys (urolithiasis, uroperitoneum) (*postrenal azotaemia*). Differentiating prerenal azotaemia from renal failure due to renal diseases (*renal azotaemia*) is not always straightforward. Renal failure may occur acutely or result from progressive disease (chronic renal failure).

8.2 *Prerenal azotaemia*

Prerenal azotaemia represents a decrease in GFR due to renal hypoperfusion. The condition is rapidly reversible.

Aetiology

The cause is usually *intravascular volume depletion* due to haemorrhage, diarrhoea, endotoxaemia, inadequate water consumption, etc.

Pathogenesis

Systemic hypotension stimulates the renin–angiotensin–aldosterone axis, release of antidiuretic hormone, and the sympathetic nervous system. As a result, blood flow is redistributed away from the renal cortex, and water is conserved.

Clinical signs

- In the horse, signs of gastrointestinal crisis (such as colic or diarrhoea) are often evident.
- Tachycardia.
- Oliguria.
- Dehydration (loss of skin turgor).

Clinicopathologic signs

- Haemoconcentration (increased packed cell volume (PCV) and/or albumin).
- Azotaemia with a urine specific gravity >1.030.
- Urine to plasma ratios of urea, creatinine, and osmolality may help distinguish prerenal from renal azotaemia.
- $FE_{Na} > 1\%$ is indicative of renal azotaemia especially if there is concurrent hyponatraemia.

Diagnosis

The diagnosis is based on clinical and clinico-pathological signs and rapid decrease in SUN and Scr in response to appropriate therapy.

Treatment

- Correction of the initiating cause. Usually involves treatment of gastrointestinal crisis.
- Fluid therapy.

8.3 *Acute tubular necrosis resulting in acute renal failure*

Aetiology

Acute renal tubular necrosis (RTN) resulting in acute renal failure (ARF) is usually due to *sustained* or *severe hypoperfusion*, or nephrotoxins, or a combination of both.

- Haemodynamic causes are most often initiated by endotoxaemia associated with some types of colic and acute diarrhoeal syndromes.
- Nephrotoxins.
  - Plants – include red maple and oak trees, onions, and white snake root. Plants containing oxalates are potentially nephrotoxic, but oxalate-induced nephropathy is rare in horses. Deposition of oxalate crystals in kidneys, however, may occur secondary to renal disease.
  - Heavy metals – mercury, lead, arsenic, and others.
  - Antibiotics – aminoglycosides (gentamicin, neomycin, amikacin), tetracycline, sulphonamides, cephaloridine, amphotericin B, and others.
  - Non-steroidal anti-inflammatory drugs – (NSAIDs) phenylbutazone and flunixin meglumine. NSAIDs are more likely to cause ARF when there is concurrent dehydration or shock.
  - Pigments – myoglobin and haemoglobin. Haemoglobinuria and myoglobinuria are an unlikely cause of ARF unless there is concurrent dehydration, shock, or acidosis.
- Acute septic pyelonephritis – most likely to occur in septicaemic neonates. *Leptospira* sp. and other bacteria can cause acute tubular necrosis in adults.

Pathogenesis

Renal tubular necrosis is induced by:

- Direct effect of nephrotoxins.
- Ischaemia caused by sympathetic constriction of renal vessels during circulatory shock.
- Inflammatory response to bacteria.

Clinical signs

Clinical signs of ARF due to RTN are *non-specific* – anorexia, depression and weakness. These clinical signs can also be attributed to a precipitating haemodynamic cause such as colic, colitis and myositis. Toxins that induce acute renal failure are often not renal specific, and clinical signs associated with organ damage of other systems may predominate.

Diagnosis

Acute renal failure due to RTN is usually diagnosed on the basis of clinical signs, physical examination, ultrasonography and laboratory evaluation.

- Caudal pole of left kidney may feel enlarged when palpated *per rectum*, or kidneys may appear enlarged on ultrasonic examination.
- Dilute urine (USG < 1.020) with concurrent dehydration and/or azotaemia.
- Granular urinary casts.
- Measurement of urinary enzymes. The UGGT/Ucr ratio is most commonly used.
- Fractional excretion of sodium and phosphorus may be increased.
- Glycosuria without hyperglycaemia.
- Urine to plasma ratios of urea, creatinine, or osmolality and FE_{Na} may help distinguish pre-renal from renal azotaemia.

Treatment

1. Treatment of predisposing disease process (e.g. endotoxaemia, myositis).
2. Removal of suspected nephrotoxins.
3. Correction of fluid balance, serum electrolyte concentration, and acid–base abnormality.
   - Intravenous fluid therapy if anuric or oliguric. Use balanced electrolyte solution. Isotonic fluid can be administered orally if the horse is polyuric. If oliguric, overhydration can be avoided by:
     - measuring central venous pressure,
     - monitoring for increases in body weight,

– auscultating lungs for oedema,
– observing for subcutaneous oedema,
– monitoring for marked decrease in PCV.
• If anuric or oliguric after rehydration, convert to polyuria with:
– 10% dextrose solution IV,
– 20% mannitol (0.25 to 1 g/kg IV),
– Furosamide (frusamide) (1 mg/kg, IV every two hours),
– Dopamine (1 to 5 mg/kg/min) in 5% dextrose IV.
4. Antimicrobial therapy is based on culture and sensitivity and ability of antimicrobial drug to concentrate in renal tissue and urine. Suggested drugs include trimethoprim-sulfonamide, aminoglycosides (monitor for nephrotoxicity) and penicillin G. Alternative drugs include cephalosporins, ticarcillin, ampicillin, tetracyclene and chloramphenicol.

Prognosis

• Toxin-induced nephrotoxicosis has a more favourable prognosis than does haemodynamic-induced nephrotoxicosis. Reason: the tubular cell basement membrane is more likely to be left intact in toxic nephritis, and cellular regeneration is more likely if the basement membrane is intact.
• Prognosis is fair to good if:
– Predisposing causes can be successfully treated.
– Creatinine stabilizes within 24 hours of therapy and then progressively declines over several days.
– The horse is polyuric.

8.4 *Chronic renal failure (CRF)*

Once thought to be a rare condition in horses, CRF is now considered to account for a significant proportion of horses presented for weight loss and anorexia.

Aetiology and pathogenesis

• Chronic glomerulonephritis – *most frequent cause of CRF* (does not always cause CRF. In one study 40% of equine kidneys examined at necropsy had microscopic glomerular lesions); there are two types of lesions:
– Antiglomerular basement membrane glomerulonephritis: due to antibodies directed against the glomerular basement membrane.
– Immune complex glomerulonephritis (most common type): due to deposition of immune complexes along the glomerular basement membrane. Immune complexes may be associated with upper respiratory infections caused by *Streptococci*.
With either type, the glomeruli become inflamed. The glomerular membrane becomes thickened from invasion of fibroblasts.
• Tubulointerstitial disease – (chronic interstitial nephritis) frequent cause of CRF; a sequel to acute renal tubular necrosis (induced by toxins or haemodynamic causes).
• Chronic septic pyelonephritis – an uncommon cause of renal failure in adult horses. The most frequently reported cause is ascending infection of the urinary tract, which is a consequence of urinary stasis caused by urolithiasis, neurological disease affecting the urinary tract (e.g. sorghum cystitis, herpes virus-1 myeloencephalitis), or trauma (e.g. from foaling). Renal infection can also occur by haematogenous spread. In adult horses, left-sided endocarditis is a cause.
• Bilateral renal hypoplasia – probably a congenital lesion; disease becomes evident when the horse is young.
• Chronic oxalate nephrosis – thought to be a consequence rather than a cause of CRF.
• Renal neoplasia – uncommon in horses. Three types reported: squamous cell carcinoma, adenocarcinoma and primary renal cell carcinoma (most common).
• Polycystic renal disease – very rare; probably a congenital disease that becomes evident at maturity.

Clinical signs

Signs vary depending upon the aetiology (i.e. chronic glomerulonephritis vs. tubulointerstitial disease vs. pyelonephritis, etc.).

• *Cachexia.*
• Anorexia and depression
• Dehydration.
• Polyuria/polydipsia (PU/PD). A differential list for PU/PD also includes Cushing's disease, psychogenic water-drinking or salt-eating, and diabetes insipidus.
• Peripheral oedema. Seen in chronic glomerulonephritis; due to extensive loss of plasma proteins through damaged glomerular capillaries. Triad of

oedema, hypoproteinaemia, and proteinuria is referred to as the *nephrotic syndrome*.
- Oral ulceration and dental tartar – occasionally observed.
- Fever – may be seen with pyelonephritis.
- Palpation *per rectum* and/or ultrasonic examination may reveal shrunken, firm kidney(s) with an irregular surface.
- Endoscopic visualization of ureteral discharge of blood or pus may be noted in horses with pyelonephritis.

Clinicopathological signs

Laboratory findings vary depending on the aetiology, stage of disease, and management factors.

- Anaemia – due to decreased renal erythropoietic factor and shortened RBC lifespan. Horses with pyelonephritis may have severe renal haemorrhage.
- Leucocytosis.
- Proteinuria – if glomerulonephritis is the cause of CRF, proteinuria is a consistent finding. Tubulointerstitial disease and pyelonephritis cause minimal proteinuria.
- Urine USG is usually in the isosthenuric range.
- Horse is usually azotaemic.
- Concentrations of serum electrolytes may be abnormal.
  - Hypochloraemia and hyponatraemia
  - Normo- or slight hyperkalaemia
  - Hypercalcaemia. Some horses with CRF on high calcium diets become hypercalcaemic.
- Pyuria and haematuria may accompany pyelonephritis.

Diagnosis

The diagnosis is based on clinical and clinicopathological signs, endoscopic and ultrasonic examination and renal biopsy.

Treatment

Chronic renal failure is progressive. Clients should be advised that treatment is aimed at prolonging life rather than resolving the condition.

- Supplementation of electrolytes based on periodic evaluation of serum concentrations of sodium, potassium, calcium and bicarbonate. (If oedema develops, sodium should be restricted from the diet, even if the horse is hyponatraemic.)
- Dietary supplementation with carbohydrates and fat.
- Restriction of dietary protein to less than 10%.
- Forced feeding in cases of anorexia.
- Anabolic steroids.
- Glucocorticosteroids – used in humans with glomerulonephritis, but no evidence for efficacy in the horse; may promote muscle wasting.
- Antimicrobial therapy for pyelonephritis. Selection of drug is based on culture and sensitivity and ability of antimicrobial drug to concentrate in renal tissue and urine.

8.5 *Cystitis*

Aetiology

- Primary (i.e., no easily discernible cause) is very rare.
- Secondary – also rare; secondary to urinary stasis with subsequent bacterial proliferation. Caused by:
  - Cystic calculi.
  - Neurologic disease of the urinary tract such as sorghum cystitis, herpes virus I myelo-encephalitis, polyneuritis equi, etc.

Clinical signs

- Pollakiuria (unduly frequent urination) that may resemble signs of oestrus, dysuria (difficult urination), and urine dribbling.
- Perineal scalding in the mare and soiling of hind legs in the male.
- Gross haematuria in some cases of pyelonephritis. (A differential list for haematuria also includes urolithiasis, renal and vesicular neoplasia, and urethral defects into the corpus spongiosum penis.)

Clinicopathological findings

Examination of urine sediment for:

- White blood cells (WBCs).
- Red blood cells (RBCs).
- Large number of bacteria.

Diagnosis

Clinicopathological findings confirm the presence or urinary tract infection, and physical examination (thickened bladder palpated *per rectum*) and/or cystoscopic examination (thickened, hyperaemic, or ulcerated mucosa) localize the infection to the bladder.

Treatment

● Correction of a predisposing cause if possible, such as removal of cystic calculi.
● Antimicrobial therapy based on culture and sensitivity and ability of antimicrobial drug to concentrate in urine.

8.6   *Urolithiasis*

Uroliths or calculi can form in the kidney (nephrolithiasis), ureters (ureterolithiasis) or bladder (cystic urolithiasis). Cystic uroliths, if small, may be voided on urination or cause urethral obstruction. Uroliths are usually composed of calcium carbonate.

Aetiology

● High urinary concentration of insoluble complexes (i.e. calcium carbonate) – unlikely cause in the horse.
● Mineralization of a nidus. Renal disease may provide the nidus for nephro and ureterolithiasis. NSAID-induced nephropathy has been speculated to be the cause of nidus formation in horses with nephrolithiasis and ureterolithiasis.
● Abnormally low concentration of natural inhibitors of mineral complexes in urine. High content of mucus produced by glands in the renal pelvis may prevent crystal aggregation.

Clinical signs of nephrolithiasis and ureterolithiasis

Clinical signs of chronic renal failure (cachexia, anorexia, depression, dental tartar, oral ulcers, etc.). Calculi may cause or be the result of renal disease.

Clinical signs of cystic and urethral calculi

● Urine dribbling, dysuria or pollakiuria. A differential list for diseases causing similar signs includes cystitis, urethritis and abdominal pain.
● Prolonged periods of penile protrusion. A differential list for diseases causing similar signs includes cystitis, urethritis and abdominal pain.

● Haematuria, especially after exercise.
● Stilted hindlimb gait.

Clinicopathological examination

● Evidence of renal failure may be found in a high percentage of horses with nephrolithiasis or ureterolithiasis.
● Haematuria.
● Evidence of cystitis (increased concentration of WBCs and RBCs, large number of bacteria).

Diagnosis

● Examination *per rectum* – cystic calculi are easily palpated. Ureteroliths or dilated ureters can be palpated *per rectum*.
● Ultrasonic examination – percutaneous or *per rectum*.
● Cystoscopic examination.
● Inability to pass urinary catheter may indicate the presence of a urethral calculus.

Treatment

● Renal function of both kidneys should be assessed before nephrolithiasis or ureterolithiasis is treated because bilateral renal failure is a common finding.
● Surgical removal of the calculus:
  – coeliotomy and cystotomy or ureterotomy;
  – pararectal cystotomy;
  – urethral sphincterotomy (in mares);
  – ischial urethrotomy (for removal of small cystic calculi of males);
  – urethrotomy at any site (for removal of urethral calculi).
● Electrohydraulic lithotripsy.
● Antimicrobial therapy for concurrent bacterial infection.

Prevention of recurrence

Rate of recurrence of cystic calculi has not been assessed for large numbers of cases. It is probably low and may not justify preventive measures, such as urinary acidification with:

● Ammonium chloride – commonly used, but results vary.
● Ascorbic acid – unpalatable at the high dose needed.

Providing 1% salt in the concentrate ration and an unlimited supply of water has also been recommended.

8.7 *Uroperitoneum*

Aetiology and pathogenesis

- Adults – bladder rupture:
  - during parturition or after parturition (due to bladder necrosis);
  - urethral obstruction by calculi (males).
- Foals – bladder rupture and urachal tears, ureteral defects.
  - Prenatal distension of the bladder (perhaps caused by partial torsion of the umbilical cord) coupled with pressure on the full bladder during parturition leads to rupture of bladder or urachus. Affected foals are usually male.
  - Congenital bladder defects may be responsible for uroperitoneum of some foals.
  - Bladder and urachal rupture may occur due to lesions caused by urinary tract infections.
  - Tenesmus associated with gastrointestinal disease may cause urachal tears.
  - Leakage of urine through a thin bladder wall.

Clinical signs (foals)

Usually occur within the first week postpartum.

- Abdominal distension; fluid can be balloted.
- Tachycardia and tachypnoea.
- Anorexia and depression.
- Pollakiuria, anuria, urine dribbling, straining to urinate, or normal urination may be noted.
- Outward bulging of vaginal mucosa may be seen in fillies with rupture of the ureter.

Clinicopathological findings

- Concentration of creatinine in peritoneal fluid containing urine is usually double that of serum creatinine (exception is foals evaluated early after bladder rupture).
- Hypochloraemia, hyponatraemia, and hyperkalaemia in foals. These electrolyte abnormalities may not be noted in the adult.
- Foals are usually, but not necessarily, azotaemic.
- Calcium carbonate crystals may be seen in peritoneal fluid.

Diagnosis

- Clinical signs and clinicopathological findings.
- Ultrasonography.
- Dye (methylene blue or fluorescein) placed into the bladder and subsequently recovered in peritoneal fluid.
- Positive contrast cystography (do not use barium).
- For diagnosis of suspected ureteral defects, exploratory laparotomy and cystotomy are performed. The ureters are infused with dye such as methylene blue, and examined for leakage. Intravenous pyelography is not very useful.

Treatment

Cystorrhaphy and/or resection of urachus. Preoperative stabilization is very important to minimize risks associated with anaesthesia. Therapy might involve:

- Measures to lower the potential for cardiac arrhythmia caused by high serum concentration of potassium.
  - Isotonic or hypertonic saline, IV.
  - 5% dextrose, IV and insulin.
  - Calcium, IV.
  - Enemas of sodium polystyrene sulphonate (a potassium removing resin).
  - Mask induction and anaesthesia with isoflurane, which is less arrythmogenic than halothane.
- Peritoneal drainage.
- Antimicrobial drugs.

8.8 *Patent urachus*

The urachus, which connects the foal's bladder with the allantoic cavity, normally closes at or shortly after birth.

Aetiology

The urachus may fail to close or it may reopen due to:

- Excessive traction on the umbilicus at birth.
- Infection of umbilical cord remnants.
- Abdominal straining.

Clinical signs

- Moist navel.
- Urination from the navel.

- Navel region may be enlarged from infection of umbilical cord remnants. (Infection may be the cause or result of a patent urachus.)
- Clinical signs of infection, such as joint-ill.

Diagnosis

- Clinical signs.
- Umbilical ultrasonography – umbilical cord remnants are scanned for evidence of infection.

Treatment

- If uncomplicated, cauterizing agents (silver nitrate, phenol, Lugol's iodine) are applied to the fistula for several days.
- Resection of the urachus and antimicrobial therapy are indicated as treatment of patent urachus if there is:
  - lack of response to conservative therapy;
  - evidence of infection of umbilical cord remnants;
  - evidence of sepsis of any distant site (such as joint-ill).

8.9 *Diagnosis of diseases of the testis and associated structures*

History and physical examination

History may include:

- Evidence of fertility/infertility.
- Presence of testicular retention.
- Changes in testicular size – *insidious increase in size* suggests neoplasia or hydrocele. *Rapid increase in size* suggests torsion, inguinal herniation or orchitis.
- Inguinal or scrotal swelling.
- Testicular pain (neoplasia is usually painless).
- Previous urogenital surgery.
- Previous illnesses.

Physical examination of the genitalia should include inspection and palpation of the testes.

- The left testis is usually larger and more pendulous than the right.
- Body of epididymis should be located on the dorsolateral surface of testis, and tail of epididymis should be located on the posterior pole of testis.

- Changes in testicular size or texture may indicate: orchitis, torsion, herniation or neoplasia. A neoplastic testis is usually insensitive to compression and heavier than normal. *Hydrocele* should be suspected if the scrotum is fluid-filled, and the testis is smaller than normal.
- If a testis is absent from the scrotum, the horse can be sedated to relax the cremaster muscles.

The scrotum should be examined for scrotal scars. A scar means only that orchidectomy was attempted – not that it was accomplished.

- Only the distal half of the inguinal canal can be palpated. The epididymis descends before the testis, and an epididymis that lies within the canal can be mistaken for an inguinal testis.
- Inguinal hernia may appear as an enlargement in the spermatic cord or scrotum. Palpation of a scrotal hernia may elicit crepitus, and peristalis may be evident. Skin over a strangulated hernia may be cold and oedematous. Fluid-filled, enlargement of the cord following castration is indicative of a hydrocele.

Examination *per rectum*

This is helpful in diagnosis and evaluation of cryptorchidism, inguinal herniation, and other urogenital conditions, but the risk of rectal tear should be weighed against the value of information to be gained. Small size and fractious nature of young horses predisposes them to rectal damage. Vaginal rings should always be palpated for inguinal incarceration of intestine when examining a colicky stallion *per rectum*.

- In average-sized horses, the *vaginal rings* can be palpated 6 to 8 cm cranial to the ilio-pectineal eminence and 10 to 12 cm abaxial to the midline.
- Vaginal rings are palpable in geldings as a slight depression, but, in stallions, the rings can accommodate a finger.
- For horses with unknown history of castration that display sexual behaviour but have no discernible testes examination *per rectum* may be useful in determining whether testes have entered the inguinal canal.
- Identification of an *abdominal testis, per rectum,* is difficult, so inability to rectally palpate an abdominal testis is diagnostically unreliable.
- Vaginal ring of a *complete abdominal cryptorchid* (i.e. one in which both the testis and epididymis are within the abdomen) cannot be palpated. If the vaginal ring can be palpated, the testis, or at least its epididymis, has probably descended through the ring into the inguinal canal.

Distinguishing a *partial abdominal cryptorchid* (i.e. one in which the testis is in the abdomen, but the epididymis is descended into the canal) from a horse whose testis and epididymis have entered the inguinal canal is difficult.

Hormonal assays

Hormonal assays are used to determine if a horse with persistent masculine behaviour has a retained testis.

Determination of concentration of testosterone in the plasma or serum

Stallions, including cryptorchids, have significantly greater concentrations of testosterone in the serum than do geldings. Concentration of testosterone in geldings is generally less than 40 pg/ml of serum and that of stallions is greater than 100 pg/ml. Concentration of testosterone of stallions varies seasonally (reaching its highest levels in the spring and summer) and with age. Concentration of testosterone is lowest in horses under 3 years of age.

Testosterone stimulation test

Concentration of testosterone in response to stimulation by human chorionic gonadotrophin (hCG) is determined. The test may be more accurate in determining whether a horse has testicular tissue than is evaluation of the horse's basal concentration of testosterone. The test is based on the fact that administration of hCG elicits a rise in concentration of serum testosterone. Following collection of serum for evaluation of basal concentration of testosterone, 6000 or 12 000 units of hCG are administered intravenously, and serum is again collected after 30 minutes (or up to 2 to 3 days later). A rise in the concentration of serum testosterone indicates that the horse has testicular tissue. Response to hCG, however, may be poor in horses less than 18 months old.

Concentrations of conjugated oestrogens

There is a high correlation between presence of testicular tissue and concentration of conjugated oestrogen. Exceptions are cryptorchid horses under 3 years of age and cyptorchid donkeys of any age. Horses with less than 50 pg of oestrone sulphate/ml of plasma or serum can be considered geldings and horses with concentrations in excess of 400 pg/ml can be considered to have testicular tissue.

Because a laboratory may have different standards from those listed above, it is important to know the laboratory's standards for normal hormonal concentrations of geldings and stallions when evaluating hormonal assays.

Other diagnostic tests

- Seminal evaluation. May aid in diagnosis of inflammatory testicular disease.
- Scrotal thermography. To detect variation in temperature between testes.
- Ultrasonography. To locate cryptorchid testes or detect other testicular abnormalites.
- Karyotyping. To determine sexual identity if intersexuality is suspected.
- Testicular biopsy. Seldom performed on horses.

8.10 *Castration*

Synonyms include *orchidectomy*, *emasculation*, *gelding* and *cutting*.

Indications

- To eliminate masculine behaviour and managerial problems that arise from this behaviour. Horses can be castrated at any age, but most are castrated when objectionable masculine behaviour begins, usually between 1 and 2 years of age.
- Indications for unilateral castration include:
  - Testicular neoplasia.
  - Testicular trauma.
  - Torsion of the spermatic cord.
  - Inguinal herniation.

Preoperative considerations

Physical examination should be performed before castration. The scrotum should be palpated, if the horse allows, to ensure that the horse is not a cryptorchid and that it has no inguinal hernia. Presence of either condition may change anaesthetic protocol or surgical approach.

Methods of restraint

Castration can be performed with the horse sedated and standing, after the spermatic cord is anaesthetized. Or, the horse can be anaesthetized and castrated in recumbency.

Advantages of standing castration
• Expense and risk of general anaesthesia are avoided.
• No need to wait for the horse to recover from anaesthesia.
• A clean, safe area to anaesthetize the horse is not required.

Disadvantages of standing castration
• Can be difficult and dangerous for the surgeon. Only docile stallions with well-developed testes should be castrated standing.
• Primary closure of scrotum is difficult.
• Risk of hernia/prolapse.

Common agents used to anaesthetize horses for castration include:

• Thiobarbiturates following sedation with xylazine.
• Ketamine HCl following sedation with xylazine, detomidine or romifidine.
• Guaiphenesin (5–10%) in combination with ketamine HCl or a thiobarbiturate.

Suxamethonium (succinylcholine) can be used to immobilize horses, but it provides no analgesia, and its use to restrain horses for castration is inhumane.

Techniques of castration

Regardless of whether the horse is castrated standing or anaesthetized and recumbent, the testes can be removed using one of three techniques.

1. Closed technique
Using this technique, each testis is isolated and removed while still encased by its parietal tunic. Removing the parietal tunic may decrease the incidence of postoperative complications such as infection of the cord and hydrocele. The closed technique is indicated when the testes are removed because of disease such as testicular neoplasia or infection.

2. Open technique
With this technique, the parietal tunic of each testis is opened, and the testis is removed. The parietal tunic of each testis remains within the horse. This technique requires less dissection than the closed technique and is often preferred when performing a standing castration. Open technique allows components of the cords to be examined before the cord is severed.

3. Half-closed technique
Each testis is isolated while still enclosed within its parietal tunic (as in the closed technique), but the parietal tunic is incised and the testis and cord are exteriorized from the parietal tunic before the tunic and testis are excised.

Scrotal incisions are usually left unsutured to heal by second intention, but they can be primarily closed. Sutured scrotal wounds heal with less complication, but primary closure increases anaesthetic time and must be performed under strict aseptic conditions.

Aftercare

• If previously vaccinated against tetanus, the horse should receive a tetanus toxoid booster.
• If not previously vaccinated against tetanus, the horse should receive both tetanus toxoid booster and tetanus antitoxin.
• Antimicrobial therapy and fly control are usually unnecessary.
• Horse should be exercised daily to prevent preputial and scrotal swelling. The horse should not be exercised for 24 hours after surgery, however, to prevent haemorrhage.

Postoperative complications of castration

Oedema

Some oedema is inevitable, especially on the 4th or 5th postoperative day, but excessive oedema is usually caused by insufficient exercise. Excessive oedema can be treated by increasing the horse's exercise and opening the scrotal wound if it is sealed.

Haemorrhage

The usual source of excessive haemorrhage is the testicular artery. Causes of excessive haemorrhage are:

- Improperly applied emasculators. Emasculators should be applied to the cord so that the crushing part of the emasculator's jaws is proximal to the cutting part.
- Emasculators that are too sharp causing the cord to be cut before it is properly crushed.
- Attempting to crush and cut a cord that is too large for the emasculator. Large cords should be separated into two sections and each crushed and cut separately.
- Heavy exercise of the horse before castration.

Treatment of excessive haemorrhage:

- If the horse has been castrated standing, the cord may still be anaesthetized with local anaesthetic, and, with the horse standing, the cord can be grasped and recrushed with the emasculator. Or a haemostat can be applied to the cord and removed the following day. If the horse was castrated under general anaesthesia, the horse may need to be reanaesthetized to recrush the cord.
- The scrotum can be packed with gauze, and temporarily closed with sutures or towel clamps.
- Fluid therapy and blood transfusions may be necessary.

Evisceration

Evisceration may follow castration if the horse has an inapparent inguinal hernia. May occur after several days, but most often occurs within several hours. Intestine that has entered the canal rapidly becomes strangulated. The horse should be immediately anaesthetized, and exposed intestine cleaned and replaced into the abdomen. The superficial inguinal ring should be sutured, or the canal packed with gauze. Devitalized and damaged intestine should be resected, and this is usually most easily accomplished through a ventral midline coeliotomy. If only omentum is visible at the scrotal wound, the horse's vaginal ring should be palpated *per rectum* to ensure that no intestine has entered the canal, and the omentum can be transected at the scrotum.

Funiculitis

Funiculitis, or infection of the cord, can occur from extension of scrotal infection or may arise from contaminated emasculators or ligature, especially braided non-absorbable sutures. A cord chronically infected with pyogenic bacteria is commonly called a 'scirrhous cord'. Abscessation of the stump of the cord caused by *Strepto-*

coccus spp. is sometimes referred to as 'champignon'.

Clinical signs of funiculitis include pyrexia, swelling in the inguinal region with discharging tracts and lameness. The swelling may or may not be painful. Clinical signs may not become apparent for months after castration. Treatment consists of:

- Antimicrobial therapy.
- Re-establishment of drainage.
- Surgical excision of the infected cord – only sure method of treatment.

Peritonitis

Subclinical, non-septic peritonitis probably occurs in many horses following castration, because the vaginal and peritoneal cavities communicate. Non-septic peritonitis may result from irritation of the peritoneal cavity by blood. Nucleated cell counts in excess of 10 000 cells/μl in the peritoneal fluid can frequently be found following castration and indicate peritoneal inflammation. If high nucleated cell counts are unaccompanied by degenerate neutrophils or bacteria, the peritonitis should be considered non-septic.

Signs of septic peritonitis following castration may include:

- Pyrexia.
- Signs of colic.
- Diarrhoea.
- Reluctance to move.

Treatment of septic peritonitis may include:

- Antimicrobial drugs.
- Non-steroidal anti-inflammatory drugs.
- Fluid therapy.
- Peritoneal lavage.
- Removal of source of peritoneal contamination, such as contaminated ligatures on the cord.

Penile damage

This is an uncommon complication of castration and usually occurs when the surgeon is unfamiliar with genital anatomy and the surgical procedure. The penis can be mistaken for an inguinal testis. Laceration of the urethra may result in urethral stricture and urethral fistulas.

Hydrocele (vaginocele)

A hydrocele or vaginocele is an idiopathic, pain-less, fluid-filled enlargement in the scrotal area that may occur weeks or months after castration. Fluid fills the vaginal cavity previously occupied by the testis. It should not occur if the horse was castrated using a closed or half-closed technique. Treatment is removal of the vaginal sac through an inguinal or scrotal incision.

Continued stallion-like behaviour

Horses that continue to display stallion-like beha-viour after castration are sometimes called 'false rigs'. Purported causes include:

• Psychic causes. Stallion-like behaviour in geld-ings should be attributed to psychic causes. Twenty to 30 per cent of horses may display some stallion-like behaviour regardless of the age at which they were castrated.
• Improper castration resulting in retention of epididymal tissue. Geldings that display stallion-like behaviour and contain epididymal tissue are sometimes said to be 'proud-cut'. The epididy-mis, however, contains no cells capable of pro-ducing androgens, and there is probably no such thing as a proud-cut horse.
• Heterotopic testicular tissue. Heterotopic testi-cular tissue has been found in pigs, but never in horses.
• Production of high concentrations of andro-gens by the adrenal cortex. This has never been shown to be responsible for stallion-like beha-viour of geldings.

8.11 *Congenital monorchidism*

Cryptorchid horses with one descended testis are sometimes improperly referred to as monorchids. Congenital monorchidism (i.e. agenesis of a testis) is extremely rare in horses.

8.12 *Cryptorchidism*

Cryptorchidism is failure of one or both testes to descend into the scrotum. Horses with this condi-tion are termed cryptorchids. Horses may be affected unilaterally or bilaterally. Colloquial

terms for the condition include 'rigs' and 'ridg-lings'. Cryptorchids may be classified as:

• *Complete abdominal cryptorchid.* Both the epidi-dymis and testis are located within the abdomen.
• *Partial abdominal cryptorchid.* The epididymis, but not the testis, has descended into the inguinal canal.
• *Inguinal cryptorchid.* The epididymis and testis have descended into the inguinal canal, but not into the scrotum. Inguinal cryptorchids are some-times referred to as 'high flankers'.

A cryptorchid testis produces androgens but is incapable of producing sperm. Bilaterally affected horses are sterile.

Aetiology

Cryptorchidism may result from improper func-tion of the gubernaculum, a mesenchymal cord that extends between the caudal pole of the testicle and scrotum and guides the foetal testis from the caudal pole of the kidney to the scrotum. Or, the testis may not descend from the abdomen if it is too large to pass into the inguinal canal. The condition is inheritable, but mechanisms of inheritance are complex and have not been clearly defined.

Incidence

Approximately 15% of 2- to 3-year-old colts are cryptorchid. Horses most commonly affected are Quarter horses, Percherons, American Saddle horses, ponies and crossbred horses. The breed least commonly affected is the Thoroughbred.

• Failure of right and left testicular descent occurs with nearly equal frequency.
• Seventy-five per cent of left undescended testi-cles are retained within the abdomen.
• Forty per cent of right undescended testicles are located abdominally.
• About 10 to 15% of cryptorchids are bilaterally affected.

Diagnosis

Diagnosis of cryptorchidism is based on history, palpation (both external and *per rectum*), hormo-nal assays and surgical exploration of the inguinal canal.

1. External palpation

The testes of prepubescent stallions are often difficult to palpate because they are small and retractile. To aid palpation, a sedative or tranquillizer can be administered to relax the cremaster muscles. Inguinal testes can sometimes be palpated, but, because the inguinal canal of the average-sized stallion is about 10 cm deep, inguinal testes high in the canal often cannot be palpated. The epididymis of a partial abdominal cryptorchid lies in the inguinal canal and can be mistakenly identified, by palpation, for an inguinal testis.

2. Palpation per rectum

Because palpation *per rectum* of an abdominal testis is difficult, and, because most horses presented for cryptorchid castration are young and fractious, the risk of rectal injury should be weighed against the value of diagnostic information to be gained. For an apparent gelding that displays stallion-like behaviour and whose history of castration is unknown, examination *per rectum* may be helpful. Failure to palpate an abdominal testis *per rectum*, however, should not be considered diagnostic.

Vaginal rings of geldings are palpable as a slight depression, but vaginal rings of stallions are large enough to accommodate a finger. A partial abdominal cryptorchid (i.e. one whose epididymis has descended into the canal) cannot be distinguished by examination of the vaginal rings from a horse whose testes have descended through the vaginal ring.

3. Hormonal assay

When history and physical examination are inadequate to determine whether a horse possesses a retained testis, hormonal assays can be used to distinguish between psychic or hormonal causes of persistent stallion-like behaviour. Concentration of serum testosterone or conjugated oestrogen in the plasma or serum can be used to distinguish between geldings and cryptorchids (see p. 166: 'Hormonal assays').

4. Surgical exploration on the inguinal canal

Finding the severed ends of the spermatic cords identifies the horse as a gelding.

Treatment

● If the horse is to be used for breeding purposes (possible only in the case of unilateral cryptorchidism), no treatment is necessary. Breeding is generally not recommended because the condition is hereditary.

● Hormonal or surgical treatment to effect descent is considered unethical and is usually ineffective. Retained testes become incapable of spermatogenesis, so bringing about their descent may not increase fertility.

● Because cryptorchidism is hereditary, affected horses are usually castrated. The scrotal testis should be removed only after the cryptorchid testis has been removed!

  – If the descended testis has been removed, and the cryptorchid testis cannot be found, the owner may misrepresent and sell the horse as a gelding.
  – Removal of only the descended testis may cause the retained testis to enlarge, via negative hormonal feedback, making future cryptorchidectomy difficult.
  – Future surgery to find the testis may be difficult if there is no written record of which testis was removed.

A cryptorchid testis can be removed through an inguinal, parainguinal, paramedian or flank approach. Except for the flank approach, the horse must be anaesthetized. Only an abdominal testis can be removed through a paramedian or flank approach because an inguinal testis cannot be retracted into the abdomen. Often the location of a testis cannot be determined prior to surgery. Because both abdominal and inguinal testes can be removed through an inguinal approach, determining the location of the testis prior to surgery is not necessary when this approach is used. Using an inguinal approach, an abdominal testis can be extracted through the vaginal ring or through a small incision adjacent to the medial crus of the superficial inguinal ring.

Incomplete cryptorchid castration

Occurs when the tail of the epididymis of a partial abdominal cryptorchid is mistakenly identified as a small inguinal testis and removed (Figure 1). The abdominal testis remains retained within the abdomen, and the horse's stallion-like behaviour persists.

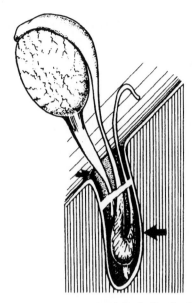

Figure 1 Failure to remove the abdominal testis of a partial abdominal cryptorchid can occur when the descended epididymis is mistaken for a small inguinal testis. If only the epididymis is removed, the horse retains stallion-like behaviour. Reproduced from article by Gayle Troffer, *Journal of the AVMA*, 1981, **178**, 246.

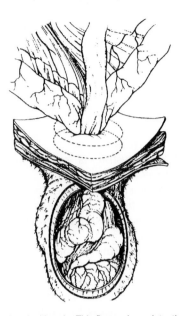

Figure 2 Inguinal hernia. This figure shows intestine protruding through the vaginal ring into the vaginal sac. Inguinal hernias of horses are sometimes inappropriately referred to as indirect hernias. Reproduced from Auer (Ed.) Equine Surgery, with permission (WBS, Philadelphia).

8.13 *Inguinal herniation and rupture*

- Inguinal herniation – protrusion of viscera through the vaginal ring into the vaginal sac (Figure 2). If the viscera descends to the scrotum, the condition is sometimes referred to as scrotal herniation. Inguinal hernias are sometimes referred to as indirect hernias, a term borrowed from a similar condition in man.
- Ruptured inguinal herniation – protrusion of herniated viscera through a rent in the vaginal sac (Figure 3).
- Inguinal rupture – protrusion of viscera through a rent in the peritoneum and musculature adjacent to the vaginal ring. Inguinal ruptures are sometimes inappropriately referred to as direct hernias. Direct hernias in man are caused by weakening in the inguinal musculature and are lined by peritoneum.

Aetiology

Inguinal herniation may be *congenital* or *acquired*. Inguinal hernias of foals are congenital and are caused by an enlarged vaginal ring. Inguinal hernias of adult stallions are usually acquired and often occur during breeding or exercise.

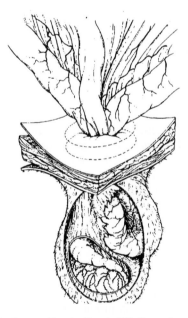

Figure 3 Ruptured inguinal hernia. This figure shows protrusion of herniated intestine through a rent in the parietal tunic. Reproduced from Auer (Ed.) Equine Surgery, with permission (WBS, Philadelphia).

Incidence

Congenital and acquired inguinal hernias may occur more frequently in Standardbreds. Congenital inguinal hernias may occur unilaterally (usually the left side) or bilaterally. Ruptured inguinal hernias occur much more commonly in foals.

Clinical signs

- Congenital hernias.
  - Herniated intestine is rarely strangulated and reduces easily.
  - Palpation of a scrotal or inguinal hernia may elicit a sensation of crepitus, and peristalsis beneath the scrotal skin may be visible.
- Acquired hernias.
  - Herniated intestine becomes strangulated, which leads rapidly to severe signs of colic. It cannot be easily reduced.
  - Vasculature of the cord becomes obstructed, which leads to scrotal and testicular oedema.

Diagnosis

- Scrotal enlargement may suggest inguinal herniation.
- Congenital inguinal hernia may become apparent only following castration when horse eviscerates. Inguinal area of foals should be closely examined for presence of congenital herniation prior to castration.
- Because acquired hernias are nearly always strangulated, skin over an acquired inguinal hernia may be cold and oedematous.
- Examination *per rectum* reveals that intestine has entered a vaginal ring.

Treatment

- Congenital.
  - Most congenital inguinal hernias cause no problem and spontaneously resolve by the time the foal is 6 months old.
  - Application of a truss may hasten resolution.
- Acquired inguinal hernias demand immediate attention because hernial contents are nearly always strangulated.
  - Reduction by external manual manipulation or rectal traction on incarcerated intestine – rarely successful.
  - Surgical reduction of hernia and removal of affected testis are usually required.

8.14 *Torsion of the spermatic cord*

Aetiology

This condition occurs when the testis rotates on its vertical axis. It may be caused by an excessively long scrotal ligament or caudal ligament of the epididymis, which allows the testis to rotate within the scrotal fascia or parietal tunic. These ligaments are part of the gubernaculum. Rotation of cord causes constriction of testicular blood supply.

Incidence

Torsion of spermatic cord is uncommon but is most often seen in Standardbreds.

Clinical signs

- Rotation of less than 180° causes no clinical signs. A tail of the epididymis located at the cranial pole of the testis indicates torsion of 180°.
- Rotation of 360° causes signs of pain and swelling of affected testis. A swollen testis and cord with the tail of the epididymis located at the caudal pole of the testis indicates torsion of 360°.

Treatment

- Torsion of the cord that causes no clinical signs (i.e. torsion of <180°) requires no treatment.
- If torsion causes irreversible strangulation of the cord, removal of affected cord and testis is indicated.
- If the cord is not irreversibly strangulated, testis can be permanently held in its proper position by a suture.

8.15 *Testicular neoplasia*

See Chapter 14.

8.16 *Intersex*

Definition

An intersex is an individual whose sexual identity is confused because of congenital anatomical

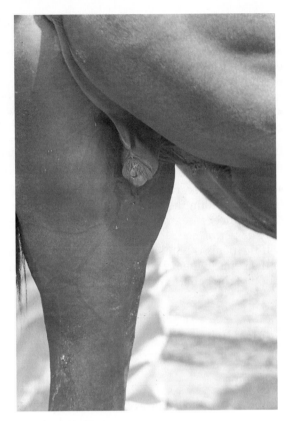

Figure 4 This male pseudohermaphrodite has a rudimentary penis and prepuce positioned caudal to the area where the scrotum should be.

abnormalities of the genitalia. An intersex may possess genitalia common to both sexes. Sexual identity can be defined by an animal's genetic makeup, its type of gonads, or the appearance of its accessory sex organs. A normal animal is the same sex in all three categories, but an intersex is different in one of the categories.

Types

• True hermaphrodite has both testicular and ovarian tissue. Not common.
• Pseudohermaphrodite has gonads of one sex, but external genitalia resemble that of the opposite sex.
    – Female pseudohermaphrodite. Has ovaries.
    – Male pseudohermaphrodite. Has hypoplastic, cryptorchid testes and a rudimentary penis and prepuce, which may resemble a clitoris, that are usually positioned caudal to the area where the scrotum should be (Figure 4). It is the most common intersex of horses. Most male pseudohermaphrodites are genetic females (64, XX).

8.17 Diagnosis of diseases of the penis and prepuce

History pertaining to penile and preputial disease should include previous injuries, illnesses, or urogenital surgery, conception rates, drug therapy, and duration of disease.

Physical examination of a horse with penile or preputial disease may include the following:

• Observation of urination. Urination can be stimulated by placing the horse in a freshly bedded stall or by administering furosemide.
• Visual inspection. Penis of a stallion can be protruded by administering xylazine or by causing sexual arousal. Phenothiazine-derivative tranquillizers probably should not be administered to stallions because they have, on rare occasion, caused penile paralysis or priapism.
• Palpation.
• Observation of erection and ejaculation.
• Ultrasonography.
• Cavernosography.

8.18 Penile and preputial injuries

Aetiology

The penis and prepuce can become damaged from:

• Failed attempts at jumping barriers.
• Masturbation.
• Kicks.
• Attempting to breed a mare over a fence, or from breeding a mare with a loosely tied breeding stitch.
• Improperly fitted or dirty stallion rings.
• Poor technique of castration.

Unsutured preputial and penile lacerations become infected, and cellulitis and swelling of the preputial and penile integument ensues. The penis and internal lamina of the prepuce may prolapse through the preputial orifice, and if left untreated, paralysis and permanent paraphimosis can result.

Treatment

• Fresh penile and preputial wounds should be sutured.
• Infected wounds should be cleansed and treated with antimicrobial ointment.

• If the penis has prolapsed, it should be replaced into the external prepuce and secured. If the penis is so swollen that it cannot be replaced, it should be wrapped against the ventral abdomen.
• Penile haematomas should be treated with compression wraps and hydrotherapy.
• If the penis is severely damaged, the most expedient treatment may be amputation, particularly if the horse is a gelding.

8.19 *Paraphimosis*

Aetiology

Paraphimosis, or inability of a horse to retract its penis into the prepuce, is caused by:

• Preputial oedema caused by genital trauma or systemic disease (e.g. dourine and purpura haemorrhagica).
• Damage to penile innervation. Can occur with spinal disease, trauma and infectious diseases.
• Debilitation.
• Phenothiazine-derivative tranquillizers (generally not a problem in geldings).

Pathophysiology

• Prolapse impairs venous and lymphatic drainage.
• Penis and internal preputial lamina swell from oedema, and preputial ring constricts distal penis.
• Oedema makes tissues fragile, and penile and preputial integument become excoriated.
• Excoriated integument becomes infected.
• Fibroblasts invade penile integument and fascia, permanently impairing the normal invaginating action of the prepuce.
• Pudendal nerves become stretched and damaged causing penile paralysis.
• Urination is unaffected, but impotence usually accompanies paralysis.

Treatment

Penile and preputial oedema and further trauma should be prevented by:

• Replacing the prolapsed penis within the external preputial lamina and retaining it with sutures, or towel clamps, or nylon netting placed across the preputial orifice.
• Compressing the prolapsed penis against the abdomen with wraps if it cannot be replaced within the external preputial lamina.
• Applying antimicrobial ointments to prevent epithelial excoriation and infection.
• Administering non-steroidal anti-inflammatory drugs to reduce swelling.
• Performing a *preputiotomy* if the inelastic preputial ring prevents penile retraction.

If paraphimosis is longstanding, the following measures must be taken:

• If preputial scarring prohibits replacement of the penis within the external preputial lamina of the prepuce, a segmental posthectomy (reefing) may be performed.
• If the penis is paralysed, permanent placement of the penis in the prepuce (phallopexy) or amputation of the penis may be indicated.

8.20 *Phimosis*

Aetiology

Phimosis (i.e. the inability of the horse to protrude its penis from the prepuce) can occur from congenital or acquired stricture of the preputial orifice or preputial ring.

• Congenital phimosis – rarely occurs in horses. (Fusion of the internal lamina of the prepuce to the free part of penis is normal during first month after birth.)
• Acquired phimosis – can be caused by tumors or damage at the preputial orifice or preputial ring.

Treatment

A triangle of external preputial fold based toward the preputial orifice is removed if the preputial orifice is constricted. If the preputial ring is constricted, a similar wedge is removed from the internal preputial fold.

8.21 *Priapism*

Aetiology

Priapism (i.e. persistent erection without sexual arousal) is uncommon in stallions but is economically significant because impotence is the usual outcome. Occurs when disturbances in arterial inflow or venous outflow prevent detumescence of the erect corpus cavernosum penis (CCP). Vascular stasis and oedema occur, leading to fibrosis of the CCP and irreversible occlusion of the collecting veins. The condition in horses usually occurs following administration of phenothiazine-derivative tranquillizers.

Treatment

Because penile protrusion may damage the pudendal nerves, the problem should be resolved as rapidly as possible.

- Further damage to the penis should be prevented with massage, emollient dressings, and slings.
- Cholinergic blockade to bring about detumescence – usually unsuccessful.
- Irrigation of CCP. If medical treatment is unsuccessful within 6 to 8 hours, the CCP should be irrigated with heparinized lactated Ringer's solution (LRS) to evacuate coagulated blood.
- Anastomosis of the CCP and CSP (corpus spongiosum penis). If erection recurs after several cavernosal evacuations, the CSP can be anastomosed to the CCP because the CSP is not involved in erection and can serve as an outlet for stagnant blood.

8.22 *Neoplasia*

Incidence

By far the most common neoplasm of the penis and prepuce is the *squamous cell carcinoma*.

- Occurs most commonly in old horses and breeds with non-pigmented genitalia.
- Has a low grade of malignancy and grows surprisingly slowly for a carcinoma.
- Metastasis to inguinal lymph nodes occurs late in the disease.

Treatment

- Cryosurgery.
- Hyperthermy.
- Excision.
- Segmental posthectomy (reefing) or phallectomy.
- En bloc resection of penis, prepuce and superficial inguinal lymph nodes.

8.23 *Cutaneous habronemiasis (or 'summer sore')*

Aetiology

- Granulomatous disease caused by cutaneous migration of the larvae of the equine stomach worm, *Habronema*. Not endemic in the UK but common in the USA.
- Preputial ring and orifice and urethral process are common sites of larval infestation.
- Lesions appear in spring and summer when flies, which are the intermediate host, are prevalent. Lesions usually disappear with appearance of cold weather.
- Lesion may recur yearly on some susceptible horses.

Clinical signs

- Lesions are *pruritic*.
- Lesions are characterized by exuberent granulation tissue that contains numerous, small, yellow, sand-like, caseous granules.
- Mucous membrane of affected urethral process may be hyperaemic and protrude from the urethral orifice.
- Lesions of the urethral process may cause horse to spray urine on its limbs during urination.
- Erosions into the CSP of the urethral process may result in haemospermia.

Diagnosis

The diagnosis is based on:

- Appearance and clinical signs.
- Marked circulating eosinophilia of affected horses.
- Identification of larvae microscopically in exudate extruded from lesions.
- Histological identification of eosinophils, granules and larvae.

Treatment

Medical treatment is aimed at:

- Eliminating larvae:
  - Ivermectin *per os*.
  - Organophosphates (administered topically, orally or intravenously).
- Decreasing the horse's hypersensitivity to the larvae:

– Prednisolone administered for several weeks.
– Diethylcarbamazine administered for 1 to 2 weeks.

Surgical treatment:

• Elliptical resection of small, isolated preputial lesions.
• Segmental posthectomy for large lesions.
• Amputation of affected urethral process.
• Cryotherapy.

8.24 *Haemospermia*

Aetiology

Haemospermia (i.e. blood in ejaculate) causes infertility, and has been attributed to:

• Bacterial urethritis, usually at the area of ejaculatory ducts.
• Urethral lacerations of unknown origin that communicate with the CSP on the convex surface of the urethra at the level of the ischial arch (Figure 5).
• Habronemiasis of the urethral process.
• Stallion rings.
• Seminal vesiculitis.

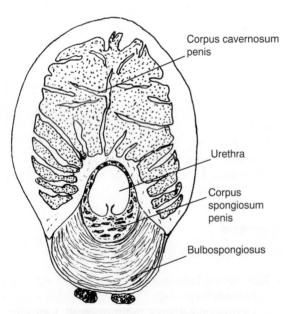

Figure 5 A urethral rent that communicates with the CSP. Urethral rents are usually found at the convex surface of the urethra at the level of the ischial arch. Reproduced from *Vet. Surg.* 1995, **24**, 231–234, with permission (WBS, Philadelphia).

Diagnosis

• Gross and microscopic examination of ejaculate.
• Clinical signs.
  – Affected stallion may require several mounts to ejaculate.
  – May exhibit pain on ejaculation.
• Urethroscopy can be performed to locate the source of haemorrhage.
• Culture and cytological examination of haemorrhage obtained by uretheral swabs.

Treatment

• Sexual abstinence.
• Medical treatment:
  – Formalin (IV)
  – Methenamine (by mouth) produces antibacterial concentrations of formaldehyde in the urine.
  – Antimicrobial drugs administered systemically.
• Temporary perineal urethrostomy combined with sexual rest has been most effective in eliminating haemospermia. Success of temporary urethrostomy has been attributed to decreased pressure in the CSP during ejaculation and urination because the CSP is probably the source of haemorrhage.

8.25 *Diagnosis of diseases of the female reproductive tract*

History

It is necessary to accurately describe the mare's reproductive status. Information is needed about previous uterine infection and treatment, abortions, twinning, neonatal deaths and treatment history.

Examination

Examination may include the following:

• Determination of general health of the mare.
• Assessment of conformation of the perineum and pelvis.
• Identification of vulvar discharge or lesions.
• Palpation *per rectum* of the ovaries, uterus and cervix.

- Ultrasonography.
- Uterine culture. A culture taken during oestrus is more meaningful. Positive cultures are meaningless without evidence of endometritis (vaginal discharge or histological or cytological evidence).
- Histologic examination of endometrial biopsy. A biopsy taken during dioestrus is more meaningful.
- Vaginoscopy.
- Digital palpation of the vagina and cervix.
- Endometrial cytology.

Less common procedures include:

- Endoscopic examination of the uterus (hysteroscopy).
- Laparoscopy.
- Determination of serum concentrations of hormones.
- Karyotyping in cases of unexplained infertility.

8.26 *Pneumovagina*

See Chapter 14.

8.27 *Perineal lacerations and fistulas*

Aetiology and incidence

- These occur at parturition when the foal's front foot or nose catches the annular fold of the hymen at the vaginovestibular junction.
- They occur predominately in primiparous mares because their annular fold at the vaginovestibular junction is more prominent than that of pluriparous mares.

Classification

- *First degree perineal lacerations.* Involve the skin and mucous membrane of the dorsal commissure of the vestibule.
- *Second degree perineal lacerations.* Constrictor vulvae muscle is also disrupted.
- *Third degree perineal lacerations.* These are a complete disruption of tissue between the rectum and vestibule (Figure 6). Injury creates a common rectal and vestibular vault. The condition is referred to as a rectovaginal, or rectovestibular, or R-V laceration. Most are recto-

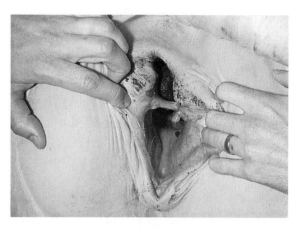

Figure 6 A third degree rectovestibular laceration. These occur during foaling and result in a common rectal and vestibular vault.

vestibular rather than rectovaginal. Third degree rectovestibular lacerations usually allow faecal contamination of the mare's vagina with subsequent bacterial infection of the vagina, cervix and uterus.

- *Rectovestibular fistulas.* Tissue between the rectum and vestibule is completely perforated, but the perineal body, or caudal portion of it, remains intact.

Treatment

First degree perineal lacerations
Mares with first degree perineal lacerations can be treated with a Caslick vestibuloplasty (Figure 7).

Second degree perineal lacerations
Require more extensive treatment because of disruption of the constrictor vulvae muscle. If only a Caslick vulvoplasty is used to repair second degree perineal lacerations, the perineum sinks, predisposing the mare to pneumovagina and urine pooling. Repair is sometimes called a vestibuloplasty. The aim of vestibuloplasty is to reduce the diameter of the vestibule by 30–50%.

- Usually best to wait 4 weeks before repairing second degree perineal lacerations.
- Repair is similar to reconstruction of the perineal body in repair of R-V lacerations and is the same technique used to treat pneumovagina caused by faulty perineal conformation.
- Repair involves removal of two right triangles of mucosa whose base is the cutaneous perineum and whose hypotenuse is the new dorsum of the

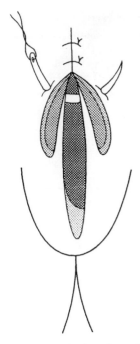

Figure 7 The Caslick operation is performed to prevent pneumovagina and to repair perineal lacerations. The labia should be apposed with sutures, except for those portions that lie below the level of the pelvic floor.

vestibule. Fresh tissue exposed by removal of the triangles is apposed, thus lowering the roof of the vestibule.

Third degree perineal lacerations

Mares require more preoperative preparation and more postoperative care because the rectum is involved in the injury. Attempts to repair the laceration immediately after injury are usually unsuccessful because the lacerated tissue rapidly becomes inflamed and oedematous. Contraction of the muscles of the rectum and vagina widen and lengthen the wound. Usually best to wait 4 to 6 weeks before attempting repair. For acute injuries, the following treatment should be considered:

- Tetanus prophylaxis.
- Broad-spectum antimicrobial drugs for 2 or 3 days.
- Stool-softeners, such as mineral oil, for several days to prevent painful defecation.
- Debriding the wound of devitalized tissue.

Preparation for surgery of third degree lacerations includes:

- Weaning the foal before the laceration or fistula is repaired. Prevents exposing foal to nosocomial disease.

- Palpation of the reproductive tract per vaginum and rectum to detect cervical lacerations, pregnancy, uterine adhesions and pyometra.
- Histological examination of the endometrium. May be indicated if the mare has gone through more than one reproductive season with an R-V laceration, especially if the mare has faulty perineal conformation. Urine and faeces in the vagina may gravitate toward the uterus if the mare suffers from poor perineal conformation. If the mare has severe fibrosis of the endometrium, surgery may be ineffective in returning the mare to reproductive soundness.
- Softening the mare's stool and decreasing its bulk. Ration should allow the mare to maintain weight. Administering 1 gallon of mineral oil *per os* by stomach tube the day before surgery assures that the stool is soft and unformed at surgery. Raw linseed oil, administered in the feed, is an effective stool softener.
- Administration of a broad-spectrum antibiotic several hours prior to surgery.

The R-V laceration or fistula can be repaired with the mare sedated and standing or anaesthetized and in dorsal recumbency. There are two stages to the procedure:

1. Rectovestibular reconstruction.
2. Anoperineal reconstruction.

Both stages may be performed during the same operation, or the anoperineal reconstruction may be completed 3 weeks or more after rectovestibular reconstruction. If anoperineal reconstruction is postponed until the rectovestibular reconstruction is healed, less stress is placed on the rectovestibular reconstruction during defecation. Perfoming both procedures during the same operation, however, minimizes hospitalization time, dietary changes and expense.

Rectovestibular fistulas

- R-V fistula can be converted into a laceration for repair. The fistula should be converted into a laceration only if it is exceptionally large.
- Fistula can be repaired using the Forssell technique, which spares the intact perineal body. The skin of the perineum is incised in a frontal plane between the anus and the dorsal commissure of the labia. The incision is deepened cranially beyond the fistula. This separates the rectovestibular hole into two holes: a rectal hole and a vestibular hole. The rectal hole is closed in a transverse plane (because the musculature of the

rectum is primarily circular, and sutures placed perpendicular to the muscle fibres are subject to less stress than sutures placed parallel to the direction of the muscle fibres). The vestibular hole is closed in a sagittal plane. The horizontal plane of dissection is quilted closed.

● Preoperative and postoperative management of mares with an R-V fistula is similar to that of mares with an R-V laceration.

Postoperative care

Postoperative treatment of the mare following repair of an R-V laceration or fistula usually includes:

● Broad-spectrum antimicrobial drugs administered for several days.
● Tetanus prophylaxis, if not previously administered.
● Faeces should be kept soft and scanty for at least 8 days by modifying diet and administering faecal softeners (e.g. mineral oil or raw linseed oil).
● Non-steroidal anti-inflammatory drugs may be indicated if the mare shows signs of discomfort after surgery.
● Repair should not be evaluated until the 8th or 9th postoperative day.
● Mares that strain excessively following surgery should be treated by epidural anaesthesia and sedation. Causes of straining include faecal impaction of the rectum and cystitis.

Other postoperative considerations

Mares are reproductively healthy before acquiring third degree rectovestibular lacerations, and reproductively healthy mares are usually able to eliminate bacteria from the tubular genital tract within one estrous cycle. Not all mares develop endometritis after third degree rectovestibular injury. Some even become pregnant. Those that do develop endometritis appear to be capable of rapidly resolving chronic inflammation after perineal repair.

Natural breeding should not be allowed for at least 3 months after repair of a third degree perineal laceration, but mares may be bred by artificial insemination within 2 weeks of perineal repair. After 2 weeks of convalescence, sufficient healing should have occurred to permit safe examination of the reproductive tract *per rectum* and passage of an insemination pipette through the cervix.

8.28 *Urovagina*

See Chapter 14.

8.29 *Cervical lacerations*

See Chapter 14.

8.30 *Neoplasia*

Perineal neoplasms

Common perineal neoplasms include melanomas of grey mares and squamous cell carcinoma of mares with non-pigmented genitalia (i.e. cremellos, Appaloosas, paints and palominos).

Treatment

● Melanomas. Genital melanomas of grey mares are often not treated because they usually develop slowly and do not interfere with intromission. Melanomas on horses of other colours tend to be malignant. Small tumours can be excised or removed with cryotherapy. If tumours are too numerous or too large to be treated in this manner, cimetidine may stop progression and decrease the size and number of tumours.
● Squamous cell carcinomas:
  – Surgical excision.
  – Cryotherapy.
  – Hyperthermy.

Tumours of the tubular genital tract

Neoplasms of the tubular genitalia are rare, but leiomyomas have been most frequently reported. Partial or total hysterectomy may be indicated.

Ovarian neoplasia

See Chapter 14.

8.31 *Uterine torsion*

See Chapter 14.

8.32 *Retained placenta*

See Chapter 14.

8.33 *Dystocia*

Causes

• Relative undersize of mare compared to foetus is an uncommon cause of dystocia but can occur in primiparous mares or in mares allowed to graze tall fescue pasture infected with endophyte (*Acremonium coenophalum*) during late gestation.
• Abnormal presentation, position, or posture. Often the result of foetal death. A dead foal does not assume proper birthing position. Long limbs of foetus predispose to dystocia.
• Uterine torsion – estimated to cause 5 to 10% of dystocias.
• Pelvic fracture.
• Prepubic tendon rupture.

Treatment

• Vaginal delivery after repositioning the foetus. Most easily accomplished with the mare anaesthetized and the hindquarters elevated with a hoist. If the foal is dead, fetotomy may be required.
• Caesarean section. Indicated when vaginal delivery is not possible or is proceeding too slowly to result in birth of a live foal.
  – The incised uterine wall of the horse bleeds more profusely than does that of other species, and the edges must be sutured to achieve haemostasis before the uterine incision is closed.
  – Incidence of retained placenta is high following caesarean section.

8.34 *Ovariectomy (oophorectomy)*

Indications

• The most common indication for unilateral ovariectomy of the mare is removal of a granulosa cell tumour.

• Other indications for unilateral ovariectomy include other, less common, ovarian neoplasia.
• Bilateral ovariectomy may be indicated for mares with a congenital defect that prohibits breed registration without bilateral ovariectomy.
• Most common indication for bilateral ovariectomy is to alleviate undesirable behaviour attributable to a hormonal influence.

Approaches

Approaches for ovariectomy:

1. Flank.
2. Ventral midline.
3. Oblique paramedian (Figure 8).
4. Vaginal (colpotomy approach). This is a standing approach often used for bilateral removal of non-tumorous ovaries. Advantages of this approach are:
   • Ovariectomy is performed without general anaesthesia, so ovariectomy using this approach is less expensive, and because the incision is usually not sutured, the technique is quickly performed.
   • Mare can be returned to athletic function sooner with this approach than with ovariectomy performed using other approaches.

Disadvantages of this approach are:

• Requires the use of a chain ecraseur (Figure 9).
• Surgeon is at some risk of injury.

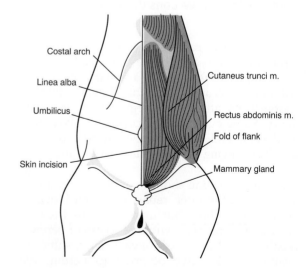

Figure 8 Paramedian approach to removal of a neoplastic ovary. Reproduced from Moll, Sloane *et al.* (*Vet Surg.* 1987, **16**, 456) with permission (WBS, Philadelphia).

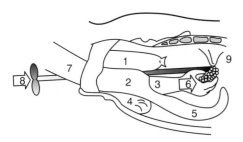

Figure 9 Vaginal approach to ovariectomy via colpotomy. Lateral view and important anatomical areas are identified. Rectum (1); vagina (2); colpotomy incision (3); bladder (4); uterine horn (5); ovary (6); operator's arm (7); ecraseur (8); mesovarium (9).

- Because the ovarian pedicles cannot be ligated, the horse is at greater risk of haemorrhage than with ovariectomy performed using an approach that allows for ligation of the pedicles.
- Extracting large, neoplastic ovaries through the colpotomy site is impossible.

Further reading

Bayly, W. (1991) A practitioner's approach to the diagnosis and treatment of renal failure in horses. *Veterinary Medicine* **86**, 632–639.

Brown, C.M. (1986) Equine nephrology. In *The Veterinary Annual* (Eds C.S.G. Grunsell, F.W.B. Hill and M.E. Raw). John Wright and Sons, Bristol, pp. 1–16.

Cox, J.E. (1987) *Surgery of the Reproductive Tract in Large Animals.* Liverpool University Press, Liverpool.

Divers, T.J. (1996) Equine renal system. In *Large Animal Internal Medicine* (Ed. B.P. Smith). C.V. Mosby, St Louis, pp. 953–974.

Kohn, C.W. and Chew, D.J. (1987) Laboratory diagnosis and characterization of renal disease in horses. *Veterinary Clinics of North America: Equine Practice* **3**, 3. W.B. Saunders, Philadelphia, pp. 585–615.

Varner, D.D., Schumacher, J., Blanchard, T.L. and Johnson, L. (1991) *Diseases and Management of the Breeding Stallion.* American Veterinary Publication. Goleta, CA.

Vaughan, J.T. (1980) Surgery of the testes. In *Bovine and Equine Urogenital Surgery* (Eds D.F. Walker and J.T. Vaughan). Lea & Febiger, Philadelphia.

9 Endocrinology

9.1 Anhidrosis (dry coat syndrome)

An *inability to sweat* (anhidrosis) is a common problem of horses, particularly racing horses, in warm, humid climates. Impaired thermoregulatory function causes decreased athletic performance. As many as 25% of racing horses in the southern United States are affected to some degree. The severity of the condition varies considerably – from mild to complete inability to sweat. Anhidrosis tends to occur in the summer and regress during cooler seasons. There appears to be no breed, sex, or colour predisposition. Onset may be abrupt or gradual. *Hyperhidrosis* may be noted before the onset of anhidrosis.

Aetiology

The cause of anhidrosis is unknown, but a warm humid climate is a predisposing cause. Contrary to previous belief, horses imported from cool to warm climates do not appear to be predisposed.

Pathogenesis

The horse and primate are unique in that their primary means of heat loss is by vaporization of sweat. Equine sweat glands are predominately under β-adrenergic control and are stimulated by circulating catecholamines or by direct postganglionic adrenergic innervation. The most likely explanation for the syndrome is decreased glandular sensitivity to catecholamines. Glandular cells subsequently undergo degeneration, and ducts become blocked with cellular debris. If thermal stress is absent, glandular regeneration may occur.

Clinical signs

- Decreased or absence of sweat in response to stimulus such as exercise or heat. Residual sweat production occurs in most affected horses and is seen at the crest of the neck, pectoral region, and perineum. Sweat does not lather.
- Tachypnoea.
- Fatigue and decreased athletic performance.
- Dry, flaky hair coat, alopecia (especially of the face).
- Decreased water consumption.
- Fever associated with exercise.

Diagnosis

- History and clinical signs.
- Intradermal epinephrine response test. Epinephrine solutions of 1:1000; 1:10 000; 1:100 000, and 1:1 000 000 are injected intradermally along the neck or ribs. Expect sweating at all four injection sites within minutes in a normal horse. Anhidrotic horses usually sweat only at the 1:1000 site and only after an extended period (hours). Caution: White hair may grow at the injection sites.
- Clinicopathology – haematologic and biochemical values (including electrolytes) are not changed.
- Triiodothyronine (T_3) and thyroxine (T_4) concentration – contrary to some reports, these are usually normal.

Treatment and prevention

- An artificially cooled environment or relocation to a more temperate climate. Stall fans and cold water baths during the hottest period of the day are useful. Glands usually regenerate in the absence of thermal stress.
- Intravenous or oral electrolytes – occasional response is claimed.
- T_4 therapy – based on older reports that anhidrotic horses are hypothyroid. Likely to be of no benefit.
- Avoidance of exercise during heat of the day.
- Dietary changes. Body heat produced by digestion can be minimized by feeding the maximal recommended amount of concentrate and minimal amount of forage. Feed early morning and late evening.

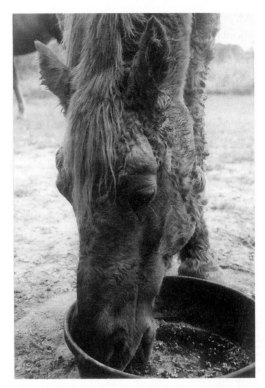

Figure 1   An aged gelding with Cushing's disease. Note the long curly hair-coat and periorbital bulges. This photo was taken in late summer.

highest in old horses (not reported in immature horses).

9.2   *Cushing's disease (CD)*

An uncommon condition caused by a pituitary tumour. Dramatic clinical signs are often multiple but variable and include laminitis, weight loss, polyphagia, polyuria, polydipsia, hyperhidrosis, bulging orbital fat, behavioural changes, chronic infection (often respiratory), and an unnaturally long hair coat (*hirsutism*) (Figure 1). Many of the clinical signs and most of the clinicopathological findings in horses with CD are the result of excess cortisol production by the adrenal cortex.

The disease occurs in either sex and all breeds of horses, ponies and donkeys. The incidence is

Aetiology

The cause is nearly always an adenoma of the pars intermedia. Loss of dopaminergic innervation of the pars intermedia may cause the tumour to develop. Tumours of the pars distalis are a rare cause. Because adrenal cortical neoplasia is so rarely reported in the horse, it deserves little consideration as a cause of Cushing's syndrome.

Clinical signs and proposed pathogenesis

The normal equine pituitary gland and adenomas of the pituitary gland synthesize a large peptide, *pro-opiomelanocortin* (POMC). POMC is a precursor of the following hormones: adrenocorticotrophin (ACTH), α- and β-melanocyte stimulating hormones (αMSH, βMSH), corticotrophin-like intermediate lobe peptide (CLIP), β-endorphin (βEND), and β-lipotrophin (βLPH). Clinical signs observed in horses with CD probably vary due to the variable increases in plasma concentrations of

POMC peptides produced by the pituitary adenoma.

- Laminitis – occurs commonly in horses with CD. Increased production of cortisol secondary to high concentration of ACTH enhances catecholamine vasoactivity, which affects laminar circulation. Increased production of cortisol may also initiate an insulin insensitivity. Because insulin induces capillary vasodilation, insulin insensitivity may decrease laminar blood flow.
- Hirsutism – occurs in over 90% of affected horses. The cause is unknown but may be due to thermoregulatory dysfunction caused by tumour pressure on the hypothalamus, or to increased production of androgens by the hyperplastic adrenal cortex.
- Polyuria/polydipsia – noted in a majority of affected horses. Increased production of cortisol causes *diabetes insipidus* (by antagonizing antidiuretic hormone (ADH) at the collecting duct) or *diabetes mellitus* (by initiating insulin insensitivity). Diabetes insipidus may also result from reduced ADH secretion by the posterior pituitary gland due to expansion of the intermediate lobe tumour into the posterior pituitary.
- Chronic infections – immunosuppression caused by increased production of cortisol.
- Behavioural changes (depression, lethargy, docility) – seen in a majority of affected horses – may be due to increased concentration of endorphin in the cerebrospinal fluid (CSF).

Diagnosis

1. Signalment and clinical signs are often sufficient for diagnosis.
2. Direct measurement of POMC peptides (especially MSH and ACTH) – few laboratories can perform these tests.
3. Measurement of endocrine and biochemical changes induced by POMC peptides. Most tests are based on the effect of increased cortisol production secondary to increased ACTH production. There is no endocrine or biochemical test that always verifies a diagnosis of equine CD.
   - Cortisol – single measurements of cortisol are of no value; cortisol concentration is usually within a normal range in cushingoid horses. (Diurnal variation in cortisol production is replaced by steady production to cause an increased production of cortisol not reflected by single determinations.)

- Dexamethasone suppression test – dexamethasone given to normal horses causes a subsequent drop in plasma cortisol concentrations. Expect cortisol concentration to remain high in a cushingoid horse. (The tumour is not under negative feedback control by glucocorticoids.) One method to perform the test is to collect a pre-dexamethasone blood sample (for cortisol measurement) and then inject dexamethasone IV at 40 μg/kg of body weight. Collect a post-dexamethasone sample 15 to 19 hours later. Normal post-dexamethasone cortisol concentration is less than 1 μg/dl (27 mmol/l); abnormal is >1 μg/dl.
- ACTH stimulation test – expect an enhanced cortisol response due to adrenal cortical hypertrophy in horses with CD. This test, however, has very little diagnostic value because the adrenal cortex of many cushingoid horses is already maximally stimulated by endogenous ACTH.
- Thyroid-releasing hormone (TRH) stimulating test – normal horses have no significant increase in cortisol concentration after being given TRH. Cushingoid horses given TRH do have an elevation in cortisol concentration.
- Insulin – concentrations are almost always elevated in horses with CD. Multiple samples are useful. Avoid sampling soon after feeding.
- Triglycerides – some cushingoid horses develop hypertriglyceridaemia (see section on hyperlipaemia).
- Intravenous glucose tolerance test – normal horses demonstrate an insulin response to a glucose load. This response is feeble in the cushingoid horse.
- Serum glucose – cushingoid horses may be normoglycaemic or hyperglycaemic (glucose >150 mg/dl or >8.3 mmol/l); hyperglycaemia is more likely.
- Urine glucose – occurs if the renal threshold for glucose (>180 mg/dl or >10.0 mmol/l) is exceeded.
- Complete blood count (CBC) – excessive cortisol concentration causes neutrophilia, lymphopenia, eosinopenia and polycythaemia. Expect to see anaemia if chronic infection is present.

Treatment

Treatment is often not appropriate, especially if signs are mild and progression is slow. Age of the horse and economic considerations may dictate that no treatment is given. Laminitis may be so severe that euthanasia is necessary.

Treatment involves use of either a *serotonin antagonist* or *dopamine agonist*. The neurotransmitter, serotonin, stimulates hormonal secretion of the tumour whereas the neurotransmitter, dopamine, inhibits secretion. Therapy involves use of:

- Cyproheptadine – a serotonin antagonist – effective in about 35% of cases (i.e. improvement noted). Improvement may not be noted for the first 6 weeks of treatment.
- Pergolide mesylate – a dopaminergic agonist; early reports indicate that this drug is more effective than cyproheptadine.
- Bromocriptine mesylate – a dopaminergic agonist; has been used alone or combined with cyproheptadine therapy.
- Insulin therapy – may be of some value in hyperglycaemic cushingoid horses.
- Laminitis therapy – corrective trimming or shoeing and analgesics.
- Antibiotic therapy for secondary infections.
- Mitotaine (Lysodren) – an adrenocorticolytic drug effective in treatment of canine CD – ineffective in treatment of equine CD.

Clinical signs

- Depression and lethargy.
- Anorexia and weight loss.
- Exercise intolerance.
- Diarrhoea.
- Mild colic.

Diagnosis

- History and clinical signs.
- Low morning cortisol concentration (normal is $>1\ \mu g/dl$).
- Decreased response to ACTH stimulation using either ACTH gel or synthetic ACTH (cosyntrophin).

Treatment

- Withhold corticosteroid therapy (tapered doses of glucocorticosteroids are *not* indicated as even small doses may cause prolonged adrenal suppression).
- 'Turn out' for 1 to 3 months.
- Decreasing alternate day doses of ACTH.

9.3 *Hypoadrenocorticism (adrenal exhaustion, turn-out syndrome, steroid let down syndrome)*

This is a poorly documented cause of poor performance in racing horses usually attributed to withdrawal of exogenous corticosteroid. Corticosteroids are commonly administered to racing horses as a stimulant (by causing euphoria) and to reduce musculoskeletal pain.

Aetiology and pathogenesis

Prolonged corticosteroid therapy causes decreased secretion of ACTH by the pituitary, which results in adrenal atrophy. Withdrawal of exogenous corticosteroid may result in low concentrations of plasma cortisol. Another cause of turn-out syndrome may be 'adrenal exhaustion' caused by chronic stress of training. In addition, long term use of anabolic steroids may lead to adrenal insufficiency.

9.4 *Phaeochromocytoma*

This tumour is found in the adrenal medulla. Functional, catecholamine secreting phaeochromocytomas cause clinical signs, but most are *non-functional* and are only an incidental finding at necropsy.

Clinical and clinicopathologic signs

Signs are non-specific; there may be sudden onset of hyperhidrosis, dilated pupils, tachycardia, tachypnoea, muscle tremors, anxiety, and abdominal pain. *Hyperglycaemia* is a consistent finding.

Diagnosis

Definitive ante-mortem diagnosis is unlikely because measurement of concentration of catecholamines in the plasma or urine is not routinely performed by most veterinary endocrine laboratories.

Treatment

Treatment of phaeochromocytoma in the horse has not been reported. Treatment in humans is surgical, but short-term management involves drugs that inhibit catecholamine synthesis.

9.5 *Diabetes mellitus (DM)*

DM is a chronic state of hyperglycaemia caused by a lack of insulin or by factors that inhibit the action of insulin. DM in the horse is almost always caused by excessive production of hormones that counter the action of insulin. Pancreatic disease in the horse is rare.

Aetiology and pathogenesis

Categorization of equine DM is similar to categorization of the disease in humans. In humans, three types of DM are recognized:

1. Primary DM – further categorized as type I or II:
   - Type I or insulin dependent – associated with low blood concentration of insulin due to islet cell destruction by viral or autoimmune disease. Type I DM has not been reported in the horse.
   - Type II or non-insulin dependent – serum insulin concentration is normal or elevated. Causes of type II DM include deficiency of insulin receptors or inability of receptor-bound insulin to cause glucose uptake. Type II DM has been reported in the horse. Ponies, especially those that are fat or laminitic, may be type II diabetics.
2. Secondary DM – DM associated with other endocrine disorders. Hormones that antagonize the action of insulin include growth hormone, cortisol, catecholamines and progesterone. By far, the most common cause of DM in the horse is tumour of the pars intermedia of the pituitary (Cushing's disease).
3. DM associated with generalized pancreatic necrosis. Several cases in the horse have been reported, possibly associated with strongyle migration.

Clinical signs

Because nearly all equine cases of DM are secondary, clinical signs of primary disease predominate (e.g. Cushing's disease or phaeochromocytoma).

Treatment

- Treatment of secondary DM involves treatment of primary disease (i.e. Cushing's disease). Insulin therapy of some hyperglycaemic cushingoid horses (those that do not have a massive insulin response) may be indicated.
- For rare cases of DM caused by pancreatic necrosis, insulin therapy has caused temporary improvement in clinical signs of weight loss and polyuria/polydipsia (PU/PD).

9.6 *Hypoglycaemia*

Hypoglycaemia is common in the septicaemic foal and accounts for the severe depression or coma seen.

Hypoglycaemia is rare in adult horses. Causes include pancreatic neoplasia, athletic exertion, malicious injection of insulin (insurance fraud), liver disease, and pseudodata (*in vitro* glycolysis by blood cells). Clinical signs may not be obvious until glucose concentration is below 20 mg/dl (1.1 mmol/l) or even 10 mg/dl (0.6 mmol/l).

Signs include staggers, blindness, depression or seizures. Hyperinsulinaemia due to pancreatic neoplasia can be suspected on the basis of insulin concentration obtained during an oral glucose tolerance test. Diagnosis of hypoglycaemia caused by injection of exogenous insulin can be made with pressure liquid chromatography (because equine insulin is not commercially available).

9.7 *Hyperlipaemia (hypertriglyceridaemia syndrome)*

A disease of ponies (particularly Shetlands) and burros characterized by mobilization of lipid into blood, which leads to fatty infiltration of body tissues. Organ failure results, most notably hepatic and renal failure. The mortality rate in ponies is high, around 75%. There is a significant difference between ponies and horses in regulation of lipid metabolism by insulin, and the syndrome rarely occurs in horses.

Aetiology

- Negative energy balance – anorexia, starvation, severe parasitism, lactation, gestation.
- Any condition that exacerbates the pony's innate insensitivity to insulin:
  - Obesity.
  - Pregnancy – progesterone antagonizes insulin.
  - Stress (infection, transportation, Cushing's disease) – cortisol antagonizes insulin.

Pathophysiology

Obese, stressed ponies are commonly insulin insensitive (the biologic response to insulin is decreased). Because insulin inhibits lipolysis of adipose tissue, mobilization of fatty acids is poorly regulated in these ponies. Fatty acids are normally mobilized as an energy source during periods of negative energy balance, but the process is inappropriately accelerated in insulin insensitive ponies. Released fatty acids stimulate hepatic synthesis and secretion of triglycerides to cause hypertriglyceridaemia. Insulin also plays a positive role in lipogenesis or removal of triglycerides from plasma. Lipogenesis, however, appears to be increased in ponies with hyperlipaemia.

Clinical signs

- Anorexia.
- Depression, lethargy.
- Ataxia.
- Diarrhoea is common, possibly due to anorexia.
- Opaque, milky appearance of plasma or serum.

Diagnosis

- Signalment, history, clinical signs.
- Triglyceride concentration >500 mg/dl (>5.0 mmol/l) is arbitrarily defined as hyperlipaemia. Normal concentration is <100 mg/dl (<1.0 mmol/l). Hypertriglyceridaemia <500 mg/dl is termed *hyperlipidaemia*, a milder condition.
- Expect biochemical evidence of hepatocellular necrosis and hepatic dysfunction. Affected horses

often have elevated L-iditol dehydrogenase, aspartate transaminase, and bile acids.
- Expect azotaemia in some ponies and all horses. Azotaemia may be a prerequisite for development of hyperlipaemia in the horse.

Treatment

- Correction of initiating primary disease or stressor.
- Improvement of feed intake: allow grazing, offer a variety of feed, oral alimentation (by nasogastric tube), diazepam (efficacy as an appetite stimulant has been questioned).
- Fluid therapy – oral or IV for correction of azotaemia.
- Heparin – accelerates removal of triglycerides from blood by increasing activity of lipoprotein lipase. Controversial therapy because activity of lipoprotein lipase is already increased in hyperlipaemic ponies.
- Glucose – by nasogastric tube or IV.
- Insulin – combined with glucose therapy. Insulin inhibits lipolysis and promotes lipogenesis.
- Consider *abortion* of a late gestation foetus. This is a controversial therapy because it is considered to induce further stress.
- A nursing foal should be weaned.

Prevention

- Avoidance of stress in predisposed ponies (i.e. fat or lactating ponies).
- Proper nutrition – to avoid negative energy balance or obesity.
- Routine exercise of predisposed ponies – improves insulin sensitivity.

9.8 *Hypothyroidism*

Hypothyroidism is a commonly diagnosed yet poorly documented syndrome in the adult horse. A poor understanding of the response of the thyroid gland to disease may cause euthyroid horses to be erroneously diagnosed as hypothyroid. Only hypothyroidism in the foal has been well documented.

Aetiology

Excessive iodine in the feed of pregnant mares has resulted in abortion or in birth of hypothyroid foals. In many cases, the cause of hypothyroidism in foals cannot be determined, but ingestion of substances with antithyroid activity (*goitrogenic substances*) by the mare during gestation is also a possible cause.

Although *primary hypothyroidism* (i.e. dysfunction of the thyroid gland itself) has not been documented in the adult horse, *secondary hypothyroidism* (i.e. inability of the pituitary to secrete thyroid stimulating hormone, TSH) has been reported to occur in some horses with Cushing's disease and some horses chronically affected with the exertional rhabdomyolysis syndrome.

Clinical signs (foals)

- Signs associated with ongoing hypothyroidism:
  - Prematurity.
  - Hypothermia.
  - Goitre (pathognomonic; usually present).
  - Weakness, lethargy, poor sucking and righting reflexes.
  - Slow growth.
  - Respiratory distress (rare).
- Signs that may possibly be associated with hypothyroidism that occurred during critical stages of gestation, but resolved before birth:
  - Forelimb joint contracture (rupture of the common digital extensor tendon is often associated with contracture of the carpal joints).
  - Mandibular prognathism (sow mouth).
  - Collapse of tarsal or carpal bones due to incomplete ossification.

Clinical signs (adults)

Often associated, but unproven, clinical signs of hypothyroidism are:

- Obesity, laminitis, and infertility in mares.
- Poor racing performance associated with myopathy.

Diagnosis

- Clinical signs.
- Low basal concentrations of T_4 (thyroxine) or T_3 (triiodothyronine) (measured by radio-immunoassay). Concentrations of T_3 and T_4 are often not reliable indicators of thyroid disease. Euthyroid horses may be misdiagnosed as hypothyroid if the following conditions are not considered:
  - The euthyroid sick syndrome. Disease unrelated to thyroid disease can depress basal thyroid hormone concentration (and response to thyroid stimulating hormone (TSH) or thyroid releasing hormone (TRH)). This is a normal response to minimize the catabolic effects of thyroid hormones during disease.
  - Some drugs can cause a decrease in thyroid hormone concentration (most notably phenylbutazone).
  - Training tends to lower T_3 and T_4 concentrations.
  - Seasonal fluctuations.
  - Diurnal fluctuations.
  - Poorly established laboratory normals or reliance on published values of other laboratories.
- If concentrations of T_3 and T_4 are low, a TSH and/or TRH response test should be performed. Unresponsiveness to TSH stimulation indicates primary hypothyroidism. The TRH response test is more economical to administer. Failure to respond to TRH (by elevation of low T_4 concentration) indicates that either primary or secondary hypothyroidism exists. The possible effect of drugs or disease on the TRH response test has not been established.
- Thyroid gland biopsy – of particular value in foals. Expect to see thyroid hyperplasia secondary to elevated TSH in hypothyroid foals. Because hyperplasia persists even after thyroid hormone concentrations return to normal, biopsy is valuable in diagnosis of resolved gestational hypothyroidism as a cause of neonatal skeletal disease.
- Measurement of free T_4 by dialysis. This test has not been thoroughly evaluated for diagnostic use in horses. However, measurement of free T_4 by this method is very useful in dogs, cats and humans suspected with thyroid disease.

Treatment

Treatment consists of once daily administration of thyroid hormone, usually T_4 as synthetic L-thyroxine. Dose in adult horses is $20\,\mu g/kg$ or 10–20 mg per 500 kg.

There appears to be a *wide margin of safety* with administration of T_4, but administration of *tapered doses* is advised if the drug is discontinued in case excessive doses have inhibited TSH production.

9.9 *Hyperthyroidism*

The condition has not been documented in the horse. Hyperthyroidism has been diagnosed, but only based on clinical signs (fractiousness) and treated with variable results by thyroidectomy with subsequent T_4 supplementation.

9.10 *Thyroid adenoma*

This is a *non-functional* tumour of the thyroid gland of old horses, which is usually solitary, but can be bilateral (Figure 2). The tumour can be removed for cosmesis without altering thyroid function. Bilateral removal necessitates supplementation with T_4 daily.

9.11 *Hyperparathyroidism*

Parathyroid hormone (PTH), secreted by the chief cells, plays a major role in calcium homeostasis by controlling fine, minute to minute regulation of blood calcium. PTH increases serum calcium by increasing intestinal absorption, kidney reabsorption, and bone resorption of calcium. Excessive secretion of PTH causes excessive bone resorption, which eventually results in skeletal disease. Excessive secretion of PTH in the horse may be the result of primary parathyroid diseases (rare),

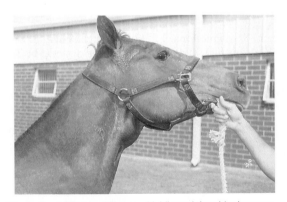

Figure 2 A 26-year-old horse with bilateral thyroid adenomas.

nutritional imbalances (common) or neoplasms of nonparathyroid origin (rare).

Aetiology

- *Primary hyperparathyroidism*. Tumours of the parathyroid gland secrete PTH.
- *Pseudohyperparathyroidism*. Neoplastic secretion of PTH-like hormone by malignant tumours of non-parathyroid origin – lymphosarcoma, squamous cell carcinoma and mesothelioma.
- *Secondary nutritional hyperparathyroidism* (SNH). Hyperparathyroidism secondary to nutritional imbalances (also called big head, bran disease or miller's disease). Diets high in phosphorus and/or low in calcium (usually high grain, poor roughage diets) stimulate secretion of PTH to maintain normal serum calcium concentration.

Pastures with high oxalate content can induce SNH even though Ca and P intake is normal. High concentration of oxalate in the diet makes Ca unavailable for absorption. (Reported from Australia.)

Clinical signs and clinicopathologic findings

- Primary hyperparathyroidism. So rare as to deserve little consideration as a differential diagnosis of hypercalcaemia in the horse.
- Pseudohyperparathyroidism. A rare cause of hypercalcaemia. Clinical signs are often referable to the body system affected by neoplasia.
- SNH. Occurs in *young horses*, usually less than 2 years of age.
  - Intermittent, shifting lameness is often the first sign.
  - Stilted gait.
  - Joint pain – react to flexion.
  - Bilaterally symmetrical thickening of the facial bones lateral to the nasomaxillary notch. The mandible may also thicken. Thickening of the facial bones is a late occurrence in the course of the disease.
  - Difficult mastication. Alveolar bone is resorbed.
  - Serum calcium and phosphorus concentrations are usually normal.

Diagnosis

- Signalment, clinical signs, and ration analysis (by laboratory analysis or reference to published values for Ca and P content of feed).

- Creatinine clearance ratio (%Cr) of phosphorus >4% suggests excessive dietary phosphorus, and %Cr of calcium >2.5% indicates adequate dietary calcium. (It has been claimed that %Cr Ca is difficult to interpret because large amounts of calcium carbonate crystals precipitate in the bladder. It is unlikely, however, that these crystals form when intake of calcium is low.)

The formula for determination of % Cr P or Ca is:

$$\% \text{ Cr P or Ca} = \frac{\text{Urine Ca or P concentration}}{\text{Serum Ca or P concentration}} \times \frac{\text{Serum creatinine concentration}}{\text{Urine creatinine concentration}} \times 100$$

- Radiographic loss of the dental laminae durae – an early and pathognomonic finding.
- PTH concentration – the value of this determination in diagnosis of SNH has not been proven.
- SNH can not be diagnosed by serum concentrations of Ca or P.

Treatment

Correction of the dietary imbalances by feeding:

- Alfalfa hay – high in calcium.
- Calcium carbonate (ground limestone) (avoid calcium supplements that contain phosphorus).

Lameness is expected to resolve within 2 months; facial swellings usually remain.

Prevention

Prevented by maintaining a calcium phosphorus ratio of 1:1 to 3:1.

9.12 *Submission of samples for endocrine testing*

Endocrine diagnostic laboratories vary in their recommendations regarding sample collection, storage and shipping. Each laboratory should also provide protocols to follow regarding their preferred testing procedure for specific clinical evaluation and the normal range of values expected. In general, plasma or serum is recommended for hormone measurement, and whole or clotted blood should never be submitted. Avoid submission of samples in glass tubes or in envelopes. Serum should be collected into plain glass (red-top) tubes, and, after allowing the blood to clot for 15–20 minutes, the sample should be centrifuged. To collect plasma, blood should be collected into EDTA-containing tubes (e.g. purple-top vacutainers). Plasma should be obtained from the blood as soon as possible (15–30 minutes of collection). Endocrine tests are affected by severe haemolysis or lipaemia.

For mailing, samples should be placed into snap-top plastic (polypropylene) tubes. It is best to refrigerate or freeze the sample until shipment.

Instructions for specific hormones

Cortisol, progesterone, testosterone and insulin: a minimum of 1 ml of serum or plasma should be submitted. In general, plasma from blood collected into EDTA is preferable. The sample should be securely packaged in an insulated container with at least one frozen refrigerant pack. Ideally, the sample should be posted using next-day or second-day delivery service (avoid more than 3 days in transit).

Thyroid hormones, thyroxine (T_4) and tri-iodothyronine (T_3): One millilitre of plasma or serum is sufficient to measure both T_4 and T_3. Thyroid hormones are quite stable at room temperature for several days, so samples for T_4 and/or T_3 analysis can be shipped by regular mail service. Measurement of full T_4 by dialysis may be useful. Serum samples should be submitted for this test.

Further reading

Mair, T.S., Freestone, J., Hillyer, M.H., Love, S. and Watson, E.D. (1995) The endocrine system. In *The Equine Manual* (eds. A.J. Higgins and I.M. Wright), Chapter 11. W.B. Saunders, London.

Sojka, J.E. and Levy, M. (1995) Evaluation of endocrine function. *Veterinary Clinics of North America, Equine Practice* (Clinical pathology) **11** (3), 415–436.

10 *Haematopoietic and immune systems*

10.1 *Diagnostic approach to haematopoietic and immune system diseases*

The clinical signs associated with diseases of the haematopoietic and immune system can be extremely varied. Alterations in blood parameters are often reflective of primary disease of other body systems. Because of this, evaluation of the blood is included in the diagnostic plan for investigation of many abnormalities identified on physical examination.

History

- Age – congenital abnormalities of the haematopoietic and immune system are most likely to become apparent in horses <1 year of age.
- Breed – congenital abnormalities are also more likely in purebred horses, although they can occur in mixed breed animals.
- In-contact horses – a history of similar clinical signs in other horses may suggest an infectious or toxic aetiology. A history of *Streptococcus equi* infection on the premises might suggest purpura haemorrhagica in a horse with vasculitis.
- Season – red maple leaf toxicity is more common in the late summer and autumn.
- Environment – fallen trees or poor pasture management might predispose to ingestion of toxic plants.
- Routine herd health records – weight loss, ventral oedema, and unexplained recurrent fever in an untested horse might indicate equine infectious anaemia. Recent vaccination against *Streptococcus equi* might suggest a diagnosis of purpura haemorrhagica in a horse with vasculitis.
- Previous illnesses – repeated infectious diseases may be suggestive of an immune dysfunction. *Cryptosporidia* spp., adenovirus infections, *Candida* spp. and *Pneumocystis carinii* infections have been diagnosed in horses with immunological disease.

Physical examination

A complete physical examination is imperative for identification of clinical signs suggestive of haematopoietic and/or immunological disease or to identify underlying disease conditions.

Non-specific systemic signs
- Pyrexia
- Weight loss
- Depression
- Pain
- Tachycardia, tachypnoea

Mucous membranes
Pale mucous membranes accompanied by tachycardia, tachypnoea, and a systolic heart murmur are highly suggestive of anaemia. In contrast, congested mucous membranes with prolonged capillary refill time are consistent with polycythaemia. Petechial or ecchymotic haemorrhages occur with thrombocytopenia or vasculitis.

Haemorrhage
Often the source of blood loss is clearly evident and a result of trauma. Prolonged bleeding from venipuncture sites, petechial or ecchymotic haemorrhages, or melaena occur with severe thrombocytopenia or vasculitis. Vasculitis may also cause severe pitting oedema of the distal extremities, ventral abdomen, and/or head. Severe haematoma formation following relatively minor trauma, or internal haemorrhage into the thorax or abdomen are more indicative of coagulation factor abnormalities or severe disseminated intravascular coagulation.

Palpation
Jugular veins should be palpated to assess their patency. Thrombosis may occur secondary to disseminated intravascular coagulation, traumatic venipuncture or infection.

Pitting oedema of the distal extremities, ventral abdomen or head may be an indication of vasculitis.

Submandibular and prescapular lymph nodes should be palpated for size, consistency, and pain. Generalized lymph node enlargement occurs with cutaneous or multicentric lymphoma. Single lymph nodes may be enlarged because of abscessation or in reaction to localized inflammatory processes.

Peripheral blood evaluation

A complete blood count (CBC) can give invaluable information about the erythron (red cell mass), the leukon (white cell mass) and platelets.

Erythrocytes

The RBC count, haemoglobin, haematocrit and packed cell volume (PCV) are the most frequently measured parameters of erythrocyte quantitation. Haemoglobin concentrations should be approximately one-third of the PCV. This will be increased with intravascular haemolysis. Anaemia is a decrease in the circulating red blood cell (RBC) mass (decreased RBC count, haemoglobin and packed cell volume) as a result of decreased rate of erythrocyte production or increased rate of erythrocyte destruction or loss. Polycythaemia is an increase in the circulating RBC mass. Red blood cell indices can be used to characterize anaemia:

- Mean corpuscular volume (MCV) – sometimes increased in horses with regenerative anaemia; decreased with iron deficiency anaemia.
- Mean corpuscular haemoglobin (MCH) – increased with intravascular haemolysis; decreased with iron deficiency anaemia.
- Mean corpuscular haemoglobin concentration (MCHC) – increased with intravascular haemolysis; decreased with iron deficiency anaemia.

The appearance of the erythrocytes should be evaluated on a stained blood smear. Examples of abnormal RBC morphology and its interpretation include:

- *Poikilocyte* – any abnormally shaped erythrocyte.
- *Anisocytosis* – varying sizes of erythrocytes are observed.
- *Polychromasia* – varying colours of erythrocytes are observed, usually due to variable haemoglobin and RNA content.
- *Spherocyte* – spherical erythrocytes occasionally observed in horses with immune-mediated anaemia.
- *Howell–Jolly bodies* – basophilic nuclear remnants occasionally observed in the cytoplasm of erythrocytes of normal horses.
- *Heinz bodies* – oxidized precipitated haemoglobin observed as round structures extending from the edge of the RBC membrane. Indicative of oxidative damage to the RBC with subsequent intravascular or extravascular haemolysis.

Leucocytes

The total WBC count and differential WBC counts are generally reported.

- *Neutropenia* – decreased neutrophil count – most often a result of a shift of neutrophils from the circulating to the marginating pools. This may occur with endotoxaemia, septicaemia, and a wide variety of acute bacterial, rickettsial or viral disorders. Chronic neutropenia may occur with severe infectious or inflammatory diseases or bone marrow suppression.
- *Band neutrophils* – are immature neutrophils released prematurely into the circulation as a response to high tissue demand ('left shift'). A *degenerative left shift* occurs when the number of immature cells exceeds the number of mature neutrophils because of an inability of the bone marrow to keep pace with demand. It is considered a poor prognostic indicator.
- *Neutrophilia* – increased neutrophil count – may occur in response to stress, excitement, exercise, glucocorticoid or adrenaline (epinephrine) administration, or almost any infectious or inflammatory condition. May be accompanied by a *regenerative left shift*.
- *Eosinopenia* – decreased eosinophil count – may be normal or may occur in response to stress or glucocorticoid administration.
- *Eosinophilia* – increased eosinophil count – occurs in response to some parasitic infections or allergic reactions. It may also occur as a primary myeloproliferative disease, or in response to systemic neoplasia.
- *Basophilia* – increased basophil count – may be observed in response to allergic, inflammatory, or neoplastic diseases or in association with lipaemia. (Basopenia is not clinically significant.)
- *Monocytosis* – increased monocyte count – occasionally observed in association with chronic inflammation. (Monocytopenia is not clinically significant.)
- *Lymphopenia* – decreased lymphocyte count – occurs in response to stress, glucocorticoid administration, many viral infections, and in foals with severe combined immunodeficiency (CID).
- *Lymphocytosis* – increased lymphocyte count – associated with excitement, exercise, adrenaline (epinephrine) administration, lymphocytic leukaemia, and chronic immune stimulation.

Platelets

Total counts in the horse are usually less than in other species. Platelets may clump if they have become activated *in vivo* or *in vitro*. Clumped platelets may be observed at the feathered edge of a stained blood smear. If platelets have clumped, automated counts are not accurate. A repeat sample may be obtained in sodium citrate and counted for more accurate data.

Miscellaneous tests

- *Autoagglutination* – agglutination of erythrocytes that is not eliminated by diluting blood in sterile saline is indicative of immune-mediated haemolytic disease.
- *Coombs test* – direct Coombs test detects antibody and/or complement on the surface of erythrocytes; indirect Coombs test detects the presence of circulating anti-erythrocyte antibodies. Either or both may be positive in immune-mediated haemolytic disease.
- *Osmotic fragility test* – assay assesses stability of erythrocytes in saline solutions of decreasing tonicity. Increased fragility is associated with immune-mediated haemolytic disease.
- *Platelet factor 3 test* – platelet factor 3 is a platelet membrane phospholipid. Patient plasma is added to platelet-rich plasma from a normal horse and monitored for accelerated clotting. A positive test is indicative of immune-mediated thrombocytopenia, but results are difficult to interpret.
- *Cross-matching* – *major cross-match* checks for compatibility between blood donor erythrocytes and any alloantibody present in patient serum. The *minor cross-match* checks for compatibility between donor serum and patient erythrocytes. Both tests are important prior to whole blood transfusion. The minor cross-match is most important prior to plasma transfusion.
- *Iron status* – may be important in characterization of some anaemias. *Serum ferritin* concentration is indicative of stored hepatic and splenic iron. *Prussian blue stain* of bone marrow aspirates also allows assessment of iron stores. *Serum iron concentration* reflects total quantity of transport iron in the plasma (iron bound to transferrin). *Total iron binding capacity (TIBC)* is the amount of iron that plasma transferrin could bind if fully saturated. *Percentage transferrin saturation* is calculated from TIBC and serum iron concentration and should normally be approximately 30%.

Bone marrow evaluation

Bone marrow aspirates and core biopsies may be obtained from the sternebrae on the ventral midline between the forelimbs, from the tuber coxae with the needle directed toward the opposite coxofemoral joint, or from the proximal ribs. The area is clipped and surgically scrubbed. A small amount of local anaesthetic is deposited in the subcutaneous tissues and periosteum. A stab incision is made with a small surgical blade. A 16-gauge or larger bone marrow needle is inserted and forced into the marrow cavity with constant pressure and rotational movement. The stylet is removed and a sterile syringe containing a small amount of EDTA or sodium citrate as anticoagulant is used to aspirate material. Smears may be made immediately and stained for cytologic analysis. Core biopsies are similarly obtained using a 10-gauge Jamshidi needle and fixed for routine histopathologic analysis.

Total body *iron stores* may be estimated by examining marrow specimens with a Prussian blue stain. Bone marrow myeloid to erythroid ratio (M:E ratio) should be approximately 1–2. An M:E ratio of <0.5 is indicative of erythrocyte regeneration or myeloid suppression.

Evaluation of haemostatic function

Evaluation of haemostatic function should include a total *platelet count*, tests to evaluate the function of extrinsic and intrinsic coagulation cascades, and assays to estimate fibrinolytic activity.

Prothrombin time or *one-stage prothrombin time (OSPT)* measures the function of the extrinsic and common coagulation cascades.

Activated partial thromboplastin time (APTT) measures the function of the intrinsic and common coagulation pathways.

Fibrin degradation products (FDPs) are increased with excessive fibrinolysis, which commonly occurs in horses with disseminated intravascular coagulation (DIC).

Antithrombin III (ATIII) activity is increased in some acute inflammatory disorders or hepatic diseases. Decreased with DIC or protein-losing nephropathy or enteropathy.

Platelet count <10 000/μl is associated with haemorrhage. Platelet function may be evaluated with *template bleeding time* assays or *platelet aggregation* tests.

Ancillary diagnostic tests

- *Urinalysis* – haemoglobinuria occurs with intravascular haemolysis. Haematuria with erythrocytes in urine sediment occurs with urinary tract haemorrhage and/or inflammation.
- *Thoracocentesis* – may be useful for identification of intrathoracic haemorrhage. Abnormal

lymphocytes observed on cytology is compatible with a diagnosis of thoracic lymphoma.

• *Abdominocentesis* – may be useful for identification of intra-abdominal haemorrhage.

• Testing of faecal occult blood may help to indicate if gastrointestinal or respiratory tract haemorrhage has occurred.

Immune function evaluation

Immunoglobulin assays
Screening tests to assess for gross alterations in serum IgG concentration include zinc sulphate turbidity, glutaraldehyde coagulation, latex agglutination, or enzyme linked immunosorbent assay (ELISA). More accurate quantification is available with radial immunodiffusion (RID) or laser nephelometry techniques. RID test kits are available to accurately quantitate serum IgG, IgM, IgG(T) and IgA. Production of antibody in response to vaccination with a specific antigen may be used to assess responsiveness of the humoral immune system.

Lymphocyte typing
Peripheral lymphocyte counts are extremely low in Arabian foals with combined immunodeficiency (CID). Dramatically increased counts with abnormal cell morphology may be observed in horses with lymphocytic neoplasias. Monoclonal antibodies are available for identification of lymphocyte subsets (CD4, CD8, pan T cell, B cell) in peripheral blood by flow cytometry.

Blood typing
Several laboratories perform erythrocyte alloantigen typing and alloantibody detection for prevention and diagnosis of *neonatal isoerythrolysis*. These laboratories will also perform lymphocyte typing for progeny verification.

Cellular immune function
Intradermal skin testing with phytohaemagglutinin (PHA) may be used to assess delayed type hypersensitivity. A crude estimate of T cell function may be obtained with lymphocyte blastogenesis assays using PHA, concanavalin A or pokeweed mitogen. More specific tests may be available in some research laboratories.

10.2 Diagnostic features of common haematopoietic and immune disorders of horses

See Table 1.

10.3 Polycythaemia

Polycythaemia is a real or apparent increase in the circulating RBC mass. It is usually recognized as an increase in RBC count, PCV and haemoglobin concentration.

Classification

• *Relative polycythaemia* – a decrease in the relative plasma volume due to haemoconcentration or splenic contraction.

• *Absolute polycythaemia* – a real increase in RBC numbers due to an increase in erythropoiesis.

Aetiology and pathogenesis

Relative polycythaemia is commonly a result of dehydration secondary to decreased fluid intake or excessive water loss in diarrhoea, urine or sweat. Endotoxaemia may cause fluid shifts from plasma to interstitial space. Excitement, exercise or adrenaline may increase PCV by up to 50% due to splenic contraction and release of sequestered erythrocytes into the circulation.

Primary absolute polycythaemia occurs as a primary myeloproliferative disease (polycythaemia vera).

Secondary absolute polycythaemia is a result of increased circulating erythropoietin concentrations. It may accompany severe right-to-left shunting of blood through the heart or great vessels (e.g. tetralogy or pentalogy of Fallot), chronic hypoxia associated with severe pulmonary disease, or as an adaptation to high altitudes. Eythropoietin-like substances can be released from some tumours (e.g. renal or hepatocellular neoplasms).

Clinical signs

Mucous membranes are muddy red to blue. Capillary refill time is prolonged and horses appear weak or lethargic. Despite the increased RBC numbers, oxygen delivery to peripheral

Table 1 Diagnostic features of haematopoietic and immune diseases

Relative polycythaemia	CBC – increased PCV, haemoglobin, RBC count; increased plasma protein if due to dehydration PaO_2 – normal Erythropoietin – normal Bone marrow – normal
Absolute polycythaemia	CBC – increased PCV, haemoglobin, RBC count PaO_2 – decreased if secondary to hypoxaemia; normal if primary Erythropoietin – normal or increased Bone marrow – increased erythropoiesis
Acute haemorrhage	CBC – PCV, RBC count, plasma protein may be normal Thoracocentesis – haemorrhagic if bleeding into thorax Abdominocentesis – haemorrhagic if bleeding into abdomen
Chronic haemorrhage	CBC – PCV, RBC count, plasma protein decreased Iron stores – decreased if chronic external blood loss Bone marrow – increased erythropoiesis (unless iron deficient)
Red maple leaf toxicity	CBC – Heinz body anaemia Methaemoglobin – increased as a percentage of total haemoglobin Urinalysis – haemoglobinuria
Immune-mediated anaemia	CBC – autoagglutination; anaemia; normal serum protein Coombs test – positive Urinalysis – may have haemoglobinuria RBC fragility – increased
Immune-mediated thrombocytopenia	CBC – thrombocytopenia PT, PTT, FDP – within normal limits Bone marrow – normal or increased numbers of megakaryocytes
Equine infectious anaemia	CBC – may be normal AGID (Agar gel immunodiffusion) or C-ELISA – positive
Equine babesiosis	CBC – anaemia; organisms may be observed in erythrocytes Urinalysis – haemoglobinuria
Disseminated intravascular coagulation	CBC – thrombocytopenia PT, PTT, FDP – increased ATIII – decreased
Purpura haemorrhagica	CBC – inflammatory leucogram; normal platelet count PT, PTT, FDP – normal
Combined immuno-deficiency	CBC – persistent severe lymphopenia Presuckle serum IgM – decreased
Generalized bone marrow suppression	CBC – thrombocytopenia; anaemia; neutropenia Bone marrow – all cell lines decreased; may observe fibrosis, fat infiltration, or abnormal (neoplastic) cell populations

tissues is decreased because of increased blood viscosity. In cases of *relative polycythaemia* clinical signs of dehydration, endotoxaemia, underlying disease conditions, and/or excitement may be observed.

Diagnosis

Relative polycythaemia is diagnosed in horses with increased PCV, haemoglobin, or RBC count in conjunction with clinical signs of dehydration, excitement, or exercise. In dehydrated horses, the total serum protein concentration is often increased. *Absolute polycythaemia* is characterized by a persistently increased PCV, haemoglobin and RBC count in the face of normal hydration and relaxed attitude. Primary absolute polycythaemia is confirmed by bone marrow evaluation, normal serum erythropoietin concentrations, and normal PaO_2. Secondary absolute polycythaemia is accompanied by increased serum erythropoietin concentrations, decreased PaO_2 and clinical signs of an underlying disease process that would produce chronic hypoxia. Absolute polycythaemia secondary to neoplasms is characterized by normal to increased serum erythropoietin concentrations and normal PaO_2.

Treatment

Relative polycythaemia due to excitement or exercise will resolve spontaneously as the horse relaxes. Relative polycythaemia due to dehydration should be treated by correcting fluid losses and treating any underlying disease condition. In horses with absolute polycythaemia, the underlying condition must be identified and treated, if possible. Periodic phlebotomy may provide some symptomatic relief.

10.4 *Haemorrhage*

Aetiology and pathogenesis

Blood loss or haemorrhage may be external or internal, acute or chronic.

• *External blood loss* is often a result of trauma and easily recognized and diagnosed with a visual examination. An exception to this is haemorrhage into the gastrointestinal tract. Significant haemorrhage into the gastrointestinal tract may occur with no melaena or haematochezia.
• *Internal blood loss*, into the thorax or abdomen, allows the body to reuse (*autotransfuse*) up to two-thirds of the erythrocytes lost.
• *Acute blood loss* – often associated with normal RBC parameters because all blood components have been lost in equal volumes. Over next 24 hours, interstitial fluid redistributes into the vascular space with resulting decreased RBC numbers (anaemia) and total protein in peripheral blood. *Bone marrow* exhibits increased erythropoiesis by 3 days post haemorrhage; maximal by 7 days. Horses *do not* release reticulocytes into circulation during a *regenerative response*. PCV should increase by 0.5–1% per day during maximum regeneration. Serial bone marrow aspirates must be examined if regenerative responses are questionable.

Clinical signs

The source of haemorrhage is often clearly evident. If haemorrhage is internal, diagnosis may be less obvious.

Diagnosis

If the haemorrhage is acute all red blood cell parameters may be within normal limits. If the

Table 2 Signs of acute and chronic blood loss

Acute blood loss	Chronic blood loss
Hypovolaemic shock	Tachycardia
Tachycardia	Tachypnoea
Tachypnoea	Pale mucous membranes
Pale mucous membranes	Systolic heart murmur
Poor venous distension	Weakness, lethargy
Weakness, lethargy	
Oliguria	

haemorrhage occurred more than 24 hours prior to presentation, RBC count, PCV, haemoglobin and plasma protein concentration should be decreased.

• *External haemorrhage* – clinical signs and/or history.
• *Intrathoracic haemorrhage* – ultrasonography, radiography, and/or thoracocentesis.
• *Intra-abdominal haemorrhage* – abdominocentesis, ultrasonography.
• *Gastrointestinal haemorrhage* – melaena, haematochezia, endoscopy, faecal occult blood test.

Treatment

1. Stop the haemorrhage.
2. Acute severe blood loss – consider:
   • Isotonic crystalline intravenous fluids.
   • Hypertonic saline.
   • Blood transfusions from a compatible donor.
3. Chronic blood loss – consider iron supplementation:
   • Ferrous sulphate at 2 mg/kg body weight.
   • Iron cacodylate IV if you must.
   • *Never* administer parenteral iron dextran to a horse (potential severe anaphylactoid reactions).
4. Whole blood transfusions.
   • *Major* and *minor* cross-matches should be compatible. Or, use previously untransfused gelding as donor.
   • Collect 5–10 litres of blood from adult 450 kg donor.
   • Use *sodium citrate* as anticoagulant; one part 2.5–4% sodium citrate per 9 parts blood.
   • Administer through an *in-line filter*. Give first 25–50 ml very slowly to monitor for adverse reactions. If safe, continue at 15–25 ml/kg/h.
   • *Adverse reactions:* increased heart rate, increased respiratory rate, dyspnoea, fever, trembling, weakness, hypotension, diarrhoea,

abdominal pain, anaphylaxis, shock, pulmonary oedema. In case of reaction *discontinue transfusion*. Hypotension treated with intravenous crystalline fluids. Anaphylaxis treated with IV adrenaline (1:1000 solution at 4.5–9 ml per 450 kg horse).

10.5 *Immune-mediated haemolysis*

Lysis of circulating erythrocytes due to attachment of antibody and/or complement to the surface of the cells. Intravascular haemolysis is generally complement-mediated. Extravascular haemolysis occurs when opsonized erythrocytes are removed from circulation by tissue macrophages.

Pathogenesis

- Alteration of erythrocyte membrane during systemic disease, with subsequent formation of antibodies against new antigens.
- Production of antibodies against normal erythrocyte antigens (true primary autoimmune disease).
- Immune complex deposition on erythrocyte membranes, usually via Fc or complement receptors.
- Drug combines with erythrocyte membrane to create new antigen.
- Drug combines with a carrier molecule and antibody is deposited as an immune complex on erythrocyte membranes.
- Drug induces true autoantibody production.
- Neonatal isoerythrolysis – discussed in Chapter 20.

During *intravascular haemolysis*, haemoglobin is released and combines with haptoglobin prior to removal from circulation by tissue mononuclear phagocytes. If the binding capacity of haptoglobin is exceeded, free haemoglobin accumulates in the plasma and is eliminated via the kidneys. Excessive free haemoglobin can be nephrotoxic. As haemoglobin is degraded in phagocytic cells, the haem moiety is converted enzymatically to biliverdin and then bilirubin. Unconjugated bilirubin is released into the circulation and binds to plasma albumin. Hepatocytes take up the bilirubin, conjugate it, and release it into the gastrointestinal tract via the bile. *Intravascular* and *extravascular haemolysis* are associated with increased serum concentrations of unconjugated (indirect) bilirubin. Excess bilirubin imparts a yellow colour to mucous membranes and other tissues (icterus or jaundice).

Clinical signs

- Tachycardia, tachypnoea.
- Weakness, lethargy.
- Systolic heart murmur.
- Icterus.
- Discoloured urine.
- Signs referable to underlying disease process.

Diagnosis

- History, clinical signs.
- Decreased RBC count, PCV.
- Haemoglobinaemia, haemoglobinuria (if intravascular haemolysis).
- Increased serum bilirubin.
- Positive *Coombs test* or autoagglutination.
- Increased erythrocyte *osmotic fragility*.

Treatment

- Treat underlying disease condition if possible.
- Discontinue current drug therapy if possible.
- Parenteral corticosteroids, e.g. dexamethasone at 0.04–0.1 mg/kg IV or IM. (Corticosteroids have been associated with an increased risk of laminitis in horses.)
- Blood transfusion if severe, life-threatening anaemia.
- Fluid diuresis to protect against pigment nephropathy if intravascular haemolysis is occurring.

10.6 *Heinz body haemolytic anaemia*

Heinz bodies are oxidized, precipitated haemoglobin visible in Wright's stained or new Methylene blue stained blood smears.

Aetiology and pathogenesis

If ferrous (Fe^{2+}) iron in haemoglobin is oxidized to ferric (Fe^{3+}) iron, methaemoglobin is formed. Methaemoglobin is incapable of carrying oxygen. If oxidative stress overwhelms normal protective mechanisms in erythrocytes, methaemoglobin accumulates and imparts a brownish discoloration to blood. Simultaneously, sulphydryl groups are oxidized, resulting in haemoglobin denaturation and precipitation, Heinz body formation, and intravascular haemolysis.

Familial methaemoglobinaemia and haemolytic anaemia have been described in Trotter mares with decreased erythrocyte glutathione reductase activity.

Toxins that can cause oxidative haemolytic anaemia include:

- Wilted red maple leaves (*Acer rubrum*)
- Onions (*Allium canadense*)
- Phenothiazine

Clinical signs

- Peracute death with brownish discoloration of blood.
- Haemolytic syndrome – icterus, brown blood (methaemoglobinaemia), haemoglobinuria, bilirubinaemia, bilirubinuria, Heinz body anaemia, death.

Diagnosis

- Clinical signs.
- History of access to toxin or familial predisposition.
- *Increased blood methaemoglobin* as a percentage of total blood haemoglobin (normal = 1–2%).

Treatment

- Remove all horses from access to toxins.
- *Activated charcoal* to decrease toxin absorption (even if no clinical signs).
- *Fluid diuresis* to protect against pigment nephropathy.
- Dexamethasone.
- *Ascorbic acid* as an antioxidant – 30 mg/kg twice daily in intravenous fluids.
- Transfuse if life-threatening anaemia.

10.7 *Equine infectious anaemia*

See Chapter 19.

10.8 *Equine babesiosis (piroplasmosis)*

This disease occurs predominantly in *subtropical regions*.

Aetiology

Aetiological agents are *intraerythrocytic parasites*, *Babesia caballi* and *Babesia equi*.

Clinical signs

- Fever, depression, pale mucous membranes, ecchymoses, colic, constipation, ventral oedema.
- Anaemia, haemoglobinaemia, haemoglobinuria, increased serum bilirubin concentration.

Diagnosis

- Identify aetiologic agents on stained blood smears.
- Complement fixation test.

Treatment

- To suppress clinical signs: imidocarb dipropionate at 2.2 mg/kg IM once.
- To eliminate organism – imidocarb dipropionate at 2 mg/kg IM once daily for 2 days.
- Imidocarb is very *toxic to donkeys*.

10.9 *Iron deficiency anaemia*

Rarely associated with deficiencies of dietary iron or abnormal iron absorption.

Usually a result of *chronic external blood loss*, often due to gastrointestinal tract haemorrhage.

Diagnosis

- Decreased serum ferritin and bone marrow iron stores.
- Microcytic, hypochromic anaemia (decreased MCV and MCHC).
- Decreased percentage saturation transferrin.
- Increased TIBC.

Treatment

• Identify and eliminate the source of haemorrhage.
• Oral supplementation with product containing *ferrous sulphate*.
• Do not give parenteral iron dextran because of risk of anaphylactic reaction.

10.10 *Anaemia of chronic disease*

Mild to moderate normocytic, normochromic, non-regenerative anaemia associated with chronic inflammatory conditions or neoplasia.

Pathogenesis

• Prevention of iron release from storage pools and so iron is unavailable for haem synthesis.
• Defective bone marrow response to erythropoietin.
• Decrease in erythrocyte lifespan.

Diagnosis

• Normocytic, normochromic anaemia of mild to moderate severity.
• Chronic inflammatory or neoplastic disease.
• Normal to increased TIBC.
• Normal to increased serum ferritin and bone marrow iron stores.
• Normal to decreased percent saturation of transferrin.

Treatment

Treat the primary disease process. Oral iron supplementation is not indicated because systemic iron stores are usually normal to increased.

10.11 *Generalized bone marrow suppression or failure*

Bone marrow suppression or failure usually affects all cell lines with resulting pancytopenia (decreased circulating erythrocytes, leucocytes and platelets).

Aetiology

• *Aplastic anaemia* – may be secondary to viral, bacterial or neoplastic disease, but in most cases a predisposing factor is not identified. An autoimmune pathogenesis has been proposed for some cases.
• *Phenylbutazone* toxicity – rare; recovery reported with discontinuation of drug administration.
• *Chronic renal disease* – decreased erythropoietin results in moderate to severe non-regenerative anaemia.
• *Haematopoietic neoplasia* – almost any cell line may be affected. Neoplastic cells crowd out normal cell development. Neoplastic cells may be observed in circulation.
• *Myelofibrosis*.

Diagnosis

Bone marrow aspirate and/or *core biopsy* will usually confirm diagnosis. In horses with aplastic anaemia, the marrow is devoid of recognizable stem cells. Hypoplastic marrow is yellow due to fat infiltration; myeloid, erythroid and megakaryocytoid cells are decreased.

Treatment

Usually no treatment is recommended. Prognosis is poor. Any prior drug therapy should be discontinued if possible. Idiopathic aplastic anaemia may respond to parenteral corticosteroid therapy.

10.12 *Immune-mediated thrombocytopenia*

Immune-mediated thrombocytopenia (IMTP) frequently occurs secondary to bacterial, viral or neoplastic diseases, but may occur occasionally as an idiopathic or true autoimmune condition.

Pathogenesis

Pathogenesis is similar to that described for immune-mediated haemolytic anaemia.

Clinical signs

Clinical signs are most commonly observed when platelet counts are $<10\,000/\mu l$.

- *Petechial and ecchymotic haemorrhages* of mucous membranes.
- Prolonged bleeding following venipuncture.
- Epistaxis.
- Melaena.
- Hyphaema.

Diagnosis

- Platelet factor 3 – difficult assay to perform with consistent, reliable results.
- Rule out other causes of thrombocytopenia; low platelet count with normal PT and PTT.
- Bone marrow aspirate or core biopsy usually shows normal to increased megakaryocytes.

Treatment

- Treat underlying disease.
- Corticosteroids – dexamethasone at 0.1 mg/kg IM or IV once or twice daily. Gradually taper the dose to once daily in the morning. Do not abruptly discontinue therapy.
- Fresh whole blood or platelet rich plasma if life-threatening haemorrhage is occurring.
- If refractory to corticosteroids, azathioprine at 3.0 mg/kg by mouth once daily.

10.13 *Disseminated intravascular coagulation*

Disseminated intravascular coagulation (DIC) is a pathologic activation of coagulative and fibrinolytic systems, ultimately leading to microvascular thrombosis and secondary ischaemic organ failure. Utilization of coagulative factors in widespread inappropriate coagulation leads to a deficiency of factors available for appropriate coagulative functions and haemorrhage is the result.

Pathogenesis

- Coagulative and fibrinolytic cascades are often triggered by circulating *endotoxin* during *gastrointestinal diseases* or *sepsis*. Endotoxin is the *lipopolysaccharide* component of the external cell wall of Gram negative bacteria.
- Other potential initiating factors include intravascular haemolysis, bacteraemia, viraemia, neoplasia, immune complex disorders, burns, hepatic

or renal disease, or severe dystocia with foetal death in utero.
- *Procoagulant inflammatory mediators* are released from activated macrophages during DIC. These include tissue factor, tumour necrosis factor, platelet activating factor and interleukins 1 and 6.
- In early stages, *thrombotic tendencies* may be observed. However, DIC is recognized more commonly as a *haemorrhagic disease* because consumption of coagulative factors leads to an inability of the blood to continue normal haemostatic function.

Clinical signs

- Thrombosis after venipuncture.
- Petechia, ecchymoses, prolonged bleeding following venipuncture, epistaxis.
- Signs referable to organ dysfunction, including acute renal failure or laminitis.
- Signs referable to the primary underlying disease process.

Diagnosis

The diagnosis of DIC is usually justified in a horse with multiple haemostatic abnormalities and thrombotic or haemorrhagic tendencies.

- In very early stages, PT and PTT may be decreased.
- Later, PT and PTT will be prolonged.
- Increased concentration of circulating FDPs.
- Thrombocytopenia.
- Decreased plasma ATIII activity.

Treatment

- Treat the underlying disease process.
- Maintain peripheral perfusion and systemic acid/base/electrolyte status with appropriate fluid therapy.
- Heparin is useful only if plasma ATIII activity is adequate.
- Non-steroidal anti-inflammatory drugs are beneficial if the horse is endotoxaemic. Appropriate antibiotic therapy must be administered if the horse is septic.
- Fresh platelet-rich plasma may be administered if life-threatening haemorrhage is occurring.

Prognosis

Early recognition of DIC and aggressive therapy are critical. Resolution of any underlying disease process will improve the prognosis. Clinical signs of haemorrhage are associated with a poor prognosis.

10.14 Hereditary defects of haemostasis

Most common in purebred horses. Many are inherited as autosomal recessive traits. Although they may be treated symptomatically, they cannot be cured. Affected horses should not be bred.

Clinical signs and diagnosis

- Von Willebrand's disease – defective platelet adhesion; reported in one Quarter Horse filly. Oral bleeding, conjunctival haemorrhage, prolonged bleeding after injections.
- Abnormalities of contact phase of coagulation – prekallikrein deficiency in Belgian horses and Miniature horses. Prolonged PTT with a normal PT. Affected horses may or may not have clinical signs of a bleeding tendency.
- Classic haemophilia – factor VIII deficiency; diagnosed in Thoroughbreds, Standardbreds, Arabians, and Quarter horses. Present with severe spontaneous haemorrhage or excessive haemorrhage following minor trauma or surgery. Prolonged PTT and normal PT. Factor VIII activity is >10% of normal equine plasma.
- Factor IX and XI deficiency – diagnosed in one Arabian with concurrent factor VIII deficiency.

10.15 Purpura haemorrhagica

An immune-mediated vasculitis that usually occurs secondary to a streptococcal or viral respiratory tract infection.

Pathogenesis

Purpura haemorrhagica after *Streptococcus equi* infection occurs because of deposition of circulating immune complexes in small subcutaneous vessels. Immune complexes activate complement with influx of leucocytes and release of inflammatory mediators. Vascular permeability is increased with resultant oedema, haemorrhage, ischaemia and *necrosis*.

Clinical signs

- Fever, depression.
- Petechial haemorrhages of mucous membranes.
- Painful swelling, oedema, serum exudation of distal limbs.
- May progress to ischaemic necrosis with sloughing of skin.
- Usually not thrombocytopenic.

Diagnosis

- History and clinical signs.
- *Cutaneous biopsy* of affected areas will reveal *neutrophilic infiltrates* around small dermal and subcutaneous vessels.

Treatment

- Immunosuppressive doses of *corticosteroids* – dexamethasone at 0.05–0.2 mg/kg IV or IM once daily.
- Support wraps for oedematous limbs; hydrotherapy.
- Non-steroidal anti-inflammatory drugs.
- Procaine penicillin G at 22 000 IU/kg IM twice daily or sodium penicillin at 22 000 IU/kg IV four times daily if ongoing *Streptococcus* spp. infection.
- Supportive care with intravenous fluids as indicated.

10.16 Vitamin K deficiency

- Rare in horses. Clinical signs of inappropriate bleeding.
- Vitamin K is essential for production of coagulation factors II, VII, IX and X.
- May occur secondary to chronic intestinal malabsorption or chronic cholestatic disorders.
- Similar syndrome produced with warfarin toxicity. Warfarin is a vitamin K antagonist.
- Early in disease only PT is prolonged. Later, PT and PTT are prolonged.
- Treat with parenteral vitamin K1 (phylloquinone) at 0.3–0.5 mg/kg subcutaneously. Do not administer vitamin K3 (menadione sodium bisulphite) as it is nephrotoxic.

10.17 Combined immunodeficiency

A severe, inherited stem cell defect that prevents maturation of B and T cells. Described in Arabians and Arabian crossbred horses. It is transmitted as an *autosomal recessive* trait.

Clinical signs

Affected foals appear normal at birth but clinical signs usually develop by 2 months of age. Most affected foals die by 5–6 months of age. A wide variety of *opportunistic infections* (bacterial, viral, fungal, or protozoal) may be diagnosed including cryptosporidiosis, *Pneumocystis carinii* pneumonia or adenoviral pneumonia.

Diagnosis

- Clinical signs and pedigree.
- Persistent lymphopenia (<1000/μl).
- Absence of serum IgM in presuckle samples or sample collected after 3 weeks of age.
- Thymic hypoplasia with characteristic histopathologic changes in lymphoid tissue.

Treatment and prognosis

Affected foals die despite intensive therapy for opportunistic infections. Both parents of an affected foal are carriers. Confirmed carriers should not be bred.

10.18 Agammaglobulinaemia

Agammaglobulinaemia is rare. It is observed in male Thoroughbreds and Standardbreds, suggesting it is an X-linked disorder. Present with recurrent bacterial infections. Serum concentrations of IgM, IgG, IgG(T) and IgA are persistently low or absent. Lymphocyte counts are within normal limits, but thymic architecture is abnormal. Horses may respond transiently to appropriate antimicrobial therapy but long-term prognosis is poor.

10.19 Selective IgM deficiency

Absent or decreased serum IgM concentration with normal or increased concentrations of other serum immunoglobulins. Three clinical scenarios:

- *Foals* with severe bacterial infections non-responsive to therapy.
- *Weanlings* or *yearlings* that present with recurrent bacterial infections and poor growth.
- *Older horses* that may have recurrent infections and/or lymphoma.

The mode of inheritance is undetermined. It is frequently reported in Arabians and Quarter horses. Lymphocyte counts are within normal limits and lymphoid architecture is normal. The prognosis is generally poor; rarely, a horse may recover.

10.20 Transient hypogammaglobulinaemia

This is a rare disorder. There is delayed onset of immunoglobulin production in the neonate. IgG and IgG(T) concentrations in foals are decreased between 2 and 4 months of age. Reported in Arabians. There are recurrent bacterial and viral infections, which should be treated until the immune system matures.

10.21 Failure of passive transfer

The most common immunological disorder of horses is failure of passive transfer of maternal antibodies from a mare's colostrum to her foal. This disorder and its potentially serious consequences are discussed in detail in Chapter 20.

10.22 Neonatal isoerythrolysis

Alloantibodies in a mare's colostrum will occasionally react with her foal's erythrocyte alloantigens, resulting in severe haemolytic anaemia. This condition is discussed in detail in Chapter 20.

10.23 *Amyloidosis*

Amyloidosis is a term used to describe a series of diseases characterized by deposits of an extracellular proteinaceous material (amyloid) in tissues. Both systemic and localized forms have been described. In secondary reactive amyloidosis, fragments of serum amyloid AA (an acute phase protein) are deposited in tissues. Thus, any chronic inflammatory condition can predispose to this form of amyloidosis. Amyloid L (AL) proteins are monoclonal immunoglobulin light chains (or fragments of these) and are associated with primary idiopathic amyloidosis and the amyloidosis occasionally observed in animals with multiple myelomas.

Systemic amyloidosis

Usually of the AA type and occurs secondary to chronic immune stimulation. In horses, has been associated with chronic pleuropneumonia, peritonitis, chronic parasitism and hyperimmunization. Amyloid is deposited primarily in the liver and spleen, ultimately impairing the function of those organs. Diagnosis is confirmed by biopsy or at necropsy.

Nasal amyloidosis

May be AA or AL type. Present with amyloid deposits in the subcutaneous tissues of the head, neck and trunk or in the nasopharyngeal submucosa and ventral turbinates. Nasal amyloidosis has been associated with epistaxis. Diagnosis confirmed by biopsy with special stains.

10.24 *Lymphoma*

Lymphoma is the most common haematopoietic neoplasm of horses. Leukaemia (neoplastic cells in circulation) is rare. There is no sex or breed predilection. Horses of any age may be affected. Low serum IgM concentrations have been reported in some affected horses.

Clinical signs

Clinical signs are variable, depending on primary site of lesions. Often there is weight loss and depression. Peripheral lymphadenopathy may or may not be observed.

- *Generalized or multicentric form:* most common. Generalized lymphadenopathy and ventral oedema. Other clinical signs depend on specific organ involvement. At necropsy, lesions are often observed in multiple internal organs.
- *Intestinal (alimentary) form:* weight loss, ventral oedema, intestinal malabsorption, intermittent abdominal pain and/or fever. Mesenteric lymph nodes may be palpably enlarged on rectal examination. Diarrhoea may or may not be observed. Hypoalbuminaemia. Occasional immune-mediated haemolytic anaemia and/or thrombocytopenia.
- *Mediastinal or thymic form:* adult horses with ventral thoracic oedema, respiratory difficulties. Pleural effusion. Enlarged thoracic lymph nodes. Bilateral jugular vein distension if masses occlude venous return.
- *Cutaneous form:* multiple subcutaneous nodules. May regress and reappear. Generalized lymphadenopathy is uncommon but individual local lymph nodes may be enlarged.

Diagnosis

Demonstrate neoplastic cells in aspirates or biopsies. In the intestinal form, xylose and glucose absorption tests are often markedly abnormal. Exploratory laparotomy and biopsy of intestine or mediastinal lymph nodes is required for definitive diagnosis. With the mediastinal form, neoplastic cells are often observed in pleural fluid.

Treatment and prognosis

Treatment is not generally recommended and prognosis is poor. The cutaneous form may transiently respond to corticosteroid therapy but lesions often recur when therapy is discontinued. The cutaneous form is the most benign form of this neoplasm and lesions may progress only very slowly.

10.25 *Sporadic lymphangitis ('Monday morning leg'; 'Monday morning disease'; 'Weed')*

An acute lameness with swelling of one or occasionally both hindlegs associated with inflamation of the lymphatics.

Aetiology and pathogenesis

The aetiology is uncertain in many cases. A nutritional basis is assumed in some cases, since the disease may occur in horses receiving full rations while taking little or no exercise (hence 'Monday morning leg'). Some cases may develop following an infection, e.g. from a puncture wound.

Inflammation of the lymphatic tracts and inguinal lymph nodes leads to lymph statis and swelling of the limb. In protracted cases, subcutaneous fibrous tissue may be laid down and normal lymphatic drainage may be impeded; these cases may be affected by recurrent bouts of lymphangitis, and permanent thickening of the soft tissues of the limb may result.

Clinical signs

There is usually an acute progressive swelling of one hindlimb and associated lameness. The limb appears painful, and the foot is 'pointed' or held off the ground. A pain response can be elicited by palpation over the ascending lymphatic tracts proximal to the medial hock and adjacent to the saphenous vein. In severe cases, the skin of the leg appears tight and may ooze serum. The body temperature is elevated.

Diagnosis

Diagnosis is based on the typical clinical signs. Ultrasonography may reveal numerous dilated lymphatics in the subcutaneous tissues. A wound may or may not be found in the leg.

If the horse has not already been treated with antibiotics, bacterial culture of a needle aspirate or of a swab taken from an area oozing serum may be attempted.

Treatment

The aims are to provide pain relief, and to treat the inflammatory reaction and infection, so that the leg is returned to mobility as soon as possible.

1. Systemic antibiotics. The antibiotic should be effective against *Staphylococcus aureus*, since this organism is frequently involved. The antibiotic may need to be changed depending on the results of culture.
2. Anti-inflammatory therapy with non-steroidal anti-inflammatory drugs. Some clinicians advocate the use of a single dose of corticosteroid early in the course of the disease.
3. Hydrotherapy with cold water is helpful in reducing the swelling.
4. The opposite leg should be supported with a bandage, and observed closely for laminitis.
5. Gentle exercise should be provided as soon as the horse is comfortable enough to be walked/exercised.
6. Provide tetanus toxoid or antitoxin if necessary.

Further reading

Divers, T.J., George, L.W. and George, J.W. (1982) Hemolytic anemia in horses after the ingestion of red maple leaves. *Journal of the American Veterinary Medical Association* **180**, 300.

Feldman, B.F. (1981) Disseminated intravascular coagulation. *Compendium of Continuing Education for the Practicing Veterinarian* **3**, 46.

Meyers, K.M., Menard, M. and Wardrop, K.J. (1987) Equine hemostasis: Description, evaluation, and alteration. Clinical Pathology, *Veterinary Clinics of North America, Equine Practice* **3**, 485.

Morris, D.D. (1987) Cutaneous vasculitis in horses: 19 cases (1978–1985). *Journal of the American Veterinary Medical Association* **191**, 460.

Perryman, L.E. and McGuire, T.C. (1980) Evaluation for immune system failures in horses and ponies. *Journal of the American Veterinary Medical Association* **176**, 1374.

Russell, K.E., Sellon, D.C. and Grindem, C.B. (1994) Bone marrow analysis in the horse. *Compendium of Continuing Education for the Practicing Veterinarian* **16**, 1359–1367.

Sellon, D.C. (1993) Equine infectious anemia. *Update on Infectious Diseases, Veterinary Clinics of North America, Equine Practice* **9**, 321.

Sellon, D.C. and Grindem, C.B. (1994) Quantitative platelet abnormalities in horses. *Compendium of Continuing Education for the Practicing Veterinarian* **16**, 1335–1347.

Tyler, R.D., Cowell, R.L., Clinkenbeard, K.D. and MacAllister, C.G. (1987) Hematologic values in horses and interpretation of hematologic data. *Clinical Pathology, Veterinary Clinics of North America, Equine Practice* **3**, 461.

van Andel, A.C.J., Gruys, E. and Kroneman, J (1988) Amyloid in the horse: a report of nine cases. *Equine Veterinary Journal* **20**, 277.

van den Hoven, R. and Franken, P. (1983) Clinical aspects of lymphosarcoma in the horse: a clinical report of 16 cases. *Equine Veterinary Journal* **15**, 49.

Appendix. Differential diagnosis of conditions presenting with haematopoietic or immunological signs

1. Epistaxis
Exercise-induced pulmonary haemorrhage
Ethmoid haematoma
Guttural pouch mycosis
Trauma
Thrombocytopenia
Disseminated intravascular coagulation
Rhinitis/sinusitis
Neoplasia
Pneumonia/pulmonary abscess
Foreign body
Nasal amyloidosis

2. Gastrointestinal blood loss
Parasites
Ulcers
Inflammatory bowel disease
Neoplasia
Coagulopathy

3. Intra-abdominal haemorrhage
Parasites
Trauma
Neoplasia
Abdominal abscess
Ruptured uterine artery
Aortic aneurysm
Coagulopathy

4. Intrathoracic haemorrhage
Trauma
Ruptured pulmonary abscess
Aortic aneurysm
Neoplasia
Coagulopathy

5. Haematuria
Cystitis/urolithiasis
Pyelonephritis
Urinary tract neoplasia
Coagulopathy
Trauma

6. Haemolysis
Neonatal isoerythrolysis
Immune-mediated haemolytic anaemia
Red maple leaf toxicity
Equine infectious anaemia

Babesiosis
Disseminated intravascular coagulation
Severe hepatic disease
Hypotonic fluid administration
Intravenous DMSO
Phenothiazine toxicity
Onion toxicity
Familial methaemoglobinaemia

7. Thrombocytopenia
Immune-mediated thrombocytopenia
Lymphosarcoma
Disseminated intravascular coagulation
Bone marrow failure (pancytopenia)
Equine infectious anaemia
Equine granulocytic ehrlichiosis

8. Petechia/ecchymoses
Disseminated intravascular coagulation
Thrombocytopenia
Purpura haemorrhagica
Vasculitis
Equine infectious anaemia
Equine granulocytic ehrlichiosis

9. Pancytopenia
Myeloproliferative disease
Aplastic anaemia
Radiation
Phenylbutazone toxicity
Myelophthisis
Metastatic neoplasia

10. Non-regenerative anaemia
Chronic inflammatory disease
Neoplasia
Chronic renal disease
Iron deficiency
Hypothyroidism
Bone marrow failure (pancytopenia)
Chronic hepatic disease
Acute haemorrhage or haemolysis
Nutritional deficiency

11. Recurrent infections
Inappropriate therapy
Failure of passive transfer of antibody
Combined immunodeficiency
Selective IgM deficiency
Transient hypogammaglobulinaemia
Agammaglobulinaemia

11 *Neurology*

CONTENTS

11.1 *Diagnostic approach to neurological diseases*

History

Important points that should be recorded include:

- Age, breed, sex, use.
- Duration and progression of signs.
- History of trauma.
- History of other disease.
- Health of in-contact horses.
- Diet and recent changes in diet.
- Sudden or insidious onset of signs.
- Medication.
- General management and environment.

Physical examination

The objects of the physical examination are to first identify the anatomical site of the lesion, and second to diagnose the cause of the disease (although this may not always be possible). The examination should start at the head, and then progress to the spinal cord and limbs, and finally to the tail and peripheral nerves.

Examination of the head

1. *Behaviour*, e.g. seizures, head pressing, circling, aggressiveness, etc.
2. *Mental status*, i.e. level of consciousness and awareness, e.g. coma (complete unresponsiveness to normal stimuli), semicoma (partial responsiveness to stimuli), somnolence, depression, etc.
3. *Head posture and coordination*, e.g. head tilt, head swaying, jerking.
4. *Cranial nerves*. The cranial nerves and their nuclei are spread along the entire brainstem, and lesions of the brainstem frequently cause abnormalities of cranial nerve function. The nerves are examined by starting with the most rostral ones and proceeding caudally.

- *Olfactory nerve (I)* is responsible for the sense of smell. Function of this nerve is difficult to assess, but may be evaluated by testing the horse's ability to smell the hand or food.
- *Optic nerve (II)* is responsible for vision. The *menace response* is assessed by making a threatening gesture with the hand to each eye (avoiding air currents or touch) and observing eyelid blinking or movement of the head away. This reflex also relies on cranial nerve VII. Depressed or excited horses, and neonatal foals, may have deficient menace responses. Further assessment of vision may be made by creating an *obstacle course*. Unilateral vision deficits can be assessed by blindfolding each eye prior to walking through the obstacle course. An ophthalmoscopic examination should be performed in addition to assessment of vision.
- *Oculomotor nerve (III)* is responsible for the control of the pupil (constriction) via parasympathetic fibres (this is opposed by dilator tone controlled by sympathetic pathways). The pupils are assessed for size and symmetry. The *pupillary light reflex* is performed by shining a bright light into each eye and observing

immediate constriction of the pupil in the same eye (*direct reflex*) and in the opposite eye (*consensual reflex*). *Strabismus* (abnormal eye position) may be caused by disease of cranial nerves III, IV or VI, or damage to the extraocular muscles.

• *Trochlear nerve (IV)* is responsible for normal eye position (along with cranial nerves III and VI). Moving the head slowly from side to side causes a rhythmic horizontal movement of each eyeball known as *normal vestibular nystagmus*. Extending the head on the neck causes the eyeballs to rotate ventrally within the orbit. The eyeballs return to a central position as the head is lowered. These normal eye movements require an intact vestibular system, intact cranial nerves III, IV and VI, and the connections between these structures.

• *Trigeminal nerve (V)* contains motor fibres to the muscles of mastication, and sensory fibres from much of the head. There are three branches – mandibular, maxillary and ophthalmic. Sensory function is tested by assessing *facial reflexes* (observed flicking of ear, closure of eyelid, flaring of nostril and withdrawal of the labial commissure in response to touch of these areas); these reflexes also require an intact facial nerve. *Facial sensation* is tested by observing a cerebral response (e.g. head jerk) in response to pricking areas on the face. Loss of motor function of the trigeminal nerve results in a dropped jaw, and inability or difficulty in chewing, and drooling of saliva.

• *Abducens nerve (VI)* is responsible for normal eye position (with cranial nerves III and IV).

• *Facial nerve (VII)* supplies motor innervation to the muscles of facial expression via the auricular, palpebral and buccal branches. The function of the facial nerve is tested by *facial reflexes* (which also test the function of sensory fibres of the trigeminal nerve as described above) and observation of the ability to move the ears, blink the eyelids and move the lips during feeding. The facial nerve also innervates the lacrimal and salivary glands. Facial paralysis results in drooping of the ear, ptosis, decreased tear production, and paralysis of the upper lip causing it to be pulled towards the unaffected side.

• *Vestibulocochlear nerve (VIII)* is responsible for hearing (cochlear division) and balance (vestibular branch). Input to the vestibular system also comes from the cerebellum and other brainstem centres. Signs of vestibular

disease include a rhythmic *nystagmus* (fast phase usually directed away from the side of the lesion), *strabismus* and *head tilt* (towards the side of the lesion). The nystagmus may occur when the head is in a normal position (resting nystagmus) or when the head is placed in an unusual position (positional nystagmus). Central vestibular disease results in additional signs including proprioceptive deficits, ataxia, weakness and depression.

• *Glossopharyngeal nerve (X), vagus nerve (XI)* and *accessory nerve (XI)* contain sensory and motor fibres that innervate the pharynx, larynx, oesophagus and many other viscera. The normal swallowing reflex can be assessed by observing the horse eating or drinking, or by passing a nasogastric tube. The pharynx and larynx can be examined by endoscopy. The *laryngeal adductor response (slap test)* is tested by gently slapping one side of the chest just caudal to the dorsal scapula, while observing the larynx endoscopically. In normal horses the contralateral arytenoid adducts briefly. This reflex involves afferent pathways in the thoracic nerves and cervical spinal cord, and an efferent pathway via the recurrent laryngeal branch of the vagus (Figure 1). Pharyngeal paralysis results in dysphagia and nasal return of food.

• *Hypoglossal nerve (XII)* supplies motor innervation to the tongue. Weakness of the tongue is assessed by observing the resistance to pulling the tongue out of the mouth.

A summary of cranial nerve function tests is given in Table 1.

Examination of gait and posture

Abnormalities of gait may arise with either musculoskeletal or neurological problems, and the former must be ruled out before proceeding with the neurological examination.

Lesions affecting *descending motor pathways* result in *paresis* (weakness) caudal to the lesion. Such lesions can also cause overactivity of reflexes (due to damage to inhibitory pathways) resulting in *spasticity* (stiffness or hypometria). Damage to *ascending proprioceptive fibres* in peripheral nerves or white matter of the spinal cord results in *ataxia* (incoordination) in the limbs caudal or distal to the lesion. Interference with the transmission of proprioceptive information to the cerebellum can result in poor control of

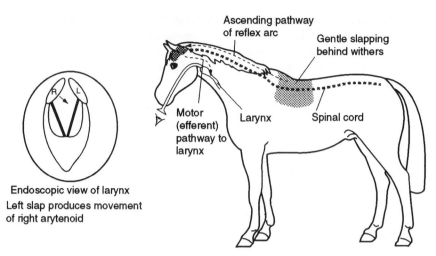

Figure 1 Laryngeal adductory function test ('slap test').

Table 1 Summary of cranial nerve function tests

Cranial nerve	Major function	Reflex/response/assessment
1 Olfactory	Sense of smell	–
2 Optic	Afferent pathway for vision and light	Menace response Pupillary light reflex
3 Oculomotor	Pupillary constriction Extraocular muscles	Pupillary light reflex Medial movement of globe
4 Trochlear	Extraocular muscles	Ventrolateral rotation of globe
5 Trigeminal	Sensory to side of face Motor to muscles of mastication	Ear, eyelid and lip (facial) reflexes Pain perception from head Chewing, jaw tone, muscle mass
6 Abducens	Extraocular muscles	Eyeball retraction Lateral movement of globe
7 Facial	Motor to muscles of facial expression	Ear, eyelid and lip (facial) tone, reflexes, and movement Facial symmetry
8 Vestibular	Afferent branch of vestibular system	Head posture Induced eyeball movement Normal vestibular nystagmus Normal gait Blindfold test
Cochlear	Sense of hearing	Response to noise
9 Glossopharyngeal 10 Vagus 11 Accessory	Sensory and motor to pharynx and larynx	Swallowing Gag reflex Endoscopy Slap test
12 Hypoglossal	Motor to tongue	Tongue size and symmetry

voluntary movements and *hypermetria* (over-reaching).

Gait and proprioceptive deficits are assessed by observing the horse walking, trotting, turning, backing, walking up and down a slope, and moving with a blindfold on. Proprioception can be assessed by walking the horse over a step or through an obstacle course, by crossing its forelegs and by forcing the horse to adopt a base-wide stance.

The degree of gait abnormality can be graded on a scale from 0 (normal) to 5 (recumbency).

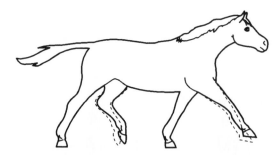

Figure 2 Diagram of a horse showing fore- and hindlimb hypermetria ('goose-stepping').

- *Ataxia* causes an unstable, swaying gait with abnormal foot placement, which becomes worse when the horse is walked on a slope. The limbs may be circumducted, especially on turning. The horse may pivot on the affected limbs when turning or backing.
- *Paresis* causes dragging the feet and stumbling. These signs may be exacerbated by walking the horse in a tight circle or up a slope.
- *Spasticity* causes a stiff movement of the limbs with reduced flexion of the joints. Spasticity can be exaggerated by walking up and down a slope with the head elevated.
- *Hypermetria* results in overstepping with excessive joint movement (Figure 2).

A summary of the neuroanatomical localization of lesions that result in gait abnormalities is given in Table 2.

Examination of the neck and forelimbs

- The neck and forelimbs are inspected for symmetry, malformations, muscle atrophy, patchy sweating and the degree and strength of voluntary effort.
- *Skin sensation* and spinal reflexes over the neck and forelimbs are assessed using a pen or probe to prod the skin. This results in flinching of the cervical musculature as well as a behaviour/cerebral response such as head or body movement away from the stimulus. The *cervicofacial reflex* is tested by prodding caudal to the ear, which results in twitching of the ear, blinking and movement of the labial commissure on the side being tested.
- The neck should be manipulated dorsoventrally and laterally to assess the range of movement and presence of pain.
- Pushing against the shoulders (*sway test*) assesses the capacity of the horse to resist lateral force, and is helpful in defining paresis and/or ataxia.

Examination of the trunk and hindlimbs

- The trunk and hindlimbs are observed for musculoskeletal malformations, vertebral column deviations and muscle atrophy.
- *Skin sensation* is assessed as for the neck and forelimbs. Prominent skin flicking over the thorax and flank in response to prodding is known as the *panniculus response*.
- A *sway test* is performed by providing lateral force to the pelvis (Figures 3a and 3b). A *tail pull test* is performed by pulling laterally on the tail when the horse is standing still and walking (Figure 3c).
- A *loin pressure test* is performed by pressing down firmly with the fingers on the loin and dorsal hip region.

Examination of the tail and anus

- The caudal body region is assessed for asymmetry of bone or muscle. Holding the tail elevated

Table 2 Summary of neuroanatomical localization of lesions resulting in gait abnormalities

Lesion location	Abnormal posture	Paresis	Ataxia	Hypometria	Hypermetria
Cerebrum	+++				
Brainstem	++	++	++	++	++
Vestibular	+++		++	++	
Cerebellum	++		+++	+	+++
Spinal cord UMN	++	++	++	++	++
Peripheral nerve/LMN	++	+++	+	(++)*	(+++)*
Musculoskeletal	+	++		+	

* Usually only with very selective sensory fibre involvement.
UMN, upper motor neuron. LMN, lower motor neuron.

(a)

(b)

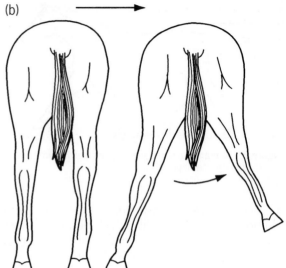

(c)

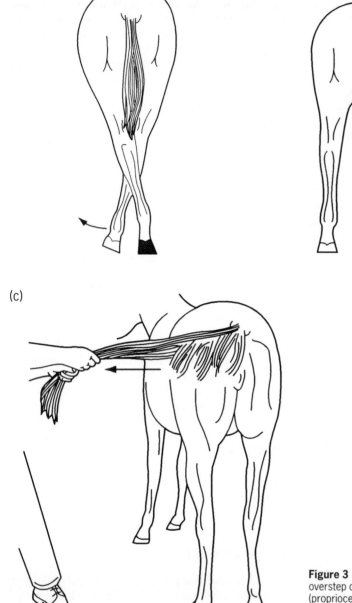

Figure 3 Sway response. (a) Push from quarters results in overstep of hindfoot across the midline and unsteadiness (proprioceptive deficit). (b) Response for comparison in normal horse. (c) Pulling tail laterally at walk shows weakness of hindquarters (paresis) in horses with CVM.

or to one side might be normal or abnormal for an individual horse.

- *Tail tone* is assessed by manoeuvring the tail.
- The *perineal reflex* is tested by gently prodding the perineum and observing a reflex contraction of the anal sphincter and clamping down of the tail.
- *Rectal palpation* is performed to evaluate rectal and urinary bladder content and tone.

Neurological examination of foals

See also Chapter 20.

Some important differences in reflex activity and neurological function exist between foals and adult horses:

- Menace response is commonly reduced or absent in normal foals.

- Jerky head movements are commonly seen in normal foals.
- Dysmetria and mild incoordination are common in normal foals.
- Response to the slap test is variable up to one month of age.

Ancillary diagnostic tests

Cerebrospinal fluid (CSF) collection

Atlanto-occipital (AO) space
With the horse under general anaesthesia, the head is flexed at right angles to the axis of the neck. Using aseptic technique, a needle is inserted at the middle of a line drawn between the cranial borders of the wings of the atlas. The subarachnoid space is entered at a depth of 2.5 to 7 cm with an 18–20 G, 9 cm spinal needle. A palpable 'give' in resistance is felt as the subarachnoid space is penetrated. Ten millilitres of CSF can be safely withdrawn.

Lumbosacral (LS) space
Collection from the LS space can be performed in the standing horse. The site of needle insertion is the palpable depression on the dorsal midline just caudal to the sixth lumbar spinous process (between the paired tuber sacrale). Using aseptic technique, a 15–20 cm, 18 G spinal needle is inserted to a depth of 11–13 cm until a change in resistance is appreciated; the horse often flinches as the subarachnoid space is entered.

CSF analysis

Bacteriologic and cytologic examinations can be performed. Normal CSF is clear and colourless, and has a nucleated cell count less than $6/\mu l$, of which all are mononuclear cells. There are normally no red blood cells, and the total protein is 0.5–1.0 g/l.

Pink discolouration results from the presence of red blood cells due either to blood contamination during collection or from central nervous system (CNS) trauma. *Xanthochromia* (yellow discolouration) results from the presence of blood pigments or breakdown products, and is seen as a result of CNS trauma or leakage from damaged vessels (e.g. equine herpesvirus (EHV) 1 vasculitis).

Increased numbers of white blood cells occurs in traumatic, infectious, neoplastic and other diseases. Bacterial infection generally results in a neutrophilic reaction, whereas viral infection results in a mononuclear reaction. Diseases causing tissue damage may result in the appearance of macrophages (some containing phagocytic vacuoles). Parasitic infections can result in an eosinophilic response.

Leakage of blood or plasma into the CSF results in an elevation of protein concentration. This is observed in traumatic, vascular, inflammatory and some degenerative diseases.

Radiology

See p. 222: 'Radiological examination of the cervical spine'.

Electromyography

Needle electromyography (EMG) can be used to detect disruption of the nerve supply to selected muscles. Damage to motor neurons in the ventral grey column or in peripheral nerves causes abnormalities of the electrical characteristics of the affected muscles.

Necropsy

THE BRAIN

11.2 *Congenital conditions*

See also Chapter 20.

Anencephalopathy

In this rare developmental condition the cerebrum and cranial vault of the skull are absent. The pituitary may also be absent. Parturition often requires to be assisted. Affected foals are not viable.

Hydrocephalus

Hydrocephalus is uncommon. It may cause dystocia due to gross enlargement of the cranium. Mildly affected foals may present with a congenital dummy syndrome with slow learning ability.

Cerebellar malformations

Cerebellar abiotrophy of Arabs

This condition affects purebred or partbred Arabian foals of either sex. The onset of clinical signs is usually between 1 and 6 months of age, but rarely at birth. It is probably inherited. There is a presumed deficiency of a vital trophic substance in cerebellar neurons that results in degeneration of neurons with depletion of Purkinje and granular cells. The cerebellum is usually small (less than 8% of total brain weight).

Clinical signs

- Sudden onset.
- Tremor of the head.
- Intention tremors (nodding movements of the head when trying to carry out a specific manoeuvre eg. moving towards the mare's udder to suckle).
- Deficit of menace response but normal vision.
- Hypermetric or hypometric ataxia; some foals show a hypometric gait at a walk that becomes hypermetric at faster gaits; there is no weakness.
- Foal may rear and fall over backwards when startled.
- Neurological deficits are exaggerated by turning sharply or blindfolding.
- Ataxia may progress to inability to stand.

Sometimes, the clinical signs stabilize, but they usually progress, and euthanasia is required.

Other cerebellar conditions

A disorder very similar to the Arabian disease is seen in Gotland ponies. Also, 1–2 month old Oldenberg foals may show signs referable to a rapidly progressive cerebellar disorder. Occasionally, degenerative cerebellar lesions are seen in newly born Thoroughbred foals when the foal begins to walk or at 2–3 days of age.

Neonatal maladjustment syndrome (NMS) (barkers, wanderers, dummies)

See Chapter 20.

Idiopathic seizures

Young growing foals, 1–10 months old, can have periods of *repeated seizures* that usually abate with or without long-term treatment. This may be more frequent in adolescent Arabian foals and possibly reflects a relatively low seizure threshold that allows expression of fits in response to many temporary toxic, infectious, metabolic and physical cerebral perturbations.

Residual behavioural changes (dementia) may occur following an episode of anoxia or hypoxia as in *anaesthetic accidents*, but blindness is more common.

11.3 *Trauma*

CNS injury can be caused by kicks or from running into a tree or fence post, rearing, somersaulting backwards and striking the poll. Signs depend on the area of the cranium and brain affected.

Forebrain trauma

Trauma to the frontal area is usually associated with a depressed fracture, often compounded, with direct laceration and haemorrhage. In some instances, there may be subdural haemorrhage.

Clinical signs

- Coma for up to several hours.
- Depression.
- Wandering in circles.
- Weakness and ataxia.
- Seizures.
- Blindness.
- Decreased facial sensation on opposite side of lesion.

Midbrain trauma

Clinical signs

- Coma.
- Depression.
- Abnormal gait and weakness.
- Asymmetric pupils and decreased pupillary light reflex (but no blindness).

Base of skull trauma

Fractures of the base of skull usually involve the region of the basilar part of the occipital and basisphenoid bones with local haemorrhage or a *contra coup* type lesion. This damage results in vestibular and facial nerve signs.

Clinical signs

- Head tilt towards the lesion.
- Facial paralysis (ipsilateral).
- Horizontal or rotatory nystagmus.
- May be central signs (depression, ataxia, weakness).
- May be other cranial nerve deficits if medulla is affected.

Vestibular signs with facial paralysis can occur without history of trauma. This may be due to otitis media or involve periosteal bony proliferation of the stylohyoid bone at its articulation with the temporal bone. Such cases may respond to antibiotic therapy.

Treatment of brain trauma

- *Sedation* with acetyl promazine or glycerol guaiacolate (guaiphenesin). If seizures continue, diazepam at 5 mg for a foal and up to 25 mg for an adult should be repeated as necessary. In some cases, general anaesthesia is necessary.
- *Corticosteroids* should always be given to decrease intracranial pressure and CNS oedema. Treatment is repeated every 4–6 hours for 1–4 days.
- *Hyperosmolar fluids* IV (e.g. 20% mannitol) are indicated in coma.
- *Dimethyl sulphoxide (DMSO)*.
- NSAIDs.
- *Surgical decompressive craniotomy* is indicated when there are bone fragments penetrating the cerebrum from an open skull fracture or when the horse fails to respond to medical management.

11.4 *Toxic conditions*

Hepatoencephalopathy

See Chapter 3.

Hepatoencephalopathy may be caused by any form of acute or severe hepatic necrosis, but is particularly associated with pyrrolizidine alkaloids in *Senecio* and *Crotolaria* spp. In foals, it can be associated with Tyzzer's disease.

Plant poisons

Locoweed and Darling pea toxicity

Locoweed (*Astragulus* and *Oxytropus* spp.) in the USA and Darling pea (*Swainsona* spp.) in Australia can produce a syndrome of dementia and periods of aggression and hyperaesthesia, along with cerebellar ataxia. The alkaloid toxins in these plants induce a lysosomal storage disease (alpha-mannosidosis) in affected horses.

Removal from exposure to the toxic plants can result in some alleviation of signs, but behavioural changes may be permanent. Reversal of signs with apparent permanent cure has been claimed using combinations of mood elevators (e.g. tranylcypromine and protriptyline) and reserpine.

Mouldy corn poisoning – leucoencephalomalacia

Associated with the ingestion of mouldy corn over a period of about 1 month, leucoencephalomalacia (LEM) develops from the mycotoxin produced by *Fusarium* spp., which affects the subcortical white matter.

Clinical signs

- Sudden onset.
- Dementia.
- Drowsiness.
- Blindness.
- Circling.
- Ataxia.
- Muscle fasciculations over neck and withers.

Signs can be asymmetric, and there may be brainstem involvement with pharyngeal paralysis and other cranial nerve deficits. The horse may also have signs of mild liver disease (e.g. jaundice).

The disease is usually progressive, terminating in coma and death. Many cases are fatal within a few hours to days from the onset of signs. Removal from the source of toxin in mild cases leaves the horse with residual brain damage.

Yellow star thistle poisoning

Nigropallidal encephalomalacia occurs in USA, South America and Australia in horses eating yellow star thistle (*Centaurea solstitialis*) or Russian knapweed (*Centaurea repens*). The toxicity results in necrosis of the substantia nigra and globus pallidus (i.e. nigropallidal encephalomalacia). Horses must eat the weeds for several weeks.

Clinical signs

- Sudden onset.
- Weight loss, depression, yawning.
- Excessive muscle tone (dystonia) of jaws, resulting in a grinding movement of the jaws without the ability to close the mouth completely.
- Inability to prehend food, chew or drink.
- Tongue may be drawn into a longitudinal trough.
- Lips retracted.
- Fasciculations of affected muscles.
- Sometimes circling, aimless wandering or ataxia.

Signs stabilize after several days, but the condition is fatal as there is no known treatment.

Birdsville horse disease

This disease is caused by toxicity to *Indigophera enneaphylla*, which contains alkaloids (i.e. indospicine and canavanine) that are arginine antagonists. It occurs in desert areas of Australia in the spring and summer.

Clinical signs

- Weight loss.
- Progressive ataxia.
- Weakness.
- Dyspnoea.
- Exaggerated hackney-type action in front.
- Reduced flexion with toe-dragging behind.
- Head and tail are held high.
- May gallop frantically on the spot, eventually the hindlimbs spreading and sinking as the animal becomes recumbent.
- May progress to convulsions and death.

In mild cases, complete recovery can occur but toe-dragging may persist.

The toxicity can be prevented by feeding a diet rich in arginine such as alfalfa or peanut meal.

Gomen disease

Gomen disease occurs in adult horses in one part of New Caledonia. Horses show progressive incoordination, debility and death. The disease is thought to be environmental in origin and likely to be caused by a toxic plant.

Lead poisoning

Lead poisoning is usually caused by the ingestion of lead acetate found in lead paint, used oil, old batteries, etc. Lead oxide and lead sheeting are less toxic. The other common source is industrial contamination or accidental feeding (e.g. boiled linseed oil). Although chronic exposure is most common, signs can be acute in onset.

Acute form
- Cerebral depression.
- Blindness.
- Partial then complete paralysis.

Subacute form
- Pharyngeal paralysis and dysphagia.
- Regurgitation of food down the nose.
- Choke.
- Aspiration pneumonia.
- Paralysis of lips.
- General muscle weakness.
- Stiff gait.
- Ataxia.

Chronic form
- Recurrent laryngeal nerve paralysis (roaring).
- Ill-thrift.

Treatment

- 1–2% calcium versenate (Ca disodium ethylene diamine tetra-acetic acid) in 5% glucose given IV.

Prognosis

The prognosis is guarded, and poor if pneumonia is present.

Snake bite

In North America, venomous snakes are members of the families Crotalidae (pit vipers), Elapidae and Viperidae (vipers). *Rattlesnake* bites are most common. Horses are usually bitten on the nose and face, and the principal clinical signs are oedematous swelling and local tissue necrosis. Neurological signs are usually slight.

In Australia, bites from the *tiger snake* may result in sudden onset of incoordination with dilation of the pupils, and gross muscle tremors. There is apparent foot pain, and the horse behaves as if 'walking on hot bricks', and lies down repeatedly. Tiger snake antivenom works well, but many horses would probably recover anyway. There is usually a good response in 12 hours and complete recovery in 24 hours. *Brown snake* bite is similar, but paralysis is usually more marked with an inability to swallow and withdraw the tongue. Treatment is by antivenom.

11.5 *Infectious conditions*

Equine viral encephalitides

The most important neurotropic viral infections of the horse are the arthropod-borne encephalitides. These include *Venezuelian encephalitis* (*VE*), *eastern encephalitis* (*EE*) and *western encephalitis* (*WE*), which are found in the Americas, and *Japanese B encephalitis*, which occurs in the Far East. All the viruses cause encephalitis in humans.

A high titre viraemia occurs with VE virus in the horse, and epidemics are maintained by a mosquito/horse cycle; infection of humans and other species is incidental. EE and WE have been recognized as separate diseases since 1933, and in the USA, horses are protected by routine vaccination. Epidemics of these diseases are now uncommon. In contrast to VE, both EE and WE viruses are maintained by a bird/mosquito cycle. The viraemia in the horse is generally considered insufficient to infect mosquito vectors; the horse is a 'dead end host'.

Several species of mosquito can act as vectors of VE, WE and EE. The extension of other arthropod-borne diseases to areas originally outside their geographical distribution (e.g. bluetongue in sheep) serves to illustrate the potential of VE, WE and EE to cause disease on other continents.

Clinically there is progressive onset of severe depression, fever, and peracute to subacute diffuse brain signs. These include dementia, head pressing, ataxia, blindness, circling and seizures. Rarely, signs of spinal cord disease are seen first.

Japanese B encephalitis (JE)

Infection by JE has been recorded in humans, but also in horses throughout the Far East. The virus is a flavivirus (previously arbovirus Group B) and is transmitted by mosquitoes, notably *Culex tritaeniorhynchus*. JE is a significant problem, but the mortality rate in the horse is usually low (less than 5%). The natural life cycle involves birds, probably wading birds, such as egrets and herons. The horse is probably a 'dead end host', although mosquitoes have been shown to transmit infection between horses.

Clinical signs

These are variable:

1. *Mild form*
   - Pyrexia (39.5°C).
   - Anorexia.
   - Jaundice.
   - Lethargy for 2–3 days.
   - Usually recover in 4–5 days.
2. *Moderate form*
   - Pyrexia (38.5–42.0°C).
   - Jaundice.
   - Petechiation of mucous membranes.
   - Somnolence.
   - Dysphagia.
   - Incoordination and falling over.
   - Temporary blindness.
   - Rigidity of neck.
   - Radial and labial paralysis.
   - Usually recover in 5–10 days.
3. *Severe form* – as above, but with tremors, excitability and sweating. This form is fatal.

Diagnosis

Diagnosis is confirmed by serology or by transmission of the disease to a normal horse.

Control

Formalized vaccine gives excellent immunity.

Borna disease

Borna, which takes its name from a town in Saxony, has been recognized in Germany for over 200 years. Comparatively little is known about the disease, but it is probably transmitted by ticks such as *Hyalomma anatolicum*. It is possible that the virus survives by a tick/bird cycle and infection of the horse is incidental. The incubation period of the disease is at least one month, and the encephalitis is indistinguishable from VE, EE or WE. Mortality is 80–90%. A characteristic inclusion, the Hoest–Degen body, may be found in the brain cells of the hippocampus and olfactory lobes of horses that die.

Clinical signs

- Fever.
- Pharyngeal paralysis.
- Hyperaesthesia.
- Lethargy.
- Flaccid paralysis.
- Course of disease 1–3 weeks.

A formalin-inactivated vaccine is available.

Rabies

Epidemiology

Neurotropic *rhabdovirus* can cause disease in any warm-blooded species. Horses are susceptible, and are usually infected via a bite wound from a rabid wild animal.

Equine rabies has been reported from most countries where the virus is endemic; at present, Great Britain, Ireland, New Zealand, Australia and Hawaii are free from the disease.

The incubation period varies from hours to months (usually 2 to 9 weeks), because the rabies virus can remain latent at the site of wound for varying lengths of time. The incubation period, sequence of clinical signs and survival period vary with the dose and pathogenicity of the virus strain, and the site of bite wound relative to the brain.

Clinical signs

Three forms of disease: furious (cerebral) form, dumb (brainstem) form and spinal cord (paralytic) form. Dumb and spinal cord forms are commonest in horses.

The clinical signs associated with the classical forms of rabies are:

Furious form
- Convulsions.
- Aggressiveness.
- Photophobia.

- Hydrophobia.
- Hyperaesthesia.

Dumb form
- Pharyngeal paralysis.
- Drooling.
- Depression.
- Ataxia.

Spinal cord form
- Ascending paralysis.

Clinical signs in individual cases are extremely variable, making the antemortem diagnosis difficult. Most cases show a rapid progression of disease, with death occurring in 4–5 days.

Diagnosis

- Clinical signs
- CSF analysis – pleocytosis with predominance of lymphocytes (occurs late in the disease)
- Necropsy
  - Histological identification of Negri bodies (intracytoplasmic inclusion bodies) in hippocampus and Purkinje cells of cerebellum.
  - Fluorescent antibody test on brain tissue.

Other viral encephalitides

Arboviruses

These include encephalitis associated with *West Nile, Semliki Forest, Near East Equine Encephalitis* (*NEEE*) and *louping ill* viruses. The clinical signs vary with each virus, but are essentially referrable to diffuse cerebral disease. In louping ill, signs of spinal cord disease predominate.

Equine herpesvirus 1 (EHV 1)

See Chapter 19.

Brain abscess

Brain abscesses are very rare and are usually associated with *Streptococcus equi* (strangles) or *Actinobacillus mallei* (glanders) infections.

Cerebral abscesses may be present without clinical signs, or be associated with septic meningitis, or cause signs of an expanding, asymmetric space occupying mass.

Clinical signs

These are variable, including:

- Depression.
- Head-pressing.
- Aimless wandering.
- Excitement.
- Circling.
- Contralateral blindness.
- Decreased facial sensation.

Diagnosis

- History (e.g. strangles).
- Haematology – neutrophilia and hyperfibrino-genaemia.
- CSF analysis – variable; xanthochromia and elevated protein.

Treatment

Treatment is with prolonged antibiotic therapy.

Meningitis

Meningitis may be due to bacterial, viral, protozoal or fungal infection, or rarely as an immune-mediated process. It is principally seen in young foals with poor immune status or secondary to septicaemia/suppurative polyarthritis (see Chapter 20). It may also be associated with a wound near the calvarium or vertebrae in adults.

Clinical signs

- Hyperaesthesia.
- Stiff neck.
- Depression – somnolence, seizures.
- Blindness.
- Pyrexia.
- Anorexia.
- Ataxia/paresis.
- Wandering, star-gazing, barking and seizures in foals.

Diagnosis

- Leucocytosis.
- CSF analysis – large numbers of neutrophils and increased protein concentration.
- Blood and CSF cultures.

Treatment

- Appropriate antibiotics.
- Control of seizures as necessary (e.g. diazepam, pentobarbitone).

Prognosis

The prognosis is poor.

11.6 *Parasitic lesions*

Encephalitis

Occurrence is sporadic, although endemic in some areas, e.g. Kumri in India due to *Setaria* spp. It is most commonly associated with *Strongylus vulgaris*, *Hypoderma* spp. and *Micronema deletrix*. Clinical signs are extremely variable depending on the number, size and location of the parasites. Progressive forebrain, brainstem or cerebellar signs may occur.

Parasitic cerebral thromboembolism

Occurs mainly in young adults due to *S. vulgaris* thromboarteritis in great vessels leading to embolic shower via carotids to cerebrum.

Clinical signs

- Acute onset of seizures.
- Depression.
- Violent or passive behaviour.
- Circling.
- Wandering towards the side of the lesion.
- Blindness.
- Subtle gait abnormality on opposite side of the lesion.

Diagnosis

- Eosinophilia.
- CSF analysis – increased neutrophils, eosinophils, erythrocytes and xanthochromia.

Treatment

- Anthelmintics (larvicidal doses).
- Anti-inflammatory drugs.

Equine protozoal myeloencephalitis (EPM)

See p. 226. EPM is more commonly a cause of spinal cord disease but occasionally there are cerebral signs alone. This disease can mimic many other neurological diseases of the horse.

11.7 *Neoplasia*

Tumours of the CNS are very rare in the horse. The most common tumour is pituitary adenoma, which usually causes Cushing's disease (see Chapter 9), although it may rarely induce blindness and severe depression.

Cholesterol granulomas are commonly found in the choroid plexuses of old horses, and are usually clinically silent. Large granulomas are sometimes associated with intermittent circling, blindness and depression.

11.8 *Miscellaneous conditions*

Epilepsy

Recurrent seizures occur due to a state of excessive and abnormal nervous discharge in the brain. It may be idiopathic or occur secondary to areas of cerebral cortex damage due to ischaemic, traumatic, infectious or neoplastic diseases. The clinical signs and intervals between attacks are highly variable.

Clinical signs

Clinical signs may include some or all of the following:

- Loss of consciousness.
- Tonic and clonic muscular activity.
- Abnormal movements of head and eyes.
- Jaw clamping.
- Opisthotonos.
- Paddling.
- Urination, defecation.
- Sweating.
- Salivation.

Treatment

Treatment with diphenylhydantoin (phenytoin) may be effective in idiopathic cases.

Narcolepsy

Abnormal sleep tendency characterized by periods of muscle relaxation and collapse (cataplexy). A familial occurrence has been noted in Miniature horses.

Clinical signs

- Cataplexy (muscular weakness), which usually affects the head and neck (head hangs low and may rest on the ground); sometimes collapse occurs.
- Attacks last from a few seconds to several minutes.
- Trigger for attack varies between horses.

Diagnosis

- Clinical signs and absence of other diseases.
- Pharmacological testing – physostigmine salicylate IV induces narcoleptic attack in 3 to 10 minutes (this test sometimes gives inconsistent results).

Treatment

Imipramine hydrochloride IM relieves narcolepsy for 5 to 10 hours.

Intracarotid drug injections cause intense vasospasm and endothelial damage which may result in cortical ischaemia and necrosis.

Clinical signs are observed immediately on injection of the drug. The horse may rear, or lunge backwards, or run wildly. Some may collapse and become comatose. Some die after a variable period, whereas others recover. Residual CNS or sympathetic trunk damage may cause blindness, Horner's syndrome, head tilt, etc.

THE SPINAL CORD

11.9 *Ataxia*

Ataxia is the result of reduced kinaesthesia, or lack of sense of motion or position of the body or limbs in space. This results from a *loss of proprioception* and is frequently accompanied by some degree of *weakness* (*paresis*). General proprioceptors (GP), which are sensitive to movement, are located in the internal mass of the body in the muscles, tendons and joints. The pathways for segmental reflex activity and transmitting proprioceptive information principally involve the spinocerebellar tracts. It may be difficult clinically to differentiate proprioceptive deficit from paresis caused by upper motor neuron (UMN) damage. The UMN and GP systems accompany each other through most of the CNS. The UMN is responsible for the initiation of voluntary movements, body support and posture regulation.

Clinical features of ataxia

The physical condition of the horse in the acute stages is usually good, and clinical signs are essentially those of proprioceptive deficit. The degree of ataxia can be graded:

Grade 0   Deficit not detected.
Grade +   Deficit not detected at normal gait or posture.
Grade ++   Deficit easily detected, and posture exaggerated by backing, turning, swaying, loin pressure and neck extension.
Grade +++ Deficit very prominent at normal gait with a tendency to buckle or fall with backing, turning, swaying, loin pressure, neck extension.
Grade ++++ Signs of stumbling, tripping and falling spontaneously at normal gait, and more severe deficits.

Clinical signs

- When standing at rest, the ataxic horse often adopts a *base-wide stance*.
- Usually, some unsteadiness is noted even when in the stable, but no distress is seen nor any awareness of the proprioceptive deficit.
- In mild cases, signs in the hindlimbs are more easily recognized.
- At the walk and trot, some swaying of the hindquarters and dragging of the toes are seen.
- They seem to be unaware of the position of their limbs and lack smooth coordinated movements (Figure 4).
- They exhibit exaggerated lifting of the hindlimbs, hesitate slightly and then stab the feet back onto the ground.
- Knuckling of the fetlock and stumbling are seen in severe cases.
- On turning in a tight circle, the outer hindlimb may circumduct with poor foot placement and a tendency to tread on the other toe (Figure 5).
- Signs are usually most noticeable at the slower paces; the horse improves at the canter, but often lacks impulsion from the hindquarters.

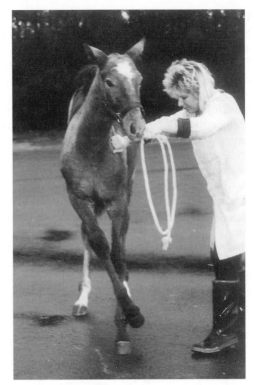

Figure 4 Abnormal placement of a forelimb in a yearling with Grade 3 ataxia due to CVS (proprioceptive deficit).

- They show difficulty in coming quickly to a halt, and the hindfeet seem to slip or may interfere with the heels of the forefeet. This is usually best demonstrated by observing the horse's gait when turned loose in a small paddock.

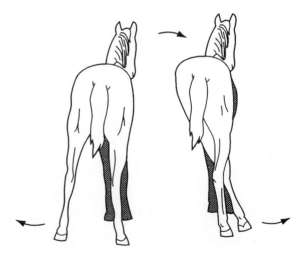

Figure 5 Turning horse in a tight circle with a proprioceptive deficit demonstrates circumduction of outer limb and abnormal placement.

- The signs of hindlimb ataxia are usually, but not always, symmetrical and can vary in severity from day to day.
- The horse often backs awkwardly due to a widening of the hindfeet position, dragging of the toes and unsteadiness (Figures 6a and 6b).
- Blindfolding rarely exacerbates the signs of proprioceptive deficit, but exercising on a mild incline usually does.
- The sway reaction, particularly on the hindlimbs, is abnormal, and pressure on the loins can cause them to nearly go down.
- Examination of the neck for stiffness, pain and muscle wastage is usually helpful only in cases of trauma.
- There may be involvement of the forelimbs, and this is usually seen as hypermetria (or goose-stepping action) due to a prolonged flexor phase of the gait.

(a)

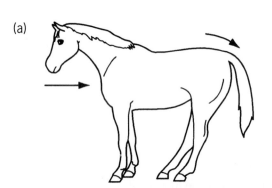

(b)

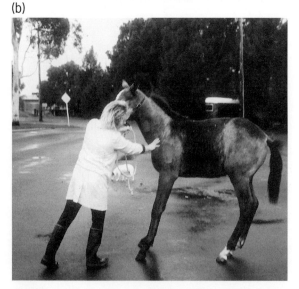

Figure 6 Backing: (a) and (b) difficulty backing with lowering of the quarters in a horse with myelitis of the lumbar region (e.g. EPM).

Epidemiological features of ataxia in horses

The clinical background of affected horses is variable, but some diagnostic clues may be obtained from a general comparison of the history, signalment and pathology of the five major causes of spinal cord diseases in horses (see Table 3).

Clinical aids to diagnosis

The following clinical aids to diagnosis may be helpful:

1. *Radiography*:
   - Lateral views in standing position (C1–T1).
   - Neutral, flexed and extended views under general anaesthesia; also ventrodorsal positions to about C4–C5 level.
   - Myelography – lateral views in neutral, flexed and extended positions.
2. *Slap test*: For evaluation of laryngeal adductory reflex as confirmation of cervical spinal cord damage.
3. *Clinical pathology*:
   - CSF analysis (from AO or LS sites).
   - Haematology – WBC count and differential.
   - Biochemical profile.
   - Serology.
4. *Electromyography*: For detection of subtle neurological problems by evaluating the entire motor unit.

Radiological examination of the cervical spine

Plain radiography performed with the horse standing has definite advantages over that carried out under general anaesthesia. A dynamic visualization of the cervical vertebrae is obtained, which makes evaluation of cervical stenosis easier. However, sophisticated equipment involving a powerful generator or overhead mounted tube and linked cassette holder is necessary to achieve this. Low output portable equipment is probably inadequate for the caudal neck and always requires general anaesthesia. Rare-earth intensifying screens and a cross hatch (8:1) grid are helpful in providing good radiographic quality.

A full radiographic survey from C1–T1 in the lateral plane is necessary in all cases because lesions may be present at multiple sites. Ventrodorsal views are possible with the horse placed in dorsal recumbency, although caudal to C4–5, the

Table 3 Some features of five major causes of ataxia in horses

	CVS	EPM	EDM	EHV 1	Trauma
Incidence					
Sporadic	+	+	±	−	+
Age at onset	3mnth to 14y	6mnth to 14y	0–24mnth	>24mnth	all ages
Sex	male	either sex	either sex	preg.mares	either sex
Breed	Tb	Stb	Arabian	none	none
Onset	variable	variable	variable	acute	acute
Clinical signs					
Neck stiffness	±	−	−	−	+
Lameness/pain	−	+	−	−	+
Muscle wastage	±	+	−	−	+
Ataxia asymmetric	±	+	−	−	−
Ataxia progressive	±	+	±	−	−
Response to DXMS	−	±*	±	−	−
HL ataxia only	+	+	+	+	+
+ FL involvement	+	+	+	−	±
+ CNS involvement	−	+	±	+	+
Other clinical signs	−	−	−	+	±
Clinical aids					
Radiol. changes	+	−	−	−	+
CSF	−	±	−	+	−
Serology	−	−	−	±	−
Pathological lesions	Focal	Diffuse and multifocal	Diffuse	Diffuse	Focal
White matter	+	+	+	+	+
Grey matter	−	+	±	+	±
Site: Cervical	+	+	+	+	±
TL	±	+	+	+	±
Brain	−	+	+	+	−
Any clinical improvement likely	±	±	−	++	variable

*Corticosteroid treatment of EPM may exacerbate the disease.
CVS = cervical vertebral stenosis. DXMS = dexamethasone. EPM = equine protozoal myeloencephalitis. EDM = equine degenerative myeloencephalopathy. EHV 1 = equine herpesvirus 1 myeloencephalopathy.

X-ray quality is usually very poor because of the large amount of soft tissue involved. For myelography, a suitable dose of contrast agent (e.g. metrizamide, iopamidol or iohexol) is injected slowly (i.e. over 2–3 min) into the atlanto-occipital (AO) space. It is important to inject the contrast agent with the head and neck raised to prevent any going forward into the lateral ventricles of the brain. Recovery from anaesthesia may be prolonged, but serious untoward sequelae (e.g. convulsions, or meningitis) are not usually encountered.

Some experience is required in interpreting cervical radiographs because there are individual variations in radiographic anatomy and differences in age, site and neck position. There are also some incidental anomalies that cannot always be differentiated from significant radiological findings. The most important one is the appearance of ventral lipping of new bone with buttressing of the articular processes from C5–T1 that is seen in many normal adult horses as well as young ataxic Thoroughbreds.

Slap test

The presence of a laryngeal adductory reflex can be demonstrated in horses by slapping the saddle region with the palm of the hand. The normal response can be seen using an endoscope, and involves a slight adductory flicker of the contra-lateral arytenoid cartilage that coincides with each slap. The adductory movement may also be palpated externally as an alternative to using endoscopy.

The degree of adductory movement elicited varies among normal horses. Some horses react to gentle slapping while in others the reflex is only observed after a more vigorous stimulus. For this reason, the optimal strength of the slap administered has to be determined for each individual horse, and varies according to the type and size of the animal. If too soft a slap is used, no response is elicited even in normal horses. If the slap is too forceful, the horse adducts both arytenoid cartilages simultaneously, which is regarded as a fear response.

In tense or excited horses, fixed bilateral abduction of the larynx occurs, and this precludes assessment of the reflex. Some horses relax after the endoscope has been *in situ* for a few minutes, and, in some instances, removal of the twitch tends to encourage relaxation of the larynx. Chemical restraint does not appear to affect the reflex.

The slap test response is often abolished from the left arytenoid in horses with laryngeal hemiplegia. In horses with cervical spinal cord damage (e.g. compressive lesion of vertebral stenosis), the slap response on both sides is absent. The test provides valuable confirmatory evidence of a cervical spinal cord lesion in horses exhibiting forelimb as well as hindlimb incoordination. In those cases where only hindlimb ataxia is present, it can help differentiate cervical from thoracolumbar (TL) spinal cord damage. Finally, the slap test has been found to be considerably more reliable as a diagnostic aid than plain radiography.

Clinical pathology

CSF can be collected from both atlanto-occipital (AO) and lumbosacral (LS) sites and should be examined for colour, clarity, cytology (i.e. red and white cell counts) and total protein. Results are usually within normal limits for most conditions apart from mild xanthochromia possibly reflecting some previous haemorrhage. In equine protozoal myeloencephalitis (EPM), an LS tap is more likely to be abnormal and may show a mild increase in white cell count. The CSF of horses with EHV 1 may have raised total protein, white cell count and xanthochromia.

The haemogram and biochemical profile are largely to provide eliminative information; serological tests (EHV 1, toxoplasma titres) are frequently unrewarding.

Specific conditions of spinal cord disease

The following list of conditions should be considered in horses showing signs of ataxia:

1. Congenital lesions
   - Occipitoatlantoaxial malformations in Arabians
   - Vertebral synostosis with meningocele
   - Cervical vertebral anomalies of development
2. Trauma
   - Fracture – vertebral body/neural arch
   - Dislocation – vertebral subluxation
   - Haematoma, soft tissue damage and other vascular accidents
3. Cervical vertebral stenosis (CVS)
   - Cervical vertebral displacement
   - Medial impingement of articular processes
   - Functional stenosis of the vertebral canal
   - Arthropathy of articular processes
   - Synovial cyst at interneural articulations (C5–T1)
4. Inflammatory conditions
   - Equine protozoal myeloencephalitis (EPM)
   - Equine herpesvirus 1 vasculitis/myeloencephalopathy
   - Migrating parasite
   - Spinal abscess
   - Vertebral osteomyelitis
5. Degenerative conditions
   - Equine degenerative myeloencephalopathy (EDM)
   - Fibrocartilaginous embolism
6. Neoplasia
   - Glioma, sarcoma, lymphosarcoma
7. Toxic conditions
   - Sorghum grass ataxia
   - Rye grass staggers

11.10 *Congenital lesions*

Occipitoatlantoaxial malformation (OAAM)

This uncommon condition, usually seen in Arabians, is probably inherited. Lesions involve developmental abnormalities of the occipital condyles, atlas and axis, with fusion and hypoplasia of the odontoid process and additional bony pieces.

Foals are either born dead, or are ataxic at birth, or show signs of progressive ataxia in the first few months of life. They may have an extended neck posture with reduced range of flexion of the atlanto-occipital joint. Vertebral abnormalities may be palpable externally. Diagnosis can be confirmed radiographically. There is no treatment.

Other vertebral and spinal cord malformations

Rare cases of block vertebrae (synostosis), spina bifida, cavitated vertebrae and myelodysplasia occur. Congenital kyphosis, scoliosis and torticollis may be associated with arthrogryposis, including the contracted foal syndrome.

11.11 *Trauma*

Cervical vertebral trauma can affect all types, breeds and ages of horses.

The severity of clinical signs of proprioceptive deficit depends on the degree of trauma to the spinal cord and the site of the damage. Signs include sudden onset of ataxia, reluctance to move or recumbency. The signs are not usually progressive, and improvement often occurs unless haemorrhage, joint instability or callus formation is present. Not all cases of vertebral damage result in discernible radiographic changes, but usually the horse has a stiff painful neck with patchy sweating.

The area most frequently affected in young foals is the occipitoatlantal region. Trauma to this area causes mild signs of tetraparesis and recumbency, but the foals usually improve with time. Vertebral fractures with spinal cord involvement carry a very poor prognosis. Radiography is essential for specific diagnosis because an incomplete or crush fracture of the thoracolumbar spine can cause hindlimb ataxia and look clinically very much like a cervical lesion. Conservative treatment includes dexamethasone, dimethyl sulphoxide (DMSO), phenylbutazone or flunixin meglumine.

11.12 *Cervical vertebral stenosis (CVS)*

Clinical features

'Wobbler' syndrome is seen principally in 18–30 month old male Thoroughbreds. The horses are usually well grown and in excellent body condition.

Clinical signs

- Onset of signs may be sudden following some traumatic incident or may be insidious.
- Severity of signs ranges from only just detectable (+) to the horse being unable to stand (++++).
- Signs may be progressive, but often plateau and then vary from day to day.
- Hindlimb ataxia always seen.
- Forelimb dysmetria may be seen, especially in young horses.
- Incoordination is usually symmetric, but, when due to a caudal cervical arthropathy, can appear more unilateral.
- Slap test is usually abnormal.

The proprioceptive deficit is caused by one or more sites of compression of the cervical vertebral canal resulting from vertebral malformation or malarticulation. This stenosis may be caused by a static lesion encroaching on the vertebral canal or by dynamic compression when the neck is in flexion or extension. Cervical vertebral stenosis, when mild, causes only hindlimb ataxia by interruption of general proprioception. As the degree of compression increases, the signs progress to spasticity and paresis as the deep motor neuron pathways are affected. The hindlimb signs are more obvious because the hindlimb spinocerebellar tracts in the lateral funiculi are more superficially positioned than those of the forelimb.

The underlying pathogenesis of the condition is unknown, but it is probably multifactorial in origin. A number of different lesions are recognized.

Pathogenesis

1. Cervical vertebral displacement

This is seen radiographically as pronounced dorsal displacement of the vertebral head of C3 to C6 resulting in narrowing at the intercentral joint space. It is not apparently a traumatic lesion, and it occurs mostly in the younger age group (9–18 months). It may be similar to the cervical instability seen in large breeds of dogs.

2. Abnormalities of vertebral development

- Symmetric overgrowth of the cranial articular processes of C3–C5 resulting in vertebral canal stenosis, which is exacerbated during neck flexion.
- Narrowing of the cranial entrance to the neural canal producing severe stenosis of the vertebral

canal. This deficit often accompanies the vertebral displacement lesion.

- The dorsal prominence of the caudal epiphysis (i.e. 'ski slope' appearance) producing a ventral stenosis of the vertebral canal in some young horses (12–24 months). This is not usually a primary lesion, but is seen in association with the others listed.

3. Functional dynamic stenosis

Narrowing of the normal vertebral canal causes spinal cord compression by flexion of the mid neck (C3–C5) or extension of the caudal neck (C5–T1).

4. Arthropathy of the interneural articulations

This is associated with asymmetric overgrowth of the articular processes, usually in the caudal cervical spine (C4–C7), and is essentially a static lesion. In young, rapidly growing horses (<24 months) the underlying problem may be associated with osteochondrosis, but older horses (>3 years) have degenerative joint disease whose pathogenesis is obscure. There may be associated damage to the ligamentum flavum and joint capsule, presumably caused by stretching and tearing of these structures. This results in local fibrosis, osteosclerosis of the dorsal lamina and osteophyte formation on the articular facets. Radiographically, there is new bone formation with ventral overgrowth obliterating the intervertebral space. Diagnosis should be confirmed by myelography because the radiographic changes occur quite commonly in normal horses. In this latter group, no ataxia ensues because there is no medial encroachment of the vertebral canal by the asymmetric articular processes. Clinical cases in this category can produce an asymmetric ataxia that is due to more pronounced impingement by the articular process on one side.

5. Synovial cyst

The presence of a small cyst or outpouching of the joint capsule of the interneural articulation on the roof of the vertebral canal can produce dorsal compression of the spinal cord. These lesions usually occur in the older age group in the caudal neck (C5–T1) and are exacerbated by extension. The pathogenesis is equivocal, but is assumed to be due to continued movement or overriding of the articular process leading to distension of the joint, which then protrudes as an outpouching ventrally into the roof of the vertebral canal.

Pathology

The symmetry of the clinical signs reflects damage to the ascending proprioceptive pathways causing ataxia, and the descending upper motor neuron pathways causing paresis. The gross lesions are associated with a flattening of the spinal cord at the site of compression with local haemorrhage and softening due to malacia.

Histologically at the site of compression there is malacia, usually with cavitation, haemorrhage, loss of myelin in all funiculi and variable axonal degeneration. Proximal to the compressive site, there is degeneration of myelin of the ascending tracts of dorsal white and superficial dorsolateral funiculi. There may also be neuronal degeneration in the grey columns with infiltration of gitter cells and proliferation of gemistocytic astrocytes. Caudal to the compressive site, there is loss of myelin and Wallerian degeneration of axons in the descending spinal cord tracts.

Treatment

- *Glucocorticoids* can provide transient relief but do not solve the underlying problem.
- *Rest* and neck braces with correction of overfeeding has helped in limiting progression of the disease, and may provide radiographic as well as clinical improvement.
- Surgical treatment. *Dorsal laminectomy*, especially at C6–T1, is indicated for absolute stenosis associated with osteoarthrosis and proliferated soft tissue. A modified Cloward technique of ventral fusion is successful in selected horses, and is particularly useful in early cases, involving one site, usually from C2 to C6.

Prognosis

The prognosis is generally poor. Some horses improve with conservative treatment of rest and dietary manipulation.

Early surgical treatment usually provides an improvement of at least one grade of ataxia.

11.13 Inflammatory conditions

Equine protozoal myeloencephalitis (EPM)

EPM is caused by *Sarcocystis neurona* infection of the CNS.

The disease is principally seen in North America. It affects horses of all ages, but most commonly 1–6 year old horses. It is non-contagious, but clusters of disease sometimes occur.

Clinical signs

- May be sudden onset of hindlimb lameness and ataxia.
- Progressive over days to weeks.
- Weakness and spasticity of limbs.
- Muscle wastage from the quarters.
- Ataxia may involve forelimbs as well as hindlimbs.
- Ataxia is often asymmetric.
- Pronounced alteration in the sway reaction.
- On backing, the horse tends to sink back, refusing to move the hindlimbs.
- Asymmetric cranial nerve deficits may develop.
- Sensory deficits and focal sweating.

Diagnosis

- Clinical features indicate multifocal lesions with asymmetric signs.
- CSF (LS) may show slight xanthochromia, red blood cells and monocytes/PMNs.
- Antibody test (immunoblot test) on serum and CSF. Positive serum indicates exposure to the organism, but not necessarily clinical disease. Positive CSF is highly correlated with clinical EPM.
- Definitive diagnosis depends on histologic observation of the infectious agent within the CNS.

Pathology

Gross discoloration and softening of the CNS tissue. Lesions are usually multifocal within the spinal cord, brainstem and sometimes the cerebrum and cerebellum. Necrotic areas with haemorrhage are present in severe lesions. Inflammatory lesions consist of prominent lymphoid perivascular cuffing. Organisms are seen singly and in groups (schizonts or merozoites in the cytoplasm of macrophages, neurons, axons, neutrophils and pericytes).

Treatment

- Pyrimethamine (Daraprim) daily by mouth, and trimethoprim-sulphadiazine (Tribrissen) by mouth, twice daily, and folic acid IM every 3 days.

Treatment is continued for 1–2 months.

- *Corticosteroids are contraindicated* because they may exacerbate the condition.

Equine herpesvirus 1 vasculitis/ myeloencephalopathy

See Chapter 19.

Usually acute onset, and several horses may be affected. Pyrexia, respiratory disease and abortion may be observed either in the neurologically affected horses or other horses on the premises.

Clinical signs

- Fever.
- Ataxia (most severe in pelvic limbs).
- Tetraplegia/tetraparesis.
- Urinary incontinence and bladder distension.
- Flaccid anus and tail.
- Variable areas of perineal desensitization
- Stallions and geldings may develop paraphimosis.

The progression of signs is variable. Many cases stabilize rapidly and improve after a few days; others show a gradual deterioration until death. Complete recovery can take up to 18 months.

Diagnosis

- Serology to show a rising antibody titre.
- Antibodies in CSF.
- Virus isolation from CSF/nasopharyngeal swab.
- Post-mortem examination and histopathology.

Treatment

Treatment is mainly supportive. Many horses respond to large doses of *corticosteroids*. Supportive care includes provision of adequate bedding for recumbent horses and catheterization to relieve bladder distension.

The pathological changes are principally haemorrhage and malacia. Histologically, there is a diffuse non-suppurative necrotizing leptomeningeal vasculitis with multifocal ischaemia, myelopathy and encephalopathy. The vasculitis with resultant vascular insufficiency causes the infarcts, and areas of ischaemic or haemorrhagic malacia.

Other inflammatory conditions

Migrating helminths occur occasionally in all ages and types of horses. Signs are usually acute and progressive, but this varies according to the movement of the parasite. The signs reflect the tortuous, usually asymmetric, random migrations of the parasites (*Strongylus* spp., *Hypoderma* spp., *Habronema* spp., *Setaria* spp.) or diffuse brain and/or spinal cord involvement (*Setaria* spp., *Micronema deletrix*). Thus, progressive forebrain, brainstem, cerebellar or spinal cord signs may predominate. Diagnosis may be assisted by circulating eosinophilia or abnormal CSF tap. Treatment consists of antiparasitic and anti-inflammatory medication. Prognosis depends on the damage incurred, but some good recoveries from acute syndromes have been recorded. The gross lesions involve swelling of the site with haemorrhage, red-brown discoloration and soft focal areas of malacia. Histologically, there may be haemorrhagic malacic tracts in acute cases with macrophages and perivascular cuffing of lymphocytes, neutrophils and eosinophils. In older lesions, macrophages, astrocytes and proliferating capillaries predominate.

Spinal abscess is rare. Vertebral osteomyelitis (see Chapter 20) is occasionally seen in foals, and usually involves the caudal cervical/cranial thoracic spine (C6–T3). Signs include sudden onset of pain or stiffness. Progressive paresis occurs. Diagnosis can be confirmed by radiological examination and clinical pathology. There is neutrophilia, left shift, abnormal protein electrophoresis, and raised fibrinogen. Treatment is by appropriate antimicrobial medication, but prognosis is usually poor.

11.14 *Equine degenerative myeloencephalopathy (EDM)*

EDM is characterized by degenerative lesions and demyelination of the spinal cord. The clinical picture is very similar to CVS because it causes symmetrical ataxia, weakness and spasticity of the limbs. Can affect most breeds (but especially Arabians). An age range from birth to 24 months is usually seen (most commonly 6–8 months), and there is no sex predilection. More than one horse on a stud or premises may be affected.

The cause of the condition is unknown, but there may be a congenital neuronal metabolic deficit, or a nutritional deficiency (e.g. vitamin E deficiency), or plant poisoning, or familial tendency.

Clinical signs

- Symmetric ataxia: knuckling, stumbling, circumduction of limbs, abduction, interference, etc.
- Spasticity and 'stabbing' with the limbs as they are placed on the ground.
- Inability to turn sharply.
- May be unable to back.
- May fall or stumble with light pressure over the withers or tuber coxae.
- The neurologic deficit is often equal in both fore- and hindlimbs.
- Clinical signs are usually slowly progressive.

Diagnosis

- Clinical features.
- Plain and contrast radiography of cervical spine (to rule out CVS).
- CSF analysis is normal.
- Plasma vitamin E may be low.
- Absence of slap test reflex.

Lesions are characterized by neuronal fibre degeneration with loss of myelin throughout the cord, but especially in the dorsolateral and ventromedial funiculi. There is also neuroaxonal degeneration of the proprioceptive relay areas in the cervical and medullary nuclei. The lesions are usually bilaterally symmetrical, but most severe in the thoracic areas.

The signs are irreversible, and there is no effective treatment.

11.15 *Neoplasia*

Spinal cord neoplasms in horses are rare, but *lymphoma, haemangiosarcoma, melanoma, undifferentiated sarcoma* and *glioma* have been recorded causing progressive para- or tetraparesis. Signs can begin suddenly and can progress rapidly.

11.16 *Toxic conditions*

Rye grass staggers, Bermuda grass staggers and Dallas grass staggers

Tremogenic diseases associated with feeding certain fields of ryegrass, Bermuda grass, and Dallas grass. Ryegrass staggers and Dallas grass staggers have been recognized in animals in New Zealand, Australia, USA and Great Britain. Bermuda grass staggers reported mainly in the USA. Dallas grass staggers is associated with ingestion of grass infected with the ergot fungus *Claviceps paspali*. Clinical disease is more commonly observed in cattle and sheep.

Clinical signs

- Stiff, goose-stepping gait.
- Ataxia.
- Tremors of all major muscle groups.
- Intentional head tremor.
- Truncal sway.
- Base-wide stance.
- Collapse.

Affected horses should be removed from the pasture. Most animals gradually recover, but full recovery may take several months.

Sorghum grass ataxia

Sorghum grass cystitis and ataxia occurs uncommonly in horses in USA and Australia.

Clinical features

- Symmetric hindlimb incoordination.
- Urinary incontinence.
- Hypoalgesia of perineum.
- Flaccid tail.
- Weakness and stiffness of hindquarters.
- On examination *per rectum*, the urinary bladder may be distended.

The lesion is due to fibre degeneration throughout the spinal cord with degenerative neuropathy of spinal nerves. Secondary cystitis often occurs.

Signs may improve following removal from affected pastures.

11.17 *Equine motor neuron disease*

Equine motor neuron disease was first recorded in 1990. The disease is most prevalent in northeastern USA and Canada, but cases have also been recorded in South America, Japan and Europe.

Clinical signs

- Weakness without ataxia.
- Muscle tremors and fasciculations.
- Shortened length of stride.
- Occasional stumbling.
- Abnormal positioning of the feet under the body.
- Excessive periods of recumbency.
- Weight loss despite normal appetite.
- Muscle atrophy.
- Condition is usually progressive necessitating euthanasia, but in some cases, the clinical signs stabilize.

Diagnosis

- Clinical signs.
- May be moderate elevations of CK and AST.
- CSF protein concentration is elevated.
- EMG shows widespread denervation of muscles.
- Muscle biopsy of the sacrocaudalis dorsalis medialis.
- Biopsy of the ventral branch of the spinal accessory nerve.

Pathology

Motor nerve cell bodies in the ventral horn grey matter of the spinal cord and in some brainstem nuclei become swollen, and there is loss of Nissl substance. This is followed by cell shrinkage and development of intracytoplasmic inclusions. Damaged nerve cell bodies are eventually phagocytosed by microglia. There is denervation atrophy of muscles with a high percentage of type I fibres.

Aetiology

Aetiology is uncertain. Possibly vitamin E deficiency. Most affected horses are stabled with no access to grass.

THE PERIPHERAL AND AUTONOMIC NERVOUS SYSTEMS

11.18 Generalized conditions

Botulism and shaker foal syndrome

These are uncommon conditions, except for shaker foal syndrome in Kentucky. Botulism occurs in adult horses of any type, and onset of signs may be associated with some stress (e.g. racing, foaling, weaning).

Clostridium botulinum produces a neurotoxin that blocks the neuromuscular junction. In adult horses, the toxin is usually preformed and ingested, and the disease is commonly known as *forage poisoning*. *C. botulinum* grows in neutral or alkaline conditions, and produces toxin in anaerobic environments such as decaying vegetable matter and animal carcases. Silage may provide a suitable medium for toxin production if the organism is present before fermentation reduces the pH to 4.5 or less. Contamination of silage by animal carcases or spoiled big bale silage are recognized sources of toxin. Cases may occur sporadically or as outbreaks. Toxicoinfectious botulism involves the ingestion of spores that germinate and produce toxin within the gastrointestinal tract. The presence of gastric ulcers may predispose to the disease. This form of botulism is the usual cause of the *shaker foal syndrome* (see Chapter 20). *Wound infection* by the organism with the subsequent production of toxin is an unusual cause of the disease. The toxin type varies in different areas and different countries, but is usually type B, C or D.

Clinical signs

Clinical signs in adult horses include sudden death or acute onset of flaccid quadriplegia with no history of illness or trauma.

- Violent trembling.
- Progressive weakness with normal sensation.
- Pharyngeal paralysis resulting in dysphagia.
- Drooling saliva.
- Flaccid tongue.
- Flaccid tail.
- Sluggish pupillary light reflexes.
- Recumbency.

- Intercostal and phrenic nerve paralysis may result in dyspnoea.
- Death may arise from respiratory failure or complications of recumbency (e.g. pneumonia).

Diagnosis

- Clinical signs.
- Identification of toxin in serum, gastrointestinal contents or food.
- Electrophysiologic testing (EMG).

Treatment

- Botulism antitoxin (requires the specific type).
- Penicillin (not procaine), metronidazole.
- Neostigmine.
- General nursing care and nutritional support.

Prognosis for adults is good when the onset of signs is gradual, but poor when onset of signs is rapid. Complete recovery in non-fatal cases takes weeks to months. The prognosis for shaker foals is poor, with up to 90% mortality. Vaccination of mares with *C. botulinum* type B toxoid twice during the last trimester is practised in some areas where the shaker foal syndrome is common.

Tetanus ('lockjaw')

Tetanus is caused by neurotoxins produced by *Clostridium tetani*. The organism produces spores and grows in anaerobic sites to produce its toxins. The disease has a worldwide distribution, and *C. tetani* spores are found in the soil, especially soils heavily contaminated by faecal matter.

C. tetani neurotoxin interferes with interneurons in the CNS resulting in hypertonia and hyperreflexia. Affected interneurons are often inhibitory; therefore there is a lack of inhibition and consequently stimulation of lower motor neuron function. Toxin is bound to gangliosides in the CNS, and the effects wear off as these are replaced.

The most frequent sites of infection are soft tissue injuries (including surgery) and puncture wounds to the foot. Tetanus is also seen in young foals through umbilical cord infection and in mares after foaling. Under anaerobic conditions (especially in the presence of necrotic tissue and pus), *C. tetani* spores germinate into the vegetative form, which produces toxins. At least three toxins are produced. *Tetanolysin* increases the local tissue necrosis. *Tetanospasmin* binds to nerves, and is transported to the CNS where it inhibits the action of inhibitory interneurons in the ventral horn of the spinal cord. *Non-spasmogenic toxin* causes overstimulation of the sympathetic nervous system.

The incubation period varies between 7 days and one month after bacterial inoculation.

Clinical signs

- Sudden onset of stiff gait leading to generalized spasticity.
- There may be signs of colic initially.
- Extended head.
- Limbs placed in 'sawhorse' stance.
- Flared nostrils.
- Ears erect and stiff.
- Lips retracted.
- Prominence of the nictitating membranes.
- Eyeball retracts readily and nictitating membrane 'flicks' when the head is tapped or in response to a loud noise.
- Stiff jaw and firmness over the masseter muscles.
- Elevated tail head.
- Dysphagia and drooling saliva.

All signs are exaggerated with stimuli, especially a hand-clap, or tapping the head. Mildly affected horses may only show a stiff gait. Severely affected horses become recumbent with the head and legs in full extension. Severe tonic muscular activity results in pyrexia and sweating. Spastic paralysis of the respiratory muscles results in hypoxia, and death occurs as a result of hypoxaemia or aspiration pneumonia. Horses frequently die while in a terminal convulsion. Horses that recover usually start to show improvement after 2 weeks, but complete recovery may take one month or longer.

Diagnosis

Diagnosis can be difficult to confirm because demonstration of circulating neurotoxin and isolation of the organism from wounds is often not possible. Differential diagnosis includes fractured cervical vertebrae, cervical osteomyelitis, colic, pleuritis, laminitis, meningitis and myopathy.

Treatment

1. *Sedation and muscle relaxation.* Keep the horse in a quiet, dark environment, and undisturbed.

Sedate with acetylpromazine, chlorpromazine or promazine at 4–6 hour intervals. Stronger sedation may be achieved, if necessary, using chloral hydrate or sodium pentobarbitone. Diazepam, used alone or in addition to other sedatives, reduces severe muscle spasms. Other muscle relaxants can be used in combination with sedatives, including guaifenesin (given to effect by slow IV drip) and methocarbamol. A balance between the amount of sedation and the degree of muscle relaxation is important.

An intravenous catheter may be left in place to minimize stimulation when administering drugs. Packing the ears with cotton wool minimizes auditory stimulation.

2. *Provide adequate bedding* for recumbent horses to minimize decubital ulcers. Standing horses should have adequate footing. Consider the use of slings to support horses that tolerate them.

3. *Eliminate infection* by surgical debridement of wounds and parenteral administration of penicillin.

4. *Antitoxin.* Administer a large dose of antitoxin (5000–10 000 IU) intravenously at the onset of clinical signs. Local infiltration of any wound with up to 9000 IU of antitoxin has also been suggested. Tetanus toxoid may be administered simultaneously with antitoxin, but at a separate site.

5. *Fluid and nutritional support.* Intravenous fluid and electrolyte therapy may be necessary. Dysphagic horses may be fed through an indwelling nasogastric tube.

Prognosis

If the horse can still drink, the prognosis is good with nursing care. For recumbent horses, the mortality rate approaches 80%. Horses that survive for more than 7 days have a fair chance of survival.

Recovery from tetanus does not protect against the disease; therefore, the horse must still be vaccinated. Other horses at risk should be vaccinated. Decubital lesions, fractured bones and scoliosis can be lethal complications of the disease.

Organophosphorus poisoning

Organophosphates and carbamates are used as insecticides or may be accidental contaminants in food and water. Overdosing with antiparasitic preparations by owners is also a hazard. The organophosphates include trichlorfon, dermeton, malathion, dichlorvos, ronnel, rulene, parathion and diazinon. The carbamate group of insecticides includes carbaryl.

Both the organophosphorus and carbamate insecticides have their effect and cause clinical signs by binding acetylcholinesterase, thereby permitting continuous cholinergic stimulation and excessive autonomic and muscular activity.

Clinical signs

Effects are manifested within one hour of exposure.

- Anxiety and uneasiness.
- Frequent urination and defecation.
- Colic due to increased peristalsis.
- Patchy sweating, particularly on the neck, shoulders and chest.
- Excessive salivation.
- Bradycardia.
- Laboured breathing due to bronchoconstriction, pulmonary oedema and weakness of respiratory muscles and laryngeal paralysis.
- Stiff gait.
- Muscle tremors of the face, neck and other body muscles.
- Hyperactivity of skeletal muscles is followed by weakness, incoordination, ataxia and prostration.
- Respiratory failure occurs in severe toxicity.
- Death may occur within minutes to several hours after the initial signs develop.

Treatment

- *Atropine* to counteract the parasympathetic signs. Use to effect, with mydriasis and absence of salivation used as indicators of an effective dose. Repeated partial doses given subcutaneously every 2 hours as needed.
- *Oximes* (e.g. protopam chloride) to bind organophosphorus and release the inhibited acetylcholinesterase. Oximes are not indicated in cases of carbamate poisoning; so, if the precise toxic agent is unknown they should not be used.
- *Fluid and electrolyte therapy* as required.

Prognosis

The prognosis is quite good providing therapy is rapidly instituted and there is no severe respira-

tory embarrassment. In cases of oral poisoning, continuing absorption prolongs the clinical signs. In other cases, horses that survive 12 hours after exposure have a good chance of spontaneous recovery.

Lactation tetany and idiopathic hypocalcaemia

This condition is also known as eclampsia and transit tetany.

This is rarely seen today; it used to be more common when draught horses were more popular. It occurs in heavily lactating mares in the first 3 days postpartum on lush pasture, especially at around the foaling heat (i.e. approximately 10 days), or 1–2 days post-weaning; it can also arise in mares during mid gestation and during the last month of gestation. It can be seen in foals, geldings and stallions exposed to stress during transport or in rounding up feral ponies for sale. It can also occur due to alkalaemic conditions, hepatitis, urea poisoning, blister beetle (catharidin) toxicosis and pancreatic atrophy.

Clinical signs

- Rapid violent respirations with thumping sounds from the chest (spasmodic contraction of the diaphragm).
- Sweating.
- Dilation of the nostrils.
- Stiff/stilted gait, hindlimb ataxia.
- Muscle fasciculations or tremors of temporal, masseter and triceps muscles.
- Trismus (with no prolapse of the third eyelid nor hypersensitivity to sound).
- Handling and excitement exacerbate the signs.
- Pulse is normal initially, but later becomes rapid and irregular.
- Slight temperature rise.
- May be inability to swallow and salivation.
- After about 24 hours, recumbency and tetanic convulsions.
- Death after about 48 hours.

Diagnosis

The diagnosis can be confirmed by low serum calcium (4–6 mg/100 ml; 1–1.5 mmol/l). There may be a low serum magnesium in transit cases.

Treatment

Calcium borogluconate IV (given to effect) results in a rapid recovery. The heart should be monitored during therapy.

11.19 *Peripheral nerve damage*

Suprascapular paralysis

This is now uncommon (used to be a common condition in draught horses). It is usually caused by kicks or collisions against objects that damage the suprascapular nerve.

Clinical signs

- Lateral subluxation ('popping') of the shoulder when weight bearing.
- Progressive atrophy of infraspinatus and supraspinatus muscles resulting in prominence of the scapular spine ('sweeney').

Diagnosis

The diagnosis can be confirmed by EMG.

Treatment

- Controlled exercise.
- Physiotherapy (e.g. faradism).
- Surgical exploration (if no spontaneous improvement after 3 months) to free the nerve from any entrapment or to perform anastomosis if a neuroma is present.

Radial nerve paralysis

The radial nerve is not commonly damaged alone. It can be involved in humeral or first rib fractures. Lesions near the elbow result in 'high radial nerve paralysis':

- Dropped elbow.
- Failure of limb protraction with toe scuffing.
- Flexion of distal limb joints with foot knuckled over.
- Inability to bear weight on the limb.

Some cases arise due to compression of the brachial plexus and radial nerve roots between the scapula and the ribs. This is then often accompanied by sweeney. Post-recumbency 'radial paralysis' is associated with a post-anaesthetic myopathy and is usually only a transient problem.

Diagnosis

The diagnosis is based on typical clinical signs. EMG is helpful to detect involvement of more than just the radial nerve. Sensory loss over the limb is variable.

Other peripheral nerve damage

The *femoral nerve* is rarely damaged alone. Clinical signs include profound loss of weight-support, with inability to extend and fix the stifle. There is a sensory deficit on the medial thigh.

Sciatic nerve damage may arise from iatrogenic injection damage or encasement of the nerve by abscesses, especially in foals. The limb is dragged with the stifle dropped and extended, and the foot is constantly knuckled.

Peroneal nerve damage can also arise from injections, but also kicks to the lateral stifle and recumbency. The limb is held slightly caudal with hyperextension of the hock; the fetlock and pastern are flexed, and the limb is jerked caudally when the horse moves.

Tibial nerve injury is uncommon and usually traumatic. The hock is held flexed and the fetlock is knuckled. The leg is raised higher than normal on moving.

Facial paralysis

The facial nerve emerges from the skull through the stylomastoid foramen and travels across the dorsal aspect of the guttural pouch where branches leave to supply the caudal ear muscles (caudal auricular nerve), eyelid muscles and cranial aspect of the ear (auriculopalpebral branch). The remainder of the nerve becomes superficial as it courses across the lateral aspect of the mandibular ramus and the masseter muscle, and divides into dorsal and ventral buccal nerves, which supply the cheeks, nose and lips.

The facial nerve may be damaged centrally or peripherally, and the site of damage determines which muscles are affected. Damage to the upper motor neuron pathways controlling the facial nerve (i.e. *supranuclear paralysis*) (e.g. cerebral haematoma, EPM and abscesses) can result in abnormal facial expression without paralysis.

There is still muscle tone and the facial (V–VII) reflexes remain, but the expression may be bland or grimacing on one or both sides. The EMG of the facial muscles is normal.

Facial nerve lesions proximal to the vertical ramus of the mandible cause *proximal facial nerve paralysis*, characterized by:

- Deviation of the nostril towards the contra-lateral side.
- Reduced inspiratory flaring of the ipsilateral nostril.
- Ipsilateral drooping of the lip, eyelid and ear.
- Exposure keratitis.

This can arise from extension of fractures of the petrous temporal bone, otitis interna/media, arthritis of the temporohyoid joint, guttural pouch mycosis, parotid gland neoplasia/abscess, or fracture of the vertical mandibular ramus.

In *distal peripheral nerve trauma*, usually one or two branches of the nerve, not all three, are involved. Pressure on the side of the face (halter, recumbency) damages the buccal branches, paralysing the nares and lips. Ear droop may occur with direct auricular trauma.

The prognosis for peripheral trauma is quite good, with most cases recovering in 1–10 days. Central facial nerve lesions carry a much poorer prognosis.

Vestibular disease

The vestibular system is a proprioceptive system that functions to maintain the orientation of the horse in its environment. The system helps to maintain the position of the eyes, trunk and limbs in relationship to movements of the head. The receptor organs are contained within the membranous labyrinth in the petrous part of the temporal bone. Impulses from the receptors are transmitted via the vestibular nerve to the vestibular nuclei, which lie adjacent to the facial nucleus in the medulla. There is also a direct afferent connection to the cerebellum.

Signs of vestibular disease vary depending on whether the central or peripheral part of the system is damaged, and whether there is unilateral or bilateral disease.

Clinical signs

- Staggering.
- Leaning.
- Circling.
- Drifting sideways when walking.
- Head tilt.
- Change in eye position (strabismus).
- Nystagmus.

Causes

- Otitis interna.
- Head trauma.
- Osteoarthrosis and fractures of temporohyoid region (often with facial paralysis).
- Idiopathic.

Treatment

Treatment depends on the cause. Prolonged antibiotic treatment can be effective in otitis media/interna, although residual signs are common in chronic cases.

Prognosis

The prognosis is good in otitis interna if early treatment is provided. Prognosis for osteoarthrosis and temporohyoid fractures is poor. Idiopathic cases often recover.

Cauda equina neuritis

This condition is seen in horses and ponies of many breeds and both sexes, and has a wide age range. In addition to the nerves of the cauda equina, other peripheral nerves are also commonly involved. The trigeminal nerve is frequently affected, but there is no definite pattern of peripheral nerve involvement (other than cauda equina nerves). The disease has also been called *polyneuritis equi*.

Aetiology and pathogenesis

The cause of the polyneuritis is often undetermined but *immunological factors* are probably important. The original lesions involve neuritis with a component of demyelination. This evolves into a polyneuritis and pachymeningitis involving the sacrocaudal roots (rarely lumbar) of the cauda equina and some cranial nerves, which can extend out to involve peripheral nerves. Sometimes diffuse involvement of many spinal nerve roots is seen. Severe, chronic, granulomatous inflammation occurs, involving lymphocytes, macrophages, eosinophils, fibroblasts, giant cells and neutrophils. Early lesions resemble allergic neuritis. Affected horses have been found to have circulating antibodies directed against P2 myelin protein.

Clinical signs

The onset and progression may be acute and fulminating, or insidious.

Acute form
- Hyperaesthesia around the head and perineum.
- May be head-tilt and ataxia.
- With time, the hyperaesthesia lessens, progressing to hypoaesthesia or anaesthesia.

Insidious form
- Gradual onset of progressive paralysis of tail, urinary bladder and sphincter, rectum and anal sphincter.
- Urinary and faecal incontinence.
- Mares develop urine scald of the perineal area and medial parts of the hindlimbs, and the vaginal mucosa may become hyperaemic.
- In males, the penis may be relaxed and protruding.
- Weakness or paralysis of the tail.
- Constipation.
- Anaesthesia of the perineum (and other areas reflecting other affected nerves).
- Ptosis.
- Drooping lips.
- Loss of tongue-tone.
- Drooling.
- Atrophy of gluteal, temporal and masseter muscles.
- Weakness and sometimes ataxia of hindlimbs.

Diagnosis

- Typical clinical appearance (especially if cranial nerve involvement).
- Lumbosacral (and occasionally cisternal) CSF is often xanthochromic with moderately elevated protein and prominent mononuclear pleocytosis (especially chronic stage).
- Epidural biopsy.
- Serum anti-P2 antibody levels.

Differential diagnosis includes other causes of hindlimb ataxia, EHV 1 infection, sorghum grass ataxia and fracture of the sacrum.

Treatment

Treatment involves evacuation of the bladder and rectum, but no specific therapy is available. Antibiotics and corticosteroids are rarely helpful.

Prognosis

The prognosis is poor because the disease gradually progresses.

11.20 *Peripheral neuropathies*

Idiopathic laryngeal hemiplegia

See Chapter 5.

Stringhalt

This is a motor disorder of unknown aetiology.

Clinical signs

- Normal at rest.
- Involuntary hyperflexion of the hock when moving.
- Unilateral or bilateral.
- Signs are worse on turning or backing.
- May be worse in cold weather or after rest.

There appear to be three syndromes:

1. *Sporadic.*
2. *Epidemic. Australian stringhalt* refers to a syndrome that occurs in outbreaks with involvement, often profound, of both rear legs and often the forelimbs and even the neck. There is an unproven association with dandelion and flatweed intoxication. Muscle atrophy can occur in severe cases.
3. Intoxication with sweet pea plants (*lathyrism*).

These syndromes may be the result of a sensory neuropathy, a myopathy or spinal cord disease. In lathyrism and Australian stringhalt, there is a Wallerian degeneration of fibres and evidence of neurogenic muscle atrophy in severe cases.

Diagnosis

The diagnosis is based on the clinical signs and ruling out other diseases. Mild forms need to be differentiated from upward fixation of the patella, fibrotic myopathy and other musculoskeletal lamenesses. Occasionally EPM and other spinal cord diseases result in stringhalt.

Treatment

Treatment is to remove the horse from any toxic plant or area. Many cases improve slowly with time. Tenotomy or tenectomy of the lateral digital extensor tendon often helps, even in cases of lathyrism, although this does not cure severely affected horses.

Shivering

A condition of mature horses (especially draught breeds) characterized by very mild muscle tremors of the hindquarters and tail occurring with movement. The pathogenesis is unknown, but it is assumed to be a peripheral neuropathy. There is no specific treatment. It does not usually affect performance.

11.21 *Neoplasia*

Peripheral nerve sheath tumours

Neurofibromas are uncommon. Localized pain in association with nerve or nerve root (sometimes multiple) deficits are recognized when sensory nerves are affected.

Lymphoma

Lymphoma can encompass peripheral nerves.

11.22 *Conditions of the autonomic nervous system*

Horner's syndrome

Horner's syndrome can occur as a sequel to guttural pouch mycosis and surgery (i.e. postganglionic), trauma to the basisphenoid area, deep cervical injuries, and space occupying lesions in the cervical area and thoracic inlet (i.e. preganglionic). The sympathetic supply for the eye and blood vessels of the head is carried in the cervical sympathetic trunk adjacent to the cervical vagus nerve. These fibres pass up the neck to the cranial cervical ganglion on the wall of the guttural pouch adjacent to the internal carotid artery, and the postganglionic fibres follow other vessels and nerves to all parts of the head.

Clinical signs

- Ipsilateral ptosis of the upper eyelid.
- Enophthalmos.
- Mild miosis.
- Slight protrusion of the nictitating membrane.
- Congestion of nasal and conjunctival membranes.
- Sweating and regional hyperthermia over the side of the face.
- Vision and pupillary light reflexes are normal.

Grass sickness

See Chapter 3.

Further reading

DeBowes, R.M. (1992) Neurological diseases. In *Current Therapy in Equine Medicine 3* (Ed. N.E. Robinson), Section 12. W.B. Saunders, Philadelphia.

Mayhew, I.G. (1989) *Large Animal Neurology: A Handbook for Veterinary Clinicians*. Lea & Febiger, Philadelphia.

Appendix. Differential diagnoses of conditions producing neurological signs

1. Differential diagnosis of conditions that produce cortical/basal ganglia signs, i.e. changes in behaviour, mental status, etc.

Hepatoencephalopathy
Brain abscess/meningitis
Viral encephalomyelitis
Rabies
Parasite migration
Leucoencephalomalacia
Trauma
Idiopathic epilepsy
Narcolepsy
Lead poisoning
Neonatal maladjustment syndrome
Intracarotid drug injection

2. Differential diagnosis of conditions that produce brainstem and cranial nerve dysfunction

EHV-1
EPM
Brain abscess
Brain tumour
Polyneuritis equi
Parasite migration
Botulism
Lead poisoning

3. Differential diagnosis of conditions that result in spasticity/tremors

Cerebellar abiotrophy
Grass staggers
Locoweed/Swainsonia poisoning

4. Differential diagnosis of ataxia/spinal cord disease

A. *Spinal cord diseases*
    Cervical vertebral stenosis
    EPM
    EDM
    EHV-1
    Trauma
    Occipitoatlantoaxial malformation
    Parasite migration
    Neoplasia
    Grass staggers
    Sorghum grass ataxia
    Equine motor neuron disease
B. *Brain and brainstem lesions*
    Viral encephalitides (VEE, WEE, EEE, Rabies, Borna disease)
    Cranial trauma/fracture
    Cerebellar abiotrophy or other disease
    Meningitis
    Cerebrospinal nematodiasis

Space occupying lesion (tumour, cholesteatoma)
    Middle ear infection
C. *Peripheral nervous system disease*
    Tetanus
    Botulism and shaker foal syndrome
    Myotonia
    Cauda equina neuritis
D. *Systemic disease*
    Liver damage
    Acute renal disease
E. *Toxicity*
    Lead
    Monensin
    Plant poisons (yellow star thistle)
    Mycotoxins
    Others (OPs)

In addition, many other conditions need to be differentiated from genuine ataxia:

A. *Causes of stumbling and toe-dragging*
    Navicular disease
    Hindlimb lameness (e.g. bone spavin)
    Upward or partial fixation of the patella
    Hindlimb arthrosis (e.g. OCD, degenerative joint disease)
    Weakness and debility
    Low back problem
    Scirrhous cord
B. *Bilateral forelimb lameness*
    Carpal lameness/sore shins
    Navicular disease
    Stiff neck due to soft tissue injury
C. *Poor performance*
    Gait asymmetry or 'leggedness'
    Fatigue
    Back problem

12 Ophthalmology

CONTENTS

12.1 *Examination and diagnosis*

Diagnostic approach to diseases of the eye and adnexa

Examination of the equine eye and adnexa (Figure 1) is performed most frequently as part of the assessment of 'soundness'. In addition, specific examination will be required if the clinician suspects a primary abnormality in this region and because ocular manifestations are a feature of some systemic disorders.

History

An accurate history may help to make the diagnosis relatively straightforward. Important points include the following:

- Onset – sudden or gradual.
- Pain – blepharospasm and lacrimation are features of ocular pain. Photophobia (dislike of bright light) may also be present. The triad of pain, blepharospasm and lacrimation indicates anterior segment involvement. Pain is not usually a feature of posterior segment disease.
- Alteration of appearance – the owner may have noticed a difference of appearance between the two eyes, or a difference of appearance relative to other horses.

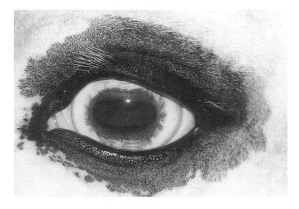

Figure 1 The normal equine eye and adnexa. There are no true eyelashes, although obvious cilia are present in the upper eyelid. The grooves which run parallel to the upper and lower eyelid margins are known as the dorsal and ventral orbital sulci; they separate the eyelids into orbital and tarsal portions. The third eyelid, caruncle and visible conjunctiva are not pigmented in this horse, although the upper and lower eyelids are quite heavily pigmented. The iris also lacks pigment and thus the darker pupillary zone can be readily distinguished from the lighter ciliary zone. The pupil is a horizontal ellipse with obvious granula iridica in the central, dorsal portion, immediately beneath the camera flash.

- Change of behaviour – the animal may become less confident under different lighting conditions, or exhibit an actual change of temperament.
- Vision – sudden blindness is easier to recognize than a gradual loss of vision. Partial visual loss is difficult to assess in horses.
- Predisposing factors – these may range from inherent factors such as a lack of local pigmentation (which increases susceptibility to squamous cell carcinoma), to external factors such as environment (exposure to ultralight light, dust etc.).

Ophthalmic examination – instruments

Ophthalmic examination is conducted in daylight (or artificial light) and in the dark. Careful observation in daylight allows comparison to be made between the two sides and enables obvious abnormalities of the adnexa or anterior segment to be identified. Artificial illumination in the dark permits bright light to fall upon the structure to be examined, making it easier to concentrate on areas of interest. The basic equipment required consists of a pen light or other light source, a means of magnification and an ophthalmoscope.

Naked eye examination
Signs that can be identified by naked eye examination include an altered appearance, pain, blepharospasm, lacrimation and an ocular discharge. Careful comparison of the two sides is essential.

Magnification
Magnification can be provided using a condensing lens, magnifying loupe, slit lamp biomicroscope, otoscope head, or ophthalmoscope. The slit lamp biomicroscope, otoscope head and ophthalmoscope have the benefit of built-in illumination, but the slit lamp is not generally available in equine practice and will not be considered further.

Magnification with or without illumination may be used to supplement naked eye examination of external ocular features.

Indirect ophthalmoscopy is an ideal and quick way of screening the fundus for abnormality. When performed with a penlight and a +20 to +30D condensing lens, monocular indirect ophthalmoscopy produces an image which is virtual, inverted and magnified. The magnification is less than that achieved with a direct ophthalmoscope, but the field of view is greater.

A commercially available monocular indirect ophthalmoscope, which provides an erect image, is also available.

For internal ocular examination, a direct ophthalmoscope will be the most generally useful instrument and provides an image which is real, erect and magnified up to $15\times$. The direct ophthalmoscope can be used to provide a magnified, illuminated, image of external detail as well as being the standard instrument for examination of the ocular fundus. In addition to being used for close direct ophthalmoscopy, the instrument can also be used for distant direct ophthalmoscopy, which is a useful means of assessing the position and extent of any opacities between the observer and the ocular fundus.

Illumination

Adequate illumination is an essential adjunct to ophthalmic examination and is of greatest benefit when used in dim or dark conditions. A variety of light sources are available, but a pen light and the light from a direct ophthalmoscope are the ones used most frequently.

Environment

A quiet environment is essential and a loose box which can be darkened completely is ideal for ophthalmic examination.

Ophthalmic examination – protocol

In daylight or artificial light

1. The general appearance of the eyes and adnexa is noted and the symmetry of each side compared.
   - The position of the globe in relation to the orbit should be assessed, especially as regards the size and position of the globe.
   - A variation from normal in the angle of the lashes of the upper lid may well indicate ptosis, enophthalmos or exophthalmos which might not otherwise be obvious.
   - Usually the eyelashes are almost perpendicular to the corneal surface.
   - The supraorbital fossa and the bony orbital rim which completely surrounds the orbit, should also be inspected both visually and manually.
2. More detailed examination of the adnexa follows.
   - The nature and quantity of any ocular and/or nasal discharge should be noted.

- The presence of the upper and lower lacrimal puncta and the nasal ostium should be confirmed.
- The margins, outer and inner surfaces of the upper and lower eyelids should be examined.
- The position of the third eyelid should be noted and its outer surface should also be inspected once the eyelid has been protruded by pressure on the globe through the upper eyelid.
- The inner surface of the third eyelid is not examined routinely, but following the application of local anaesthetic (0.5% proxymetacaine hydrochloride), may be everted using thumb forceps.
- The caruncle is an obvious feature of most equine eyes, so this too should be checked for normality.

3. The ocular surface includes the conjunctival, limbal and corneal epithelium and is defined as the continuous epithelium which begins at the lid margin, extends onto the back of the lids, into the fornices and onto the globe.
   - Naked eye examination will indicate if the appearance of the ocular surface is normal.
   - There will be variation in the amount of visible pigment of the bulbar conjunctiva, third eyelid and caruncle between individual animals and even between the two eyes of the same animal.
   - A pen light can be used to assess the corneal reflex (the light from the pen light should be reflected on the corneal surface without disruption).

The anterior chamber and iris can be examined briefly with a pen light at this stage, but it is easier to examine these regions in the dark.

In the dark

At this stage specific abnormalities detected in the first part of the examination can be looked at in more detail without distracting reflections.

The anterior segment (the internal structures of the globe up to and including the lens) is examined with a light source and magnification.

1. The limbus and cornea should be examined first.
   - In most horses there is an obvious grey line at the medial (nasal) and lateral (temporal) limbus which represents the insertion of the pectinate ligaments into the posterior cornea.
   - In shape the cornea is a horizontally elongated ellipse and the medial cornea is slightly wider than the lateral cornea.

2. The anterior chamber is filled with aqueous humour and should be optically clear. A slit beam, rather than a diffuse beam, should be used to detect subtle opacities within the aqueous. Most modern ophthalmoscopes have a slit beam as one of the beam selector options. The depth of the anterior chamber is most easily assessed by shining a beam of light across the eye from lateral to medial and the drainage angle can be examined at the same time.

3. The iris of most horses is heavily pigmented and the distinction between the pupillary zone (usually darker) and ciliary zone (usually lighter) at the collarette is not always distinct.

   • Colour variations may be present between irides and within different sectors of the same iris. Variations of pigmentation produce a range of colours; dark brown is commonest, with pale brown, gold, grey, blue, white and pink less common. In the least pigmented, genuinely albinotic iris, which is white or pink in colour, the iris is often so thin that it can be transilluminated to reveal details of the underlying lens equator and the ciliary processes of the ciliary body.

   • Persistent pupillary membrane remnants are a common feature of the equine iris. They are usually evident in the collarette region, but are of no significance unless they span the pupil or attach to the lens and cornea.

   • Darkly pigmented granula iridica (corpora nigra) are a prominent feature of the pupillary border of most horses; those of the upper (dorsal) pupillary margin are better developed than those of the lower (ventral) pupillary margin. They originate from the posterior pigmented epithelium of the iris and can be surprisingly large without obvious effect on vision.

4. The adult pupil is a horizontal ellipse with the medial area being slightly wider than the lateral area.

   • It is important to observe the size and shape of the pupil, paying particular attention to the pupillary margin.

   • The pupillary light response, which is a subcortical reflex, is evaluated in the dark with a focal light source. The normal equine pupil responds somewhat sluggishly and incompletely, unless the light is particularly bright.

5. Darkness and pupillary dilation are both necessary if the whole lens is to be examined in detail. Tropicamide 1% is the mydriatic of choice and should be applied to the eye once the pupillary light response has been evaluated.

   • After confirming the position of the lens, the light source may be used to demonstrate the anterior and posterior lens surfaces, for an image of the light source may be readily identified on the anterior cornea (corneal reflex) and with decreasing clarity on the anterior lens capsule and the posterior lens capsule. These are the Purkinje–Sanson images and their relative movement in relation to the light source (parallax) is a simple way of establishing the depth of anterior segment opacities.

   • A direct ophthalmoscope may be used at a distance (distant direct ophthalmoscopy) to silhouette any opacities in the ocular media against the fundus reflex (the light reflected from the fundus).

   • There are a number of lens opacities which may be regarded as normal variations; for example, it is quite usual to be able to visualize the anterior and posterior lens suture lines, the point of attachment of the hyaloid vessel (Mittendorf's dot), refractive concentric ('onion') rings, fine 'dust-like' opacities and sparse 'vacuoles' within the lens substance. The lens sutures are often prominent in horses and there is marked variation in their pattern, ranging from a traditional Y-suture pattern to complex meandering opaque lines. They may also have an indistinct, somewhat feathery, appearance. In old horses the suture lines and the lens capsule become slightly greyer as a normal feature of ageing.

6. The posterior segment (the internal structures of the globe beyond the lens) is next examined using some or all of a light source, indirect ophthalmoscopy (Figure 2), distant direct ophthalmoscopy and close direct ophthalmoscopy (Figure 3). The various methods are complementary rather than exclusive. Mydriasis is required for comprehensive examination of the posterior segment.

   • The adult vitreous should be free of obvious opacities. Some or all of the hyaloid system may be present at birth, but most remnants have disappeared by 9 months of age. Persistent hyaloid remnants may be associated with discrete posterior capsular lens opacities.

   • It is not uncommon in horses of any age to see vitreal condensations, usually as filamentous strands, which are especially obvious where the anterior vitreous face attaches to the posterior lens capsule.

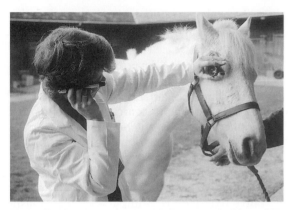

Figure 2 Monocular indirect ophthalmoscopy. A +20 to +30D condensing lens is held some 8 cm from the horse's eye with the fingers resting lightly on the animal's head. The pen light is lined up at approximately arm's length so that the beam passes throught the centre of the lens and the centre of the pupil. The technique must be performed in darkness or near darkness and useful information can often be obtained without dilating the pupil.

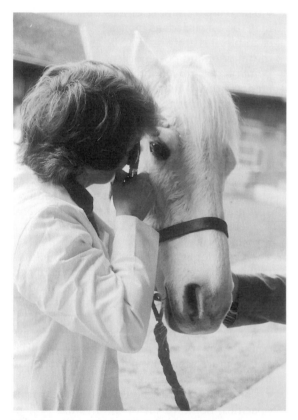

Figure 3 Close direct ophthalmoscopy. A direct ophthalmoscope may be used to provide a magnified image of, for example, focal lesions of the eyelids, corneal and lens opacities as well as being used to obtain an image of the fundus. The ophthalmoscope is placed close to the eye with a setting of approximately +20 to allow examination of external features. Without taking the ophthalmoscope away from the eye, the strength of the plus lenses is reduced successively, so that the focus of observation moves posteriorly. Thus the magnified details of the eyelids, cornea, aqueous, iris, lens and vitreous are visualized until features of the fundus are brought into focus.

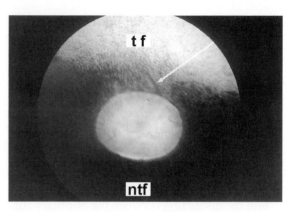

Figure 4 Normal equine fundus. This is the most typical appearance of the normal equine fundus. and shows the rather small area which is seen with a direct ophthalmoscope. The tapetal fundus (tf), non-tapetal fundus (ntf) and optic disc (papilla) are obvious. The optic disc is in the centre of the photograph and many small retinal vessels radiate a short distance away from it. In the region of the original foetal (choroidal) fissure in the 6 o'clock position there is an absence of these fine vessels. Dorsal to the disc there is less pigment than elsewhere, allowing a choroidal vessel (arrowed) to be visualized. The grey striations which are obvious accompanying the retinal vessels in the dorsal peripapillary region are myelinated retinal nerve fibres. In the tapetal fundus the 'Stars of Winslow' can be seen; these discrete black dots represent choroidal arteries viewed end on.

7. Indirect ophthalmoscopy followed by close direct ophthalmoscopy are used to examine the ocular fundus (Figure 4). Indirect ophthalmoscopy not only provides a means of surveying a large area at low power, but is particularly useful when the ocular media lack optical clarity. Direct ophthalmoscopy provides a magnified view of a relatively small area and a set routine should be adopted so that all quadrants of the ocular fundus are examined properly. In addition, any lesions identified with the indirect ophthalmoscope can be scrutinized in detail.

• With either type of ophthalmoscopy the optic disc (papilla), which is always situated within the non-tapetal fundus, is located first and its size, shape and colour should be noted.

• The retinal vasculature is next examined, paying particular attention to the number and distribution of the retinal vessels.

• If the choroidal vessels are visible, then they too should be examined.

• Finally all four quadrants of the ocular fundus are checked in whichever order the examiner finds most convenient; for example, dorsolateral, dorsomedial, ventromedial and ventrolateral. Variations, which may or may not be of clinical significance, can only be appreciated if there is an understanding of the normal range of appearances.

Ophthalmic examination – diagnostic techniques

Sampling techniques

1. Swabs and scrapes are most usefully taken from the eyelid margins, conjunctiva and cornea; the area affected is the area which is sampled. Samples should be taken before applying topical ophthalmic stains.
   - For the conjunctiva and eyelid margins local anaesthesia is unnecessary, whereas for precise sampling of corneal lesions topical anaesthesia is essential (the isolation of bacterial pathogens is not affected adversely by the bacteriostatic properties of the local anaesthetic).
   - If corneal ulcers are sampled it is the edge of the ulcer which will yield replicating bacteria and a Kimura spatula is the best instrument to use for this technique.
   - Swabs and scrapes are useful for confirming mycotic and bacterial infections, but they are not as helpful as a means of identifying viruses.
   - When keratomycosis is supected the deep corneal scrape or keratectomy specimen must include affected cornea and the sample should be processed correctly for fungal isolation and identification.
2. Impression smears can be used to establish the nature of problems which involve the ocular or adnexal surface, such as squamous cell carcinoma. A clean dry glass slide is pressed gently, but firmly, against the abnormal area and the preparation is air-dried, fixed in methanol and submitted for histopathology.
3. Biopsies may be taken from the eyelids and conjunctiva following adequate topical anaesthesia or as part of more extensive surgery under local or general anaesthesia.
   - The biopsy is taken using a biopsy needle (fine needle aspiration biopsy) or by surgical excision.
   - It is important to avoid crushing and distorting the tissue when obtaining the sample and the correct orientation is often most easily maintained if the sample is placed on very thin card before immersion in fixative.
   - The amount of fixative should be some ten times the volume of the specimen. Neutral buffered formaldehyde is acceptable for routine light microscopy and immunohistochemistry, whereas 2.5% glutaraldehyde in 0.1M cacodylate buffer is the fixative of choice for electron microscopy.
4. Aqueous and vitreous paracentesis are very rarely indicated as a means of diagnosis in horses and specialist advice should be sought if the techniques are contemplated.

Topical ophthalmic stains

1. Fluorescein sodium is an orange dye which changes to green in alkaline conditions.
   - It is primarily used to detect corneal ulceration as it is rapidly absorbed by the exposed hydrophilic stroma in such cases.
   - It does not stain the lipid-rich epithelium or Descemet's membrane.
   - Impregnated strips or single dose vials may be used and it is often simplest to place the strip or solution in the lower conjunctival sac and allow the blink to distribute the fluorescein.
   - To avoid false positives and provide sufficient moisture for adequate staining it is sometimes necessary to irrigate the eye with sterile saline.
   - It is easier to detect subtle staining with a blue light source.
2. Rose bengal is a red dye which can be used to demonstrate abnormalities of the tear film and ocular surface. It is irritant to the eye and its use should be reserved for the detection of subtle epithelial defects.

Schirmer tear test (STT)

Few disorders of the preocular tear film (ptf) have been described in horses and testing tear production is not regarded as a routine part of equine ophthalmic examination. The Schirmer 1 tear test (STT1) is the method most commonly employed. Topical local anaesthetic solution is not used for a Schirmer 1 tear test so that it is stimulated (reflex) tear production which is being assessed. The test is easily performed using commercially available test strips which are 30 mm or 40 mm in length, with a notch some 5 mm from the tip. The strip is bent at the notched region and the tip is placed just within the conjunctival sac. The strip is removed after 1 minute or 30 seconds and the value is read immediately, as measured from the notch in millimetres. Values of at least 20–30 mm per minute are obtained in normal horses. Values of less than 10 mm per minute should be regarded with suspicion and repeated values of less than 5 mm are indicative of a lack of aqueous component production, clinically manifest as keratoconjunctivitis sicca.

Investigation of nasolacrimal drainage

The upper and lower lacrimal puncta and the nasal ostium are obvious in horses and this means that investigations can be performed from the proximal (puncta) and/or distal (ostium) parts of the system.

1. Initial examination consists of visual inspection of the puncta and nasal ostium. Their presence, size and position should be checked.
2. If samples are required for culture and sensitivity they may be obtained by irrigation with sterile water following topical local anaesthesia and cannulation/catheterization of the upper punctum and canaliculus, or by retrograde flushing with sterile water after cannulation/catheterization of the nasal ostium. Local anaesthetic drops or gel can be applied to the nasal ostium and the catheter or cannula before insertion.
3. If culture is not required, patency can be tested using fluorescein drops instilled into the lower conjunctival sac, which should appear at the ipsilateral nostril within 1–5 minutes of application. Both sides should be tested.
4. Dacryocystorhinography is a useful technique for establishing the extent of congenital or acquired abnormalities and, as the technique may confirm the necessity for surgical intervention, dacryocystorhinography is best performed under general anaesthesia. It is usual to cannulate/catheterize the upper lacrimal punctum and to inject approximately 5 ml of an iodine-based contrast agent. Lateral and, if necessary, oblique radiographs are taken.

Tonometry

Tonometry is not usually required in horses as glaucoma is uncommon; it is most reliably performed with some form of portable electronic applanation tonometer such as the Proton or Tono-pen XL applanation tonometer. The normal intraocular pressure of unsedated horses is some 17–27 mmHg.

Diagnostic imaging

1. Radiography is of limited value in aiding diagnosis of soft tissue problems in and near the eye, but can be useful when there is bony abnormality, or the possibility of radio-opaque foreign material.
2. Ocular ultrasonography is a valuable technique for soft tissue imaging in horses and is best performed with a high frequency transducer of between 7.5 and 10 MHz. Ultrasonic techniques can be used in biometric studies (the size of both eyes should be compared), for the assessment of eyes in which opacity prevents complete examination, for identification of foreign bodies and for the differentiation of intraocular and orbital masses.

12.2 *Globe and orbit*

Microphthalmos and anophthalmos

Microphthalmos (small, imperfectly formed eye) or anophthalmos (complete absence of an eye) may be unilateral or bilateral. The aetiology is usually unknown, but it is probably not inherited. Associated abnormalities include cataracts and colobomotous defects. There is no treatment.

Endophthalmitis and panophthalmitis

- Endophthalmitis – severe intraocular inflammation which does not extend beyond the sclera.
- Panophthalmitis – severe intraocular inflammation which involves the sclera, Tenon's capsule and which may also involve the orbital tissues.

Possible causes include unrecognized trauma to the globe and incorrect treatment regimes.

Clinical signs and treatment

The clinical signs reflect the extent of globe and orbital involvement.

- The globe is painful, the ocular media cloudy, or frankly opaque and there is usually marked congestion of the conjunctival and episcleral vasculature.
- When panophthalmitis is present there may, in addition, be blepharoedema, swelling in the region of the supraorbital fossa and prominence of the third eyelid.
- Pyrexia and depression may be present.

Treatment consists of referral to a specialist, enucleation or exenteration, according to the extent of the inflammation. In addition to the usual precautionary measures in relation to tetanus, a course of systemic broad-spectrum antibiotics should be administered and samples should be taken for culture and sensitivity testing.

Phthisis bulbi

This is a common sequel to severe ocular damage in horses.

The globe is irreversibly blind, shrunken, but painless. There may also be an ocular discharge because of the small size of the globe relative to the orbit. If the discharge is constant, excoriation of the skin will develop with time.

The eye may be left *in situ* if its appearance is cosmetically acceptable, but should be removed if it is not.

Orbital cellulitis and orbital abscess

Inflammation involving the sinuses, guttural pouch, nose or mouth can spread to the orbit. Although an uncommon problem, such inflammation may be associated with physical damage (trauma and foreign bodies), sinusitis, guttural pouch infection and dental disease.

Clinical signs and treatment

The clinical signs include pain, pyrexia, blepharoedema, swelling in the region of the supraorbital fossa, prominence of the third eyelid and an ocular discharge. Severe inflammation can damage the optic nerve and affect vision.

Urgent treatment is required and consists of systemic broad-spectrum antibiotics, possibly combined with retrobulbar drainage or aspiration. Trephination of the maxillary sinus may also aid drainage in a proportion of cases, and topical ocular lubricant and antibiotic will be required if lid function is compromised.

The prognosis is guarded.

Orbital hydatid cysts

Hydatid cysts may be located in paraorbital regions (e.g. sinuses) and within the orbit itself. Hydatid disease is common in horses, but orbital and paraorbital involvement is rare. The clinical presentation usually mimics a slowly expanding neoplasm, resulting in a unilateral and painless exophthalmos, accompanied by periorbital swelling and possibly strabismus. Ultrasonography may help to confirm the cystic nature of the mass. Surgical evacuation can be attempted and the diagnosis should be confirmed by identifying the characteristic brood capsule histologically.

Orbital neoplasia

There are a number of possible primary tumours as there is a range of tissue types within the orbit. May also have extension of tumours from neighbouring tissues (e.g sinuses and nose) as well as metastases.

Clinical signs and treatment

Tumours can produce an exophthalmos of gradual onset and there is often an associated prominence of the third eyelid and strabismus (squint), the direction of which may help in locating the site of any mass.

Investigations include careful physical examination to try and determine the exact location of the space occupying lesion and whether the mass is of primary or secondary origin.

Exophthalmos in horses can be a consequence of space occupying lesions within the orbit (retrobulbar) and outside the orbit (retro-orbital). For example, ethmoidal haematomas and carcinomas can produce exophthalmos because of the proximity of the ethmoidal labyrinth to the orbit and this makes the differentiation of space occupying lesions in this region particularly important if invasive diagnostic techniques such as needle biopsy are contemplated. Ultrasonography can help in differentiation.

If treatment is thought to be feasible, then biopsy, or debulking, or total excision, may be attempted according to circumstances. Radiotherapy may be required in follow up so accurate histopathology is essential. Possible orbital tumours include squamous cell carcinoma, melanoma, meningioma and lymphoma; the latter being the commonest tumour to spread to the orbit.

12.3 *Eyelids*

Prominence of the third eyelid (membrana nictitans, nictitating membrane)

Aetiology

• Lack of pigment, especially if unilateral, may make a normal third eyelid appear more obvious. Non-pigmented third eyelids are more susceptible both to solar-induced inflammation and to squamous cell carcinoma, so they always merit careful scrutiny.

• Prominence may be a consequence of inflammation of the third eyelid; causes include solar-induced inflammation, conjunctivitis and parasitic granulomas.

• Prolapse of the extraorbital fat pad will make the third eyelid appear more prominent.

• Primary neoplasia of the third eyelid, notably squamous cell carcinoma (SCC), is common. Secondary tumours, most commonly lymphoma, may spread to involve the third eyelid and, rarely, can be found as an isolated, apparently primary, tumour.

• Prominence may be a consequence of orbital and paraorbital space occupying lesions (see above).

• Tetanus can produce a rapid flicking of the third eyelid as part of the clinical presentation; both third eyelids are prominent in this condition.

• The most obvious clinical signs of Horner's syndrome in horses are ptosis (drooping of the upper eyelid), localized sweating and increased skin temperature. Miosis and apparent enophthalmos are usually present, but easily missed, and third eyelid prominence is often absent.

Diagnosis and clinical signs

The clinical appearance is often diagnostic. Inflammation and neoplasia should be differentiated on the basis of clinical appearance. For example, squamous cell carcinoma in this site has a characteristic plaque-like appearance and erosions may be present. Histopathology, whilst the preferred technique for confirmation of tumour type, can also be used to distinguish different types of inflammation. Some tumours of the third eyelid can be completely excised whilst retaining third eyelid function, whereas others will necessitate partial or complete removal of the third eyelid. Prolapse of the extraorbital fat pad does not always require surgery. The choice is made on the basis of discomfort, cosmetic appearance and whether the third eyelid is permanently prolapsed. Surgery aims to excise the prolapsed fat and suture the overlying conjunctiva to prevent further herniation.

Entropion

Inversion of the eyelid margin and lashes occurs, which may be unilateral or bilateral. It can be congenital or early onset (relatively common) or acquired later in life (less common). Previous injury is the commonest reason for acquired, cicatricial, entropion.

Diagnosis and clinical signs

Entropion in foals is usually a consequence of either anatomical imperfection or of dehydration and debility. The lower eyelid is most frequently involved and the inward rotation of the eyelid allows hairs to rub against the cornea so that keratitis may result.

Later onset entropion is usually a consequence of traumatic injury and is more likely to be encountered when primary repair of eyelid lacerations has not been undertaken. Spastic entropion, as a result of pain coupled with globe retraction, is not observed with any frequency in horses.

Treatment

Entropion in foals associated with pain and corneal damage should be dealt with by manual repositioning of the eyelid or by temporary pleating sutures in a vertical mattress pattern through the skin of the affected lid to evert the lid margin. Acquired entropion may require standard skin-muscle resection techniques, or more extensive blepharoplasty, according to the cause and extent.

Ectropion

Ectropion is rare in horses and may be seen as a consequence of cicatrization or as a feature of ageing. The lower lid is usually affected. It may be unilateral (e.g. cicatricial) or bilateral (e.g. ageing).

For cicatricial ectropion excision of the cicatrix or V to Y blepharoplasty may be required.

Trauma

Traumatic injuries to the eyelids which result in bruising and laceration are common. In such cases the orbit and orbital rim should also be evaluated carefully.

Treatment

• Extensive bruising can be treated with compresses containing nitrofurazone ointment to

soften and protect the injured tissues until healing takes place.
- Full thickness eyelid lacerations should always be repaired surgically. Single or double layer closure is effected, with meticulous reapposition of the eyelid margin. For skin closure, a figure of eight suture is placed first to reconstruct the eyelid margin, followed by simple interrupted sutures for the remainder of the skin closure.

Inflammation

Inflammatory eyelid diseases are not particularly common in horses. Possible causes include bacteria (specifically *Moraxella equi*), parasitic infestations (e.g. habronemiasis, onchocerciasis and thelaziasis), mycotic disease (not in temperate climates), systemic diseases (e.g. Arabian fading syndrome), immune diseases (e.g. polyclonal gammopathies) and allergies. In addition, eyelids which lack pigment are susceptible to solar-induced inflammation.

The diagnosis of the various types of blepharitis rests on the history and clinical appearance, together with other routine diagnostic procedures such as skin scrapings, culture and sensitivity testing, skin biopsy and laboratory examination.

Neoplasia

Primary neoplasia of the eyelids is common. Abnormal tissues should be submitted for histopathology as the clinical appearance is not necessarily diagnostic. Less commonly, secondary neoplasia, usually lymphoma, may infiltrate the eyelids. Whilst primary neoplasia of the eyelids is usually unilateral, secondary neoplasia is more likely to be bilateral.

Aetiology

The three most common eyelid tumours of adult animals are squamous cell carcinoma (SCC), sarcoid and melanoma. Solar radiation, geographical location and individual susceptibility (which may relate to breed, age and lack of adnexal pigment) are probably the most important risk factors associated with SCC.

Papillomas are fairly common tumours of the eyelid and periocular tissues in young animals and usually regress spontaneously over a period of months so that no treatment is required.

Treatment of primary eyelid neoplasia

1. Squamous cell carcinoma.
   - Suitable cases can be treated by complete or partial surgical excision, according to the location and extent of the tumour.
   - Cryotherapy. A double freeze–thaw cycle using liquid nitrogen is the treatment of choice.
   - Radiotherapy. Refer to a specialist centre.
2. Melanomas can be dealt with in the same way as SCC – see Chapter 13.
3. Periocular sarcoids. The treatment of choice is immunotherapy using intralesional injections of BCG. Surgical excision is not recommended as it is associated with an unacceptably high rate of local recurrence.

12.4 *Lacrimal system*

Keratoconjunctivitis sicca (KCS)

A deficiency of the aqueous portion of the tear film is rare. KCS may be a consequence of damage (usually traumatic) to the parasympathetic fibres of the facial nerve or, less likely, due to direct damage (e.g. toxic or immune-mediated) to the lacrimal gland.

Clinical signs and diagnosis

Pain or discomfort is common and there is usually a mucopurulent ocular discharge. The cornea is dull and lacklustre and there is often a nonspecific vascular keratitis and corneal oedema. Ulceration may be present.

STT 1 readings rarely reach 10 mm per minute and in some animals may be zero. In some cases the reduction in tear production may be temporary so STT 1 should be repeated at intervals.

Treatment

Any ocular discharge should be cleaned away before applying a commercial tear replacement gel, ointment or solution. Newer generation products require less frequent applications than drops and are easier to use for long-term management. The aim should be to apply the gel, ointment or drops as often as is necessary to keep the cornea of normal appearance. Cyclosporin therapy may be used if an immune-mediated component is suspected.

Congenital dysgenesis and atresia of the lacrimal system

Congenital dysgenesis (abnormal development) including absence (atresia) of the nasal punctum (ostium) is the commonest congenital abnormality of the lacrimal system encountered in foals. Other congenital problems such as proximal dysgenesis are rare.

Diagnosis

Epiphora which is superseded by a florid mucopurulent discharge develops early on in life. There is no sign of a nasal ostium and fluorescein applied to the eye does not appear at the ipsilateral nares. A catheter passed into the drainage system via the upper lacrimal punctum may help to establish the degree of abnormality and it is often possible to palpate the tip in the rostral (distal) portion of the nasolacrimal duct. Dacryocystorhinography can also be used to determine the extent of the dysgenesis.

Treatment

The condition is treated by creating a nasal punctum ± nasolacrimal duct by cutting down on the tip of the catheter and then grasping the tubing with a haemostat and delivering it through the incision. The catheter is retained in place by sutures or superglue and left *in situ* for 2–3 weeks.

Acquired stenosis/occlusion of the lacrimal drainage system

Aetiology

Stenosis and/or occlusion of the lacrimal drainage system may be a complication of infectious, inflammatory, traumatic, or neoplastic, disease processes within the drainage system, or external to it. Internal problems include foreign bodies, parasites (e.g. habronemiasis) and neoplasia (e.g. SCC). Inflammation of the lacrimal sac and duct (dacryocystitis) is a common sequel to a variety of insults. External problems which may involve the lacrimal drainage system include traumatic damage, inflammatory disease (e.g. sinusitis, rhinitis), upper arcade dental disease and neoplasia.

Clinical signs and diagnosis

1. Epiphora (tear overflow) is typical of simple obstruction without infection, whereas a mucopurulent ocular discharge usually indicates infection.
2. Nasal discharge may also be present.

Careful examination is often all that is required in order to establish a diagnosis. On other occasions careful investigation of nasolacrimal drainage and/or radiography will be required.

Treatment

An accurate diagnosis to ascertain whether the problem is within, or outside, the nasolacrimal drainage system is essential. All forms of treatment aim to re-establish and maintain patency. Any topical preparations (e.g. antibiotics and corticosteroids) should be in liquid form. Systemic antibiotics are sometimes required in cases of suppurative dacryocystitis.

12.5 *Conjunctiva, limbus, episclera and sclera*

Dermoid (choristoma)

Dermoids are common congenital abnormalities in foals. They are skin-like tissues in an abnormal site such as the limbal conjunctiva and cornea, but they may also involve other ocular tisues such as the eyelids.

Diagnosis and treatment

The appearance is typical. Their size, position and the presence of hairs on the outer aspect may cause problems, so epibulbar dermoids are usually removed by superficial keratoconjunctivectomy. A topical antibiotic and corticosteroid preparation is given as soon as the cornea has re-epithelialized in order to minimize corneal scarring.

Conjunctivitis

Aetiology

• There are many causes of conjunctivitis which include, for primary conjunctivitis: local irritants, allergies, toxins, chemicals, parasites (e.g. onchocerciasis), bacteria (e.g. *Moraxella equi*) and mycoses in non-temperate zones (e.g. blastomycosis).

• Inflammation of the conjunctiva may also be secondary to other ocular diseases such as eyelid problems, disorders of the lacrimal system and keratitis.

• Conjunctivitis is also a non-specific feature of a number of systemic diseases, most notably respiratory viral infections (e.g. equine influenza, equine viral arteritis, adenovirus infections in foals).

Clinical signs

• The eye is often uncomfortable.
• Ocular discharge which may be serous, mucoid, purulent, or combinations of these. Occasionally there is a haemorrhagic discharge.
• The conjunctiva is reddened ('pink eye') because of active hyperaemia of the conjunctival vessels.
• Chemosis (conjunctival oedema) is usually present.
• In some cases, sometimes as a feature of chronicity, granulomatous inflammation and follicle formation may occur; the follicles are particularly obvious when they occur at the limbus and in the region of the third eyelid and caruncle.

Diagnosis and treatment

The diagnosis and treatment of conjunctivitis depends upon establishing and eliminating the cause. For bacterial and mycotic conjunctivitis a knowledge of normal conjunctival isolates is important for the correct interpretation of swabs and scrapings. Regional and seasonal variation, for example, may influence the isolates obtained and there will be a greater range of fungal organisms in the right climatic conditions and heavily contaminated environments. In normal eyes Gram positive organisms predominate, whereas in horses with any type of ocular surface disease, Gram negative organisms can be cultured with greater frequency.

Chloramphenicol is probably the most useful topical antibiotic when Gram positive organisms predominate and gentamicin is effective against Gram negative organisms. *Moraxella equi* has been isolated as a specific cause of bacterial conjunctivitis in the USA, but does not appear to be a relevant pathogen in the UK.

Granulomatous changes may be seen as a consequence of chronic non-specific conjunctival inflammation, but may also be associated with specific causes such as foreign bodies, yeasts, fungi and parasites. The cause of granulomatous swellings can be confirmed by biopsy and the condition treated with antifungal agents, oral levamisole or a single dose of ivermectin as appropriate.

Irritant-induced and allergic conjunctivitis is not uncommon in horses, especially in animals kept indoors. Affected animals tend to present with chemosis, together with a variable amount of ocular discharge and conjunctival hyperaemia. Most cases resolve if the causal agent(s) can be identified and eliminated from the environment, but in a proportion of cases, secondary bacterial conjunctivitis develops.

Conjunctival foreign bodies

The majority are caused by organic material. There is usually acute onset of, usually unilateral, ocular discomfort. Initial excessive lacrimation is soon replaced by copious ocular discharge.

The dorsal and ventral fornices must be inspected carefully as must the inner aspect of the third eyelid, and the examination is easier if performed after sedation and the application of topical local anaesthetic. An auriculo-palpebral nerve block is sometimes required.

Removal of conjunctival foreign bodies is most easily achieved using a cotton wool bud or similar to enmesh the offending material.

Conjunctival neoplasia

Aetiology, diagnosis and treatment

Of possible *primary tumours*, squamous cell carcinoma (SCC) is the most common and usually affects zones of epithelial transition, such as those found at the mucocutaneous junction of the eyelid, the limbus, the nictitating membrane and the punctal openings. The appearance is quite variable according to the site and extent of the tumour, but squamous cell carcinoma should always be considered as a possibility, especially so in horses which lack pigment in the affected area. A mild ocular discharge with minimal discomfort may be present and the appearance ranges from localized hyperaemia, with or without ulceration, to plaque-like and cauliflower-like masses. The treatment of SCC has been described previously under eyelids.

Other primary tumours of the conjunctiva are rare and include those of pigment (melanoma) and vascular derivation (e.g. haemangioma and haemangiosarcoma).

Differential diagnosis

Conjunctival neoplasia should be differentiated from conjunctival inflammation (common) and conjunctival amyloidosis (rare) by clinical appearance and histopathology.

12.6 *Cornea – keratitis*

Congenital problems of clinical significance are rare in horses. Microcornea, in association with both microphthalmos and a globe of normal size, may be seen occasionally, as may corneal melanosis, linear keratopathy (band opacities) and corneal dermoids.

Acquired corneal problems, especially as a result of trauma, are common in horses, mainly because of the relative prominence of the cornea in this species.

Keratitis accounts for a large proportion of eye cases examined in equine practice; common causes include trauma and infection.

Traumatic keratitis

Lacerations and penetrating injuries are common. In most cases of full thickness penetration, aqueous loss and iris prolapse occur and the prolapsed iris frequently seals the wound. If the wound is not repaired, the iris becomes incarcerated and restoration of normal ocular anatomy is then difficult. Complications of corneal trauma include hyphaema, iris damage (including the granula iridica), collapse of the anterior chamber, synechiae formation, lens luxation, loss of vision and phthisis bulbi. Glaucoma can occur, but is rare in horses as they have effective uveo-scleral outflow.

Diagnosis and treatment

• In most cases there is a sudden onset of pain, blepharospasm and excessive lacrimation and it may be possible to determine the specific cause of the injury from the history.

• The extent of the corneal damage can be determined from clinical examination. Fluorescein dye can be used to check the extent of ulceration. If a descemetocoele is present the ulcer will look deep, the elastic nature of Descemet's membrane will cause it to bulge outwards at the base of the ulcer and fluorescein will not be taken up.

When laceration is present, healing will be aided if any loose flaps of corneal tissue are excised. With corneal injuries which involve more than one-third of the corneal thickness a conjunctival graft (e.g. pedicle graft) will enhance healing (Figure 5).

When perforation has occurred, prolapsed uveal tissue can be returned to the anterior chamber in acute cases without gross contamination. In cases where the iris has become necrotic, or heavily contaminated, prolapsed tissue may require excision. Prolapsed or avulsed granula iridica should also be removed. The anterior

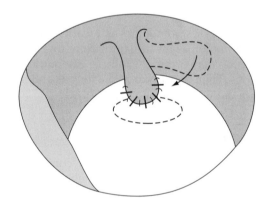

Figure 5 Conjunctival pedicle graft. This is a useful means of providing support during healing of corneal ulcers. Careful debridement of the corneal ulcer is performed with the patient under general anaesthesia. A narrow zone (1–2 mm) of corneal epithelium immediately peripheral to the ulcer is removed, so that there will be better adhesion between the graft and the corneal stroma. The bulbar conjunctiva 1–2 mm behind the limbus is grasped with Colibri forceps, a small conjunctival incision is made with tenotomy scissors and blunt dissection is used to undermine a thin piece of conjunctiva parallel to and at least 2 mm away from the limbus. Once the blunt dissection is complete the graft can be fashioned to create a pedicle of conjunctiva with a wide base. The completed graft should be under no tension and be larger than the ulcer it is to cover. The graft is sutured to the cornea using 4 to 8 absorbable sutures of 6–0 or 7–0 polyglycolic acid or polyglactin 910; fine 8–0 suture material in a continuous pattern may also be used to keep the graft in place. The exposed area of bulbar conjunctiva is usually closed with the same suture material in a simple continuous pattern. The graft may be left in place long term, but is usually trimmed close to the limbus, after applying topical local anaesthetic, once the ulcer has healed.

chamber is reformed with viscoelastic material, balanced salt solution or a small quantity of air before, during, or after, corneal repair. Apposition of the wound edges must be precise to minimize scar formation and closure is achieved under magnification using microsurgical instruments with either non-absorbable material (e.g. 9/0–10/0 nylon) or absorbable material (e.g. 7/0–10/0 polyglactin) on a cutting needle.

Symptomatic treatment for uveitis is also required for deep corneal injuries, and in all cases topical broad-spectrum antibiotic effective against Gram negative organisms (e.g. tobramycin) are needed. Anticollagenases may be required if there is any possibility of liquefactive stromal necrosis (see below). If the eye is painful, or the horse is of difficult temperament, an indwelling sub-palpebral device can be placed beneath the upper eyelid at the start of therapy (Figure 6).

Fortified topical antibiotic and/or systemic antibiotic are sometimes required in complicated cases and systemic treatment with non-steroidal

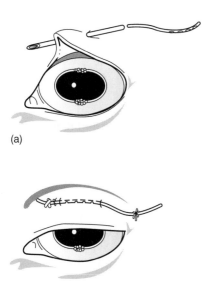

(a)

(b)

Figure 6 Sub-palpebral medication device. This is the easiest way of administering a course of topical medication to a painful equine eye. (a) Insertion. Pliable polyethylene tubing is passed through a large (12 to 14G) needle that passes through the upper eyelid to the fornix and out through the eyelid again. The needle is placed high in the fornix to avoid corneal irritation from the tube. (b) The needle is removed, and the tubing fixed in place. Fenestrations are made in the tube that lies in the conjunctival fornix, taking care that they do not allow medication to escape subconjunctivally. Usually 2 holes will be sufficient and they can be made with a hot 16 gauge hypodermic needle prior to, or following, the insertion of the tubing.

anti-inflammatories (e.g. flunixin meglumine) can be useful initially.

Liquefactive stromal necrosis ('melting' ulcer)

Liquefactive stromal necrosis is not uncommon in horses and constitutes a genuine ocular emergency because of the speed with which corneal perforation can occur. Most equine corneal ulcers are of traumatic origin and secondary infection is likely. Bacteria such as *Pseudomonas aeruginosa*, fungi, alkalis, necrotic corneal stromal cells and polymorphonuclear inflammatory cells can all induce corneal degradation resulting in stromal lysis, necrosis and liquefaction.

Diagnosis

The 'mushy' appearance of the cornea is diagnostic as is the speed with which corneal perforation can occur if the condition is not recognized.

Treatment

- Initial swabs and scrapes for culture and sensitivity. The affected area should be debrided thoroughly to remove necrotic tissue.
- A sub-palpebral medication device should be inserted.
- A pedicle graft should be applied if there appears to be any possibility of corneal perforation.
- Topical application of a fortified antibiotic solution (effective against *Pseudomonas* spp.) should be given every hour initially, with a decrease of frequency once a maintained improvement is observed.
- Anticollagenases (e.g. fresh whole serum, acetylcysteine) topically may be of value. They are given following the same regime described for antibiotics. Systemic ascorbic acid (vitamin C) can be used on an empirical basis.
- Any accompanying uveitis should be treated sympomatically.

Corneal foreign bodies

Diagnosis

These are usually organic material. Use oblique illumination, magnification and, if necessary, ophthalmic stains to aid diagnosis.

Treatment

• Superficial foreign bodies can be removed following the application of local anaesthetic, using a corneal spud or a cotton wool bud.
• Removal of penetrating corneal foreign bodies should be carried out under general anaesthesia if there is any possibility of anterior chamber collapse. They may be retrieved via their site of entry, although those of complex shape, particularly when they have impaled the iris, may require removal via a limbal-based incision to prevent further damage. Full thickness penetrations with involvement of uveal tract and/or lens carry a guarded prognosis.

Viral keratitis

Equine herpesvirus has been suggested as a possible primary ocular pathogen. At present, the diagnosis of suspected viral keratitis is based upon response to treatment rather than viral isolation.

Diagnosis and treatment

The clinical appearance of suspected equine viral keratitis is variable, with multiple, usually punctate, superficial corneal opacities, accompanied by blepharospasm and lacrimation. Most cases are unilateral. Less commonly, shallow ulcers may be present and, in others, circular stromal opacities are the most obvious clinical feature.

Treatment of acute cases consists of topical antiviral agents (e.g. idoxuridine, vidarabine, trifluorthymidine and acyclovir); only acyclovir is available in the UK. In chronic cases with stromal involvement the judicious concurrent use of topical corticosteroids should also be considered.

Bacterial keratitis

Aetiology and diagnosis

Bacterial keratitis is most commonly seen following corneal injury, particularly when ulcerative keratitis is present.

The patient usually presents with acute ocular pain and a serous discharge which can quickly become mucopurulent or purulent. Chemosis and conjunctival hyperaemia are usually prominent.

The clinical appearance is rarely diagnostic and culture and scrapings from the edge of the ulcer, where bacterial replication occurs, are both helpful diagnostic aids.

Treatment

For superficial lesions topical antibiotics (preferably after sensitivity testing) are adequate. For deeper lesions topical treatment with fortified antibiotic solution may be required.

When Gram negative organisms such as *Pseudomonas* spp. are isolated, treatment with gentamicin or tobramycin will be needed. The use of anticollagenases should also be considered because of the risk of corneal 'melting' (liquefactive stromal necrosis), a complication of keratitis which is not uncommon in horses. Any accompanying uveitis should be treated with topical atropine to relieve ciliary spasm.

Initially treatment of complicated cases must be as frequent as every 1–2 hours, and an indwelling sub-palpebral device is advisable. Treatment should be maintained until the eye is quiet and free of pain.

Mycotic keratitis

Keratomycosis is rare in the UK, but may be found as a significant cause of keratitis in other countries with a climate more supportive of fungal growth. Most cases are seen in late summer and autumn.

Aetiology, clinical signs and diagnosis

Diagnosis is based on the history, clinical appearance, demonstration of fungal hyphae and positive fungal culture. Keratomycosis may be a complication of previous corneal trauma or a consequence of inappropriate drug (i.e. corticosteroid) therapy. Clinical signs include the anterior segment triad of pain, blepharospasm and excessive lacrimation. The appearance ranges from a superficial ulcer, to more diffuse and deeper corneal involvement with satellite lesions; on occasions frank abscessation is present. An accompanying uveitis is common.

Specimens should be taken using a moist sterile swab and a Kimura spatula. As yeasts and fungi can be isolated as normal flora of the horse conjunctival sac it is important to sample from the affected cornea. On occasions, this means performing superficial keratectomy with the extra advantages of obtaining samples for histopathology and exposing affected cornea to antimycotic agents. A conjunctival pedicle graft may be required following some keratectomies. Corneal scrapings should be taken from the edge and base of lesions and, as vigorous scraping is required, local anaesthesia is necessary. Histopathology following keratectomy is the most successful means of demonstrating fungal hyphae. Sabouraud's medium and blood agar are used for culture and incubation should be for a minimum of one month when yeasts and fungi are suspected.

Treatment

Treatment may be required for weeks or months. Topical clotrimazole, miconazole, natamycin and pimaricin have all been used as treatments for equine keratomycosis.

In addition to treating with specific antifungal agents it may also be necessary to treat any accompanying uveitis symptomatically and mixed infections may require broad-spectrum antibiotic therapy. Corticosteroids, by any route, are contraindicated in the management of equine fungal corneal infections.

Topical treatment is usually maintained until good clinical healing has occurred; usually this takes a minimum of 6–8 weeks. The prognosis in keratomycosis is always guarded when stromal involvement is present and, on occasions, the eye may still be lost because of intraocular extension despite aggressive therapy.

Corneal neoplasia

Whilst primary corneal neoplasia is very rare in most animals, in horses intraepithelial carcinoma *in situ* as well as extension of squamous cell carcinoma from the conjunctiva and limbus, occurs.

Diagnosis and treatment

Intraepithelial carcinoma may resemble superficial keratomycosis, but can be distinguished by histopathology, or occasionally, from impression smears. Cryotherapy, with or without surgical excision, is the treatment of choice for both intraepithelial carcinoma *in situ* and squamous cell carcinoma. Other effective treatments include laser therapy (e.g. carbon dioxide laser) and brachytherapy (e.g. beta irradiation).

12.7 *Uveal tract*

The uveal tract consists of the iris, ciliary body and choroid. There is some variation of iris colour (heterochromia) according to the amount of pigment present and iris colour may vary between the two eyes and between different sectors of the iris in the same eye.

Persistent pupillary membrane

The pupillary membrane consists of the vascular arcades and associated mesenchymal tissue which are a normal feature of the developing eye. Persistent remnants of the pupillary membrane (ppm) represent a failure of the normal processes of atrophy. Pupillary membrane remnants are very common in horses, although there is no evidence that they are inherited. They are usually of no consequence even when they contact the posterior cornea or anterior lens capsule to produce localized opacities at the point of contact.

Pigmented filamentous strands usually arise from the mid-iris collarette; commonly they are arranged in annular fashion in this region, but they may also span the pupil, or pass anteriorly to the cornea, or posteriorly to the lens. One or both eyes may be affected and no treatment is necessary.

Coloboma

Coloboma is the term used to describe a congenital condition in which a portion of the eye is missing. In horses colobomatous defects involving the uveal tract are sometimes found in the iris and ocular fundus.

Diagnosis

Partial or complete holes may be seen in the iris and should be distinguished from acquired iris atrophy which may be seen following previous iris inflammation or as a feature of ageing. Iris hypoplasia, usually in the stroma of the mid-dorsal region of the iris, manifesting as 'cystic' swelling is also not uncommon in animals with poorly pigmented (subalbinotic) irides (e.g. Welsh ponies).

Colobomatous defects of the ocular fundus appear as clearly defined focal areas of a lighter colour than the normal surrounding tissues; they may be single or multiple. As they usually primarily affect the retinal pigment epithelium they are easiest to visualize in the non-tapetal fundus.

Aniridia

This rare condition in which there is partial or complete absence of the iris has been recorded sporadically in horses and an inherited basis has been demonstrated in Belgian draft horses.

Affected animals are usually photophobic with large, circular, unresponsive pupils. There may be other secondary changes such as cataract or keratitis.

Hypertrophy of the granula iridica

This is a common condition of unknown cause which may be unilateral or bilateral. Despite an often spectacular appearance, the large size of the granula iridica does not have any obvious effect on vision and no treatment is required.

Cystic anomalies

Cysts arising from various parts of the uveal tract are not uncommon in horses, although those anterior to the iris are most likely to be noted on casual inspection.

Diagnosis, differential diagnosis and treatment

Although the amount of pigmentation varies, most cysts irrespective of their origin (granula iridica, pigmented and non-pigmented uveal epithelium) are smooth, round, do not invade neighbouring tissues and can be transilluminated with a bright focal light source; these features help to distinguish them from uveal neoplasia. Occasionally they become free floating within the anterior chamber, their size can fluctuate and, on occasions, they rupture and the remnants become attached to the anterior lens capsule or the posterior surface of the cornea. No treatment is required except for the very rare occasions when they interfere with vision. In such cases the cysts can be evacuated and removed.

Neoplasia

Uveal neoplasia is rare, the commonest tumours being iris melanomas. These tumours are locally invasive with no cellular malignancy.

Diagnosis and treatment

Intraocular melanomas are commonest in grey horses. The majority arise from the iris and cases are presented because a dark, solid mass, which gradually enlarges, has been noticed within the anterior chamber. Examination of the eye usually indicates obvious iris and pupil distortion, and there is also localized corneal opacity if the tumour is large enough to impinge on the posterior cornea.

Local surgical excision is possible if cases are seen early enough, but enucleation is required if the tumour is extensive.

Trauma

Trauma to the iris can be caused by direct insult, from iris prolapse as a sequel to corneal perforation and by 'whiplash' injury, a partial avulsion of the granula iridica from the iris as a result of sudden and violent head movement or blunt trauma.

Diagnosis

The history can be very helpful and the clinical appearance may provide an immmediate diagnosis in cases of iris prolapse following corneal perforation. Other injuries, however, are only discovered after careful ophthalmic examination in a darkened box. Foreign bodies, especially dark objects like twigs and thorns, are not easy to identify, especially if there is corneal oedema and an accompanying uveitis. Avulsion, or partial avulsion of the granula iridica, is also easy to miss. In all cases of uveal trauma the situation may be further complicated by intraocular haemorrhage (usually hyphaema, but occasionally more extensive haemorrhage).

Treatment

Irrespective of the type of traumatic injury any accompanying uveitis is controlled medically.

- For cases of iris prolapse viable prolapsed iris which is not contaminated is returned to the anterior chamber. Non-viable and heavily contaminated iris tissue may require excision, but it is better to avoid sacrifice whenever possible.

- A foreign body which has impinged upon or penetrated the iris is best removed. It is important to check that the lens has not also been damaged as leakage of lens protein may result in a phacoclastic uveitis which is impossible to control medically. In more longstanding cases the decision to attempt foreign body removal will be largely dependent on whether the foreign body is causing problems which cannot be controlled by a course of medical treatment.
- Avulsion or partial avulsion of the granula iridica does not usually require surgical intervention and only symptomatic treatment for uveitis is required.
- Hyphaema in horses is usually left to resorb naturally, but viscoelastic material such as sodium hyaluronate can be used to evacuate haemorrhage from the anterior chamber and as a means of making iris surgery simpler.

Uveitis

Aetiology

There are many causes of uveitis in horses which include keratitis-associated, trauma, lens-associated, intraocular parasites and as part of generalized viral (e.g. equine viral arteritis) and bacterial disease (e.g. *Rhodococcus equi* septicaemia in foals). On many occasions there is no obvious cause and this category encompasses the endogenous type of imune-mediated uveitis known as equine recurrent uveitis (synonyms – recurrent iridocyclitis, periodic ophthalmia, moon blindness, lunar blindness) where the characteristic feature is hypersensitivity to a variety of antigens.

Many infectious agents have been associated with equine recurrent uveitis (ERU). In the USA, *Leptospira pomona* is commonly cited as a cause of ERU on the basis of a significant association between antibodies against *L. pomona* and ERU, whereas in the UK a small number of cases may be associated with *L. sejroe*. ERU has also been reported in association with a range of other infectious agents which include equine herpesvirus-1, the togavirus responsible for equine viral arteritis, *Borrelia burgdoferi* (Lyme disease), *Brucella* spp., *Salmonella* spp., *Streptococcus equi* (strangles), *Cryptococcus neoformans*, *Onchocerca cervicalis* and *Toxoplasma gondii*.

Bilateral involvement is uncommon and 50% of affected animals show recurrence of the acute disease. Initial episodes are commonly seen at 2–3 years of age, especially in Thoroughbreds.

Clinical features of acute uveitis

Some or all of the features listed below may be present.

- Impaired vision
- Pain
- Anterior segment triad – blepharospasm, lacrimation and photophobia
- Eyelid oedema
- Chemosis
- Conjunctival and episcleral injection, especially in the ciliary region
- Cornea dull because of mild oedema; corneal vascularization can be an early feature of uveitis in horses
- Anterior chamber changes (aqueous flare, hyphaema)
- Miosis (the pupil constriction can be intense)
- Loss of iris detail and early synechiae formation
- Low intraocular pressure
- Peripapillary retinal oedema
- Inflammatory cells in the vitreous
- Optic neuritis

Clinical features of chronic uveitis

Some or all of the features listed below may be present.

- Impaired vision or total blindness
- Corneal neovascularization and chronic corneal oedema
- Anterior chamber changes (hypopyon)
- Darkening of the iris and loss of iris detail
- Rupture of the granula iridica
- Immobile, or partially mobile, irregular pupil
- Posterior synechiae
- Cell rests (pigment deposits on the anterior lens capsule)
- Secondary cataract formation
- Lens subluxation or luxation
- Syneresis (vitreal liquefaction) and opacities (vitreal floaters)
- Fibrous traction bands within the vitreous
- Retinal detachment
- Peripapillary chorioretinopathy or more extensive chorioretinopathy
- Optic atrophy
- Hydrophthalmos and glaucoma are rare
- Shrinkage of the globe (phthisis bulbi)

Management of equine uveitis

Careful examination as early as possible in the course of the inflammation is the key to accurate symptomatic diagnosis and successful treatment.

- Affected animals should be placed in a quiet fly-free and dust-free environment, usually a darkened box.
- According to the temperament of the patient and the amount of pain which is present it may be sensible to insert some form of sub-palpebral or nasolacrimal lavage device early on as this will simplify topical drug therapy.
- Initial treament must be aggressive, with frequent topical applications (every hour) until clinical improvement is noted. The frequency and intensity of therapy can be reduced once clinical improvement is maintained, affected animals require a minimum of 3 weeks of treatment and sometimes several months of treatment are required. As a general principle it is probably sensible to maintain medical therapy for at least 2 weeks after the eye has become quiet.

Drug therapy

- Topical mydriatics (1–4% atropine sulphate $\pm$ 10% phenylephrine). These are used only as often as is required to keep the pupil dilated. The owners should be warned that it may be days or weeks before the pupil responds normally to light following therapy.
- Topical corticosteroid with good intraocular penetration (e.g. prednisolone acetate) is given provided that the corneal epithelium is intact. Topical non-steroidal anti-inflammatory (NSAID) drops (e.g. flurbiprofen sodium) can be used concurrently or, with *great care*, as an alternative to topical corticosteroids when the corneal epithelium is not intact.
- Topical antibiotic drops are given if appropriate.
- Parenteral non-steroidal anti-inflammatory drugs (e.g. flunixin meglumine or ketoprofen or phenylbutazone) are given by injection in the acute stage of inflammation. Follow-up therapy may be given with oral flunixin meglumine or phenylbutazone. In chronic cases with periodic recrudescence of inflammation, oral aspirin may be palliative.
- Parenteral corticosteroids (e.g. prednisolone) may be used as an alternative to NSAIDs. Systemic corticosteroids and NSAIDs should not be used concurrently as there is an increased risk of gastrointestinal ulceration and haemorrhage. The usual care should be exercised when administering NSAIDs and corticosteroids by any route.
- Specific parenteral therapy is indicated where a particular aetiological agent has been demonstrated.

12.8 *Aqueous production and drainage and glaucoma*

Aqueous is produced by the ciliary body, passes through the pupil and drains circumferentially via the iridocorneal angle; the 'conventional' outflow mechanism. In horses 'unconventional' low resistance aqueous outflow routes, the uveoscleral and uveovortical pathways, are thought to be important routes of aqueous drainage. The 'conventional' scleral outflow route may be of lesser importance. The design of the outflow mechanism means that there is little risk of developing glaucoma.

Glaucoma

Glaucoma (a pathological elevation of intraocular pressure) is *unusual* in horses. Primary glaucoma (which develops without antecedent eye disease) is exceptionally rare and secondary glaucoma (which develops secondary to eye disease) is uncommon and when it does occur is usually a sequel to anterior segment inflammation. The clinical signs of equine glaucoma are subtle.

Diagnosis of glaucoma

- Minimal ocular discomfort or no ocular pain
- Conjunctival and episcleral congestion are rare
- Anterior chamber may be shallower than normal
- Corneal oedema and/or corneal striae and/or neovascularization
- Lack of a pupillary light reflex
- Fixed pupil (may be mildly dilated, but likely to be constricted if glaucoma is secondary to anterior uveitis)
- Synechiae may be apparent
- Raised intraocular pressure
- Globe enlargement

- Subluxation or luxation of the lens
- Vitreal changes (inflammation, opacities, liquefaction)
- Fundus changes (cupping of the optic disc, optic atrophy, peripapillary chorioretinopathy, retinal atrophy)
- Decreased vision or blind

Treatment

Treatment can be attempted if vision is still present and aims either to increase the uveoscleral outflow (e.g. atropine), or to decrease aqueous production by means of oral or topical carbonic anhydrase inhibitors, or topical beta blockers. Cyclophotoablation (e.g. Nd:YAG laser) may be valuable in controlling intraocular pressure.

When the eye is blind it may be left without treatment if pain or excessive globe size are not causing problems; if some form of intervention is required then cyclodestruction (cryotherapy or laser ablation) or removal of the eye is the treatment of choice.

12.9 *Lens*

Horses have a large lens and minor refractive errors of no clinical significance may be apparent as already described under the protocol for ophthalmic examination earlier in the chapter.

Minor opacities associated with embryonic remnants are common and include those arising from the hyaloid system and tunica vasculosa lentis; less commonly such opacities are more obvious and merit the description of capsular cataracts, as do the opacities from persistent pupillary membrane remnants attached to the anterior lens capsule. Senile sclerosis is not an obvious ageing change in the equine lens and in horses of twenty or more years the lens may appear yellow.

Lens abnormalities may be either congenital (present from birth) or acquired. The position, size, shape and transparency of the lens may be abnormal from birth, whereas later in life disease processes are restricted to a loss of transparency or a change of position.

Cataract, an opacity in the lens or its capsule, is the commonest lens abnormality likely to be encountered in practice.

Cataract

Opacities of the lens or its capsule may be classified in various ways:

- Cause: e.g. post-inflammatory, traumatic.
- Age of onset: e.g. congenital, juvenile, senile.
- Location: e.g. capsular, cortical, nuclear, polar, equatorial.
- Stage of development: e.g. immature, mature, hypermature.

Some cataracts may progress with increasing size and density, others may remain static or, rarely, become less dense with increasing maturity. With few exceptions, it is impossible to predict the progress of a cataract at a single examination.

Most cataracts, apart from the complete cortical type, cause no obvious visual deficit. However, if they are dense and obstructing the visual axis, they will have a significant effect on vision and some affected animals may be suitable for cataract surgery.

1. *Congenital cataracts* are seen occasionally and may have a variety of causes including teratogenicity. They are more common in Arab foals than Thoroughbreds, but inheritance, although suspected, is unproven.

   The only confirmed primary inherited cataract in this species is a congenital nuclear cataract in the Morgan horse, although there are occasional reports of congenital nuclear cataracts in other breeds (e.g. Quarter horse) which may have an inherited basis. Cataracts may be seen in association with other inherited ocular defects (e.g. cataracts secondary to aniridia in Belgian horses) and other defects of uncertain cause (e.g. microphthalmos, persistent pupillary membrane, persistent primary vitreous).

2. *Acquired cataracts* include both blunt and penetrating trauma and other cataracts of post-inflammatory origin. Undoubtedly the commonest reason for acquired cataract in horses is uveitis and for this reason alone both eyes should be examined meticulously to check for indications of active or previous inflammation of the uveal tract in animals where cataracts are found. Cataracts of this type are unsuitable for surgery.

Subluxation and luxation of the lens

Subluxation and luxation of the lens is unusual in horses, but may be seen in association with multiple ocular anomalies, and also as a possible sequel to trauma, previous inflammation and globe enlargement (e.g. as a complication of glaucoma).

12.10 *Vitreous*

Anatomy

The adult vitreous is a transparent gel which is formed from the third stage of vitreal embryogenesis (tertiary vitreous). In the foal there are still vestiges of the hyaloid system which forms the primary vitreous and the hyaloid vessel can be seen traversing the vitreous from the optic nerve head to its termination at the posterior lens capsule (Mittendorf's dot). The vessel regresses in early postnatal life and only Cloquet's canal and Mittendorf's dot mark its original course in animals of more than 9 months of age.

Condensations of vitreal fibrils (the vitreal tracts) may be apparent in normal horses as may slight mobility of the vitreal components as a consequence of poor cohesion of the vitreous gel; these findings are of no clinical significance.

Congenital vitreal abnormalities

Persistence of the primary vitreous and persistent hyperplastic primary vitreous

Persistence of the primary vitreous and persistent hyperplastic primary vitreous are both uncommon in horses. The latter is rarely seen and affected foals present with obvious leucocoria (white pupil). No treatment is available for either condition.

Acquired vitreal abnormalities

Inflammation

The avascular vitreous is rarely a source of primary disease, but may become secondarily involved when there is disease of the retina and/or uveal tract.

● In the acute phase the predominant clinical finding may be vitreal haze, or more marked vitreal opacity.
● Later in the pathogenesis, cellular and/or fibrous debris ('floaters') and liquefaction (syneresis) may be apparent. Organization of inflammatory tissue (adhesions) within the vitreous can result in a traction detachment of the retina.

Management is aimed at the diagnosis and treatment of the primary source of inflammation (e.g. treatment of uveitis).

Haemorrhage

Haemorrhage into the vitreous is usually a consequence of trauma (including foreign bodies) or severe inflammation. Even if the cause can be identified and eliminated, the haemorrhage will be resorbed very slowly and often incompletely and there is a substantial risk of retinal detachment as the haemorrhage becomes organized.

Synchysis scintillans

This is an occasional finding, of no apparent clinical significance, in older horses. Small crystals of cholesterol are present within the liquefied vitreal gel; they swirl within the vitreous when the horse moves its head and settle under the influence of gravity.

12.11 *Fundus*

There is considerable normal variation in the appearance of the equine fundus and it is important to appreciate the range of normality before attempting to diagnose abnormality. The protocol outlined at the beginning of the chapter should be followed and the appearance recorded by means of annotated diagrams. In acute cases it is important to attempt to find the underlying cause of the observed retinal pathology (e.g. systemic bacteraemia or viraemia) so that treatment can be attempted. However, in most situations in which fundus changes are detected, the role of the veterinary surgeon is simply to determine whether the lesions observed are of any visual significance and thus, by inference, whether the animal is suitable for its intended purpose.

Evaluation of vision in affected animals is often subjective, but in general, the presence of a normal retinal vasculature is likely to indicate a functional retina. Thinning or loss of vasculature indicates local or generalized retinal pathology, possibly causing visual deficit. It is useful to classify fundus appearance empirically into normal variants and pathological variants.

Normal variants of fundus appearance

Partial albinism

Pigment dilution may be localized (e.g. peripapillary) or generalized, affecting either or both of the tapetal and non-tapetal fundus. The varying degrees of pigment dilution enable details of the underlying choroidal vasculature to be observed.

Albinism

Albinism is associated with absence of a tapetum and lack of pigment allowing the choroidal vasculature to be observed against the pale scleral background.

Variations of pigmentation

Hypopigmentation and hyperpigmentation may both be observed as a normal variant. The peripapillary region is commonly involved and variants include a complete circumpapillary halo, or localized peripapillary foci of hypopigmentation (relatively light) or hyperpigmentation (relatively dark). Focal and linear regions of hyperpigmentation may also be seen in the tapetal fundus and the region of the ventral tapetal/non-tapetal junction.

Retinal vessels

Normally some 30–60 inconspicuous retinal vessels radiate from the disc margin, except for a site ventral to the disc where a small notch usually marks the site of the original choroidal (foetal) fissure. There is little variation in the appearance of these vessels in normal animals.

Choroidal vessels

The extent to which choroidal vessels are visible is entirely dependent upon the amount of pigment present and the presence or absence of a tapetum.

Variations of myelination

In most horses the retinal nerve fibre layer is unmyelinated, but in some animals the nerves become myelinated as they approach the optic disc and, on examination, they may be observed as radiating greyish white striae.

Other variants

A discrete zone of yellow located as a vertical band dorsal to the optic disc and sometimes as much smaller focal opacities may indicate lipid deposition in the tapetum. Remnants of the hyaloid system of the primary vitreous are occasionally observed in adult animals.

Pathological variants of fundus appearance

Coloboma

Colobomatous defects are not uncommon (single or multiple, typical and atypical) and usually involve individual (i.e. retina, choroid, sclera) structures; they are not of significance and have no apparent effect on vision. Rarely, colobomatous defects are more extensive, involving collective anatomical structures and sometimes associated with other ocular abnormalities (e.g. microphthalmos). In these cases vision is severely affected.

Congenital stationary night blindness

See Chapter 20.

Retinal haemorrhage

These are most commonly observed as discrete or linear haemorrhages in neonatal foals. They usually resorb without complication. In foals with neonatal maladjustment syndrome they tend to be larger and more numerous. Haemorrhages may also be seen occasionally in adult horses and it is important to try and establish the cause (e.g. trauma, generalized disease).

Retinal detachment

Retinal detachment is occasionally identified as a cause of congenital unilateral or bilateral blindness in foals. In adults, it is occasionally a complication of uveitis or the result of trauma (especially blunt trauma).

Inflammation

Active inflammation

Active inflammation is rarely diagnosed. Active lesions are less striking than inactive ones and usually manifest as poorly defined focal, or diffuse areas (e.g. soft exudates at the vitreoretinal interface) in the fundus. In these cases it is important to try and establish the cause.

Chronic, inactive, chorioretinopathy

Chronic, inactive, chorioretinopathy is a frequent incidental finding at ophthalmic examination and the main point at issue in these cases is the extent of any concomitant visual deficit. The appearance and significance vary according to the extent of chorioretinal involvement. There is a wide range of appearances which include loss of pigment, proliferation of pigment, hyporeflectivity, hyper-reflectivity and abnormalities of retinal and choroidal vasculature.

1. *Focal chorioretinopathy* lesions are usually small depigmented foci in the non-tapetal fundus. Such lesions are common and do not affect vision adversely per se. They may have an apparently random distribution, or a more linear configuration. Focal chorioretinopathy lesions are observed less commonly in the tapetal fundus. Extensive focal lesions are unusual and of possible significance as they may be accompanied by attenuation of the retinal blood vessels.
2. *Peripapillary chorioretinopathy* ('butterfly' lesions) may be detected on occasions; this type of chorioretinopathy can be related to a number of non-specific insults (e.g. panuveitis, optic neuritis, optic nerve damage). The significance of peripapillary chorioretinopathy is unknown when the associated retinal vasculature is normal, but must be regarded as of significance when the retinal blood vessels are abnormal (e.g. attenuated).
3. *Diffuse chorioretinopathy* is rare in horses and must always be regarded as a lesion which is likely to be associated with gross visual impairment.

Retinal atrophy

Retinal atrophy may have a multiplicity of causes. For example, in addition to retinal atrophy as an end-stage consequence of severe inflammatory and degenerative disease of the fundus, retinal atrophy may also follow ocular ischaemia, as from surgical ligation of the carotid artery, profound systemic haemorrhage and septic embolism. Retinal atrophy may also be a result of blunt trauma, usually as a striate, localized, retinopathy. With generalized retinal atrophy the eye is blind, whereas with localized atrophy it may not be possible to detect any visual problems.

Traumatic optic neuropathy

Traumatic optic neuropathy is a possible sequel to trauma, especially in those situations where there is direct compression, stretching or avulsion of the optic nerve. Affected animals are usually acutely blind (e.g. bilateral blindness following basisphenoid and basioccipital fractures when the horse falls over backwards). Initially the optic papilla may appear normal, but sometimes there is papillary hyperaemia, oedema and extrusion of myelin at the optic nerve head. Later there is attenuation of the retinal vessels and optic atrophy. The prognosis for vision in most cases is hopeless, even when there is early and aggressive therapy with systemic anti-inflammatories.

Optic neuritis

As with other acute inflammations of the fundus, optic neuritis is rarely diagnosed in horses. It is associated with a number of systemic diseases (especially neurotrophic viruses, bacterial septicaemia and immune-mediated problems). Animals are blind or visually impaired in the affected eye, or eyes and the optic papilla appears hyperaemic and not clearly defined. There are frequently vitreal opacities in affected animals and fine grey striae radiate from the papilla into the vitreous. Management consists of establishing and eliminating the underlying cause and treating the optic neuritis symptomatically with systemic corticosteroids.

Optic atrophy

Optic atrophy is a consequence of many insults which include trauma, space occupying lesions and severe inflammatory disease (e.g. chorioretinitis, panuveitis). The papilla appears pale and the pattern of the lamina cribrosa is more obvious than usual. The retinal vesels are profoundly attenuated or absent and there is no treatment.

Proliferative optic neuropathy

Proliferative optic neuropathy, which may be focal or generalized, probably represents reactive glial cell responses to a range of insults.

• The appearance is either of a *focal* lobulated mass at the edge of the papilla which is often an incidental finding of ophthalmoscopic examination in older horses. There is no apparent effect on vision and no tendency to progress to produce clinical problems.

• *Generalized* proliferative optic neuropathy involves the entire surface of the optic disc and can sometimes be related to previous orbital trauma or profound haemorrhage; such eyes are blind and there is no treatment.

Neoplasia

Primary and secondary neoplasia of the fundus is very rare. Astrocytoma is a discrete tumour of the optic papilla and resembles focal proliferative optic neuropathy. Other tumours of the optic papilla include medulloepithelioma and neuro-epithelioma and if these involve the orbital portion of the optic nerve, exophthalmos may be part of the clinical presentation.

Further reading

Auer, J.A. (Ed.) (1992) *Equine Surgery.* W.B. Saunders and Co., Philadelphia.

Barnett, K.C., Rossdale, P.D. and Wade, J.E. (Eds) (1983) *Equine Veterinary Journal* Supplement 2.

Barnett, K.C., Rossdale, P.D. and Wade, J.E. (Eds) (1990) *Equine Veterinary Journal* Supplement 10.

Barnett, K.C., Crispin, S.M., Lavach, J.D. and Matthews, A.G. (1994) *Colour Atlas and Text of Equine Ophthalmology.* Mosby-Wolfe, London.

Davidson, M.G. (1991) Equine ophthalmology. In *Veterinary Ophthalmology* (Ed. K.N. Gelatt), 2nd Edition. Lea and Febiger, Philadelphia.

Lavach, J.D. (1990) *Large Animal Ophthalmology.* C.V. Mosby Co., St Louis.

Moore, C.P. (Ed.) (1992) *Veterinary Clinics of North America: Equine Practice 8:3 Ophthalmology.* W.B. Saunders and Co., Philadelphia.

Roberts, S.M. (Ed.) (1984) *Veterinary Clinics of North America: Large Animal Practice 6:3 Large Animal Ophthalmology.* W.B. Saunders and Co., Philadelphia.

Appendix. Differential diagnosis of common ocular and adnexal problems

In each section the diagnostic possibilities are listed following the format of the text (i.e. adnexa, ocular surface, anterior segment, posterior segment).

1. Sudden onset of ocular pain
1. Orbital trauma
2. Globe trauma (e.g. blunt and penetrating injury)
3. Eyelid trauma
4. Entropion
5. Acute, usually allergic, blepharoconjunctivitis
6. Conjunctivitis (rarely)
7. Foreign body (e.g. beneath eyelids, within cornea, involving iris and lens)
8. Corneal insult, especially ulcerative keratitis (e.g. physical and chemical trauma)
9. Uveitis

2. Gradual onset of ocular pain
1. Orbital cellulitis and orbital abscess
2. Endophthalmitis and panophthalmitis
3. Blepharitis and meibomianitis
4. Keratoconjunctivitis sicca
5. Glaucoma (rarely)

3. Sudden onset of bilateral blindness
1. Skull trauma (uncommon, e.g. basisphenoid and basioccipital fractures)
2. Cranial trauma (e.g. cerebral concussion, contusion, laceration and haemorrhage)
3. Uveitis (rare as a bilateral problem except in foals with septicaemia)
4. Optic neuritis (uncommon, but may be associated with systemic disease)

4. Sudden onset of unilateral blindness
1. Orbital injury (uncommon)
2. Globe injury (uncommon)
3. Corneal injury (common)
4. Uveitis (uncommon)
5. Intraocular haemorrhage (rare)
6. Retinal detachment (rare)
7. Optic neuritis (rare)

5. Exophthalmos (forward displacement of the globe)
1. Extraorbital space occupying lesion (e.g. ethmoid haematoma, neoplasia)
2. Orbital space occupying lesion (e.g. inflammation, cyst, neoplasia)
3. Orbital trauma (e.g. fracture, displacement of orbital contents, haemorrhage)
4. Sinus trauma (e.g. fracture, emphysema) sinusitis, sinus cysts

6. *Enophthalmos (backward displacement of the globe)*
1. Pain (active retraction)
2. Emaciation/loss of orbital fat
3. Orbital trauma (e.g. fracture, entrapment of orbital contents, chronic fibrosis)
4. Tetanus (third eyelid prominence is usually the most obvious feature)
5. Horner's syndrome (ptosis is usually the most prominent ocular sign)
6. Dehydration

7. *Ocular discharge*
1. Orbital damage and globe injuries
2. Orbital cellulitis and abscess
3. Endophthalmitis and panophthalmitis
4. Small eye (e.g. microphthalmos, phthisis bulbi)
5. Congenital atresia/dysgenesis of nasolacrimal drainage system
6. Acquired stenosis, blockage of nasolacrimal drainage system ± inflammation
7. Blepharitis and blepharoconjunctivitis (e.g. solar-induced, immune-mediated, parasitic)
8. Neoplasia (especially squamous cell carcinoma of eyelids and conjunctiva)
9. Conjunctivitis
10. Keratitis (including keratoconjunctivitis sicca)
11. Uveitis

8. *Ocular opacity*
1. Microphthalmos, multiple ocular defects, phthisis bulbi
2. Hydrophthalmos (usually as a result of chronic glaucoma)
3. Epibulbar dermoid
4. Non-inflammatory corneal opacities (e.g. pigment, band opacities)
4. Keratoconjunctivitis sicca
5. Parasitic keratoconjunctivitis (e.g. onchocerciasis)
6. Corneal oedema (e.g. idiopathic, following blunt trauma, associated with ulceration)
7. Keratitis (e.g. ulceration, cellular infiltration, neovascularization)
8. Corneal neoplasia (rare), perilimbal neoplasia encroaching on cornea (commoner)
9. Persistent pupillary membrane ± corneal and lens opacities
10. Corneal striae (e.g. as a feature of glaucoma or as an anomaly of no clinical significance)
11. Hypopyon
12. Hyphaema
13. Uveal cysts
14. Uveal neoplasia
15. Cataract
16. Glaucoma (e.g. corneal neovascularization, discoloration, striae, pigmentation)
17. Lens subluxation and luxation
18. Persistent primary vitreous and hyperplastic primary vitreous
19. Vitreal haemorrhage
20. Vitreal opacities (e.g. synchysis scintillans)
21. Retinal detachment

13 Dermatology

CONTENTS

13.1 The approach to the skin case

History

As in other diseases, history and signalment are an important first step. It may be useful to prepare a questionnaire to ensure a complete history is taken on every occasion. Important information includes: age, sex, breed, husbandry, feeding and bedding, environment, seasonality of signs, details of incontact animals, familial details, duration of signs, nature of signs (e.g. pruritus, hair loss, nodules etc.), previous disease and current therapy.

Physical examination

This should be thorough and should not be confined to the skin. Examination should assess:

- General body condition.
- Distribution of lesions – generalized or localized.
- Size and morphology of lesions – papules, nodules, wheals, alopecia, vesicles, bullae, erosion, ulceration.
- Mucous membranes – colour, petechiation, ecchymoses.
- Palpation of the skin and associated structures noting:
  - Coat character – dryness, crusting, hair loss.
  - Peripheral lymphadenopathy.

Diagnostic techniques

In many cases, a thorough clinical examination will provide grounds for instituting therapy, but confirmation of the diagnosis may require recourse to supplementary techniques.

Skin scraping

Scrapings should be taken using a scalpel and collected onto a glass microscope slide. Samples may be cleared by adding several drops of 20% potassium hydroxide (KOH) to the slide and heating gently for 20 to 30 seconds prior to microscopic examination. Useful for parasitic and fungal conditions. Acetate tape may also be used to take a surface impression and may be applied directly to a slide.

Stains

Several stains are available and may be used on air-dried impression or direct smears onto glass slides. Gram, Diff-Quick or methylene blue are all useful. They may also be added to KOH preparations.

Culture

Bacterial and fungal conditions may warrant isolation of the causal organism. Blood agar usually suffices, but special culture media may be necessary, e.g. Sabouraud's medium for fungi.

Biopsy

Often required for a definitive diagnosis, particularly in chronic cases. The skin should not be scrubbed or disinfected. Biopsies may be taken under local or regional anaesthesia using a 5–10 mm biopsy punch. Care should be taken to preserve the integrity of the specimen, as inappropriate handling can produce artefacts. It is preferable to take an excisional biopsy if possible, using a scalpel, including a representative section of the lesion, the edge of the lesion and adjacent healthy tissue. The elliptical defect can be closed with one or two simple interrupted sutures. The specimen should be blotted dry and pressed gently onto a piece of card or cork, to prevent curling, and immersed in 10% buffered formalin.

13.2 Parasitic skin conditions

Pediculosis (lice)

Horses are commonly infected, especially during late winter and early spring, with both sucking (*Haematopinus asini*) and biting (*Damalinia equi*) lice. Animals in poor condition which are kept together in large numbers and are not groomed regularly often have heavy burdens. Adult lice lay operculate eggs attached to the hairs. The nymph resembles the adult and matures through three larval stages on the host over a period of 2 to 3 weeks. Lice are host-specific and do not live for more than a few days off the horse. Transmission is by direct contact via grooming equipment, harness or bedding.

Clinical signs

- Pruritus.
- Parasites in the mane and tail–head areas, but may be anywhere on the body.
- Loss of hair – irregularly shaped bare areas with ill-defined borders, especially head, neck and thighs.
- Superficial abrasions may be caused by rubbing.
- Anaemia in extremely heavy infestations of sucking lice.

Diagnosis

This can be made by a thorough clinical examination. Biting species are fawn in colour, and sucking lice become blue-black when they are filled with blood. The eggs have a shiny appearance and are attached to the hair shafts.

Treatment

Synthetic pyrethroids (cypermethrin or permethrin) and selenium sulphide washes (unlicensed) are effective.

Cutaneous habronemiasis

Cutaneous habronemiasis or 'summer sore' is a seasonal condition characterized by variably pruritic granulomatous lesions. The occurrence of lesions corresponds with the fly season, being caused by the aberrant intradermal migration of the larvae of stomach worms, *Habronema musca*, *Habronema microstoma* and *Draschia megastoma*. Adult worms live in the horse's stomach producing larvae which are passed in the faeces. There, the worm larvae are ingested by the larvae of intermediate host flies. Infectious larvae are deposited on the horse while flies are feeding. This condition occurs in most parts of the world, especially where the climate is warm and wet. It is uncommon in the UK.

Clinical signs

The characteristic lesions are reddish-brown granulomatous masses.

- Occur at the medial canthus of the eye, the penis, prepuce and urethral process of male horses.
- Also may be found in uncovered wounds.

- Are accompanied by a serosanguinous exudate and exhibit gritty, yellow nodules on section.

Pathology

- Diffuse granulation tissue infiltrated by eosinophils.
- Cross-sections of larvae may be seen as well as foci of coagulative necrosis.

Diagnosis

Diagnosis is based on history and clinical signs, but confirm by skin biopsy or impression smear.

Treatment and control

Treatment objectives are to reduce the size of the lesion, to reduce the inflammation and to prevent reinfection. Killing larvae in tissue is unimportant but can be achieved using ivermectin. Excess granulation tissue may be removed by conventional surgery or cryosurgery, although the location of lesions often makes this difficult. Prednisolone may be administered orally or intralesional triamcinolone acetonide has proved effective.

To prevent reinfection, immediate wound care is vital, and fly control, for the animal and its environment, should be undertaken. This includes wound dressing and strict manure management and the use of fly repellents.

Chorioptic mange

This condition is often called leg mange or itchy heels, and is caused by infection with non-burrowing mites (*Chorioptes* spp.). Chorioptic mange tends to be more common in winter months, and particularly in individuals with heavy leg feather. Eggs are laid on the skin, and hatch in 1 to 5 days. The subsequent larval and two nymph stages do not penetrate below the skin surface, and the life cycle is completed in 9 to 10 days. Transmission is by direct or indirect contact.

Clinical signs

- Stamping and rubbing of the lower limbs.
- Fetlock and pastern becomes matted with dried exudate.
- Scaly patches may occur in chronic cases.

Diagnosis

Confirmation is obtained by microscopic examination of skin scrapings.

Treatment and control

Treatment is with topical synthetic pyrethroids or topical ivermectin (unlicensed).

Sarcoptic, psoroptic and demodectic mange

Sarcoptes scabei, *Psoroptes communis* and *Psoroptes equi* are rare causes of skin disease throughout the world. Lesions caused by these mites occur mainly on the body, and are associated with loss of hair and thickening of the skin. *Psoroptes cuniculi* is often found in the ear canal, and can cause head irritation and ear rubbing. Demodectic mange is a very rare follicular dermatosis of horses. Clinically, there is patchy alopecia and scaling. Squamous and pustular forms have been described.

Miscellaneous parasitic skin conditions

Cutaneous onchocerciasis

Onchocerca cervicalis is a widespread filarial nematode of horses. Adults live in the ligamentum nuchae, producing microfilariae which migrate in connective tissue to the upper dermis, particularly the skin of the ventral midline. *Culicoides* spp. act as a vector, and although many horses are infected, the majority never show evidence of clinical disease. Skin reactions are probably caused by hypersensitivity.

Clinical signs include areas of alopecia, scaling and ulceration with variable pruritus. Lesions occur most commonly on the ventral abdomen and chest, and on the face and neck. Diagnosis is confirmed by skin biopsy but this is a rare diagnosis in the UK. Treatment includes ivermectin and systemic corticosteroids.

Harvest mite infection (trombiculidiasis)

Infection with larvae of the harvest mite *Trombicula autumnalis* is common in some parts of Europe and Australia in the autumn. The larvae come off the herbage and live for a few days on an animal causing pruritus of the horse's heels, face, neck and ventral abdomen. The orange-red mites may be visible to the naked eye.

Warbles

The bovine warble flies (*Hypoderma bovis* and *H. lineatum*) are found in many countries in the northern hemisphere. Warble flies rarely lay their eggs on the horse, but larvae may migrate and reach the dorsum, and sometimes migrate to unusual sites. Diagnosis is made on the appearance of the lesion (subcutaneous nodule, often with a breathing pore). The lesions are most commonly seen over the withers, and are about 2 cm in diameter. The lesions can be poulticed or surgically lanced to express the warble fly.

Fly infestations

Horses are attacked by a variety of flies, causing annoyance and discomfort, and bites may result in allergic reactions, producing skin wheals and papules, which may be pruritic. These include stable flies (*Stomoxys calcitrans*), black flies (*Simulium* spp.), horn flies (*Haematoba irritans*) and horse flies (*Tabanids* and *Hybomitra* spp.). Control is by regular use of insect repellants applied to the animals and the environment.

Equine ventral midline dermatitis

This is a seasonal, fly-related dermatitis associated with the bites of *Haematobia irritans* (horn fly) and *Culicoides* spp. There is crusting, thickening and alopecia along the ventral midline and variable pruritus.

Parafilariasis (*Parafilaria multipapillosa*)

Parafilariasis occurs in Eastern Europe. Adult worms live in subcutaneous nodules, which open to the surface and discharge a bloody exudate containing eggs and larvae. Lesions occur over the neck, shoulders and trunk. The disease is seen in the spring and summer. The condition may recur for several years and then resolves.

Dourine (*Trypanosoma equiperdum*)

Dourine is a protozoal infection that occurs in Africa, Asia, south eastern Europe, Central and South America. Venereal infection is characterized by oedema and papules of the vulva or prepuce followed by depigmentation of these areas.

13.3 *Bacterial skin conditions*

Dermatophilosis

Dermatophilosis is an acute or chronic infection of the epidermis resulting in an exudative epidermitis. The causal organism, *Dermatophilus congolensis*, is an actinomycete, which is a bacterium, not a fungus. There is no age, breed or sex predilection for the disease, but it occurs most commonly in horses and ponies kept and/or exercised outdoors in wet/muddy conditions. In the UK, the disease is seen most frequently during the autumn and winter months. The organism resists drying and the flagellated zoospore may be transmitted from infected animals by direct or indirect contact.

Clinical signs

The disease can be generalized, affecting the dorsal aspect of the body; this form is generally known as 'rain rash' or 'rain scald'. The localized form, 'mud rash' or 'mud fever', is confined to the distal limbs and occurs commonly when the horse has been standing in flooded, muddy conditions. In both forms, the exudate mats the hairs giving a classic 'paintbrush' appearance to the lesions.

- Palpation reveals crusty lesions under the hairs.
- Scabs can be more than 0.5 cm thick, between 1 and 2.5 cm diameter.
- Scabs are grey with tufts of hair protruding from them (paintbrush effect).
- Green-grey pus may be evident on removal of the scabs.
- May be painful, but not usually pruritic.

In the chronic phase, there are plaque-like hard lesions of raised hair and flaking skin. Hair is usually retained giving the coat a rough appearance. In 'mud rash', the animal may be lame, as a result of deep cracking and heavy scabbing of skin around the coronet, heels and pastern, with secondary cellulitis in some cases.

Diagnosis

Diagnosis is usually made on clinical examination as the appearance and distribution of the clinical lesions are distinctive. Confirmation is by demonstration of the causal organism on smear and/or culture.

Treatment and control

Affected animals should be confined to dry places, and at least rugged if they cannot be stabled. Various topical treatments can be used: povidone-iodine solution, chlorhexidine solution, 0.5% chloramphenicol solution, and sometimes aluminium or zinc sulphate washes. These should be used after as many scabs as possible have been removed without causing unnecessary pain. Severe cases and cases resistant to topical therapy require parenteral antibiotics, e.g. procaine penicillin (20 000 IU/kg) intramuscularly for 3 to 5 days. Recovery usually occurs within 3 weeks, but recovered animals do not seem to be immune. Transmission from chronically infected animals via fomites should be prevented.

Folliculitis and furunculosis

A variety of organisms can cause folliculitis or furunculosis, including *Staphylococcus aureus*, *Rhodococcus equi*, and sometimes *Bacillus* spp. Ill-fitting tack, parasitic skin infection, lack of grooming and trauma are all predisposing causes. Folliculitis is most commonly seen in the saddle area of young horses in training in the summer. The lesions are painful but rarely pruritic.

Diagnosis

Diagnosis is made on the history and physical examination, direct smears of exudate and pus, KOH preparations, bacterial culture and skin biopsy.

Treatment

Treatment consists of parenteral antibiotics to which the organism is sensitive. A combination of IM procaine penicillin twice daily for 7 days and daily povidone-iodine scrubs is usually effective. If *Strep. epidermicus* is isolated or suspected, a prolonged course – up to 30 days – may be necessary to prevent abscessation.

Corynebacterium pseudotuberculosis

Subcutaneous abscesses

C. pseudotuberculosis causes deep subcutaneous abscesses. The disease is found in the western parts of the USA and Brazil. Single or multiple deep subcutaneous abscesses develop in the pectoral and ventral abdominal areas. The abscesses discharge creamy or caseous pus, and there is associated oedema, fever and lameness. Treatment involves warm soaks and surgical drainage. Complications include purpura haemorrhagica and endocarditis.

Ulcerative lymphangitis

This is a rare disease. Infection of the cutaneous lymphatics is associated with poor hygiene. Clinical signs include oedematous swelling of one or more limbs (usually hindlimbs) with the development of painful nodules (especially at the fetlock), which ulcerate and produce a purulent discharge. Individual ulcers tend to heal within 2 weeks, but new lesions continue to develop. The regional lymphatics are corded, and there is frequently lameness and debilitation. Fibrosis and disfigurement often occur.

Diagnosis is confirmed by biopsy and culture. Treatment must be early to avoid excessive fibrosis. High doses of procaine penicillin for prolonged periods may be effective.

Glanders (farcy)

Glanders is a contagious disease caused by *Pseudomonas mallei*. See Chapter 19.

Botryomycosis

Botryomycosis, an uncommon, chronic staphylococcal granulomatous disease, occurs most commonly at the site of limb or castration wounds. There are non-healing, non-pruritic granulomatous nodules. A chronic discharging sinus may develop at castration wounds (scirrhous cord – see Chapter 8).

13.4 *Fungal skin infections*

Dermatomycosis (ringworm)

Ringworm is one of the most important skin diseases of horses and is found throughout the world. *Trichophyton equinum*, *Trichophyton mentagrophytes* and *Microsporum equinum* are most common. The disease is common in riding and racing stables. Transmission may be by direct contact, or indirect spread via grooming equipment, tack, clippers or from a contaminated box. The incubation period may be as long as 4 weeks. Young horses are more susceptible due to lack of previous exposure. Resistance develops with age, although adult horses which have previously been exposed can become reinfected. Ringworm cases occur more commonly in autumn and winter in the northern hemisphere. Ringworm is a zoonosis.

Clinical signs

- Lesions are most common in the saddle, girth or neck areas (areas physically rubbed by tack).
- Appearance is variable.
- Alopecia as a result of weakened hair shafts breaking.
- Erythema, scaling and crusting due to reactions to fungal toxins.
- Hypersensitivity may lead to oedema, suppuration and necrosis.
- Pruritus is occasionally present, but in most cases the lesions are non-pruritic.

Diagnosis

Diagnosis is confirmed by microscopical examination of a skin scraping/hair sample, and isolation of the organism.

Treatment and control

Infection is usually self-limiting, with spontaneous remission occurring in 1 to 3 months. Topical treatments include natamycin or enilconazole. Tack and fomites should also be treated. Griseofulvin in feed or as a paste (10 mg/kg daily for 7 days) is arguably helpful and both treatments can be given together. As far as possible, direct or indirect contact with infected animals should be avoided.

Subcutaneous and systemic mycoses

A variety of subcutaneous fungal infections are recognized, usually occurring in specific geographical locations.

Sporotrichosis (*Sporothrix schenckii*)

Sporotrichosis occurs in southern USA, Canada, South Africa and parts of Europe. Hard subcutaneous nodules form along the line of lymphatics. Nodules may ulcerate.

Basidiobolomycosis (*Basidiobolus haptosporus*)

Basidiobolomycosis is found in tropical areas, southern USA and Mexico. Large, ulcerative granulomas occur on the head, neck, chest and trunk and also pruritus.

Conidiobolomycosis (*Conidiobolus coronatus*)

This disease occurs in tropical areas, southern USA and Mexico. There are ulcerated nodules on the external nares and in the nasal passages and intermittent serosanguineous nasal discharge.

Histoplasmosis (epizootic lymphangitis) (*Histoplasma farciminosum*)

Histoplasmosis may be found in Africa, Asia and eastern Europe. Nodules in the skin of the head and neck rupture and granulate. After 2 to 3 months, the lesions spread to the limbs and ventral abdomen.

Pythiosis (phycomycosis, swamp cancer, Gulf Coast fungus) (*Pythium* spp.)

Pythiosis occurs in tropical and subtropical areas, the Gulf Coast of the USA, South America and Australia. Large ulcerative granulomas containing white necrotic tissue, called 'leeches', form on the distal limbs, ventral abdomen and chest. There may also be pruritus.

13.5 *Allergic and immune-mediated skin diseases*

Culicoides hypersensitivity – 'sweet itch'

Equine insect hypersensitivity is a common recurring, intensely pruritic dermatitis of horses which occurs mainly during the summer months in temperate areas, but can be non-seasonal in warmer climates. It is a hypersensitivity reaction to the bites of flies and midges (gnats), including *Culicoides* spp., *Simulium* spp. and *Stomoxys calcitrans*. *Culicoides* midges appear to be the most common cause of the disease. In Britain,

C. pulicaris is usually incriminated. *C. brevitarsus* is commonly involved in Australia, whereas *C. variipenis*, *C. insignis*, *C. spinosus* and *C. stellifer* are implicated in the USA. The disease is seen particularly in ponies and donkeys with a probable familial tendency and possible predisposition in animals with dark coloured haircoat.

Clinical signs

- Predilection sites are the base of the mane, the croup and tail head.
- Intense pruritus.
- Mane and tail hairs may be broken.
- Alopecia of affected areas.
- Marked excoriation and lichenification in severe cases.
- Some cases show a ventral distribution with lesions affecting the legs, ventral thorax and abdomen, and intermandibular space.
- Although most cases may clear up after several months in temperate areas, the condition tends to recur in the same animal the following summer.

Diagnosis

This is based on the distribution and appearance of the lesions and the associated marked itching.

Treatment

Treatment is aimed at reducing inflammation and pruritus:

- topical calamine lotion to affected areas
- topical benzyl benzoate mixed with linseed or cod liver oil
- consider systemic corticosteroids (but risk of laminitis, especially with repeated administration).

Control

Control is by minimising exposure to midges (gnats) and flies.

- Frequent application of synthetic pyrethroid washes and/or attachment to braided mane/tail or head collar of insect repellant cattle ear tags. All in-contact animals as well as affected animals should receive washes/tags.
- Twice weekly tar–sulphur shampoos.
- Stable affected animal in airy but enclosed loose box during peak midge (gnat) activity, i.e. dawn and dusk.

- Hang insecticide impregnated strips in stabling.
- Utilize strong ceiling fan (midges cannot fly against strong air current).

Allergic contact dermatitis

The condition is associated with a type IV or delayed hypersensitivity, but immediate or type I hypersensitivity may also be involved. Sensitizing agents act as haptens on direct contact with the skin, conjugating with skin protein. Sensitization usually takes between 1 and 4 weeks and any subsequent contact with the allergen will result in dermatitis within 1 to 3 days.

Clinical signs

- Direct contact is necessary; head, extremities, ventral body surfaces and tail region are most commonly affected.
- Development of red, plaque-like swellings ± vesicles.
- The lesions may be painful or pruritic in the early stages.
- Alopecia and desquamation in chronic cases.

Diagnosis

Patch testing may be helpful in allergen identification. Biopsy demonstrates a reaction which is limited to the dermis and epidermis. Diagnosis can be confirmed by removal of the animal from the suspected sensitizing agent, and, once the condition has regressed, potential sensitizers are reintroduced.

Treatment and control

Treatment is avoidance or removal of the allergen, if it can be identified. Corticosteroids may be of some benefit but hyposensitization is generally unsuccessful.

Urticaria

Urticaria is an acute skin condition characterized by the rapid development of round, elevated, flat-topped, steep-sided oedematous areas on the skin surface. Although reasonably common, the causative agent is seldom found. Type I and type III hypersensitivity reactions are involved. Possible causes include: drugs (especially penicillin or phenylbutazone), vaccines, food, dusts and pollens, and infections of bacterial, fungal and parasitic origin. Bites and stings are also possible causes. Genetic predisposition to the signs may be associated with atopy. The disease may be recurrent.

Clinical signs

The clinical features of urticaria are diagnostic:

- Head, neck, shoulders and thorax are the commonest areas affected.
- Lesions appear suddenly.
- Oedematous lesions (wheals, plaques and hives) pit on pressure.
- Lesions are commonly small (2–4 cm) but may be large and extensive.
- Variably pruritic.
- Mucous membranes of the nose, mouth, anus and vulva are sometimes involved.
- Lesions usually disappear rapidly.

Treatment and control

Dexamethasone given once at a dose of 0.1 mg/kg IM usually results in recovery within 24 hours, but most untreated cases regress spontaneously. Recurrent cases may require feed elimination trials and/or environmental modification. Intradermal allergen testing may be helpful in defining the offending antigen(s).

Nodular skin disease

Nodular collagenous granuloma/nodular necrobiosis, axillary nodular necrosis, unilateral papular dermatosis, sterile nodular panniculitis and mastocytoma may be grouped together under the heading 'nodular skin disease'. Nodular necrobiosis is probably the most common of these. This is a relatively common lesion that is also known as collagenolytic granuloma, collagen necrosis, eosinophilic granuloma and eosinophilic dermatitis. The cause of these lesions is unknown, although hypersensitivity reactions to insect bites, and trauma from the saddle and tack are often implicated.

Clinical signs

- Single or multiple, firm, non-ulcerating dermal nodules of 1.0 to 2.0 cm diameter.

- Dorsum (especially in the saddle area), neck or girth region usually affected.
- Non-painful unless traumatized by tack.
- Non-pruritic.
- Lesions usually arise during the summer.

Pathology

- Superficial and deep inflammatory reaction.
- Foci of collagen degeneration surrounded by a granulomatous infiltrate which contains eosinophils as well as macrophages and sometimes multinucleate giant cells.
- Older and larger lesions may become mineralized.

Diagnosis

Diagnosis is made on inspection and biopsy.

Treatment

Biopsy may be curative and, if lesions are few, intralesional triamcinolone acetonamide (3–5 mg per nodule, total dose not to exceed 20 mg), or for single lesions, 40–80 mg methylprednisolone acetate intralesionally may be effective. The treatment of choice for multi-lesional cases is 1 mg/kg prednisolone daily for 2 to 3 weeks, orally. Mineralized lesions should be excised. Some lesions may undergo spontaneous regression; others may recur after therapy.

Pemphigus foliaceus

This is a rare autoimmune disease characterized by transient vesicles and pustules followed by crusting, scaling and oozing. There may be pruritus. Lesions commonly start on the face or limbs, but may become widespread. Systemic signs such as weight loss, depression and pyrexia also occur. Diagnosis is confirmed by skin biopsy and immunofluorescence. Treatment (which may need to be lifelong) is by systemic corticosteroids.

Bullous pemphigoid

This is a rare autoimmune vesicobullous and ulcerative disease affecting the oral cavity, mucocutaneous junctions and skin (especially the axillary and inguinal regions). Diagnosis and treatment are as for pemphigus foliaceus.

Systemic lupus erythematosus

This rare systemic autoimmune disorder is characterized by lymphoedema, panniculitis, alopecia and scaling of the face, neck and trunk. Other signs include polyarthritis, thrombocytopenia, proteinuria, fever, depression and weight loss.

Discoid lupus erythematosus

This rare autoimmune skin disease affects the head and neck. Lesions include erythema, scaling and alopecia.

Eosinophilic epitheliotrophic disease

This is a rare disease of unknown aetiology characterized by eosinophil infiltration of epithelial tissues throughout the body. Scaling, crusting and oozing begins on the face, coronary bands and chestnuts, followed by a generalized dermatitis. Pruritus is variable, but may be intense. Weight loss occurs due to intestinal malabsorption and maldigestion.

Generalized granulomatous disease (equine sarcoidosis)

Granulomatous inflammation occurs in multiple organs including the skin. Scaling, crusting and alopecia often begin on the face or limbs, followed by other areas of the body. Peripheral lymph nodes may be enlarged. Systemic involvement results in pyrexia, weight loss, inappetence and dyspnoea.

Amyloidosis

Amyloidosis is rare. Amyloid may be deposited in the respiratory mucosa or skin. Cutaneous lesions include papules, nodules or plaques, most commonly occurring on the head, neck or shoulders. See also Chapter 10.

13.6 *Environmental skin disease*

Photosensitization

The disease involves the presence of a photo-dynamic agent within the skin and exposure to a sufficient amount of UV light. Absorption of UV radiation is greatly facilitated by lack of pigment and hair coat. The major endogenous agent in the horse is phylloerythrin, a porphyrin produced by bacterial degradation of chlorophyll in the intestine. If the liver is diseased, hepatic excretion of phylloerythrin is reduced. There are also some plant species associated with photosensitization, such as rape, alfalfa and some clovers (see Chapter 22). Recent drug therapy may also be a cause; tetracyclines, chlorothiazides and sulphonamides have all been implicated.

Clinical signs

● Involvement limited to the unpigmented skin areas of distal extremities and muzzle is suggestive of contact photosensitization.
● Unilateral or bizarre patterns are suggestive of drug-induced photosensitization.
● Skin is swollen and tender with vesicle formation and a weeping surface.
● Pruritus may be observed.
● Crusting, necrotic skin often peels.
● Scarring and poor hair coat may result.

Diagnosis

Diagnosis is based upon clinical signs (distribution of lesions, evidence of liver dysfunction) and an accurate history (grazing habits, seasonality of signs, recent drug administration). Photosensitization should be differentiated from sunburn which usually occurs as thick, crusty lesions on white areas of face and dorsum.

Treatment and control

In cases of liver disease the prognosis is guarded. Otherwise, restriction of access to feed material containing photodynamic agents will usually result in full recovery if the horse is also kept out of the sun for 1 to 2 weeks. Corticosteroids are helpful in controlling inflammation and pruritus. Severely affected skin can be treated with antibiotic/emollient creams.

Contact dermatitis

Contact dermatitis can be allergic (see 13.5) or irritant in nature. Most contact dermatitis is caused by irritants damaging the skin by direct action, with no underlying immune reaction. The dermatitis usually results from continued exposure to secretions or accidental exposure to materials such as strong acids, irritant plants or the application of irritating drugs.

Clinical signs

● Extremities and the areas in contact with tack are most frequently affected.
● Erythema, exudation and vesicle formation.
● Hair loss may occur due to follicle damage or self-inflicted trauma.
● Crusting and lichenification occurs in chronic cases.
● Leucoderma and leucotrichia may be permanent sequelae.

Treatment and control

Many topical preparations used in the treatment of skin diseases may actually produce a contact dermatitis. Affected areas should be cleaned. In severe cases, systemic corticosteroids may be used (with caution), in combination with an appropriate antibiotic if secondary bacterial infection has developed. Local glucocorticoid ointment may be sufficient in mild, localized cases.

13.7 *Neoplastic conditions*

Equine viral papillomatosis

Possibly the most common neoplasm of the horse, the infectious papilloma involves the cutaneous epithelium of the young horse. The condition is caused by an equine papillomavirus.

Clinical signs

● Wart-like papillomas usually on the muzzle and head of young animals (< 5 years).
● Lesions may reach 2 cm in size.
● Immunocompromised animals may also develop lesions.

Diagnosis

A diagnosis may be reached based upon history, signalment and appearance of lesions.

Treatment

The disease is usually self-limiting and it is usually unnecessary to treat the condition. The lesions resolve in 3–4 months. If the papillomas are interfering with tack or are traumatized, they may be removed by sharp excision or by cryotherapy. Cytostatic/toxic drugs and autogenous vaccines have also been used. The application of topical antiseptics reduces secondary infection of traumatized lesions or necrotic papillomas during rejection.

Aural plaques

Aural plaques are small, light-coloured accumulations commonly seen on the underside of the pinna of the ears. The aetiology is unconfirmed, but a papillomavirus has been isolated. Lesions are grey-white plaques on the inner surface of the pinna, varying from less than 1 mm to 2 cm in size. The keratinous crust can be easily removed to reveal a pink, non-ulcerated base. The occurrence of the lesions has been linked to the presence of black flies also found feeding on the internal aspect of the pinna. A variety of topical medicaments, including corticosteroids and antibiotics, have been used without success.

Squamous cell carcinoma

This is a neoplastic condition of the older horse which has been attributed to chronic exposure to ultraviolet light and the co-carcinogenic properties of equine smegma. There is no breed and, surprisingly, no sex predilection. Papillomaviruses do not appear to be involved in this disease.

Clinical signs

The lesion is usually solitary and occurs either at the mucocutaneous junction around the eye or on the external genitalia. There are two forms:

- Non-healing ulcers with indistinct borders.
- Cauliflower-like masses.

The tumour is locally aggressive and may metastasize to local lymph nodes. The tumour may also occur at other sites such as in the maxillary sinus.

Pathology

Irregular configurations of epidermal cells extend down into the dermis with keratin pearls and atypical mitotic figures.

Diagnosis

Diagnosis is based on clinical examination but should be confirmed by histopathological examination.

Treatment

Radical surgical excision is the most common form of treatment (e.g. amputation of the penis or reefing) although cryosurgery and implantation with radioactive needles have also been used.

Equine sarcoid

A locally aggressive fibropapilloma, the sarcoid is the equine neoplasm most commonly submitted for histopathological examination. The aetiological agent most probably involved is a papillomavirus closely related to the bovine papillomaviruses. Recent work suggests a genetic predisposition to the disease. The tumour is seen most frequently in young to middle-aged animals. The lesion is very difficult to treat, frequently recurring, although metastasis to remote points does not occur. Spontaneous rejection is rare.

Clinical signs

There are dermal and epidermal components to the neoplasm (cf. papillomatosis) which is found in four main areas of the body:

- Head, especially around the eye.
- Axillae, girth and ventral abdomen.
- Ventral body, especially the paragenital region.
- Limbs.

There are four clinical manifestations:

- Type I Verrucose: poorly defined area of rough, warty skin with flaking in the superficial layers.
- Type II Fibroblastic: sarcomatous appearance. Fleshy and may be pedunculated, sessile and/or ulcerated.
- Type III Mixed I and II.

- Type IV Occult sarcoid: a slow-growing area (often circular) of alopecia and grey scaling of the skin. Commonest in the inguinal and facial areas.

Two other forms are recognized clinically:

- Nodular sarcoid: spherical, single or multiple, subcutaneous. They may or may not move freely under the skin.
- Malevolent sarcoid: unusual but more serious. Extensive tracking of the sarcoid tissue via lymphatics and direct extension.

The tumours often appear on the site of a previous injury and the lesions, which can grow to be very large, may become ulcerated and traumatized.

Pathology

Diagnosis should be confirmed by histopathological examination demonstrating rete pegging of the epidermis and spindle formation of the fibroblasts.

Treatment

Sarcoids are notoriously difficult to treat, and there are a number of therapies available.

- Surgical excision may be used on smaller lesions, removing a large margin of normal tissue. Even so, recurrence and the appearance of satellite lesions are common sequelae.
- Cryotherapy is more successful, and should be performed after debulking of large tumours. A 'quick-freeze, slow-thaw' cycle should be performed at least twice. Liquid nitrogen is the cryogen of choice and may be applied by probe or by spray. Sloughing of the lesion occurs during the following 3–6 weeks.
- The use of gold and iridium radioactive implants has been successful, but the requirement for dedicated premises and operator hazard make this difficult in the field.
- Bacillus Calmette–Guérin (BCG) may be injected intralesionally to stimulate a local cell-mediated immune response. The BCG may be adjuvanted and should be injected intralesionally on three to four occasions 2–3 weeks apart. Appropriate precautions should be taken to reduce the risk of anaphylaxis (e.g. premedication with flunixin and/or corticosteroids). Swelling, hyperaemia and sloughing may start after the second treatment. Periocular sarcoids seem to respond to this treatment better than tumours elsewhere in the body.

- Cisplatin (an antineoplastic drug with alkylating action) has recently been used to good effect.
- Cytotoxic drugs, e.g. 5-fluorouracil applied topically or injected intralesionally.

Melanoma

Melanomas are common neoplasms of the older horse. They are tumours of varying malignancy arising from the melanocytes or melanoblasts of the equine skin. The cause is unknown. The lesions may be benign or malignant, or may suddenly become malignant, metastasizing to other organs and body systems.

Clinical signs

- Hyperpigmented firm nodular lesions which may be ulcerated are found on the perineum, and periocular regions of adult to old horses.
- Nodular lesions also commonly occur within the parotid salivary glands.
- Grey horses are more frequently affected, although, very rarely, horses of other colours may develop lesions.
- The animal may present with signs referable to the site of the tumour, for example difficulty in defecating in the case of perianal lesions.
- If the tumour has metastasized, the signs may involve other body systems, for example hindlimb ataxia if there is spinal cord involvement.

Pathology

There is some debate as to whether melanomas are 'normal' accumulations of melanocytes, i.e. melanocytosis, or whether they are true tumours. Histopathological examination reveals masses of cells filled with melanotic granules. Abnormal mitotic figures may be visible in the malignant neoplasms.

Diagnosis

Due to their characteristic appearance, diagnosis is by inspection.

Treatment

As it is a disease of older animals, and because the benign lesions only occasionally cause problems, treatment is rarely undertaken. However, excision and cryotherapy have been used. Cimetidine can be used to slow down the rate of growth in rapidly growing melanomas. Melanomas on horses other than greys carry a poorer prognosis as they are usually more malignant.

13.8 Viral skin diseases

Horsepox

This rare disorder has been reported in Europe. It causes lesions (vesicles and pustules) in the oral cavity, distal limbs or vulva. There is spontaneous recovery.

Equine viral papular dermatitis

Caused by an unclassified pox virus, this disease has been reported in the USA, Australia, New Zealand and Africa. Papules develop all over the body (excluding the head). Spontaneous recovery occurs in 2–6 weeks.

Equine molluscum contagiosum

This disease is caused by an unclassified pox virus. Multiple papules develop on the penis, prepuce, scrotum, udder, axillae and muzzle. The papules develop a central pore from which a caseous plug extrudes.

Herpes coital exanthema

See Chapter 14.

Vesicular stomatitis

See Chapter 19.

Equine viral arteritis

See Chapter 19.

13.9 Congenital and developmental skin diseases

Aplasia cutis

Congenital deformity of the squamous epithelium is due to an autosomal recessive gene. Areas of abrupt absence of epithelium occur, especially on the limbs.

Linear keratosis

Linear keratosis is possibly inherited. Unilateral, linear, vertically orientated bands of alopecia and hyperkeratosis occur over the neck and thorax. It is most common in Quarter horses and develops at 1–5 years of age.

Cutaneous asthenia (cutis hyperelastica)

This is an inherited, congenital defect of connective tissue characterized by loose, hyperextensible and abnormally fragile skin.

Albinism

A congenital absence of normal pigmentation (hair, skin and eyes), albinism is most common in palominos and cremello coloured horses.

Lethal white foal disease

See also Chapter 20.

Inherited albinism in overo paint horses is associated with serious developmental defects of the digestive tract (such as colonic atresia).

Cysts

- *Epidermoid inclusion cyst* (*atheroma*) of the false nostril.
- *Dermoid cysts* of the dorsal midline, containing hair and caseous material.
- *Temporal teratoma* adjacent to the petrous part of the temporal bone (see 5.1).

13.10 *Acquired disorders of pigmentation*

Leucoderma

Depigmentation of the skin following trauma or inflammation, may be temporary or permanent.

Vitiligo

Idiopathic depigmentation with no preceding cutaneous inflammation or injury is commonly seen in Arabians (Arabian fading syndrome) but can occur in any breed. It may be hereditary. Depigmentation most commonly occurs around the eyes, and on the muzzle and lips.

Leucotrichia

In this disorder there is depigmentation of the hair following trauma or inflammation on the skin.

Reticulated leucotrichia

This is probably a hereditary disorder. It is reported in Quarter horses, Thoroughbreds and Standardbreds. Linear crusts develop over the back, followed by regrowth of white hair.

Spotted leucotrichia

This is an idiopathic disorder of Arabians in which white spots develop in the coat over the rump and sides.

13.11 *Other conditions: rare, or mentioned elsewhere*

- Actinobacillosis.
- Equine viral arteritis – see Chapter 19.
- Gangrene.
- Haematoma.
- Herpesvirus infection – see Chapter 14.
- Hyperadrenocorticism – see Chapter 9.
- Hypotrichosis.
- Purpura haemorrhagica – see Chapter 10.
- Ticks.
- Tumours.

Further reading

Scott, D.W. (1988) *Large Animal Dermatology*. W.B. Saunders, Philadelphia.

Appendix. Differential diagnoses

1. Nodular skin lesions
Fly and mosquito bites
Urticaria
Melanoma
Sarcoid
Nodular necrobiosis
Granulation tissue
Papilloma
Dermatophilosis
Dermatophytosis
Folliculitis and furunculosis
Abscess
Warbles
Botryomycosis
Tumours
Axillary nodular necrosis
Glanders
Ulcerative lymphangitis
Mycoses
Parafilariasis
Foreign body granuloma
Calcinosis circumscripta
Panniculitis

2. Granulomatous skin lesions
Exuberant granulation tissue
Sarcoid
Viral papillomas
Habronemiasis
Phycomycosis
Squamous cell carcinoma

3. Pruritic and alopecic skin diseases
Culicoides hypersensitivity
Ectoparasites
  Pediculosis
  Chorioptic mange
  Sarcoptic mange
  Psoroptic mange
  Demodectic mange
  Trombiculidiasis
Onchocerciasis
Urticaria
Pemphigus foliaceus

4. Non-pruritic and alopecic skin diseases
Dermatophilosis
Pemphigus foliaceus
Photosensitization

Seborrhoea
Exuberant granulation tissue
Pemphigus foliaceus

14 Reproduction

CONTENTS

14.1 The non-pregnant mare

The oestrous cycle is normally 21–22 days. Most mares are seasonally polyoestrus (cycle April–September). Ovarian activity usually ceases under conditions of decreasing light. Extending the photoperiod in the evening suppresses melatonin release by the pineal gland which stimulates ovarian activity.

Phases of the oestrous cycle

1. Oestrus
• Usually lasts 5–6 days with ovulation occurring 24–48 h before the end of oestrus.
• Mare is sexually receptive – stands to be mounted, seeks stallion's attention, squats, raises the tail, rhythmically everts the clitoris ('winking') and urinates, does not flatten ears or kick (Figure 1).
• The cervix is pink, moist, relaxed, open and oedematous. It lies on the floor of the vagina.
• The uterus is oedematous and flaccid. On ultrasonographic examination, the oedematous endometrial folds make the cross-section of the uterine horn resemble a sliced tomato.
• Characterized by high concentrations of oestrogen and luteinizing hormone (LH) and basal concentrations of progesterone. Follicles often soften 24 h prior to ovulation but some become turgid again prior to ovulation. The mare is frequently sensitive to ovarian palpation at this time. The preovulatory follicle increases from approximately 30 mm 6 days prior to ovulation to an average of 45 mm by the day of ovulation. At the height of the breeding season, however, it is not unusual for a mare to be in oestrus for only 3–4 days and ovulate a follicle of less than 35 mm in diameter.

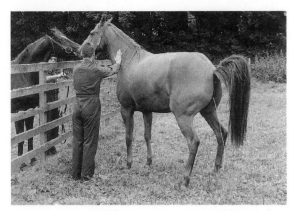

Figure 1 Mare in oestrus being teased over a fence by a stallion.

• Following ovulation, the follicular cavity fills with blood and is termed a corpus haemorrhagicum (CH). Double ovulations occur in approximately 16% of cycles with the highest incidence in Thoroughbreds, Warmbloods and Draught horses. The average interval between ovulations is 1 day with a range of 0–5 days.

2. Dioestrus
• Usually lasts 14–15 days.
• Mare actively rejects the stallion – clamps tail down, swishes tail, flattens ears, strikes, squeals, bites.
• A corpus luteum (CL) is present on the ovaries. The CL may be fluid-filled (50%) or non-fluid-filled. The CL is not normally palpable.
• The cervix is pale, firm, dry and closed. It projects into the middle of the vaginal lumen.
• Uterine tone increases and the uterine horns become tubular.
• Characterized by high circulating concentrations of progesterone. Prostaglandin F-2α, released from the uterus on day 14 or 15, causes luteolysis and return to oestrus.
• Mares can have considerable follicular growth during dioestrus. Ovulation occasionally occurs during dioestrus when progesterone concentrations are high and oestrous behaviour is absent.

3. Transitional breeding season
• Occurs before and after seasonal anoestrus.
• In spring, oestrous behaviour may be observed intermittently or continuously for several weeks. The first ovulation of the season is generally followed by normal, cyclic activity.
• Clusters of large follicles (>30 mm) are often found on the ovaries.
• The cervix does not close tightly until the mare ovulates.

4. Seasonal anoestrus
• Often the mare is passive to the stallion or may even show some mild signs of oestrus.
• The ovaries are inactive.
• The cervix is moderately closed or thin and open.
• The uterus is flaccid.
• Progesterone and oestrogen concentrations are low.

Examination of the mare for breeding soundness

1. History
1. General:
   • Age
   • Health
   • Breed
   • Management
2. Reproductive:
   • Regularity and length of oestrous cycles
   • Behaviour
   • Breeding dates – artificial insemination (AI) or natural cover, stallion fertility
   • Foaling date, normality
   • Indications of previous uterine infection and treatment

2. General physical
Check for the presence of any painful or chronic conditions.

3. Examination of external genitalia
1. Vulva: the vulvar lips should meet evenly. For maximal function the dorsal commissure of the vulva should be no more than 4 cm above the pelvic floor. There should be a cranial-to-caudal slope of no more than 10° from the vertical (Figure 2).
2. Discharge on the vulvar lips, tail or hindquarters.
3. Clitoris: can harbour contagious equine metritis (CEM) organism (*Taylorella equigenitalis*) or other venereally transmissible organisms. Use a standard hospital-type swab to sample the clitoral fossa. A narrow-tipped (paediatric-type) swab is then used for the central and, if present, lateral clitoral sinuses (Figure 3). The swabs are then placed in Amies charcoal transport medium and kept at 4°C until their arrival at the laboratory. If more than one mare is being swabbed a disposable glove should be worn on the hand used to evert the clitoris.

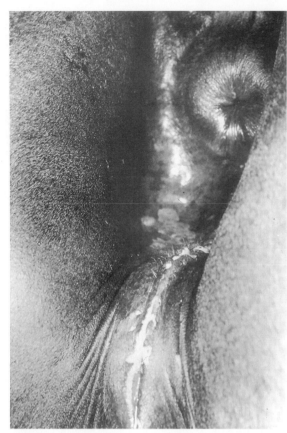

Figure 2 Poor conformation. Anus is recessed with sloping vulvar lips.

4. Mammary glands: assess capability to lactate normally.

4. Examination of internal genital tract
Transrectal palpation:

1. Cervix: correlate shape and consistency with cycle stage.
2. Uterus and endometrial folds. Check for presence of
   - Fluid.
   - Sacculations: commonly at body–horn junction.
   - Pregnancy.
3. Ovaries.
   - Size.
   - Follicles and CH (cannot palpate CL).
   - Presence of ovulation fossa.

Transrectal ultrasonography:

- Pregnancy.
- Follicles, CH and CL.
- Uterine fluid.
- Endometrial cysts.

5. Endometrial swabbings for microbiological culture
Bandage the mare's tail or place in plastic sleeve. Wash perineum three times with mild soap or povidone-iodine solution, rinse and dry. Use sterile sleeve or clean sleeve and sterile surgeon's glove. Lubricate with a small amount of sterile water-soluble lubricant. Use double-guarded swab (Figure 4). Try to avoid sampling the uterus during dioestrus because of high susceptibility to infection at this stage of the cycle.

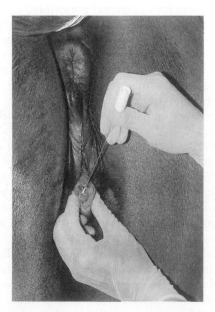

Figure 3 Swabbing the central clitoral sinus with a narrow-tipped swab.

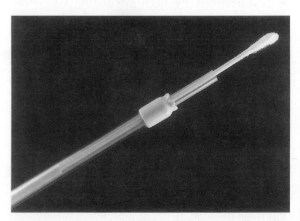

Figure 4 Double guarded swab. Once the swab is in the uterus the inner tube is advanced through the tip of the outer tube. The cotton swab is then advanced and held in apposition to the endometrium for a few seconds. The swab and then the inner tube are retracted inside the outer tube before withdrawing the swab.

6. Endometrial cytology

Obtain smear from aspirated uterine fluid or from swab. Stain with 'Diff-Quik'. The presence of neutrophils suggests uterine infection.

7. Vaginal examination

1. Speculum: the vulvovaginal fold serves as a barrier to ascending bacterial infection. This seal is best tested during oestrus using an unlubricated speculum. If the seal is effective, resistance will be met. In dioestrous mares lubricate the speculum with a sterile, water-soluble lubricant.
   - Appearance of cervix and vagina.
   - Urovagina.
   - Source of exudates.
   - Vaginal varicosities in region of vulvo-vaginal fold.
2. Digital:
   - Cervical tear or adhesions.
   - Vaginal tears, adhesions or small recto-vestibular fistulas.

8. Endometrial biopsy

Use Bouin's fixative. Endometrial biopsy is used as a prognostic indicator to evaluate ability of a mare to carry a foal to term.

- Endometritis (Figure 5).
- Periglandular fibrosis.
- Cystic glandular distension (Figure 6).

The following two items are not carried out routinely during a breeding soundness examination.

9. Endoscopy
- Endometrial cysts.
- Transluminal adhesions.

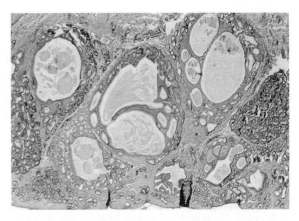

Figure 6 Endometrial biopsy showing severe cystic glandular distension with periglandular fibrosis.

10. Hormone analysis
- Progesterone – ovarian function.
- Testosterone – granulosa cell tumour.

Diseases of the mare's reproductive tract

ENLARGED OVARIES

Ovarian neoplasm

Ovarian tumours are not uncommon in mares. They may cause abdominal pain and discomfort to the mare if they reach a sufficient size.

Granulosa cell tumour: most common ovarian tumour. It originates from the sex cord stromal tissue, is usually multilocular, benign, unilateral and often secretes hormones (Figure 7).

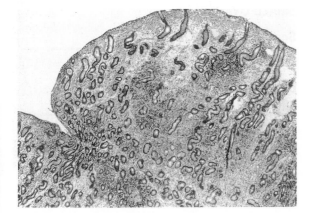

Figure 5 Endometrial biopsy showing a heavy infiltration of inflammatory cells into the endometrial stroma.

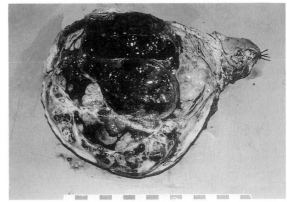

Figure 7 Cross-section of granulosa cell tumour showing numerous irregular cystic spaces.

Clinical signs

There is an enlarged ovary with no palpable ovulation fossa. The contralateral ovary is usually small and firm with no follicular activity because of:

- Inhibin production by the tumour and/or
- Pituitary suppression by ovarian steroids.

Behaviour varies depending on the predominant hormone secreted:

- Male-type behaviour – high testosterone.
- Nymphomania } not closely associated
- Anoestrus } with circulating hormones.

Diagnosis

Palpation and ultrasonography of an enlarged ovary with a small inactive contralateral ovary. Ultrasonographic findings may range from a uniformly dense structure to having one or several large cysts.

- Obliteration of ovulation fossa.
- Behavioural changes.
- Elevated plasma hormones.
- Histopathology of removed ovary.

Treatment

Treatment involves removal of the affected ovary (see Chapter 8). It may be 3–18 months before the other ovary becomes functional.

Teratoma: benign, unilateral originating from germ cells. May contain bone, cartilage, teeth and hair. Does not interfere with cyclicity and pregnancy.

Serous cystadenoma: benign, primary epithelial tumour arising from surface epithelium of the ovulation fossa. Appears to have minimal effect on the function of the contralateral ovary. Affected ovary contains palpable large cysts.

Dysgerminoma: rare, malignant tumour of germ cell origin. Rapidly metastasizes. Affected mares may or may not have chronic weight loss and abdominal discomfort. Poor prognosis. Perform thoracic radiographs and abdominocentesis for assessment of metastases.

Other tumours: melanoma, haemangioma, lymphosarcoma.

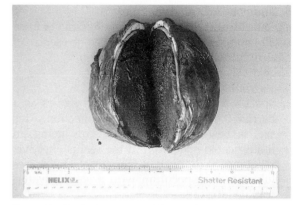

Figure 8 Ovarian haematoma. All normal ovarian tissue had been destroyed.

Haematoma

A haematoma results from the follicular cavity overfilling with blood after ovulation. It can become quite large (>10 cm), but usually regresses within 2–3 cycles, occasionally leaving a calcified nodule. The mare continues to cycle normally. Occasionally a haematoma may expand to destroy part or all of the ovary (Figure 8).

Anovulatory follicles

These may be termed persistent or autumn follicles. They can be 10–15 cm in diameter and are commonly found in autumn associated with declining concentrations of LH. They are non-pathological structures containing blood, which can be gelatinous in consistency. Ultrasonographic examination of the uterus reveals a dioestrus rather than an oestrus appearance.

SMALL OVARIES

Seasonal anoestrus

Hypoplasia – Turner's Syndrome (63XO genotype) or 64XY sex reversal

Clinical signs

- Anoestrus.

Diagnosis

- Small firm ovaries.
- Lack of follicular activity.

- Uterus and cervix lack tone – infantile.
- Karyotype analysis.

Ovarian atrophy

This may be caused by severe malnutrition, parasitism, chronic disease, anabolic steroids.

OVIDUCT

Abnormalities are rare. Hydrosalpinx has been reported to occur secondary to segmental aplasia and to external pressure from adhesions obstructing the lumen.

Cysts in the region of the ovulation fossa are relatively common. There are three types based on their origin.

1. Mesonephric origin – cysts located adjacent to the ovary. Usually called paraovarian cysts.
2. Paramesonephric origin – cysts in the region of the ovulation fossa, but are not of ovarian origin.
3. Epithelial inclusion cysts – often called fossa cysts. Originate in the ovulation fossa. Surface epithelium is disrupted at ovulation and becomes pinched off and embedded in the ovarian cortex. The cysts can become numerous in older mares and can eventually obstruct ovulation. In severe cases, most of the ovary can be destroyed.

UTERUS

Endometritis

This is probably the commonest cause of subfertility in mares.

Aetiology

Normal, resistant mares are able to clear bacteria from the uterus within 72 h. Susceptible mares appear to have defects in uterine contractility and/or uterine immune defence mechanisms, and remain infected after bacteria are introduced into the uterus. The three physical barriers to microorganisms gaining entrance to the uterus are the vulva, the vulvovaginal fold and the cervix. If any of these structures is incompetent the mare is predisposed to developing persistent endometritis.

Infection is introduced by:

- Pneumovagina.
- Parturition.
- Coitus.
- Veterinary gynaecological procedures.

Causative organisms are:

- Beta-haemolytic streptococci (most commonly isolated).
- *E. coli.*
- *Klebsiella pneumoniae.*
- *Pseudomonas aeruginosa.*
- Yeasts.
- Fungi.

Clinical signs

- May be none.
- Discharge from uterus.
- Fluid in uterus.
- Failure to become pregnant.

Diagnosis

- Fluid in uterus.
- Presence of neutrophils in endometrial cytology smear ($>10\%$).
- Cloudy uterine lavage.
- Heavy growth of microorganisms (not diagnostic unless other signs are present).
- Neutrophils migrating through tissue in endometrial biopsy sample.
- Hyperaemia of vagina or cervix.

Treatment

- Correct any predisposing conformational defects.
- Remove fluid from the uterus by lavage with sterile saline (Figure 9). Can use oxytocin (15 IU IV) to assist in fluid removal.
- Infuse uterus with antibiotic (choice depends on microorganism cultured – use IV preparation). Use 20–50 ml.
- Treat the mare daily during oestrus (short cycle with PGF-2α if necessary).
- Use hygienic techniques during examination and breeding.

If the mare is still infected at the oestrus at which she is to be bred, the following treatment regimen can help to control infection.

- If the uterus contains a large amount of fluid on the day before breeding, flush with consecutive litres of *buffered* saline (non-irritant) until the

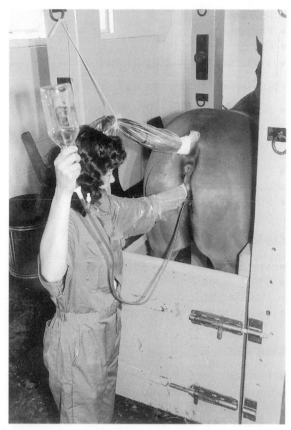

Figure 9 Flushing the uterus. Sterile saline is allowed to flow into the uterus. The bottle is then lowered and the fluid flows back into the bottle.

recovered fluid is clear. Infuse broad spectrum antibiotic. Avoid gentamicin at this time (irritant).
• Use artificial insemination if possible. Otherwise, infuse 100 ml of semen extender containing an appropriate antibiotic into the uterus immediately prior to covering.
• Flush the uterus with consecutive litres of buffered saline 4 h after breeding until the recovered fluid is clear. Infuse antibiotic.
• Repeat flushing and infusion of antibiotic for 3 days after ovulation. On the fourth day infuse antibiotic only. Oxytocin can be administered to ensure 100% fluid recovery during these flushes.

Acute metritis

Aetiology

The entire uterine wall is inflamed. Metritis occurs after parturition and is often related to trauma. It can be secondary to retained placenta. Toxins can pass through the uterine wall to the general circulation.

Clinical signs

• May be systemically ill.
• Uterine discharge may be present.
• May develop secondary laminitis.

Treatment

• Systemic antibiotics.
• NSAIDs.
• Large volume uterine lavage (several litres of sterile saline).
• Oxytocin to assist fluid recovery.

Endometrosis (formerly called chronic endometritis)

Chronic degenerative changes occur within the endometrium, increasing with age. There are three main pathological findings:

1. Periglandular fibrosis – fibrosis around the glands. Associated with reduced ability to carry a foal to term.
2. Cystic glandular distension – glands swollen. Commonly contain inspissated secretion. Fibrosis may prevent secretion from leaving glands.
3. Endometrial cysts – may interfere with pregnancy if extensive. Caused by coalescence of lymphatic lacunae (enlarged lymphatics). If large, can surgically excise via endoscope using biopsy instrument, electrocautery or laser. Some workers have advocated the use of repeated hypertonic, hot (45–50°C) saline flushes to enhance uterine contraction.

Ventral uterine sacculations are commonly palpated at the junction of the uterine horns and body in old, infertile mares. Focal myometrial atony results in lymphatic lacunae in these mares.

Intrauterine adhesions

Aetiology

• Dystocia.
• Intrauterine infusion of caustic solutions.
• Endometritis.

Diagnosis

Diagnosis is by endoscopy. There may be single or multiple bands, partial or complete sheets or tunnels between adjacent endometrial folds. They result in infertility if extensive, cause pyometra or impede movement of embryo.

Treatment

Break down manually or with endoscope and biopsy forceps. Laser or electrocautery is possible. They may recur.

Pyometra

Unlike the cow, pyometra in the mare is not always accompanied by a retained corpus luteum and anoestrus. Affected mares may cycle regularly or may have short cycles due to premature release of PGF-2α. The uterus may accumulate 0.5 to 60 litres of exudate. Mares with pyometra frequently have a fibrosed or occluded cervix. Usually there are no systemic signs.

Treatment

This is often unsuccessful.

- Break down any adhesions.
- Lavage uterus and infuse appropriate antibiotics daily for 4–7 days or longer if necessary.

Mucometra

Mucometra is rare. It can be due to a non-patent cervix.

Treatment

Repair cervix.

Uterine abscess

This is rare. It can be secondary to dystocia, AI, severe metritis or uterine therapy. In acute phase, can have systemic signs – fever, neutrophilia, peritonitis. If small, can attempt surgical drainage into the uterus; otherwise, use abdominal approach. Poor prognosis for future breeding.

Neoplasia

Leiomyomas are rare.

Clinical signs

Usually there are none.

Diagnosis

Diagnosis is by palpation.

Treatment

If small and pedunculated they can be removed using a snare. Otherwise perform hysterectomy if benign. Partial hysterectomy may preserve fertility.

Contagious equine metritis (CEM)

Aetiology

This disorder is caused by *Taylorella equigenitalis*, a microaerophilic, Gram negative coccobacillus. Transmission is venereal. The organism persists in clitoral sinuses of carriers. Stallions are inapparent carriers.

Clinical signs

Signs are severe endometritis with profuse watery, mucopurulent discharge. Mares have short oestrous cycles. Chronic infection can develop where clinical signs are less obvious. A symptomless carrier state can also exist.

Diagnosis

Isolation of organism on chocolate agar in atmosphere of 5–10% CO_2.

Treatment

Many mares recover spontaneously. If treatment is needed, use intrauterine infusions of penicillin and topical treatment of clitoris with dilute chlorhexidine.

CERVIX

Cervicitis

Aetiology

Cervicitis is usually associated with vaginitis and/or endometritis. Apart from infection, it can be associated with irritants such as air or urine in the vagina and uterine medications.

Diagnosis

Diagnosis is by speculum examination.

Treatment

Identify and treat the endometritis or vaginitis.

Cervical laceration

Aetiology

- Trauma at parturition.
- If severe, can prevent closure of the cervix resulting in uterine contamination and endometritis.
- If detected at foaling, should wait 30 days before attempting repair.

Diagnosis

Diagnosis is by digital examination of the cervix while it is under the influence of progesterone (dioestrus).

Treatment

Treatment involves surgical correction by a 2- or 3-layer closure after evaluating the endometrium by endometrial biopsy. Mares are given a sedative/analgesic combination of rimifidine or xylazine plus butorphanol or epidural anaesthesia plus sedation. Retraction of the cervix may be facilitated by infiltration of local anaesthetic dorsal to the cervix. An incision is made along the scar of the healed edges of the tear and extended 1 cm cranial to the end of the tear, to ensure separation of mucous membrane from the fibromuscular layer. The wound can be sutured in three layers (internal mucous membrane, fibromuscular, and external mucous membrane) using a continuous horizontal mattress for the outer and inner layers and a continuous suture for the fibromuscular layer, or two layers (internal mucous membrane + inner fibromuscular layer, outer fibromuscular layer + external mucous membrane) in a continuous suture pattern using absorbable suture. The lumen of the cervix should be checked for patency throughout the procedure. Give a course of antibiotics plus NSAIDs if necessary. Wait 30 days before breeding. Advise the owner that the cervix may tear again at the next parturition.

Cervical adhesions

Aetiology

- Result of trauma at parturition or after uterine therapy with irritant agents.

Diagnosis

Diagnosis is by digital and speculum examination.

- Can be transluminal or attach the cervix to the vaginal wall.
- Interfere with cervical function.

Treatment

Treatment can be very difficult. The adhesions can be manually broken down and steroid cream applied, but they tend to reform rapidly.

VAGINA

Pneumovagina (windsucking)

This is an important and relatively common condition.

Aetiology

- Poor vulvar and perineal conformation.
- Thin condition predisposes.
- <80° angle of vulva.
- <2/3 of the vulvar lips below the level of the tuber ischii.

Diagnosis

- Aspiration of air when vulvar lips are parted.
- Commonly associated with endometritis.
- Severe cases may have pneumo-uterus and urovagina.

Treatment

Treatment is by Caslick's vulvoplasty. Treat endometritis first. Infiltrate vulvar margins with local anaesthetic from just below level of the ischium to the dorsal commissure. Remove a 1 cm strip of mucosa from the mucocutaneous margin (NB: Do not remove skin). Use continuous or interrupted sutures to appose denuded tissue surfaces. Remove sutures after 10–12 days. Do not close vulva excessively – predisposes to urovagina. A 'breeder's stitch' of umbilical tape can be placed at the ventral edge of the repair to protect the suture line during coitus until the mare is confirmed pregnant. Use of a breeding roll is recommended for mares being covered by natural service. Open vulvoplasty prior to foaling. The vulvoplasty should be closed as soon as possible after foaling unless there is significant oedema or uterine lavage is necessary.

Some mares with a sunken anus and forward sloping of the vagina have both pneumovagina and urovagina. Horizontal transection of the perineal body has been used successfully in these cases.

Urovagina

Urine accumulates in the vagina (urine pooling, vesicovaginal reflux) causing inflammation. The condition is associated with poor conception rates and early embryonic death.

Aetiology

- Poor perineal conformation.
- Poor body condition.
- Relaxed ligaments – may occur only at oestrus or postpartum.

Pneumovagina and urovagina often occur concurrently.

Diagnosis

- Speculum examination reveals urine in vagina.
- Associated with endometritis.

Fluid in the vagina can be positively identified as urine by observing calcium carbonate crystals by microscopic examination, and determining the creatinine and urea concentrations.

Treatment

Treatment depends on the cause – correct poor body condition – urovagina may correct itself if it occurs after foaling. In mild cases, mares can conceive if urine is physically removed from the vagina before breeding. Intrauterine infusion of semen extender protects sperm from the deleterious effects of urine. If there is injury to the vulvovaginal fold or if the vagina has a severe cranioventral slope, surgery is required. Urethral extension appears to give the most reliable results. The mare is sedated, and epidural anaesthesia is induced. After appropriate cleansing of the region, the vulvovaginal fold is retracted with forceps. The dorsal mucosa and submucosa of the vulvovaginal fold are incised horizontally along the dorsal edge 2–4 cm cranial to its caudal border. The incisions are continued onto the middle of the vestibular wall and extended caudally to the labia. The cut edges are freed from the deep submucosa by dissection to create mucosal/submucosal flaps. The opposing edges of the flaps are joined in a Y-shape by an inverting suture line to create a tunnel from the urethral orifice to the caudal vestibule. A sterile catheter can be placed in the urethra prior to performing the procedure to prevent damage to the urethral orifice and to provide a template. Antibiotics and NSAIDs should be given post-surgery, and the reproductive tract should not be examined for at least 2 weeks.

Persistent hymen

This is more common in mares than in other domestic species.

Aetiology

The hymen may be imperforate or may present because the caudal section of the paramesonephric duct failed to fuse with the urogenital sinus.

Clinical signs

- Failure of intromission.

Diagnosis

- Manual and speculum examination.

Treatment

Treatment is by surgical excision after sedation of the mare. It is usually adequate to make a nick in the membrane with a guarded blade and then extend the incision with the operator's fingers. Secretions may accumulate cranial to the hymen. These secretions may infrequently become infected and result in infertility.

VULVA

Neoplasms

- Melanoma – common in old grey mares. Usually not treated.

- Squamous cell carcinoma.
- Leiomyoma.

Perineal lacerations

See Chapter 8.

Enlarged clitoris

Aetiology

- Intersex. Most common form is the male pseudohermaphrodite, which has testes and a 64XX karyotype.

Coital vesicular exanthema

Aetiology

- Venereal transmission of equine herpesvirus 3.

Clinical signs

- Papules, vesicles, scabby erosions on the vulva (penis and prepuce of stallion).

Diagnosis

- Examination.
- Intranuclear inclusion bodies on cytology.

Treatment

- Sexual rest for 60 days.
- Treat lesions with antiseptic cream to prevent secondary bacterial infection.

14.2 *The pregnant mare*

Ovulation
- Occurs through the ovulation fossa.
- Occurs 0 to 2 days before the end of oestrus.
- Oocyte is in metaphase II at ovulation.

Fertilization
- Occurs in the ampulla.
- The fertilized ovum enters the uterus as an early blastocyst approximately 6 days after ovulation.
- Unfertilized ova are retained in the oviduct or pass down into the uterus.

Embryonic period
- The embryo is mobile in the uterus until day 16 after ovulation. It is thought that this mobility of the embryo is necessary for maternal recognition of pregnancy by inhibiting PGF-2α release. At this time it is thought that the signal released by the embryo that inhibits PGF-2α release is a 1000–6000 mol. wt substance (α-interferon-like substances do not seem to be secreted by the equine conceptus).
- The zona pellucida is shed at day 7, and the embryo is surrounded by a glycoprotein capsule. 'Hatching' from the zona pellucida, as seen in the cow, does not occur in the mare. The capsule persists until the fourth week of pregnancy.

Placenta
1. Diffuse, non-deciduate.
2. Epitheliochorial.
3. Microcotyledonary. Attachment by microvilli does not occur until approximately 38 days. The macrovilli, which appear at day 45, are the forerunners of the microcotyledons. Maximum placental attachment does not occur until completion of the interdigitation of the placental microcotyledons at day 150.

The uterine glands secrete 'uterine milk' throughout pregnancy.

Direct apposition of the trophoblastic membrane with the endometrium is necessary before microcotyledons develop, and, therefore, they are absent at the following areas:

- Overlying the endometrial cups.
- At the cervical os (called the cervical star).
- Opposite the opening of each oviduct.
- Overlying the attachment of the yolk sac.
- Along invaginated folds of allantochorion.

Hippomanes
These are large, flat bodies composed of concentric rings of amorphous material which occur in the allantoic fluid. They originate from deposition of material from the allantoic fluid onto a nucleus of epithelial cell debris.

Endometrial cups
These are discrete, raised areas arranged in a horse-shoe or circular fashion at the caudal portion of the gravid uterine horn. The cups arise from invasion of the uterine epithelium by trophoblastic cells of the chorionic girdle. They are present between approximately day 40 and 120 of pregnancy. After sloughing, the remnants may be

enclosed by invaginations of allantochorion termed allantochorionic pouches.

The endometrial cups secrete equine chorionic gonadotrophins (eCG) formerly called pregnant mare serum gonadotrophin (PMSG). eCG has LH-like activity in the horse and may support formation of secondary corpora lutea. Endometrial cups are also thought to induce maternal immunotolerance towards the antigenically foreign foetus.

Changes in the reproductive tract during pregnancy

Ovaries
- Numerous follicles > 10 mm are present on the ovaries between days 10 and 100.
- The primary CL persists until about day 120–150.
- Secondary CL form after day 40 from ovulated follicles and from luteinized, unruptured follicles. They also persist until around day 120–150.
- After day 100 of pregnancy, the ovaries are not necessary as a source of progesterone.

Cervix and uterus
- After ovulation, the cervix closes and uterine tone increases.
- By 14–17 days, there is a marked increase in tubularity of the uterus.
- By 17–21 days, the cervix tightens and lengthens giving a characteristic pencil-like shape. The endometrial folds are no longer palpable.
- At 23–28 days, the embryonic vesicle may be palpated at the base of the pregnant horn.
- At 40 days, one half of the gravid horn is filled by the conceptus.
- At 60 days, the gravid horn is filled by the conceptus.
- At 80 days, both horns are filled by the conceptus.
- After 85 days, a decrease in tension of the allantois allows direct palpation of the foetus.

Pregnancy diagnosis

- Palpation *per rectum*: Accurate after about 28 days and optimal around day 42.
- Transrectal ultrasonography: Day 10 to term.
  - Day 9–12: Blastocoele converts to yolk sac, which is detectable as a round structure.
  - Day 18: Changes from round to triangular appearance – due to hypertrophy of dorsal uterine wall.
  - Day 21: Embryo present ventrally.
  - Day 25: Heart beat detectable. Allantois visible.
  - Day 30: Allantois occupies ventral half of vesicle.
  - Day 40: Allantois occupies most of vesicle; yolk sac has regressed.
  - Day 50: The umbilical cord has lengthened, and the foetus has descended to the floor of the allantoic sac.
- Transabdominal ultrasonography: Day 80 to term.
- Oestrone sulphate: Produced by precursors from foetal gonads and, therefore, confirms viability of foetus. Measured in high concentrations in serum from day 90.
- eCG: Day 40–120. Problem with false positives. Indicates presence of endometrial cups, not foetus.

Endocrinology of pregnancy

1. Progesterone:
   - Secreted by corpora lutea.
   - Reaches first peak around day 20, then declines until day 40–50.
   - Between day 40 and 90, secondary CL secrete progesterone resulting in increased concentration.
   - Progesterone concentration decreases to low levels by day 150.
   - The placenta secretes progestogens (progesterone and progesterone metabolites) from day 70 to term by *de novo* synthesis. Takes over from CL as source of progestogens.
2. Oestrogen:
   - Increases between day 35 and 40 (? result of stimulation by eCG). Second rapid increase after day 80. Peaks at 7–8th month gestation and then decreases gradually to term.
   - Until day 70 maternal ovaries are the major source.
   - After day 70, foetoplacental oestrogen production predominates.
   - Precursor for oestrogen derives from foetal gonads; therefore both viable foetus + placenta required.
3. eCG:
   - Secreted by endometrial cups.
   - First detected day 35–40. Peaks at day 70 and disappears by day 150.

- Does not have the FSH-like activity seen in other species.
4. Relaxin:
   - Secreted by the placenta.
   - First detected around day 70 and peaks at 5–6 months.
   - Increases again near parturition.

Complications during pregnancy

INFECTIOUS CAUSES OF ABORTION

Bacterial

Bacterial infections are responsible for approximately 30% of aborted foetuses seen at post-mortem. Many species of bacteria have been incriminated. Most commonly associated are *Streptococcus* spp., *E. coli*, *Pseudomonas* spp., *Klebsiella* spp. and *Staphylococcus* spp. *Leptospira* spp. are now also being recognized as causing abortion in mares and *Ehrlichia* spp. are suspected as well. Higher bacteria, that is bacteria resembling fungi, can cause chronic proliferative placentitis and abortion.

Frequently secondary non-pathogenic bacteria are isolated but if only one species is found in multiple organs, the stomach contents and placenta, it is likely that the organism is a primary or secondary cause of abortion. The bacteria may be considered a primary cause if inflammatory changes are seen in the foetus.

Most infections are caused by ascending infection through the cervix. This tends to occur early in pregnancy.

Fungal

Fungal infection usually occurs in second half of gestation. Abortion results from an ascending infection spreading from the cervical area. The chorioallantois is thickened and leathery and a thick mucoid exudate is often present. The foetal organs are usually not decomposed. The liver is often large, pale and mottled. *Aspergillus fumigatus* is the most frequently isolated fungus. Fungi are ubiquitous; therefore signs of an inflammatory response to the fungus should be demonstrated before the organism is considered significant. Even in these cases, fungi may only be opportunistic and secondary to another predisposing cause. The foetus is usually small and emaciated, but near-term foals generally have a good chance of surviving.

Viral – equine herpesvirus I (EHV-1)

See Chapter 19. EHV-1 is a respiratory virus which is widespread among the horse population but responsible for fewer than 15% of abortions seen at post-mortem. Mares usually abort suddenly during the last four months of gestation. It usually only affects one or two in a group but occasionally causes multiple abortions.

Foetuses are fresh with petechiation of mucosae. Excessive straw coloured fluid is present in thoracic and abdominal cavities.

Diagnosis

- Histology – intranuclear inclusion bodies in liver, and adrenals. Focal necrosis in liver, adrenals, lungs, thymus and spleen.
- Virus isolation.
- Fluorescent antibody test and immunohistology.
- Serology (may not detect an increase in antibody titre).

Prevention

- Isolate mares after the third month of gestation.
- Vaccination every 2 or 3 months during pregnancy, but protection is not complete.

Viral – equine viral arteritis (EVA)

See Chapter 19. EVA is transmitted by the respiratory route and venereally by carrier stallions. Incubation period is 3–14 days. The virus localizes in the accessory sex glands of stallions and about 34% of stallions recovered from EVA shed virus in their semen for long periods. Shedder stallions are always seropositive but not all seropositive stallions are shedders. Recovered mares do not shed the virus longer than 3 weeks. Seropositive mares with a stable or declining antibody titre are thought not to infect stallions or in-contact mares. Clinical signs vary from mild fever and conjunctivitis to severe illness comprising fever, depression, filling of the lower limbs, ventral oedema, urticarial rashes and oedematous plaques, conjunctivitis with periorbital oedema and nasal discharge. Up to 80% of non-immune mares may abort especially in late gestation. Foetuses are decomposed.

Diagnosis

- Virus detection in nasopharyngeal swabs, heparinized blood, semen, serum and possibly urine.
- Serology – rising titre in blood samples collected 2 weeks apart.

Prevention

- Test mating. Identify and isolate infected animals.
- Vaccination. Vaccinated animals will become seropositive. Animals should be serologically tested prior to vaccination to demonstrate that the animal has not previously been infected.

Because EVA virus can be secreted by mares for up to 3 weeks post-infection, newly arrived horses should be quarantined for at least 3 weeks. Identification of shedder stallions is very important in control of the disease.

Viral – equine infectious anaemia (EIA)

See Chapter 19. EIA is a systemic disease caused by a retrovirus. Signs vary from peracute to chronic, with infection in some horses being inapparent. Infected horses remain persistent carriers. The disease is usually transmitted by blood-feeding insects. On first exposure to the virus acute signs may develop including fever, anorexia and petechiation on mucosae. This phase is transient and is followed by recurrent episodes of fever, anaemia, jaundice and weight loss. It only rarely causes abortions.

Diagnosis

- Virus isolation.
- Coggin's test.

Prevention

- No vaccine available therefore identify and control movement of infected horses.

NON-INFECTIOUS CAUSES OF ABORTION

Twinning

Twinning is common in all breeds of horses, especially Thoroughbreds. It accounts for approximately 20% of all aborted foetuses examined at post-mortem. There is a high rate of natural reduction before day 40. After day 45, 65% of twins will be aborted. Abortions are due to placental insufficiency. They most commonly occur between mid-pregnancy and term. The foetuses often appear to have died at different times. When only one twin is found, diagnosis can still be made by demonstration of a large avillous area of chorion – the contact area between the chorion of the two twins.

Umbilical cord abnormalities

In Thoroughbred mares cord length should be less than 84 cm

1. Too long:
   - Can twist and compromise vascular supply to foetus. Must demonstrate evidence of ischaemic necrosis before diagnosing abortion due to a twisted cord.
   - Can become wrapped round a foetal appendage.

2. Too short:
   - May break prematurely at birth leading to perinatal asphyxia.

NB. Many normal foals are born with abnormal umbilical cords.

Placental insufficiency

- Aborted foetuses have retarded growth due to insufficient nutrients from the placenta.
- Associated with endometrial fibrosis or atrophy in older mares.
- Can also be due to infectious placentitis causing atrophy of the chorionic villi.

Uterine body pregnancy – uncommon

- Chorioallantois fails to expand, and the foetus develops in the uterine body.
- Foetal growth is retarded, and abortion usually occurs after the 7th month of pregnancy.

Luteal insufficiency

In some mares with repeated unexplained abortions in the first third of gestation, supplementation with altrenogest until day 100 has resulted in the mare carrying a foal to term. Luteal insufficiency is probably an extremely rare occurrence and there are very few documented cases.

UTERINE TORSION

- Occurs between the 5th and 11th month.
- Approximately 50% occur at foaling.
- Mare presents with colic – usually only moderate pain.
- Does not usually involve cervix.
- Torsions can be clockwise or counterclockwise. Most are 360° or more.

Diagnosis

- Signs of colic unresponsive to treatment. If intestine is entrapped by the torsion, intestinal dysfunction (nasogastric reflux, intestinal distension etc.) may be present.
- Palpation of broad ligaments *per rectum*.

Treatment

- Check for evidence of foetal death, uterine necrosis or rupture.
- If cervix is open – untwist uterus via cervix.
- If cervix is closed – roll anaesthetized mare (variable results).
- Surgical correction – high flank incision in standing mare (on side towards direction of torsion). If torsion occurs at foaling, surgical correction and caesarean section can be performed through a midline laparotomy.

VENTRAL RUPTURES: RUPTURE OF PREPUBIC TENDON AND THE ABDOMINAL MUSCLES

Late gestation

- Most common draught breeds.
- In mild cases may just present as oedematous swelling.
- Abdominal pain.

Treatment

- Support abdomen in sling if <330 days.
- Induce parturition and pull the foal out if >330 days.
- Do not rebreed.

HYDROPS

- Usually hydrops allantois.
- Excessive accumulation of allantoic fluid at 8–11 months.
- Tremendous abdominal distension.
- Foetus cannot be palpated.
- Frequently fatal.

Treatment

- IV fluid therapy while slowly draining the uterus.
- Treat shock.
- Induce parturition in the mare and assist foetal extraction. Many foals are born alive but are malformed or soon die. If mare survives can have normal fertility.

VULVAR BLEEDING

Occasionally small veins of the vestibule or vagina become distended and may bleed. Vulvar bleeding is only rarely associated with placental detachment and impending abortion.

Diagnosis

Diagnosis is by speculum examination.

Treatment

Pack the vestibule, ligate vessels or electrocautery but treatment is usually not required – varicosities often shrink when pregnancy ends.

UTERINE DORSORETROFLEXION

This is seen in the last trimester of pregnancy. It presents as acute colic. In severe cases there may be abdominal straining (foetal parts in pelvic canal) and swelling of the vulva and perineum.

Diagnosis

Examination *per rectum* reveals foetus in a tightly contracted sac-like distension of the uterus within the pelvic canal.

Treatment

Spasmolytic drugs (isoxsuprine/clenbuterol) are used. Colic rapidly disappears and the foetus can be pushed back into the abdomen. Repeated treatments may be necessary at 3–6 h intervals for 1–2 days. Restrict feed intake and encourage exercise.

PROLONGED GESTATION

Approximately 1% of pregnancies exceed 370 days. The majority of these mares have a spontaneous parturition and produce a foal of normal size (occasionally small).

Causes

- Embryonic diapause between 30 and 60 days.
- Foetal gonadal and/or placental dysfunction.
- Foetal mummification.

Treatment

Do not induce parturition if the mare and foetus appear healthy.

PREMATURE UDDER DEVELOPMENT

- Commonly seen before abortion of twins.
- Perform a complete physical examination of dam.
- Check foetal heartbeat with ultrasound.
- Depending on cause, therapy may include progesterone, NSAIDs, antibiotics.

Elective termination of pregnancy

Day 5–35
Give PGF-2α IM.

Day 35–120
If endometrial cups are present:

- PGF-2α IM once or twice/day until abortion (usually within 3–5 days).
- Uterine lavage 3 × 1 litre sterile saline. If the foetus is not expelled within 24 h, repeat the lavage. The mare will not come into oestrus until the endometrial cups have regressed.

Day 120–near term
Termination is not recommended because of the risk of uterine damage, retained placenta and dystocia.

Uterine lavage: Dilate cervix. Rupture membranes and remove foetus. Large volume lavage will help dislodge foetal membranes.

14.3 *Parturition*

Gestation length: Average 342 days (range 321–365 days).

Signs of impending parturition
1. Enlarged abdomen

2. Mammary development
   - 3 to 6 weeks prepartum. Major changes within 2 weeks of term.
   - Initially straw-coloured discharge.
   - Udder distends with colostrum 2–3 days prepartum.
   - Teat waxing in last 48 hours.
   - Increase in calcium and magnesium content of milk.
   - At term, calcium >10 mmol/l.
3. Relaxation of sacrosciatic ligaments and vulva
4. Relaxation of cervix (may occur 0 to 30 days prepartum)

Mares vary tremendously in the signs that they show, ranging from none to all.

NB. Remember to open vulva at least 2 weeks before expected foaling date if Caslick sutures are present.

The foetus is highly mobile within the uterus during the first half of gestation. During the last half of gestation, the foetus is in the dorso-pubic position with the head and forelimbs flexed.

Stages of parturition
Stage I:

- Lasts approximately 1 hour (mares have a high degree of maternal control over length of stage I).
- Uterine contractions start.
- Cervix relaxes and dilates.
- Restlessness.
- Signs of colic.
- Patchy sweating.

The end of 1st stage labour is marked by rupture of the allantochorion at an avascular area, the cervical star, and release of straw-coloured watery allantoic fluid. The foal rotates to a dorso-sacral position just before birth. The amnion should protrude through the vulvar lips within 5 minutes of rupture of the allantochorion.

Stage II:

- Lasts less than 30 min.
- Assume lateral recumbency.
- Abdominal contractions.
- Foal is delivered covered by amnion (more correctly termed the allantoamnion).
- The equine placenta separates from the endometrium rapidly and foetuses not delivered within a relatively short time of onset of 2nd stage labour are deprived of oxygen.
- Normal presentation is anterior, dorsosacral, extended.

NB. If the red allantochorion appears at the vulvar lips, rupture the membrane and extract the foal immediately. Differentiate from prolapsed bladder!

Stage III: Expulsion of placental membranes usually occurs within 1 hour. The allantochorion is turned inside out.

NB. Always examine the placenta for completeness.

The foal should be standing within an hour and should have sucked within 4 hours. As retained meconium is common, it may be advisable to give all foals an enema (saline, soapy water or lubricant) soon after birth.

Endocrinology of parturition

Oestrogens decrease during the last month of pregnancy. Progestogens increase during the last month of pregnancy. However, progestogen concentrations decrease during the 24 hour period before parturition; hence the ratio of oestradiol: progestogen increases prior to parturition.

PGF-2α and oxytocin increase dramatically at parturition. The sudden enhanced secretion of oxytocin may trigger second stage labour.

Induction of parturition

Because of the great variability in gestation length in the mare, it is impossible to arbitrarily set a gestation length at which induction can be performed. The mare must be at least 321 days pregnant (preferably >330 days), have an enlarged udder, teats distended with colostrum, and relaxed sacrosciatic ligaments. Ideally the mare's cervix should be softening, but this is not essential. Concentrations of electrolytes in the milk have been used to assess foetal maturity. Ca^{2+} concentrations $\geqslant 40$ mg/dl, Na^+ concentrations $\leqslant 30$ mEq/l and K^+ concentrations $\geqslant 35$ mEq/l generally indicate foetal readiness for birth. Commercial mare-side kits are available for measuring Ca^{2+} concentrations in mammary secretions. Do not induce if the mare shows signs of impending abortion or if foal viability is questionable. Examine the mare *per rectum* to check foal presentation as well as viability of the foetus. Place tail wrap on mare and thoroughly wash perineum. Then perform vaginal examination to evaluate cervical dilation.

- Oxytocin: Most widely used drug. Can be administered IM or IV. Dosage varies with degree of cervical relaxation. If relaxed to 2 cm can give a 40–60 IU bolus IV. Delivery of foetus within 90 min (often within 30 min). If cervix closed, give 2.5–10 IU every 15 min IV until labour commences. If cervix relaxes after 4–5 boluses but labour has not started, give 40–60 IU IV. May also give as IV infusion 60 IU oxytocin in 1 litre saline over 1 h. Larger doses of oxytocin have been associated with premature placental separation and foetal hypoxia.
- Prostaglandin: Foal survival with PGF-2α is compromised because of the strong myometrial contractions leading to premature placental separation. Analogues with less smooth muscle activity have been used, e.g. fluprostanol, and can induce parturition within 1–3 h. When this analogue was administered to mares which were not ready to foal (less than 344 days pregnant), none of the mares delivered as a result of treatment.
- Dexamethasone: Not commonly used. Need to give repeated high doses and is associated with placental retention and weak foals.

14.4 Dystocia

The incidence of dystocia in horses is low (approximately 4%). However, it represents a life-threatening situation to the foal, and the future reproductive performance of the mare is often reduced. Dystocia exists when 1st or 2nd stage labour is prolonged or not progressive. Examination of the birth canal and foetus are necessary to determine the cause of dystocia.

Examination of the mare:

1. Adequate restraint. Epidural anaesthesia may be administered to prevent straining.
2. Hygiene – bandage tail, scrub perineal region with povidone-iodine.
3. Lubrication. Assess birth canal for size, evidence of previous trauma, and degree of relaxation. Check presentation of foetus and determine viability.

Obstetric procedures

Mutation

- Repulsion – pushing the foetus back into the uterus where space is available to correct position or posture. It is always necessary to repel before attempting other mutations.

- Rotation – turning the foetus on its long axis to bring it into a dorsosacral position.
- Version – turning the foetus on its transverse axis to convert a transverse presentation into a longitudinal presentation.

To adjust extremities, it is necessary to repel the proximal portion, bringing the middle portion of the extremity laterally and the distal portion medially. If mutation cannot be accomplished successfully in less than 15 minutes, an alternative form of delivery should be used.

Forced extraction

This may be attempted after foetal malposture has been corrected. Traction snares or chains are placed around the pasterns. Traction devices should be used only to position the head, not to exert traction on the head (the bones of the skull are not as well developed as in the calf).

Limit force to 2 or 3 people.

Hip-lock is uncommon in the mare, and there is usually no need to rotate foetus.

Foetotomy

- Complete foetotomy is required only rarely in the mare. In most cases, a partial foetotomy allows removal of impediment to delivery.
- Epidural anaesthesia and sedation are required to minimize straining.
- When more than one or two cuts are anticipated, general anaesthesia is indicated.
- Sequelae to foetotomy: retained placenta, metritis, peritonitis, laminitis, vaginal and cervical lacerations and delayed uterine involution. The severity of sequelae are proportional to the number of cuts required and the duration of labour prior to presentation.

Caesarean section

Indications: transverse presentation, uterine torsion, malposture of living foetus that cannot be corrected rapidly, oversized foetus (rare because mare controls foetal size, not stallion) and maternal pelvic deformities.

The usual approach is by midline laparotomy. Until the foetus is removed, general anaesthesia should be maintained in a light plane to avoid foetal respiratory depression. The uterus is incised along its greater curvature. Uterine contents should be treated as contaminated and carefully drained to the outside. The live foal should be placed alongside the mare with the umbilical cord left intact until the foal is breathing normally and pulsations in the umbilical vessels have stopped. The cord should then be broken at the constriction a few centimetres away from the navel. If the foal is alive the placenta should be left inside the uterus. If the foal is dead the membranes should be removed and the uterine lumen medicated with antibiotics. The use of a continuous interlocking suture through all the layers of the uterine wall and around the entire margin of the incision controls intraluminal haemorrhage – a significant cause of maternal mortality. The uterus is closed with inverting sutures taking care to exclude any placenta. After surgery, administer 20 IU oxytocin IV to aid involution and assist membrane expulsion. A low dose of NSAIDs can be given to reduce colic pains caused by uterine contractions.

Postoperative complications may include metritis, peritonitis, laminitis and retained placenta. Check for early adhesions by palpation *per rectum* after 4 days – break down manually.

14.5 *The postpartum period*

1. Uterine involution:
   - Occurs by 6–10 days postpartum.
   - Little tissue is lost at parturition, therefore vaginal discharge is scant.
2. Foal heat
   - First oestrus occurs 7–9 days after foaling.
   - Fertility tends to be lower than at subsequent heats.

Postpartum complications

Retained placenta

- Treatment should be initiated if the placenta is retained more than 3 hours (2–10% of mares). Mares are likely to be less fertile at foal heat if not treated.
- Use 10–20 IU oxytocin IV or IM every 15 min or 60 IU in 1 litre of saline infused intravenously over 1 h.
- Repeat as necessary (usually expelled within 30 min).

- If retention is *prolonged* (>8 hours) the mare can develop laminitis and endometritis. Use more aggressive therapy:
  - NSAIDs.
  - Broad-spectrum antibiotics.
  - Exercise.

Alternatively: The allantochorionic space may be infused with 10–12 litres dilute (0.1%) povidone-iodine solution or saline. The opening in the foetal membranes is tied shut. The distension of the reproductive tract stimulates uterine contractions (via oxytocin release) and the membranes are usually passed within 30 min.

Haemorrhage

- May involve uterine, utero-ovarian or external iliac arteries. Can also have severe intrauterine haemorrhage.
- Mares may exsanguinate. Survival depends upon whether haemorrhage is contained within the broad ligament or whether the ligament ruptures.
- Signs of colic with weak rapid pulse and pale membranes.
- Keep mare in dark, quiet stable.
- Sedatives may help.
- Do not give oxytocin in case clot is disrupted.

Rectovaginal fistula/perineal laceration

- Caused by damage to birth canal by foal's hoof.
- Repair surgically after 30 days when damaged tissue has sloughed and swelling has resolved.

Uterine rupture

- Usually uterine body.
- May pass blood clots vaginally.
- Diagnosed by manual examination *per vaginam* and peritoneal fluid cytology.
- Mare may be depressed and ill due to blood and foetal fluids in abdominal cavity. Uterus has tense, ridged feel.
- Give oxytocin (20–40 IU) hourly to contract uterus.
- Antibiotics/NSAIDs.
- Surgical repair of uterus may be indicated.

Endometrial haemorrhage

- Uncommon.

- Usually not serious but may persist for 3–4 days.

Treatment

- Restrict exercise.
- Oxytocin to reduce size of uterus.
- Pack uterus if necessary.
- Antibiotics.
- ? Surgical repair but difficult to adequately expose uterus.
- Lavage uterus after 1 week to break down any adhesions.

Uterine prolapse

- Rare in mare. More commonly, one horn invaginates into the uterine lumen causing pain and straining.
- Usually follows placental retention or dystocia.
- May be accompanied by shock.

Treatment

- Tranquillizers (do not administer if mare is in shock).
- Epidural anaesthesia.
- Clean and replace uterus.
- Systemic antibiotics + oxytocin (IM).
- Exercise.
- If handled quickly and effectively future fertility is good.
- If only part of the horn is invaginated infuse 4–8 litres warm saline and drain.

Endometritis

Some degree of endometritis is normal after foaling. Only treat if the uterus fails to involute or the mare is systemically ill.

Treatment

- Lavage uterus with 3–5 litres of sterile saline. Recover as much fluid as possible. Repeat as necessary.
- Can give oxytocin to help drain uterus.
- Infuse uterus with appropriate antibiotic.
- Exercise.
- Laminitis is a possible complication.

Cervical tear

- Occurs not only after dystocia but after apparently normal foaling.
- Diagnosed by manual vaginal examination during dioestrus.

Treatment

- Surgical repair.

14.6 *The stallion*

Examination of the stallion for breeding soundness (BSE)

Reasons for performing a BSE:

- Prepurchase.
- Before the start of the breeding season.
- Fertility problems.

The components of the BSE are described below.

Identification

Ensure that a thorough description of the stallion is included in the BSE certificate.

History

1. General – illness, use, medications.
2. Reproductive:
   - Number of mares bred/season.
   - Number of pregnancies.
   - Fertility of mares.
   - Results of previous BSE.
   - Performance of other stallions on farm.

General physical examination

- Musculoskeletal.
- Respiratory.
- Eyes.
- Mouth.
- Body condition.

Semen collection and evaluation

If the stallion is available for only one day, collect two ejaculates one hour apart. Otherwise it is more representative to collect daily ejaculates for 5–7 days. Using this method stores of sperm in the excurrent duct system will be depleted and the last ejaculates will represent daily sperm output (DSO). This figure may be used to calculate the number of mares that a stallion can cover in a season. For semen collection, use an artificial vagina filled with hot water so that its internal temperature is 44–48°C. Use a plastic disposable liner. Lubricate with non-spermicidal water-soluble lubricant. Rinse the penis with warm water (42°C) and dry. If excessive smegma is present use a water-soluble low-residue soap and rinse thoroughly with warm water. After collection maintain semen at 34–37°C and protect from light, temperature extremes, chemicals and water.

The following features should be evaluated.

Motility
Motility should be evaluated first because it decreases with time. Because of the tendency for stallion sperm to clump, it is sometimes easier to check motility after adding extender to the semen.

Total motility = percentage of sperm that are moving.

Progressive motility = percentage of sperm that are moving forward in a relatively straight line.

Express motility as total/progressive motility.

pH
pH should be evaluated soon after collection as the metabolic activity of the sperm will increase the pH with time (normal = 7.2–7.6). High pH may be due to contamination with soap or urine, or infection in the urethra or proximal tract.

Volume and concentration
Both gel and gel-free volume. Average is 70 ml containing a total of 8×10^9 sperm (total sperm number = volume $\times$ concentration). Can measure concentration on a haemocytometer or a spectrophotometer.

Morphology
- Can be performed using phase contrast microscopy on wet mount preparation in buffered formol saline, or by staining with nigrosin eosin.
- Count 200 sperm. At least 60% should be normal.
- Abnormalities are classified according to specific type (normal sperm, abnormal head, detached head, proximal droplet, distal droplet, abnormal midpiece, abnormal tail). Morphologic abnormalities have been divided into primary (arise in testis) and secondary (arise in the excurrent ducts or during storage or ejaculation) abnormalities. As the true origin of abnormalities is not

known this classification system has been questioned. In bulls' sperm abnormalities have been categorized as major (abnormal sperm head, proximal droplet and abnormal mid-piece) or minor (detached head, distal droplet and abnormal tail) depending on their association with impaired fertility. However, in the stallion the association between specific abnormalities and reduced fertility is not clear. NB. Abaxial mid-pieces are considered normal in stallion sperm.

Number

Number of morphologically normal, progressively motile sperm = total number of sperm in ejaculate × % morphologically normal × % progressively motile.

There should be at least 1×10^9 in second ejaculate. This figure is the most important in calculating the potential fertility of a stallion. The second ejaculate should contain approximately 50% of the number of sperm in the first ejaculate.

Longevity of motility

Aliquots of raw and extended semen are kept in airtight, dark conditions at 4°C and at 23°C. Motility should be evaluated hourly for 6 h then at 24 h. At least 10% sperm should be progressively motile at 6 h in the raw semen sample and at 24 h in the extended semen. Shortened sperm longevity and increased morphological defects may suggest accumulation of extragonadal sperm from infrequent ejaculation. Evaluation of sperm longevity at 4°C is necessary if the stallion's semen is to be chilled and used in an AI programme. However, the relevance of longevity at 23°C in a laboratory is questionable.

NB. Morphology and motility of stallion semen are not affected by season, but volume of seminal fluid and total sperm numbers increase in spring and summer. Although photostimulation can hasten testicular and libidinal recrudescence early in the year, the period of time of heightened reproductive capacity is not prolonged.

Testicular size and consistency

This is highly correlated with the daily sperm output (DSO).

Length, width and height of each testicle are measured using calipers or ultrasonography. Total scrotal width should be greater than 8 cm. However, whatever the size of the testes, stallions with flabby or hard testes are potentially poor producers of sperm. Estimates of testicular

volume may improve accuracy in determining daily sperm output (DSO). DSO = mean daily yield of sperm after extragonadal reserves have been depleted. This figure enables calculation of the number of mares a stallion can breed in a season (may be limited by libido).

$$DSO = 0.024x - 0.76 \text{ where } x = \text{testicular volume}$$
$$(TV)$$

$$TV = 4/3\pi abc \text{ where } \begin{array}{l} a = \text{testicular height}/2 \\ b = \text{testicular width}/2 \\ c = \text{testicular length}/2 \end{array}$$

Venereal pathogens

NB. Rectal sleeves should be worn and changed between handling the external genitalia of different stallions.

1. Prior to rinsing the penis, swab
   - Fossa (Figure 10).
   - Shaft.
   - Sheath.

   This establishes the normal flora (*Corynebacterium* spp., fungi and small numbers of *Streptococcus* spp.).
2. After rinsing and drying the penis, swab the urethra.

   This establishes the flora of the terminal urethra. Small numbers of mixed bacteria are normal. There should not be a heavy pure growth of any one bacterial species.
3. Immediately after collecting the first ejaculate, swab the urethra. This establishes the flora of the internal genital tract. There should be no growth from this swab.

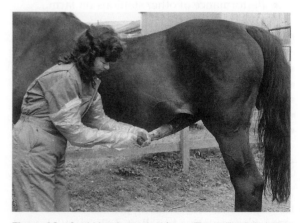

Figure 10 Swabbing the urethral fossa. The stallion is being teased with a mare to facilitate swabbing of the penis.

A pure growth of *Pseudomonas aerogenes*, *Klebsiella pneumoniae* (capsule types 1, 2 and 5), *Streptococcus* spp. or *Taylorella equigenitalis* is considered abnormal. All are potential venereal pathogens. Not all strains are pathogenic, however. Apart from *Taylorella equigenitalis*, all can be present as incidental contaminants. If a stallion is blamed for infecting a mare with *Pseudomonas* or *Klebsiella*, check capsule or serotype of isolates from both the mare and stallion for confirmation.

Code of practice for CEM and other bacterial venereal diseases (in Great Britain)

All breeding TB stallions must be swabbed on two occasions more than 7 days apart from:

- Urethra.
- Urethral fossa.
- Penile sheath.
- Pre-ejaculatory fluid.

Put swabs in transport medium and keep at 4°C during shipment. Should reach the laboratory within 24 h of collection.

Stallions should be swabbed *before* the start of the breeding season. If the cultures are positive for a venereal pathogen the stallion is designated as unsuitable for breeding until he is treated and three sets of negative swabs are obtained at intervals of > 7 days.

Treatment

Klebsiella and *Pseudomonas* are difficult to treat. Wash erect penis with povidone-iodine. Dry penis and pack with an aminoglycoside cream or 1% silver sulphadiazine daily for 1–2 weeks. Collect serial swabs over several weeks for cultural examination to monitor success of treatment. Alternatively for *Pseudomonas*, wash erect penis with dilute HCl (10 ml of 38% HCl in 1 gallon of water) daily for 2 weeks. Reduce concentration if any skin reaction is noted. Treat after each breeding. For *Klebsiella*, use dilute sodium hypochlorite. Add 40 ml 5.25% sodium hypochlorite/gallon.

Taylorella is sensitive to most antibiotics and antiseptics. Wash erect penis daily for at least 5 days with chlorhexidine solution (>2%) followed by topical application of nitrofurazone or penicillin ointment. Pay particular attention to the urethral fossa where the organism is harboured.

After treatment of infections, cultures of commensals from the penis of a normal stallion have been used to recolonize the treated stallion's penis. However, the efficacy of this technique has not been reported.

Code of Practice for EVA (in Great Britian)

All unvaccinated stallions and teasers should be serologically tested prior to the breeding season. Seropositive stallions should be isolated pending virus detection. Semen used for AI, whether fresh, chilled or frozen, can act as a source of infection of EVA. All stallions used for AI should therefore be tested negative for EVA prior to the breeding season. Mare owners should also establish the antibody status of the donor stallion before importation of semen. If the stallion is seropositive, the semen should not be used unless it can be proved that seroconversion was due to prior vaccination.

Physical examination of the reproductive tract

- Penis: examine during the washing procedure.
- Scrotum and testes:
  - Palpation.
  - Ultrasonography.
- Internal genital organs:
  - Palpation (per rectum).
  - Ultrasonography.

Abnormalities of the genital tract

SCROTUM – ACQUIRED

Any inflammation or swelling will raise the temperature and adversely affect spermatogenesis. It takes approximately 2 months after the lesion resolves for the stallion to produce normal ejaculates but can take considerably longer.

Causes of swelling
1. External:
   - Dermatitis.
   - Trauma.
   - Ventral oedema – check for EVA and EIA.
2. Internal:
   - Haematocele.
   - Hydrocele.
   - Herniation.
   - Peritonitis.
   - Haemorrhage.
3. Diagnosis:
   - Ultrasonography.

• Needle aspiration – first palpate inguinal rings to ensure that a scrotal hernia is not present. Ensure asepsis.

Acute trauma

Treatment

Cryotherapy – icepacks with simultaneous massage. Should not exceed 20 min; apply at 1–3 h intervals. Systemic anti-inflammatory and antibiotic treatment may be administered. Emollients should be applied to the skin to prevent maceration.

Intrascrotal haemorrhage or haematocele will lead to permanent testicular damage due to the insulating properties of the resultant fibrous tissue. The organized blood clot can be surgically removed in an attempt to save the testis.

Scrotal lacerations

Treatment

• Cleanse with isotonic salt solution containing antibiotic.
• Suture parietal vaginal tunic.
• Debride subcutaneous tissues.
• Skin closure with non-absorbable suture.
• Systemic antibiotics and NSAIDs.

Hydrocele

• Abnormal collection of fluid between visceral and parietal vaginal tunic.
• Usually not painful.
• Can accompany scrotal oedema.

Treatment

• Remove underlying cause.
• Exercise.
• If unilateral and persistent, remove affected testis and tunics to save contralateral testis from heat-induced degeneration.

Herniation

See Chapter 8.

SCROTUM – CONGENITAL

Defective scrotal development can occur in intersex horses.

Male pseudohermaphroditism

• Testes are usually intra-abdominal or inguinal.
• Stallion-like behaviour.
• Variable phenotype-underdeveloped penis or enlarged clitoris.
• 64XX or mosaic karyotypes.

Testicular feminization

• XY karyotype.
• Female phenotype.
• Abdominal testes – male behaviour.

X–Y sex reversal

• XY karyotype.
• Female genitalia – small inactive ovaries and hypoplastic tubular genital tract.

TESTIS

Cryptorchidism

See Chapter 8.

Haematoma

Extensive necrosis can occur leading to complete loss of testicular function.

Diagnosis

• Ultrasonography.

Treatment

• If haemorrhage is contained within the tunica albuginea, adhesions may not occur. Treat as for acute scrotal trauma.
• If haemorrhage is massive – hemicastration.

Torsion

See Chapter 8.

Neoplasia

Seminoma is the most common tumour.

• Germinal epithelial origin.
• Locally invasive.
• Metastases reported.

Teratoma is found predominantly in cryptorchid testes.

Uncommon tumours
- Interstitial cell.
- Sertoli cell.
- Embryonal carcinoma.
- Lipoma, fibroma, leiomyoma.

Small testes

Hypoplasia
- Relatively common (3% of stallions in one survey).
- Incomplete gonadal development. Usually associated with an underdeveloped epididymis.
- Possibly genetic.

Degeneration
- Major cause of subfertility/infertility.
- Acquired condition.
- Numerous causes:
  - thermal injury,
  - infection,
  - hormonal disturbances,
  - malnutrition,
  - toxins,
  - autoimmune disturbances,
  - drugs.

Both conditions can present as:

- Unilateral or bilateral (NB. Left testis tends to be larger than right in normal stallions).
- Soft or firm consistency.
- Oligo- or azoospermic.
- Round germ cells in ejaculate. May be multinucleate.
- Libido usually unaffected.

History is important in differentiating between hypoplasia and degeneration. Unlike testicular hypoplasia, testicular degeneration may be reversible by removing the factor responsible for changes. Replacement therapy with gonadotrophin-releasing hormone (GnRH) may be more useful in stallions with hypogonadotrophic hypogonadism (defect in pituitary-hypothalamic axis – low LH and follicle-stimulating hormone (FSH)) than in stallions with damage to the seminiferous epithelium (suggested by elevated concentrations of FSH). However, the use of GnRH in stallions remains controversial.

Orchitis – bacterial

This is rare.

Diagnosis

Affected testes are hot, slightly swollen, tense and acutely painful. Fever and scrotal oedema are common.

Treatment

Treatment includes antimicrobial therapy, NSAIDs, hydrotherapy. Prompt removal of a unilaterally affected testis may save the contralateral testis.

Orchitis – traumatic

Diagnosis

- Hot, tense, painful testes.
- Swelling is restricted by the tunica albuginea.
- Increased testicular pressure and temperature lead to marked testicular degeneration.

Treatment

Counteract local inflammation as described above.

EPIDIDYMIS

- *Epididymitis*. Rare. Usually secondary to orchitis.
- *Spermiostasis*. In some stallions, sperm accumulate abnormally in the epididymis and deferent ducts during sexual rest. Semen contains a large proportion of detached sperm heads. High sperm numbers in ejaculate and sperm may be clumped. Treat by frequent ejaculation. Can recur if the stallion does not ejaculate regularly.

SEMINAL VESICLES

Seminal vesiculitis is rare. There are inflammatory cells in the semen. The stallion may be infertile. Systemic treatment is often unsuccessful. Local irrigation of the glands and infusion of antibiotics via an endoscope may be tried.

AMPULLAE

When the *ampullae* are *blocked* spermiostasis occurs and the ampullae feel tense and swollen on palpation. The condition is treated by massage and frequent ejaculation. Oxytocin (10–20 IU) may be administered prior to ejaculation.

PREPUCE AND PENIS

Paraphimosis

See Chapter 8.

Haematoma

This often follows a kick from the mare at breeding. It usually results from haemorrhage of superficial vessels on the dorsum of the penis. There is rapid swelling and it can lead to paraphimosis.

Treatment

- Apply compression bandage then treat as for paraphimosis.
- Daily massage to minimize fibrosis.

Coital exanthema

- Caused by EHV-3.
- Pox-like lesions on penis.
- Venereally transmitted.
- Self-limiting.
- Complete resolution in 3–5 weeks.

Treatment

- Sexual rest.
- Daily application of protective emollients.

Squamous cell carcinoma

See Chapter 8.

Squamous papilloma

- Develop only rarely on penis or prepuce.
- Multiple proliferative cutaneous growths that usually regress spontaneously in 1–6 months.

Cutaneous habronemiasis

See Chapter 8.

Altered semen

In *urospermia* urination occurs during ejaculation.

Treatment

- Train the stallion to urinate prior to collection.
- Fractionation of ejaculate – only useful if the stallion urinates in the final stages of ejaculation.
- Centrifugation and resuspension of sperm in extender.
- Can try diazepam (100–500 mg orally twice a day).

For haemospermia see Chapter 8.

Abnormal reproductive behaviour in stallions

Behaviour-related fertility or management problems comprised over 25% (*n* = 250) of stallion fertility problems referred to a large American clinic over a 5 year period.

Low libido – causes

- Managemental.
- Musculoskeletal.
- Hormonal.

Managemental

May have preference for

- Mare.
- Handler.
- Location.

Treatment

- Keep quiet.
- Try outdoor breeding.
- Blinkers.
- Hot compresses applied to base of penis while artificial vagina on glans.
- Watch another stallion (voyeur effect).
- Use more than one mare.
- Use unrestrained mare in oestrus.

Musculoskeletal

Treatment

- Provide mount mare of appropriate height.
- Position mare on slope downhill from stallion.
- Collect semen with stallion standing on ground.
- Treat pain.
- Ensure good footing.
- Provide lateral support.

Hormonal

1. Impotent stallions tend to have lower blood concentrations of LH and oestradiol-17β whereas concentrations of testosterone tend to be similar to normal stallions.
2. Administration of low levels of testosterone (50–200 μg/kg SC every other day) does appear to help slow-starting stallions. Plasma testosterone should be monitored to avoid reaching undesirably high blood levels. Increased sexual interest should be apparent within 10 days. Novice stallions generally do not need treatment after the first ejaculation.
3. Treatment of slow stallions with 50 μg GnRH subcutaneously 2 h and then 1 h before breeding may increase sexual arousal. Typically, concentrations of testosterone in blood double after this treatment regimen.

Ejaculatory dysfunction

This is a relatively common disorder.

Discharge of semen into the urethra appears to be caused by stimulation of α-adrenergic receptors and by inhibition of β-adrenergic receptors, whereas transport of semen through the urethra is regulated by the somatic nervous system.

1. Often presents as a stallion with good libido and normal copulatory behaviour.
2. May appear to ejaculate (tail flags, urethral pulsations) but does not.
3. May ejaculate after several breeding attempts.

Causes

1. Psychogenic
   - Breeding injury.
   - Overuse.
   - Aggressive handling.
   - Unfamiliar surroundings.
2. Organic
   - Damage to the dorsal nerve of the penis.
   - Malfunction of the autonomic nervous system.
   - Blocked ejaculatory ducts.
   - Retrograde ejaculation (semen expelled into bladder).

Treatment

Treatment depends on cause.

Pharmacological aids

1. α-agonist (L-norepinephrine 0.01 mg/kg IM) 15 min before breeding + β-antagonist (carazolol 0.015 mg/kg IM) 10 min before breeding. Used to treat organic ejaculatory failure. Do not use in stallions with COPD.
2. Xylazine (α-adrenergic): In normal stallions, spontaneous ejaculation occurs 25% of the time after 0.66 mg/kg IV.
3. PGF-2α: Spontaneous ejaculation in 50% of stallions within 10 min of administering 0.01 mg/kg IM.
4. Diazepam: Used in timid stallions at a dose of 0.05 mg/kg (slow) IV 5–7 min before breeding.

14.7 Reproductive management

The official breeding season for Thoroughbreds starts on 15 February in the northern hemisphere and 1 August in the southern hemisphere. As many mares only start to cycle later in the spring, manipulation of the breeding season is frequently practised.

Artificial control of photoperiod

- Start 1 December for 15 February breeding season.
- Maintain a ratio of 16 h light:8 h dark. Add light in evening. Continuous light may delay onset of cyclicity.
- A 12 × 12 ft loose box requires a 200 W bulb.

Transitional breeding season

- Lasts 30–60 days.
- Numerous large follicles (> 30 mm) are present on the ovaries, but ovulation fails to occur.
- Mare remains in oestrus for prolonged periods.

Onset of normal cyclicity may be hastened by

- Altrenogest daily for 10 days.
- Twice daily injections of buserelin (10 μg).

Breeding season

- Mares should be teased at least three times per week (preferably daily).

- One follicle, occasionally two, becomes dominant and ovulates on the last or second last day of oestrus. Mean diameter at ovulation is 45 mm.
- Traditionally, mares are bred on day 2 of oestrus or when a 30 mm follicle is present on the ovaries, and then every other day until the end of oestrus. If it is necessary to limit the number of breedings, the ovaries should be palpated daily and the mare should be bred on the day before ovulation is anticipated. If ovulation has occurred, good conception rates may still be achieved by breeding 12–18 h after ovulation. However, the incidence of early embryonic death increases, due to fertilization of an aged ovum.

Aberrant patterns of cyclicity

Persistent oestrus

Check behaviour with stallion – many owners misdiagnose true signs of oestrus.

Causes

- Seasonal anoestrus – mares may show weak signs of oestrus in the absence of the strongly inhibiting effects of progesterone.
- Transitional breeding season.
- Granulosa cell tumour.

Treat first two with altrenogest.

Prolonged dioestrus

- Occurs in bred and non-bred mares.
- Failure of luteal regression at end of dioestrus, and therefore mare fails to return to oestrus.
- Up to 25% of cycles may be affected.
- CL may persist for 2 months or more.
- Can result from dioestrous ovulation on day 9–14 (the developing CL is unresponsive to PGF-2α) or early embryonic death.
- Treat with PGF-2α.

Pseudopregnancy

- A syndrome in which non-pregnant, bred mares do not return to oestrus or ovulate, and uterine tone is characteristic of early pregnancy.
- Thought to result from embryo loss but can occur occasionally in non-bred mares (not convincingly documented).

Split oestrus

- In oestrus for several days, then out for 1–2 days, followed by several more days of oestrus.
- Ovulation usually does not occur until the second half.
- More common early in the breeding season.

Double ovulations

- Occurs at about 16% of ovulations.
- Tends to occur repeatedly in certain mares (especially Thoroughbreds, Draught breeds and Warmbloods).
- Conception rates are higher than in single ovulating mares, therefore breed the mare.
- Check the mare for twin pregnancy by ultrasonography before day 30 (preferably before day 16) and crush one conceptus if twins are present.
- If twins have fixed in the one horn (70%) and it is not possible to crush one, natural reduction rates prior to day 40 are 89%. However, in bilateral fixation, only 11% reduce naturally.

Foaling mares

- Foal heat usually occurs at 7–9 days. Second heat around 30–35 days.
- Pregnancy rates for mares bred at the foal heat tend to be lower, and embryonic death rates higher than for mares bred at subsequent heats. Select mares with history of normal foaling and that have no fluid in the uterus at time of breeding.
- Mare must conceive by day 25 in order to foal at the same time the next year.

Lactational anoestrus

- Fifty per cent of pony mares and most Thoroughbred mares have a foal heat after foaling in the anovulatory season.
- Approximately half of these mares return to anoestrus after their first postpartum ovulation.
- The incidence of lactational anoestrus in the breeding season is low. Can stimulate ovulation within 14 days by weaning the foal.

Pregnancy losses (Table 1)

Seventy-seven per cent of all detected pregnancy losses occur before day 49.

Table 1 Pregnancy losses

	Fertile mares	Subfertile mares
Fertilization rate (%)	>90	>80
Embryonic loss rate (%)		
<day 14	9	70
day 0–40	20	>70
>day 60	9	

Manipulation of the oestrous cycle

- Progestogens: Altrenogest – synthetic, oral (Regumate). Oestrus occurs 4–5 days after a 12–15 day treatment period.
- Prostaglandin F-2α: CL must be between 6 and 14 days old to respond. Come into oestrus in 2–5 days. Ovulation is variable (3–12 days) depending on follicular development at time of treatment. Causes colicky side effects (sweating, trembling, muscle cramping) that subside in 30 min.
- Progesterone/oestradiol: 150 mg progesterone + 10 mg oestradiol IM for 10 days followed by PGF-2α (10 mg) on day 10. Oestrus occurs on approximately day 16 with ovulation on day 20–22.
- Human chorionic gonadotrophin (hCG): Hastens ovulation of a mature follicle; 2500 IU IV or IM will cause ovulation of a 35 mm follicle in 36–48 h.
- Gonadotrophin-releasing hormone (GnRH): Buserelin does not hasten ovulation unless given twice daily during oestrus. Deslorelin is a GnRH analogue that induces ovulation of a 35 mm follicle at 36–48 h. It is administered as a short-term implant.

Teasing programmes

Mares should be teased daily through oestrus. Teasing after breeding is a good method of detecting early pregnancy loss.

The teaser stallion should be an intact male horse with the following characteristics:

- Good libido.
- Easy to handle.
- Not easily frustrated.

Teasing systems are designed to suit the farm's management.

- The stallion teases the mare over a teasing board or teasing stocks.
- The stallion is placed in a small pen in the mares' pasture.
- The stallion is led to the fence of the mares' pasture.
- The stallion is brought to the door of the mare's loose box.
- The mare is brought to the door of the stallion's loose box.

It is important that each mare is given the chance to exhibit oestrous behaviour – watch for subordinate mares in group-housing situations.

Breeding management

Preparation of the stallion for breeding

- A breeding bridle or a headcollar with a chain through the mouth or over the nose should be placed on the stallion.
- Tease the stallion with a mare in oestrus until he achieves a full erection.
- The penis may be rinsed with warm water and dried with a soft paper towel. Avoid antiseptics.
- Allow stallion to tease the mare, and then mount. Usually a groom holds the mare's tail out of the way and another inserts the stallion's penis into the mare's vagina.
- At time of ejaculation, the stallion's tail flags and 7–9 pulsations are detected at the base of the penis.
- A dismount sample can be collected to check for the presence of sperm.
- After the stallion dismounts, the penis may again be rinsed with warm water.

Preparation of the mare for breeding

- Use a bridle or headcollar plus twitch.
- Place padded boots on the hindfeet. Can use breeding hobbles but the stallion can catch a foot in these. Can tie a foreleg up before stallion mounts (should be released after intromission).
- Bandage tail or place in plastic sleeve.
- Wash vulva, perineal region and hindquarters with mild soap. Rinse and dry.

Minimum contamination technique

In mares susceptible to endometritis, artificial insemination minimizes antigenic challenge to the mare's uterus. If AI is not permissible, then the mare should be bred once only. Scrupulous hygiene should be applied to both the stallion and the mare. Semen extender containing antibiotic (100 ml) can be infused into the mare's uterus immediately prior to breeding. The mare's uterus can either be flushed with buffered saline 4 h after breeding to physically remove contaminants, or the mare can be scanned 12 h later. If fluid is present, she can be treated with an injection of oxytocin followed by daily intrauterine antibiotic infusions for 4 days after ovulation, possibly in combination with uterine lavage.

Semen collection and preparation for AI

Artificial vagina

- CSU Model – expensive, heavy, well insulated.
- Missouri – inexpensive, light, easy to use (Figure 11).
- Nishikawa – moderately expensive, tends to leak water.

1. Artificial vagina must be clean and dry. A disposable plastic liner should be used.
2. To clean:
   - Soak for 20 min in 70% alcohol.
   - Hang up to dry.
   - Rinse with distilled water.
   - Dry
3. Fill with water so that internal temperature is 45°C.
4. Use non-spermicidal lubricant, e.g. K-Y jelly.

Semen treatment

1. Filter to remove gel.
2. Protect from cold shock, water, sunlight.
3. Evaluate:
   - Motility (total and progressive).
   - Volume.
   - Concentration.
4. Extend 1:1 or 1:2, or, optimally, dilute to 25–50 million per ml for chilled semen.

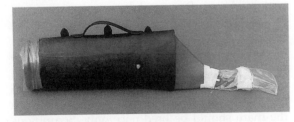

Figure 11 Missouri AV assembled ready for use.

5. Most commonly used extender is non-fat skim milk powder containing glucose and antibiotics.
   - Non-fat dry skim milk: 2.4 g.
   - Glucose: 4.9 g.
   - Make up to 100 ml with sterile distilled water.
   - Add penicillin (150 000 units) + streptomycin (150 000 μg),
     - or ticarcillin (100 mg),
     - or reagent grade gentamicin (100 mg) + $NaHCO_3$ (2 ml, 7.5%).
6. Mares should be inseminated with a minimum of 300 million progressively motile, morphologically normal sperm.
7. Use insemination volumes under 50 ml (usually 10–20 ml) containing 1 billion progressively motile sperm.

AI of the mare

Advantages
- Mares can be bred by a stallion that is geographically inaccessible.
- Mares with young foals are not transported from home.
- Mare can still be ridden.

Disadvantages
- High veterinary expenses.
- If the mare is to remain at home, mare owners must tease mare and communicate with vet and stud farm.
- Semen shipment costs.

Preparation of the mare
- Wrap tail in sleeve or bandage.
- Empty rectum.
- Wash perineal region three times with mild soap, dry.
- Draw semen into Air Tite syringe.
- Wear a clean plastic sleeve and a sterile glove.
- Lubricate hand with sterile, non-spermicidal lubricant (K–Y jelly).
- Introduce plastic insemination pipette into the uterus; the tip is covered by the hand as it is passed through the vagina. Deposit the semen in the uterine body. Hold cervix shut as the pipette is withdrawn.

Cooled semen
- Before committing a stallion to an AI programme, the stallion's semen must be checked to

ensure that it withstands the cooling process satisfactorily.
- Semen should be evaluated for motility and concentration. Extend to 50 million progressively motic sperm/ml.
- Prepare three packages of semen. Send two to the mare owner and keep one at the stud for evaluation 24 h later.
- Semen is double-bagged in whirlpak bags or placed in plastic containers. The samples are placed in a polystyrene cup. Excess space inside the cup is filled with ballast bags containing a blue dye. The cup is then loaded into the Equitainer.
- Should be used within 48 h of collection.
- Do not open Equitainer until mare is prepared for insemination.
- Inseminate mare (the semen does not need to be pre-warmed).
- Check motility of sperm by placing on a slide at 37°C. Motility improves over a few minutes.
- For optimum pregnancy rates the mare should have ovulated when she is checked on the day after AI.
- Check mare for pregnancy before day 18 so that she can be rebred at the next oestrus.
- Pregnancy rates as good as, or better than, natural service.

Frozen semen
- Most commonly stored in 0.5 ml straws or 4 ml macrotubes in liquid nitrogen.
- Quality of semen after freeze–thaw process varies markedly between stallions (only approximately 30% of stallions produce semen that has good motility after thawing).
- Pregnancy rates variable depending on semen quality. The mare must be checked at least every 12 h and inseminated at the examination before and after ovulation. Alternatively scan every 6 h and inseminate at the first examination after ovulation

Embryo transfer

Advantages
- Embryo can be collected from performance mares and transferred to recipient mare. This means that the donor mare can remain in training.
- Embryos can be collected from mares that are unable to carry a foal to term. NB. Recovery rate of embryos is very poor from mares with endometritis.

- A number of embryos can be collected from a valuable mare over one breeding season.
- It is possible to chill embryos in Equitainers and transport them. At this time embryo freezing is producing poor results.

Problems
- The mare is resistant to superovulation. However, recent work in which mares are immunized against inhibin is producing promising results.
- Due to problems with precise synchronization of ovulation it is necessary to have two recipient mares.
- Embryo transfer is expensive due to mare and veterinary costs.

Procedure
- The oestrous cycles of donor and recipient mares are synchronized.
- The donor mare is bred at oestrus.
- Ovulation is monitored in all mares. Recipients can be used only if they ovulate between 3 days before and 2 days after the donor ovulates.
- The uterus of the donor mare is flushed with 3×1 litre of buffered saline 7 or 8 days after ovulation.
- The embryo is identified microscopically and transferred to the recipient mare via an insemination pipette.
- Scrupulous hygiene must be maintained to prevent introduction of infection.
- The donor mare is given PGF-2α to bring her back into oestrus.

Further reading

Ginther, O.J. (1992) *Reproductive Biology of the Mare*, 2nd Edn. Equiservices, Wisconsin.

Horserace Betting Levy Board. *Common Code of Practice for Control of Contagious Equine Metritis and Other Equine Bacterial Venereal Diseases and Equine Viral Arteritis*. HBLB, 52 Grosvenor Gardens, London SW1W 0AU.

McKinnon, A.O. and Voss, J.L. (1992) *Equine Reproduction*. Lea & Febiger, Philadelphia.

Varner, D.D., Schumacher, J., Blanchard, T.L. and Johnson, L. (1991) *Diseases and Management of Breeding Stallions*. American Veterinary Publication, Goleta, CA.

Appendix 1. Differential diagnoses of reproductive problems in the mare

1. Anoestrus
Season
  autumn
  winter
Failure to tease adequately
Ovarian acyclicity
  granulosa cell tumour
  atrophy
  hypoplasia
Prolonged dioestrus
Pregnancy
Pseudopregnancy
Lactational anoestrus

2. Excessive signs of oestrus
Misdiagnosis of signs of oestrus
Season
  transitional
  winter anoestrus
Granulosa cell tumour

3. Failure to conceive
Breeding at the wrong time
Endometritis
Intrauterine adhesions
Cervical laceration
Cervical adhesions
Urovagina
Poor quality semen
Chromosomal abnormality
Anovulation
Hydrosalpinx

4. Abortion
Infectious
  bacterial
  viral
  fungal
Non-infectious
  twinning
  umbilical cord abnormalities
  placental insufficiency
  uterine body pregnancy

5. Vulvar bleeding
Prepartum
  vestibular/vaginal varicosity
  placental detachment
Postpartum
  uterine rupture
  endometrial haemorrhage
  vaginal or vestibular damage

6. Vulvar discharge
Endometritis
Cervicitis
Vaginitis
Urovagina
Urological problem

Appendix 2. Differential diagnosis of reproductive problems in the stallion

1. Enlarged scrotum
Dermatitis
Trauma
Ventral oedema
Haematocoele
Hydrocoele
Varicocoele
Herniation
Peritonitis
Haemorrhage

2. Defective scrotal development
Male pseudohermaphroditism
Testicular feminization
X–Y sex reversal

3. Enlarged testis
Haematoma
Torsion
Neoplasia
Orchitis

4. Small testis
Hypoplasia
Degeneration

5. Poor quality semen
Season
Urospermia
Haemospermia
Contamination with disinfectants etc.
Poor handling
  heat
  cold
  light
  oxygen
  agitation
Infection
Testicular hypoplasia/degeneration
Chromosomal abnormality
Impaired epididymal function
Blocked ejaculatory ducts
Elevated scrotal temperature
Hormonal imbalances
Malnutrition

Ageing
Overuse

6. *Low libido*
Managemental
Musculoskeletal
Hormonal

7. *Ejaculatory dysfunction*
Psychogenic
Nerve damage or malfunction
Blocked ejaculatory ducts
? Retrograde ejaculation

8. *Erection failure*
Psychogenic
Local vascular or neurological damage

15 Orthopaedics 1. Diagnosis of lameness/diseases of joints and bones

CONTENTS

15.1 Diagnostic approach to lameness

Diagnosis of orthopaedic problems involves a number of basic steps namely:

- Defining the problem to be investigated.
- Localizing the site or sites of abnormality.
- Characterizing the nature of the pathological change.

The following two chapters describe disorders of the lower and upper limbs of the horse.

However, it is worth noting from the outset that lameness in most horses is most commonly a result of abnormalities in the distal limb, i.e. the carpus or hock and distally, particularly the foot. The distal limb should therefore always be carefully evaluated first to eliminate it as the source of lameness.

History

1. Essential information includes:
   - Breed.

- Age.
- Sex.
- Duration of ownership.
- Use (or intended use) of the horse.
2. Details of recent management may be relevant including exercise, shoeing, housing and feeding.
3. Previous locomotor problems known to the owner should be noted.

Physical examination

Provided that the routine adopted for physical examination is comprehensive in its detail and scope, the precise order in which it is performed is not critical. Every effort should be made to examine the entire musculoskeletal system even in the presence of obvious abnormalities at one site. The examination at rest logically falls into two stages:

1. Overall inspection of the horse from all angles noting particularly:
   - General body condition.
   - Conformation of body, limbs and feet.
   - Posture and weight bearing on the limbs.
   - Skeletal and soft tissue symmetry.
   - Any localized swellings or thickenings.
2. Detailed evaluation of all individual regions of the limbs by:
   - Inspection.
   - Palpation.
   - Manipulation.

All three procedures should involve comparison of the region under examination with the contralateral limb to detect asymmetries.

- Inspection should reveal deformity, swelling or thickening, skin wounds and muscle wasting.
- Palpation is helpful in detecting heat and pain as well as characterizing the precise location and consistency of any swellings or thickenings.
- Manipulation of joints allows evaluation of their range of movement – detecting restriction, instability, pain or crepitus.

Gait evaluation

The aim should be to identify:

1. The presence or absence of a gait abnormality.
2. The limb or limbs involved.
3. The character of any abnormality present.
4. The degree of abnormality.

- The gait is usually best evaluated on a hard level surface. Ideally this should be done in a safe, enclosed area free of distractions and dangers such as traffic and other horses.
- Some forms of lameness are best examined immediately after taking the patient out of its stable (i.e. 'cold lameness'). Chronic low-grade lameness may require a period of sustained exercise to become more obvious.
- Horses should be stripped of all tack, rugs and blankets and should be held by a loose rope that is fixed to a headcollar or bridle.
- Abnormalities of gait are usually most apparent when the horse is moving at the walk and slow trot. Variations in foot placement and limb movement, e.g. shortening of one phase of the stride on one limb, are generally easiest to appreciate at the walk when limb movement is slower.
- Abnormalities in head and hindquarter movement resulting from pain during weight bearing are usually most apparent at the slow trot.
- The horse should be observed moving in a straight line and at an even pace from in front, the side and behind.
- Forelimb lameness is best observed while the horse is trotted towards and past the examiner. Hindlimb lameness is best observed while the horse is trotted past and away from the examiner. Observation from the side is easier if the observer is on the side of the lame limb.
- Lunging the horse in tight circles is helpful in demonstrating more clearly lameness that is subtle or inapparent when the horse is moving in a straight line. If circumstances do not permit such an examination, trotting the horse around sharp corners may accentuate lameness in a similar, though more transient, way.
- It is rare for horses to have to be ridden or driven to make a lameness noticeable. Lameness in Standardbreds is an exception to this rule, and can often only be observed on the track at full racing speed.
- Canter or gallop is only occasionally of value in the observation of lameness.
- Horses with forelimb lameness due to pain on weight bearing shift the distribution of weight from the affected limb across to the contralateral forelimb and back to the hindlimbs. This is achieved, at least in part, by raising the head and neck as the lame forelimb takes weight, the head being lowered again as the sound forelimb strikes the ground. This downward nodding of the head as the sound forelimb strikes the ground is generally the easiest abnormality of movement to

appreciate and allows identification of the lame (or lamer) forelimb. The sound limb may also be heard to strike the ground with greater force, particularly if the horse is shod.

- In hindlimb lameness the normal symmetrical vertical movements of both quarters, as observed from behind the horse, is disturbed. The quarter on the lame side will rise and fall through a greater range of motion than that of the sound limb. This is usually characterized by a long downwards drop during the swing-phase of the stride, followed by a fast, sudden, upwards flick during the weightbearing phase of the stride.
- Head movements are less helpful in the recognition of hindlimb lameness. With moderate to severe lameness, the horse may attempt to shift its centre of gravity forward when the lame hindlimb starts to weightbear, which can give the misleading impression of a head nod during the support phase of the contralateral forelimb.
- Bilateral forelimb or hindlimb lameness is often very difficult to recognize when the horse moves in a straight line. The horse usually shows a stiff, stilted gait with bilaterally shortened stride length. More pronounced unilateral signs of lameness are usually observed when the limbs are subjected to uneven stresses (e.g. by lunging in tight circles).
- Abnormalities of limb movement may also be appreciable in the lame horse:
  - *Alteration in the relative lengths of phases of the stride*. The cranial phase of the stride is that part which occurs in front of the footprint of the contralateral limb, while the caudal phase occurs behind it. If the horse is moving in a straight line, the overall stride length in a pair of contralateral limbs must be even; therefore a reduced cranial phase must always be accompanied by an increased caudal phase. Overall reductions in stride length frequently accompany bilateral orthopaedic conditions leading to a 'pottery' or restricted gait.
  - *Alteration in the arc of foot flight*. Lowering of the arc of foot flight may occur as a compensation to reduce impact when the foot lands or to reduce limb flexion during protraction. If severe, it may lead to dragging of the toes. Exaggerated elevation of a foot due to hyperflexion of the limb joints is occasionally seen, e.g. in 'stringhalt'.
  - *Variations in the path of foot flight and in foot placement*. These may occur for similar reasons to those that cause alterations in the arc of foot flight. The foot may be swung medially or laterally during protraction of the limb. The foot may land asymmetrically contacting the ground first at the toe, heel or on one or other side.

Certain gait characteristics may be indicative of the site of pain:

- Swinging limb lameness often originates from the proximal limb.
- Supporting limb lameness usually reflects pain in the distal limb.
- In bilateral lameness, the cranial phase of the stride is bilaterally shortened, even in distal limb lameness. This results in a stiff, stilted gait.

It is useful to examine the horse on both soft and hard ground.

- Lameness in the distal limb is often exacerbated on hard ground.
- Proximal lameness may be exacerbated on soft ground.
- Lunging or circling the horse provides further information for the observer:
  - Proximal lameness may be exacerbated with the affected limb on the outside of a circle.
  - Distal lameness is usually worse with the affected limb on the inside of a circle.

These 'rules' are certainly not absolute. For instance, one must take into account whether the painful locus is located on the medial or lateral aspect of the limb.

Records of a lameness evaluation should contain some assessment of the severity of the problem. A variety of scoring systems are employed, e.g. 0 to 5 or 1/10th to 10/10ths, with higher scores representing more severe grades of lameness.

Provocative tests

Provocative tests may be utilized for three basic reasons:

1. To demonstrate occult lameness in a horse that appears 'sound' on initial gait evaluation.
2. To exacerbate a mild lameness.
3. To aid localization of the abnormality causing the lameness.

A variety of manoeuvres are employed. The most commonly used are *'flexion tests'*:

- A flexion test is performed by holding the joint under consideration in a firmly flexed position for a period (usually 1 or 2 minutes) and then immediately watching the horse move, usually at the trot, to detect any change in gait compared to that observed before performing the test. The response to a flexion test should be interpreted in the light of other findings, and it is wise to avoid using it as the sole criterion upon which to base a firm diagnosis.

- As far as possible, the examiner attempts to flex the suspected joint only. Since some joints are inherently linked together in flexion and extension (i.e. hock and stifle; phalangeal joints and fetlock), exact differentiation of pain responses between these joints is not possible.
- Extension of the distal interphalangeal (DIP) joint may be performed using a wedge-shaped piece of wood with a 20° inclination, which is placed under the weightbearing foot to raise the toe and increase the load on the deep digital flexor tendon (DDFT), the navicular bone and its ligaments. After 2 minutes, the animal is trotted away. Unfortunately, the response to this test is inconsistent, even in confirmed cases of navicular syndrome.
- Response to localized pressure over exostoses, tendon swellings, splints, etc., can be assessed. Localized pressure is maintained for 2 minutes over the suspected site of pain, after which the horse is immediately trotted away.
- In all tests, the examiner looks for any significant exacerbation of lameness. Only by experience can one learn where the boundaries of normality lie for the amount and duration of tension applied. A sound horse should not show consistent lameness following any of these tests.

Regional analgesic techniques

'Nerve blocking' is time consuming, invasive, and sometimes hazardous to both horse and examiner. It relies on subjective evaluation of gait for its interpretation. Despite these disadvantages, it is often the only way to determine the answer to the question 'where does it hurt?'.

Local analgesic solutions can be used in a variety of ways to localize the source of pain responsible for lameness.

- The use of local analgesia depends on accurate placement of local analgesic into or around the structure to be desensitized, followed by evaluation of its effect on the gait.
- The results of regional analgesia are most easily and reliably interpreted when the horse shows an adequate and consistent degree of lameness in the first instance.

- Interpretation is more difficult and less reliable if the initial lameness is slight or inconsistent.
- Techniques for accentuating the degree of lameness, such as lunging the horse in tight circles on hard ground, have been described previously.
- If the lameness is chronic and low grade, it may be helpful to exacerbate the problem by exercising the horse for a few days to make the lameness more apparent prior to the use of local analgesia.

Conversely, caution should be exercised with the use of regional analgesia in acutely lame horses if there is a possibility that the cause may be an injury which could be exacerbated by injudicious use of a limb rendered pain free by the use of local analgesia. An example would be a horse with an undisplaced fracture that may displace with increased weight bearing. Initial radiographic and/or scintigraphic examination may be prudent if such injuries are suspected.

Local analgesia may be used for:

1. Perineural infiltration around specific nerves to desensitize the limb regions supplied by that nerve distal to the site of injection.
2. Intrasynovial analgesia of joints, tendon sheaths or bursae.
3. Direct local infiltration over suspect superficial lesions.
4. Field analgesia, performed by circular injection around the suspected site of pathology, thereby blocking all nerve fibres entering the area.

- All local analgesics prevent depolarization of the nerve by changing the permeability of the cell membrane to sodium ions (Na^+). The analgesic cation binds to the nerve cell membrane anion. This results in blocking of the Na^+ channels in the membrane.
- The preparations used for nerve blocks in lameness examinations should be intermediate in duration of action (60 to 90 minutes). Lignocaine hydrochloride is commonly used, but may produce more soft tissue swelling than mepivacaine which is somewhat more expensive, but causes minimal tissue reaction and has a slightly longer duration of action.
- The site of injection should be clean. The hair need not be clipped for nerve blocks, but the site of injection should always be clipped when performing intrasynovial injections. Strict adherence to antiseptic technique is required for all intrasynovial injections.

For perineural analgesia a minimal volume that will still reliably block the nerve is deposited as accurately as possible adjacent to it. The more proximal nerve trunks are thicker and more deeply situated within the limb tissues making accurate placement more difficult. The volume of local analgesic solution used is therefore generally greater for more proximal nerve blocks. For proximal blocks requiring long, and therefore relatively wide gauge, needles it can be helpful to place a small bleb of local analgesic subcutaneously first using a fine gauge needle before positioning the larger needle.

The peripheral nerves generally run in association with an artery and a vein as a neurovascular bundle. If a needle inadvertently enters a blood vessel on initial placement it should be withdrawn slightly and repositioned (usually slightly more caudally).

Distal limb blocks will usually take effect within 5 to 10 minutes; because of the increased thickness of proximal nerve trunks, more proximal blocks take longer to become effective and should generally be given at least 20 minutes to act. The efficacy of distal perineural analgesia can be tested to some extent by evaluating skin sensation distal to the block. This is best done using a blunt point such as a ball point pen. The response should be compared to that in the equivalent region of the contralateral limb, assuming that this limb has not been previously blocked.

Perineural analgesia should be carried out in a sequential manner starting distally and working proximally if the lameness is still present. If a specific joint is suspected to be the source of the lameness from the initial physical examination, it is better to perform an intra-articular block of this joint first, rather than a regional block proximal to the joint, as this will not interfere with subsequent more distal regional blocks if the response is negative.

When performing intrasynovial analgesia the most reliable sign that the needle has been accurately placed within the synovial cavity is the appearance of synovial fluid in the hub of the needle. This will not, however, always occur immediately for a number of reasons:

1. Some of the smaller joints and bursae contain only a very small amount of synovial fluid (e.g. the navicular bursa or the distal intertarsal joint).
2. Synovial villi may be sucked into the end of the needle and prevent any synovial fluid escaping through it.

There is no reliable way of testing whether an intrasynovial block has been effective and thus it is important to be sure that needle placement is accurate in the first instance. In those cases where a positive response is seen, the time taken to achieve soundness varies from as little as 5 minutes for small distal joints such as the distal interphalangeal joint to up to an hour for large complex joints such as the stifle.

Peripheral nerve blocks of the lower limb

Anatomy

Two separate systems of innervation have been identified in the lower limbs: the superficial and deep innervation systems.

- The superficial innervation of the forelimb is supplied by the lateral and medial palmar nerves, which course distally between the suspensory ligament (SL) and the DDFT. These nerves are a continuation of the median and ulnar nerves.
- The deep innervation of the forelimbs originates from the lateral palmar nerve (palmar branch of the ulnar nerve) which forms the lateral and medial palmar metacarpal nerves. These nerves course distally between the splint bones, the SL and the metacarpus. Distal to the button of the splint bone these nerves come to the surface, turn to the dorsal aspect of the fetlock, and end halfway down the pastern.
- The pattern of distribution of the deep and superficial innervation of the lower hindlimb is similar to the forelimb, apart from one major difference – the presence of a dorsal deep innervation system that originates from the deep peroneal nerve. The lateral and medial dorsal metatarsal nerves course distally all the way down into the laminar corium of the foot.
- Variations on this pattern of nerve distributions are commonly found in the front limbs.
  - In 30% of horses, an intermediate branch originates from the dorsal digital nerve, and forms the intermediate digital nerve.
  - In up to 50% of horses, the medial palmar metacarpal nerve continues down to the coronary corium.

Perineural analgesia of the lower limb

Palmar digital nerve block (PDNB) (Figure 1)
The palmar digital nerve is palpated along the borders of the DDFT, palmar to the accompanying artery. Two millilitres of local analgesic solu-

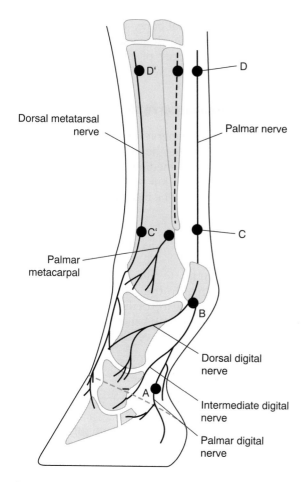

Figure 1 Schematic representation of the nerve blocks of the lower limb. A, B, C and D mark the sites for the palmar digital, abaxial sesamoid, low 4 point and high 4 point injections. C' and D' mark the additional sites for the low and high 6 point injections in the hindlimb.

tion is injected in the angle between the cartilages of the third phalanx and the palmar/plantar aspect of the pastern, on the palmar/plantar border of the neurovascular bundle. This results in desensitization of the navicular bone, the navicular bursa, the suspensory ligaments of the navicular bone, the distal part of the DDFT, the digital cushion, the corium of the frog, the palmar/plantar half of the solar and laminar dermis, the palmar/plantar half of the DIP joint and the palmar/plantar half of the third phalanx.

Absence of skin sensation over the heels indicates that the block has taken effect.

Abaxial sesamoid nerve block (ASNB) (Figure 1)

The dorsal and palmar/plantar digital nerves are part of the neurovascular bundle which is easily palpated over the abaxial surface of the proximal sesamoid bones. The needle is inserted in a distal direction, just palmar/plantar to the neurovascular bundle, by the base of the proximal sesamoid bone, and 3 ml of local analgesic is injected on both sides. Correct injection leads to desensitization of the entire foot, the DIP joint, the distal sesamoidean ligaments and flexor tendons distal to the site of injection, the proximal interphalangeal (PIP) joint, and often part of the fetlock joint. The skin around the coronary band should be entirely desensitized. A ring block of the pastern may be a useful alternative, because it avoids the sometimes confusing partial desensitization of the fetlock joint achieved with an abaxial sesamoid nerve block.

Low 4 point nerve block (palmar and palmar metacarpal nerve block) (L4PNB) (Figure 1)

The palmar nerves are desensitized by injection of 3 ml of local anaesthetic solution subcutaneously on either side of the limb, between the SL and DDFT at the level of the distal buttons of the splint bones.

Two millilitres of local analgesic is injected over each palmar metacarpal nerve where these emerge to a subcutaneous location, just distal to the buttons of the splint bones.

This nerve block desensitizes all structures distal to the level of injection, although some skin sensation may still be present over the dorsal fetlock due to additional innervation of this area by branches of the cutaneous antebrachii medialis nerve, which is a dorsal branch of the ulnar nerve.

In the hindleg, this block is referred to as the low 6 point nerve block, because some local analgesic solution has to be injected further dorsally from the plantar metatarsal nerves in order to desensitize the dorsal metatarsal nerves.

High 4 point nerve block (high palmar and palmar metacarpal nerve block) (H4PNB) (Figure 1)

The palmar nerves are situated between the SL and the DDFT, beneath the heavy fascia of the flexor retinaculum, 2 cm distal to the level of the carpometacarpal joint.

These nerves tend to be closely associated with the dorsal surface of the DDFT, although occasionally the lateral palmar nerve is found further palmarly, between the superficial digital flexor tendon (SDFT) and the DDFT. The palmar metacarpal nerves lie between the SL, the palmar surface of the cannon bone and the axial surface of the splint bones.

Since the local analgesic solution must be deposited deep to the retinaculum, the skin should not bulge during or after injection. Three millilitres of local analgesic is injected over each of the four sites, which should lead to desensitization of all structures distal to the level of injection, apart from the skin over the dorsal cannon bone, the most proximal part of the suspensory ligament and the proximal ends of the splint bones.

Proper desensitization is monitored by probing the skin over the palmar aspect of the flexor tendons, and squeezing the SL.

For reasons mentioned before, this nerve block becomes a 6 point block in the hind leg.

Desensitization of the proximal SL

To desensitize the most proximal part of the SL, the following techniques can be used:

- The lateral palmar nerve block, performed just below and halfway down the palmar border of the ligament between the accessory carpal bone and the proximal end of the lateral splint bone.
- Direct infiltration from both medial and lateral over the proximal SL with the limb raised.
- The ulnar nerve block (see below).

Peripheral nerve blocks of the upper limb

Median and ulnar nerve block

Median and ulnar nerve blocks will desensitize the carpus and most structures distal to it. As with tibial and peroneal blocks in the hindlimb, skin desensitization is not complete distal to the block but only affects certain areas (see below). This makes it advisable to perform these proximal limb blocks on a different occasion to the more distal regional blocks in order to be able to demonstrate that appropriate skin desensitization has occurred.

Median nerve
- Needle: 19G × 2 in (5 cm).
- Volume: 15 ml.
- Site: The caudomedial border of the radius just distal to the superficial pectoral muscle. The nerve lies cranial to the median artery and vein. Skin desensitization involves only the medial aspect of the pastern.

Ulnar nerve
- Needle: 20G × 1 in (2.5 cm).
- Volume: 10 ml.
- Site: In the groove on the caudal aspect of the antebrachium between the ulnaris lateralis and the flexor carpi ulnaris muscles, 10 cm proximal

to the accessory carpal bone, at a depth of one to two centimetres. Skin desensitization occurs on the dorsolateral aspect of the proximal metacarpus.

Tibial and peroneal nerve block

Tibial and peroneal nerve blocks will eliminate deep sensation from the hock and structures distal to it. As with median and ulnar block in the forelimb, loss of skin sensation is limited to certain areas and may be inconsistent.

Tibial nerve
- Needle: 20G × 1 in (2.5 cm).
- Volume: 15–20 ml.
- Site: Just caudal to the deep digital flexor tendon and cranial to the achilles tendon about 10 cm proximal to the top of the tuber calcis on the medial aspect of the limb beneath the fascia. Skin sensation is usually lost over the bulbs of the heel.

Peroneal nerve
- Needle: 19G × 2 in (5 cm).
- Volume: 15 ml total (10 ml deep and 5 ml superficially).
- Site: Between the long and lateral digital extensor tendons on the lateral aspect of the crus, 10 cm proximal to the lateral malleolus. The peroneal nerve has deep and superficial branches. Ten millilitres is injected around the deep branch, about 2–3 cm deep and 5 ml around the superficial branch during withdrawal of the needle. Skin desensitization usually occurs on the lateral aspect of the proximal metatarsus.

Intrasynovial analgesia

Navicular bursa
- Needle: 20G × 3.5 in (9 cm).
- Volume: 5 ml.
- Site: The needle is inserted 1 cm proximal to the coronary band in the midline between both heel bulbs, along the sagittal plane of the foot, towards an imaginary point, situated halfway along and just distal to the coronary band. The needle hits the flexor surface of the navicular bone at this point, and 3 to 5 ml of local analgesic solution is injected.

Distal interphalangeal joint
- Needle: 23G × 1 in (2.5 cm).
- Volume: 5 ml.
- Site: The needle is inserted 1 cm proximal to the

coronary band in the dorsal midline, at an angle of 45° to the horizontal, and advanced through the common digital extensor tendon.

Extra-articular structures (e.g. the navicular bone) may also be desensitized by this injection even though the DIP joint and the navicular bursa do not physically communicate.

Proximal interphalangeal joint (PIP)
- Needle: 20G × 1 in (2.5 cm).
- Volume: 5 ml.
- Site: This joint can be difficult to locate, but deep palpation may reveal the level of the dorsal joint margin. A needle is introduced through the skin, common digital extensor tendon and joint capsule, in the dorsal midline to enter the dorso-proximal synovial pouch of the joint.

Metacarpo/metatarsophalangeal (fetlock) joint
- Needle: 23G or 21G × 1 in (2.5 cm).
- Volume: 10 ml.
- Site: The dorsal approach is very similar to the PIP joint but easier. Because of the prominence of the sagittal ridge of the distal metacarpus/meta-tarsus, the needle is introduced lateral to the common digital extensor tendon, 1 cm proximal to the dorsoproximal margin of the first phalanx.
  - An alternative approach can be made through the palmaroproximal pouch, which is located between the SL, apex of the proximal sesamoid bone, distal button of the splint bone and palmarodistal surface of the cannon bone.
  - A third approach, which reputedly causes the least synovial haemorrhage, involves intro-ducing the needle through the collateral sesa-moidean ligament, between the palmar surface of the metacarpal condyle and the dorsal articular surface of the proximal sesamoid bone, with the limb flexed.

Digital synovial sheath
- Needle: 20G × 1 in (2.5 cm).
- Volume: 10 ml.
- Site: The digital synovial sheath extends a few centimetres proximal to the proximal sesamoids. Synoviocentesis is best performed between the DDFT and the SL, close to DDFT. This may be very difficult if synovial effusion is absent.

An alternative approach, which is most suc-cessful when the sheath is distended distally, is to introduce a needle into the distal pouch of the sheath, between the bifurcating branches of the SDFT. The point of the needle must remain super-ficial to the palmar surface of the DDFT.

A third approach involves entering the sheath in the triangular space bordered by the upper part of the proximal digital annular ligament, the base of the sesamoid, the flexor tendons and the palmar aspect of the first phalanx.

Midcarpal joint
- Needle: 20G × 1 in (2.5 cm).
- Volume: 10 ml.
- Site: With the carpus flexed, on the dorsal surface of the joint just lateral to the extensor carpi radialis tendon, between the proximal and distal rows of carpal bones. The midcarpal joint usually communicates with the carpometacarpal joint, which will, therefore, also be desensitized by this procedure.

Antebrachiocarpal joint
- Needle: 20G × 1 in (2.5 cm).
- Volume: 10 ml.
- Site: With the carpus flexed, on the dorsal surface of the joint just lateral to the extensor carpi radialis tendon, between the distal radius and the proximal row of carpal bones.

Elbow
- Needle: 19G × 2 in (5 cm).
- Volume: 15 ml.
- Site: Just cranial or caudal to the lateral collat-eral ligament. The joint space can usually be appreciated by careful palpation.

Shoulder
- Needle: 19G × 3 in (8 cm) spinal needle.
- Volume: 20 ml.
- Site: Advance the needle between the cranial and caudal prominences of the lateral tuberosity of the humerus, at a 45 degree angle to the long axis of the horse and slightly proximodistally.

Tarsometatarsal joint
- Needle: 20G × 1 in (2.5 cm).
- Volume: 5 ml.
- Site: Over the proximal end of the fourth meta-tarsal bone between it and the 4th tarsal bone. Needle angled at 45 degrees distally and slightly axially.

Distal intertarsal joint
- Needle: 20G × 1 in (2.5 cm).
- Volume: 5 ml.
- Site: Advance the needle in a mediolateral direction in the proximal extent of the interosseus space between the second and third tarsal bones and the central tarsal bone.

Tarsocrural joint
- Needle: 20G × 1 in (2.5 cm).
- Volume: 15 ml.
- Site: Into the dorsomedial pouch of the joint, just medial or lateral to the saphenous vein.

Femoropatellar joint
- Needle: 20G × 2 in (5 cm).
- Volume: 20 ml.
- Site: Medial or lateral to the middle patellar ligament just distal to the distal border of the patella. The needle is directed caudoproximally. The femoropatellar joint communicates with the medial femorotibial joint in at least 65% of horses.

An alternative approach involves injection into the lateral cul-de-sac of the femoropatellar joint just caudal to the lateral patellar ligament and 5 cm proximal to the lateral condyle of the tibia.

Medial femorotibial joint
- Needle: 20G × 2 in (5 cm).
- Volume: 20 ml.
- Site: Between the medial patellar ligament and the medial collateral ligament just proximal to the tibial plateau.

Lateral femorotibial joint
- Needle: 20G × 2 in (5 cm).
- Volume: 20 ml.
- Site: Between the tendon of origin of the long digital extensor and the lateral collateral ligament of the femorotibial joint, just proximal to the tibia.

Arthrocentesis and analysis of synovial fluid

Joint fluid is a dialysis product of plasma to which hyaluronic acid (HA) is added. Its composition is determined by the permeability of the joint membrane. Inflammation of a joint leads to depolymerization of normal HA, and the permeability barrier is disturbed resulting in joint effusion. Changes in joint fluid reflect the degree of synovial membrane inflammation.

1. *Gross appearance of fluid.*
   - Normal: pale yellow, translucent and free of debris.
   - Trauma: haemorrhagic, dark yellow or amber, with flocculent material.
   - Infection: serofibrinous, fibrinopurulent, turbid, cloudy.
   - Degenerative joint disease (DJD): minimal changes.
2. *Volume.*
   - Trauma: increased.
   - Chronic DJD: increased, or rarely decreased.
   - Infection: increased.
3. *Clotting test in plain tube.*
   - Normal: no clot formation because lack of fibrinogen.
   - Abnormal: speed of clot formation relates to the degree of inflammation.
4. *Total protein.*
   - Normal: 18 ± 2 g/l.
   - Inflammation: 20–40 g/l.
   - Infection: >40 g/l.
5. *Viscosity.*
   - Normal: 5 to 7 cm string from syringe; 2.5 to 5 cm string between fingers.
   - Abnormal: from reduced viscosity to watery.
6. *Cytology.*
   - WBC count.
   Normal: 0.2×10^9/l; $<10\%$ neutrophils, some lymphocytes and mononuclear cells.
   Trauma: 0.5–10×10^9/l; neutrophils increased.
   DJD: 0.5–1×10^9/l.
   Infection: $>50 \times 10^9$/l; $>90\%$ neutrophils.
7. *Culture.* In approximately 50% of cases of septic synovitis, no organisms are found in synovial fluid because bacteria are sequestrated in the synovial membrane, joint fluid is bactericidal, or antibiotics have been previously administered. A higher culture rate can be obtained by using enrichment broths, anaerobic as well as aerobic cultures, and culturing synovial membrane biopsies as well as synovial fluid samples.
8. *pH.* The pH is the only factor in infectious joint disease that will remain unaffected by previous administration of intra-articular corticosteroids.
   - Normal: >6.9.
   - Infection: <6.9.
9. *Markers of cartilage degeneration.* The search for a quantitative marker of DJD has led to the attempt to analyse joint fluid for the presence of cartilage particles after filtration of the synovial fluid sample. Although this has proved to be an inconsistent technique, new promising biochemical markers of proteoglycan and collagen breakdown are presently under investigation.

Radiography

Following identification of the site of pain during the clinical examination, the next step in a logical sequence is to image this area with radiography, ultrasonography and/or scintigraphy.

Foot

A complete radiographic examination of the equine foot usually consists of four different views:

- Lateromedial (LM).
- Two dorsoproximal-palmarodistal oblique (DPr-PaDiO) ('upright pedal' or 'high coronary route') (i) centred and exposed for the distal phalanx (ii) centred and exposed for the navicular bone.
- Palmaroproximal-palmarodistal oblique (PaPr-PaDiO) ('flexor' or 'skyline' view).

Other oblique views can be useful when fractures of the wings of the third phalanx are suspected, or abnormalities of the hoof wall are investigated.

Pastern

- Lateromedial (LM).
- Dorsopalmar (DPa).

Oblique views are occasionally obtained to highlight the palmarolateral and palmaromedial borders of the first phalanx, onto which the distal sesamoidean ligaments insert.

Fetlock

- Dorsopalmar (DPa).
- Lateromedial (LM).
- Dorsolateral-palmaromedial oblique (DL-PaMO).
- Palmarolateral-dorsomedial oblique (PaL-DMO).

These four standard projections can be supplemented with different specialized views if a particular area of the fetlock requires further highlighting.

Carpus

- Lateromedial (LM).
- Dorsopalmar (DPa).
- Dorsolateral-palmaromedial oblique (DL-PaMO).
- Palmarolateral-dorsomedial oblique (PaL-DMO).
- Flexed lateromedial (flexed LM).
- Dorsoproximal-dorsodistal oblique (skyline) (DPr-DDiO) – taken at varying angles to skyline the distal radius or proximal or distal rows of carpal bones.

Elbow

- Flexed mediolateral (flexed ML).
- Craniocaudal (CrCa).

Shoulder

- Extended mediolateral (extended ML).
- Craniomedial-caudolateral oblique (CrM-CaLO).

Hock

- Lateromedial (LM).
- Dorsoplantar (DPl).
- Dorsolateral-plantaromedial oblique (DL-PlMO).
- Plantarolateral-dorsomedial oblique (PlL-DMO).

Additional view: Plantaroproximal-plantarodistal oblique (PlPr-PlDiO) – 'skyline' of the sustentaculum tali.

Stifle

- Lateromedial (LM).
- Caudocranial (CaCr).

Additional views:
- Cranioproximal-craniodistal oblique (CrPr-CrDiO) – 'skyline' of the patella.
- Oblique variations on the CaCr.

Hip

- Ventrodorsal.

Ultrasonography

Principles

Ultrasonography involves the use of high frequency sound waves to image the soft tissues of the body. Sound waves of frequencies usually in excess of 2 MHz are emitted from a transducer. Sound is reflected from interfaces between tissues of different physical characteristics (acoustic impedance). The percentage reflected varies in proportion to the degree of difference in acoustic impedance of the regions. Reflected sound is received either by separate transducers in the emitting equipment (or 'probe'), or more commonly periods of emission are followed by periods of 'listening' by the same transducer.

The most commonly used equipment for examining equine tendons and joints is 7.5 MHz sector or linear array probe.

Technique

Ultrasonographic examination of tendons and ligaments in the distal fore- and hindlimbs must follow a methodical approach that allows comparative views to be taken of contralateral limbs and for follow-up examination.

Metacarpal region (Figure 2)
The probe is applied to the palmar aspect of the metacarpus in a horizontal (transverse) fashion. Seven equidistant levels are chosen between the accessory carpal bone and the ergot of the fetlock (levels 1 to 7). This allows sequential identifica-

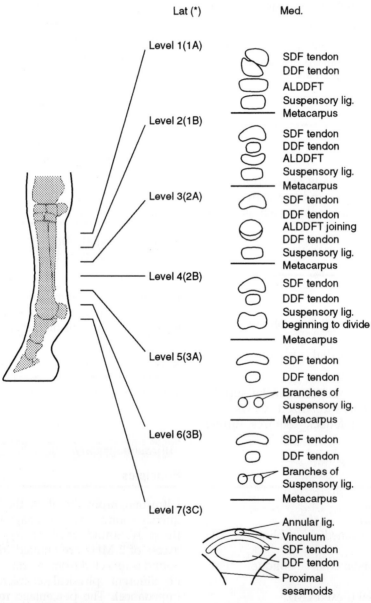

Figure 2 Ultrasonographic appearance of the soft tissues on the palmar aspect of the distal limb (courtesy of R.K. Smith and P.M. Webbon. *The Athletic Horse, Principles and Practice of Equine Sports Medicine* 1994. Editors D.R. Hodgson and R.J. Rose. W.B. Saunders Co, Philadelphia. pp. 300–302).
SDF – superficial digital flexor; DDF – deep digital flexor; SL – suspensory ligament; ALDDFT – accessory ligament of the deep digital flexor tendon (inferior check ligament).

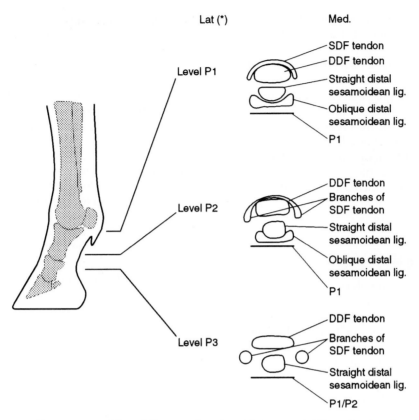

Figure 3 Ultrasonographic appearance of the soft tissues on the palmar/plantar aspect of the pastern (courtesy of R.K. Smith and P.M. Webbon. *The Athletic Horse, Principles and Practice of Equine Sports Medicine* 1994. Editors D.R. Hodgson and R.J. Rose. W.B. Saunders Co, Philadelphia. pp. 300–302).
SDF – superficial digital flexor; DDF – deep digital flexor.

tion of the SDFT, the DDFT, the accessory ligament of the DDFT (inferior check ligament), the SL and its branches, and the annular ligament of the fetlock.

Three longitudinal views (levels 1 to 3) are then taken with the probe in line with the tendons.

Pastern region (Figure 3)
The probe is applied to the palmar/plantar aspect of the pastern and three transverse views are assessed (levels 1 to 3).

Identifiable structures are the proximal digital annular ligament (if enlarged), the branches of the SDFT, the DDFT and the distal sesamoidean ligaments (middle and straight).

One longitudinal view (PL) is also usually assessed.

Interpretation

Significant alterations in the ultrasonograms of tendons may involve:

1. Changes in echogenicity:
   - Hypoechoic/anechoic areas ('black holes') in acute tendon injuries represent the presence of fluid, granulation tissue, or young fibrous tissue (in order of increasing echogenicity).
   - Hyperechoic ('brighter') areas in a healed tendon injury represent fibrosis.
   - Calcification may cause acoustic shadowing. The calcified area reflects almost all of the sound.
2. Changes in cross-sectional size of tendons/ ligaments. The size should be compared to that of the same structures in the unaffected leg.
3. Changes in shape/position.
4. Changes in margination/outline which may indicate the formation of peritendinous adhesions.

Indications for the use of ultrasonography

1. Diagnosis. Ultrasonography of swollen palmar metacarpal soft tissues allows identification of

the structure(s) involved, and enables more accurate assessment of the severity of the damage.

2. Prevention of more severe injury. Ultrasonography allows an accurate assessment of the subtle signs that are harbingers of severe injury. If these are recognized the horse can be withdrawn from strenuous exercise and treated before the tendon fails.
3. Ultrasonographic monitoring of healing is useful in the management of tendon injuries.
4. Ultrasonography is increasingly used to assess joint disease.

Nuclear scintigraphy

Nuclear scintigraphy involves administration of a radioactive nucleotide that is conjugated to a compound that becomes preferentially located in a particular body system or lesion. The level of uptake at a particular site can then be determined using a detecting or imaging system to record the radiation emitted from that site at a particular time after administration.

The isotope most commonly employed in evaluation of the skeletal system is technetium 99m which emits gamma radiation at 140 keV with a half-life of 6 hours. This is usually linked to methylene diphosphonate or hydroxymethane diphosphonate, which is taken up into the mineral lattice of bone at a level dependent on the rate of bone turnover at a particular site. Sites that have a high rate of bone turnover for physiological or pathological reasons, therefore, accumulate more of the nucleotide than normal, and this is reflected in increased gamma radiation being emitted from that particular site.

The use of bone scintigraphy in the horse lies mainly in the recognition of stress injuries to the skeleton (i.e. fatigue fractures).

Thermography

Thermography is a non-invasive diagnostic technique that allows quantitative visualization of changes in skin surface temperature. The infrared radiation that is emitted from the skin is converted into electrical impulses, which are converted into computer images. The major diagnostic value of thermography is its ability to detect early soft tissue inflammation (e.g. early tendinitis) before clinical signs develop.

Diagnostic arthroscopy

Arthroscopy allows direct inspection of synovial cavities including joints and tendon sheaths. It allows evaluation of the non-osseous tissues of the joint, i.e. the cartilage, the synovial membrane and the intra-articular ligaments and menisci, all of which may be difficult to assess by other means.

- The equipment consists of a 4 mm wide telescope with a 25° forward angle of view. The telescope is connected to fibreoptic light. This scope is inserted into the joint through a 5 mm arthroscopic sleeve. This sleeve has a connection for fluid inflow into the joint.
- The technique (Figure 4) relies on distension of the joint with sterile balanced electrolyte solution

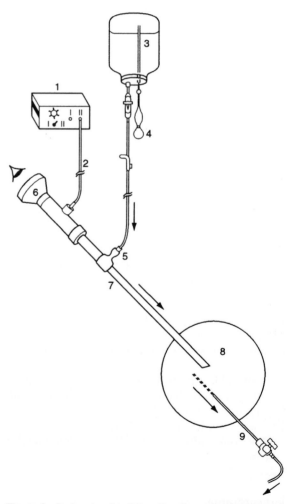

Figure 4 Basic set-up for diagnostic arthroscopy. 1. Light source. 2. Light transmitting cable. 3. Fluid source. 4. Pressure bulb. 5. Inflow stop cock. 6. Telescope (4 mm). 7. Telescope sleeve (5 mm). 8. Distended joint. 9. Drainage cannula.

(Hartmann's solution). Once distended, it becomes possible to push the narrow sleeve through a stab incision in the tense joint capsule with a conical trocar with little risk of damaging the intra-articular structures (i.e. cartilage). Only a small stab incision in the skin is needed, which is later closed with a single suture. Once the position of the sleeve is ascertained inside the joint, the trocar is exchanged for the telescope. Inflow of fluid is necessary to maintain joint distension during the procedure. This allows for better visualization.

- Applications in the horse are numerous. All equine joints are fully or partially amenable to arthroscopic examination.
- Indications for diagnostic arthroscopy in the horse include persistent intra-articular pain and/or pathological changes seen in radiographs. The technique is now widely regarded as the preferred method for most joint surgery.

15.2 *Joint diseases*

Idiopathic synovitis

Definition

Chronic synovial effusion of a joint or tendon sheath of uncertain pathogenesis and often unassociated with pain or lameness. Examples include articular and tendinous 'windgalls' at the fetlock (distension of the metacarpo/metatarsophalangeal joint or digital synovial sheath respectively) and 'bog spavin' in the hock (distension of the tarsocrural joint).

Aetiopathogenesis

Presumed to be due to a low grade synovitis as a result of minor trauma or abnormal stresses due to poor conformation. May be self-perpetuating once present, due to stretching of the synovial membrane and joint capsule. Usually no radiographic abnormalities are present.

Treatment

- Treatment is usually unnecessary if there is no functional disturbance or evidence of an underlying problem (e.g. osteochondrosis in young horses).

- In young horses the swellings may spontaneously resolve as the horse reaches maturity.
- Drainage of the synovial fluid is possible but must be done under aseptic conditions – rapid refilling of the synovial cavity with excess fluid is common.
- Drainage may be followed by attempts to prevent recurrence by bandaging or injection of corticosteroids or hyaluronic acid. However, recurrence is still common.

Traumatic arthritis

Aetiology

- Single event trauma.
- Chronic repetitive trauma.

Pathogenesis

See osteoarthritis – the dividing line between traumatic arthritis and osteoarthritis is really one of degree, chronicity and reversibility, i.e. if the disease becomes persistent and progressive it should be referred to as osteoarthritis.

Pathology

The following pathological conditions may be present individually or in varying combinations.

- Synovitis.
- Capsulitis.
- Articular cartilage damage.
- Articular fracture.
- Ligamentous injury.
- Luxation/subluxation.
- Subchondral bone sclerosis or lysis.

Clinical signs

- Lameness.
- Joint swelling.
- Synovial effusion.
- Periarticular soft tissue swelling.
- Pain on joint manipulation – particularly forced flexion.
- Heat – increased surface temperature over joint.
- Instability/crepitus – if severe ligament or bone damage are present.
- Later – chronic thickening and reduced range of movement.

Further tests

- Radiography.
  - For fractures.
  - Immediately and 7–10 days later if results inconclusive.
  - For evidence of pre-existing or secondary osteoarthritis.
- Synovial fluid analysis.
  - White blood cell total and differential.
  - Total protein.
- Diagnostic arthroscopy – for synovitis, cartilage damage, intra-articular fractures and ligamentous injury.

Treatment

- Box rest and later a progressive programme of controlled exercise.
- Cold application locally over first 24–48 hours.
- Support bandaging.
- Non-steroidal anti-inflammatory drugs (NSAIDs).
- Single dose of short acting corticosteroid in selected cases of synovitis/capsulitis.
- Polysulphated glycosaminoglycan.
- Hyaluronic acid.
- Joint lavage.
- Specific surgery for fractures etc.

Osteoarthritis (degenerative joint disease)

Definition

Progressive destruction of the articular cartilage of a joint accompanied by changes in the bones (marginal osteophytes, subchondral sclerosis or lysis) and soft tissues (capsular fibrosis, villous hypertrophy) of a joint.

Classification

Equine osteoarthritis (OA) has been classified in a variety of ways.

1. Primary OA
   - Probably due to chronic repetitive trauma in most cases.
   - Risk factors may be inherent e.g. breed, age, sex, conformation; or external, e.g. occupation.
   - Systemic predisposition may relate to properties of the tissues involved, e.g. cartilage and bone; while expression, site and severity may be determined by use etc. (i.e. local biomechanical factors).

2. Secondary OA – the consequence of other joint diseases including:
   - Traumatic arthritis.
   - Articular fracture.
   - Osteochondrosis.
   - Septic arthritis.

Pathogenesis

The pathogenesis of OA involves both *mechanical* disruption of the articular surface and the destructive effects of a number of *chemical mediators*.

Chemical mediators of OA:

1. Cytokines, e.g. interleukin 1 (IL-1), tumour necrosis factor (TNFα).
   - May act as messengers from synoviocytes or leucocytes to activate chondrocytes to produce enzymes.
   - Reduce proteoglycan synthesis by chondrocytes.
2. Enzymes
   - Extracellular neutral metalloproteinases, e.g. proteoglycanase (stromelysin).
   - Collagenase.
   - Gelatinases.
   - Lysosomal enzymes – cathepsins, glycosidases etc.
3. Inflammatory mediators
   - Eicosanoids (prostaglandins, thromboxane).
   - Leukotrienes.
   - Kinins.
   - Histamine, 5HT.
   - Nitric oxide.
4. Free radicals
   - Superoxide.
   - Hydroxyl.
5. Antibodies – complement factors.

The initial result of these mechanical and chemical insults is breakdown and loss of proteoglycans from the articular cartilage. The cartilage thereby loses its stiffness and becomes soft which predisposes it to further mechanical disruption. It also increases its permeability to destructive enzymes and impairs chondrocyte nutrition. Proteoglycan loss *per se* is probably reversible provided the chondrocytes and collagen framework remain intact. Collagen disruption is only seen at a later stage accompanied by gross evidence of fibrillation.

The causes of pain in OA are unclear, and possibly include raised intramedullary bone pressure and synovitis.

Osteophytes form at the marginal transition zone, i.e. at the junction of articular cartilage, synovial membrane and periosteum. They are probably produced by mesenchymal cells in response to substances released in inflamed or degenerate joints. They may represent an attempt by the joint to extend its surface area to reduce concussion and improve stability but at the expense of loss of range of movement.

Pathology

1. Cartilage
   - Gross.
     - Yellow discoloration.
     - Softening.
     - Dullness.
     - Surface fibrillation.
     - Erosion and ulceration.
   - Histological.
     - Chondrocyte death.
     - Fibrillation.
     - Reduced metachromasia.
   - Biochemical.
     - Proteoglycan depletion.
     - Increased water content.
     - Collagen disruption.
2. Soft tissue
   - Congestion and thickening.
   - Mononuclear infiltration.
   - Villous hypertrophy.
   - Capsular oedema and later fibrosis.
3. Bone
   - Marginal osteophytes and remodelling.
   - Subchondral sclerosis or lysis.
   - Articular fractures.
   - Increased subchondral bone pressure.

Although articular cartilage changes are the primary pathological characteristic of OA they are poorly correlated to the severity of either clinical signs or radiographic changes. As in other systems and diseases the pathological changes seen are a combination of the effects of the primary insult and the body's reactions and attempts at repair.

Clinical signs

- Lameness.
- Pain on manipulation.
- Positive response to joint flexion.
- Thickening.
- Reduced range of movement.
- Crepitus.

Note – there are frequently few localizing clinical signs in chronic OA in horses and local analgesia to eliminate the lameness is often the only way to identify the joint concerned. Scintigraphy may also be of use in this regard.

Diagnosis

Imaging techniques
- Radiology.
  - Periarticular new bone formation (osteophytes).
  - Subchondral sclerosis/lysis.
  - Narrowed joint space (only in very severe cases).
  - Radiological changes occur relatively late and may correlate poorly with clinical signs.
- Scintigraphy.
  - Increased nucleotide uptake may predict radiographic changes.
- Magnetic resonance imaging. Can see changes in cartilage and other soft tissues. Not generally available yet.

Biochemical markers
A variety of substances have been measured in synovial fluid, blood or urine as markers of OA. These include:

- Fragments released on matrix degradation, e.g. keratan sulphate.
- Products of attempted repair.
- Mediators of matrix degradation, e.g. proteases, cytokines.
- Byproducts of inflammation.

Treatment

Treatment of established OA is often unrewarding in terms of sustained return to athletic activity.

- Controlled light exercise/swimming etc.
- Correct overweight and any foot imbalance.
- Intra-articular.
  - PSGAGs.
  - Hyaluronic acid.
- NSAIDs.
- Surgical arthrodesis of low motion joints, e.g. small intertarsal and pastern joints.

Osteochondrosis

Osteochondrosis involves defective endochondral ossification leading to failure of conversion of cartilage into bone. In dogs and horses the condition particularly affects the articular surface resulting in a specific manifestation of osteochondrosis referred to as osteochondritis dissecans (OCD). As the articular surface cartilage fails to ossify in its deepest layers, it becomes thicker than normal and the chondrocytes become further away from their source of nutrition – the synovial fluid. Eventually they die. The deep layers of cartilage then undergo necrosis and fissures form, which may then extend to the articular surface to form a cartilage flap. The flap may undergo partial ossification to form an osteochondral fragment.

Osteochondrosis is one of a number of conditions (including angular and flexural limb deformities, physitis and the 'wobbler' syndrome) that have been grouped together under the heading of 'developmental orthopaedic disease' because of potential similarities in their aetiopathogenesis. Because the initial lesion of 'osteochondrosis' occurs in cartilage rather than bone the term 'dyschondroplasia' has been suggested as a potentially better name.

The aetiology of osteochondrosis is poorly understood and probably multifactorial. Important factors probably include rapid growth, dietary energy levels and mineral imbalances, endocrinological dysfunction, biomechanical trauma and heredity.

1. Rapid growth rate – particularly spurts of growth which may follow a growth setback for example caused by a period of poor nutrition.
   Growth rate is in turn determined by:
   • Genetic factors.
   • Intensive feeding (especially excess soluble carbohydrates).
2. Mineral imbalance
   • High phosphorus diets.
   • Copper deficiency.
   (Possibly high zinc and cadmium diets).
3. Mechanical trauma
   • May account for site specificity within joints.
   • May cause separation of already defective cartilage (pathological fracture).
   • Excessive weight will increase use trauma.
   • Conversely exercise may have a protective effect against osteochondrosis in the face of high energy diets.
4. Hormonal factors
   • Growth hormone, insulin, thyroid hormone, sex hormones.

   • High postprandial insulin concentrations may inhibit growth hormone which is necessary for cartilage maturation.
5. Heredity
   • There are reported increases in incidence in the offspring of some stallions. However, clinically and radiologically normal stallions may produce affected foals making the implementation of screening programmes difficult.

Epidemiology

Clinical signs usually arise during the growth period, from birth to 2–3 years of age. Sometimes the condition may not become clinically obvious until affected horses are put into work.

Most case series show a predominance of male animals (2:1 male:female).

There are breed variations in overall and individual joint incidence, e.g. OCD of the distal intermediate ridge of the tibia in the hock seems to be most common in Standardbreds. Ponies seem to have a low incidence of osteochondrosis.

Clinical signs

• Lameness, stiffness, positive response to flexion.
• Joint effusion is common especially in the stifle and the hock.

Diagnosis

• Radiography.
• Arthroscopy.

Treatment

Both conservative and surgical methods of treatment are utilized. Conservative treatment consists primarily of rest and correcting dietary input to achieve even and appropriate growth rates.

Surgery comprises debridement and removal of separated or partially attached osteochondral fragments and abnormal subchondral bone. This is usually done under arthroscopic visualization.

Subchondral bone cysts (osseous cyst-like lesions)

Radiographically detectable cystic lesions in the subchondral bone which often communicate with the articular surface have been reported in a number of joints including the medial femorotibial, carpus, pastern, coffin, fetlock, elbow, shoulder and hock.

Aetiopathogenesis

There are conflicting opinions as to the cause of subchondral bone cysts.

1. They may be a manifestation of osteochondrosis with thickened necrotic cartilage persisting as a localized defect within the subchondral bone.
2. They may result from localized trauma damaging primarily either
   - The articular cartilage.
   - The underlying subchondral bone.

Clinical signs

- Lameness localisable to a joint cavity – often few other signs.

Diagnosis

- Radiography.

Treatment

Both conservative (rest) and surgical treatment have been described.

Surgery usually consists of debridement of the cyst via an articular or extra-articular approach depending on the joint involved. Additional procedures such as forage of the bone surrounding the cyst or packing the cyst with an autogenous cancellous bone graft are sometimes performed.

Septic arthritis

Aetiology

Organisms involved include:

- Coliforms.
- *Staphylococcus aureus*.
- *Streptococci*.

In foals *Salmonella*, *Rhodococcus equi* and *Actinobacillus* are also found.

Pathogenesis

In adult horses infection is usually the result of a penetrating wound involving the joint or extension from a site of local infection close to a joint.

Kick wounds adjacent to the hock or elbow are a common cause. Infection may be iatrogenic following arthrocentesis or surgery.

In foals infection may spread to joints via the haematogenous route and multiple joints may be involved. The initial source of infection may be the umbilicus, pneumonia or enteritis. Failure of passive transfer of immunoglobulins may predispose. The same organisms may also colonize metaphyseal or epiphyseal bone leading to osteomyelitis.

Articular cartilage is rapidly destroyed by enzymes from bacteria, white blood cells and inflamed synovial membrane. These cause proteoglycan and collagen breakdown. Cartilage nutrition is compromised by extensive fibrin clots that form in the joint.

Clinical signs

- Lameness – often severe especially in adult horses.
- Joint swelling, heat and pain.
- May be an accompanying regional cellulitis that may mask the specific joint effusion.
- Variable systemic signs of pyrexia, leucocytosis, neutrophilia etc. – not always present.

Diagnosis

1. Synovial fluid analysis
   - Increased volume, turbid, clots, low viscosity.
   - Increased WBC count $>50 \times 10^9/l$; $>90\%$ neutrophils.
   - Protein $>40 \, g/l$.
   - Culture – into blood culture medium initially.
2. Radiography
   - Soft tissue swelling.
   - Subchondral bone destruction and periarticular new bone (in adult horses these changes occur late and the joint is usually beyond redemption by this stage).
   - Osteomyelitis of the epiphysis or metaphysis accompanying septic arthritis is quite common in foals.

Treatment

1. Drainage and lavage of the joint, with several litres of sterile polyionic fluid (e.g. Hartmann's solution). The use of continued drainage via implanted suction drains or open arthrotomies remains controversial but has been reported to

be successful. It may be particularly applicable to chronic or recurrent cases. It may be combined with repeated lavage via a tube drain or separate arthrocentesis puncture.

2. Synovectomy and removal of fibrin clots. (Both of these can be done arthroscopically in many joints – synovial membrane biopsies can also be obtained for culture at the same time. These procedures may need to be repeated if the response to initial treatment is unsatisfactory.)

3. Prolonged intensive antibiotic therapy preferably based on culture and sensitivity. Initial therapy with penicillin/gentamicin IV is often used. Local intrasynovial antibiotic therapy may also be used, e.g. gentamicin or amikacin.

4. Analgesia with NSAIDs, e.g. flunixin meglumine or phenylbutazone.

Treatment should be monitored in terms of improvement in clinical signs i.e. reduction in lameness, joint swelling, heat, pain on palpation/manipulation and reduction in discharge where appropriate. Sequential synovial fluid sampling may also be helpful in determining whether the inflammatory response is diminishing due to elimination of the infection.

Prognosis

The prognosis for established synovial infection is usually regarded as guarded. If treated *early* and *aggressively* the results can be rewarding particularly in adult horses where survival of up to 85% of cases has been recorded. The prognosis in foals is generally less good.

15.3 *Fractures*

Classification

Fractures may be classified in a variety of ways with reference to the characteristics listed below. This allows a concise description which has relevance in relation to management and prognosis.

1. Direction and anatomical location of fracture line
   - Transverse.
   - Oblique.
   - Longitudinal.
   - Spiral.
   - Comminuted – three or more major fragments present.
   - Multiple – more than one bone fractured.
   - Diaphyseal.
   - Metaphyseal.
   - Physeal/epiphyseal (Salter-Harris subclassification).
   - Articular – involving a joint surface.

2. Relative displacement of fragments.
   - Overriding.
   - Distracted.
   - Impacted.
   - Compression – usually applied to vertebral fractures.
   - Folding.
   - Depression – usually with reference to skull fractures.

3. Complete/incomplete.

4. Open (compound)/closed.

5. Stable/unstable.

6. Monotonic/fatigue/pathological.

7. Complicated – involving damage to other organs or systems.

Clinical signs

- Pain (and therefore lameness).
- Swelling.
- Deformity.
- Abnormal mobility.
- Loss of function.
- Crepitus.

It is important to note that incomplete undisplaced fractures, which are relatively common in the horse compared to other domestic species, will not cause evidence of deformity, instability or crepitus and that in some situations the degree of swelling may also be minimal. In these cases signs are therefore confined to lameness. If this is of acute onset and severe the possibility of a fracture should not be dismissed merely because the other signs are not present.

Fracture healing

Healing by callus

1. Inflammatory phase.
   - Vascular damage results in haemorrhage and haematoma formation.
   - Osteocytes at the bone ends are deprived of nutrition and die.
   - An acute inflammatory response ensues
     - Fibrin plug.
     - Platelet adherence.
     - White cells phagocytose debris.

2. Repair phase
   - Haematoma organizes as granulation tissue and serves as a scaffold for repair.
   - Pluripotential mesenchymal cells found perivascularly and from the periosteum, endosteum and muscle differentiate to form:
     - Fibrous tissue.
     - Cartilage.
     - Bone.
   - Cartilage progresses to form bone by endochondral ossification.
   - Reparative phase ends when the callus forms a rigid functional union.
3. Remodelling
   - Resorption and replacement of bone to restore normal architecture.

Primary bone healing

No fibrous tissue or cartilage is formed – repair is directly with bone.

1. Gap healing – newly formed bone lamellae are at right angles to original and remodelling with aligned osteones occurs later.
2. Contact healing – primary osteonal repair across the fracture site.

Complications of fracture healing

1. Infection – particularly following open reduction and internal fixation.
2. 'Fracture disease'.
   - Muscle atrophy.
   - Soft tissue adhesions.
   - Joint stiffness.
   - Osteoporosis.
3. Delayed union/malunion/non-union.
4. Laxity of the supporting soft tissues in immobilized limbs in foals.
5. Growth disturbance – in young animals – angular limb deformities in the contralateral limb due to excessive weight bearing.
6. Laminitis of the contralateral foot in adult horses.

Evaluation of equine fractures

Equine fractures vary in their severity and implications from catastrophic comminuted proximal limb bone fractures for which the only recourse may be euthanasia to small chip fractures that are candidates for routine elective surgery with a good prognosis for return to full athletic activity. Certain fractures appear to be occupational hazards, particularly in the racehorse, and may be a consequence of pre-existing physiological or pathological processes that predispose to failure. These fractures often have a predictable location and configuration and examples might include third carpal slab fractures and sagittal fractures of the first phalanx. Direct external trauma is another common cause of fractures. In small animals road traffic accidents are by far the commonest cause of such injuries. However, in horses, falls, collisions with fences and kicks from other horses account for the majority.

Before embarking on treatment it is important to have a clear idea of the likely prognosis in terms of the intended use of the horse, the likelihood of achieving that endpoint and whether fallback positions are acceptable. This requires a thorough evaluation of the fracture, the patient and also of the owner's aspirations. The financial implications of major surgical intervention and the attendant costs in aftercare in the short- and long-term also need to be discussed at an early stage.

Initial evaluation should attempt to answer the following questions:

1. Is a fracture present?
2. Which bone is fractured?
3. What is the likely configuration of the fracture? Try to evaluate the degree and direction of instability if this is present. Knowledge of the common fracture configurations in specific locations is useful.
4. Is the location and likely configuration of the fracture such that the prognosis is definitely hopeless and euthanasia should be performed without delay?
5. Are there any additional injuries that need to be taken into account – in particular are there associated wounds that might, or definitely have, resulted in contamination of the fracture site?

If treatment is still a possibility then priority should be given to *emergency stabilization* of the fracture followed by *comprehensive radiographic examination* to allow full evaluation.

Emergency stabilization

Objectives

1. Minimize additional damage to
   - Soft tissues – skin, blood vessels, nerves. (It is essential to preserve soft tissue cover to

prevent contamination and preserve potential blood supply to the fracture site).
- Bone ends – (movement between fracture ends causes bone eburnation which makes accurate reduction more difficult at surgery).
2. Allow horse to regain control of limb thereby reducing tendency to panic.
3. Provide a degree of pain relief.
4. Limit soft tissue swelling.

If skin penetration has occurred, clean the wound and cover with water soluble antibiotic ointment and a sterile dressing before immobilizing.

Forelimb

1. *Phalanges and distal metacarpus*. Stable (e.g. incomplete) fractures are probably best immobilized in a normal weight bearing position.

   Unstable fractures tend to bend at the fracture site rather than the fetlock and so should be stabilized with the fetlock straight by splinting along the dorsal surface of the limb from carpus to toe so that the dorsal cortices of the bones are in a straight line. This ensures axial loading and negates the tendency to bending at the fracture site. A splint should be taped to the dorsal surface of the limb over a light bandage and the limb cast or substantially bandaged to just below the carpus.
2. *Metacarpus, carpus and distal radius*. Splint from elbow to ground caudally and laterally over a substantial Robert Jones bandage.
3. *Mid and proximal radius*. As above but extend lateral splint up side of chest to prevent abduction of the distal limb and consequent penetration of the skin by bone fragments on the medial aspect of the radius (where there is little protective muscle).
4. *Elbow and proximally*. In the proximal limb the bones are generally well covered with muscle and splinted by the body wall. Attempts at additional splinting are often ineffective and possibly counterproductive by increasing the weight (and thus pendulum like effect) of the distal limb. Lightly splinting the carpus in extension has been suggested to help by enabling the horse to use the leg for balancing.

Hindlimb

1. *Distal metatarsus and phalanges*. As for forelimb.
2. *Mid and proximal metatarsus*. Caudal and lateral splints over a Robert Jones bandage. Caudal splint placed to top of tuber calcis.

3. *Hock and tibia*. Contoured lateral splint (e.g. aluminium tubing) from foot to lateral thigh applied over a Robert Jones bandage. As with radius, try to prevent abduction and consequent skin penetration medially.
4. *Femur*. No splinting.

Medication

1. Start intravenous broad-spectrum antibiotic therapy.
2. Analgesics.

Preferably do not sedate.

Radiography

Try to obtain at least two views of the whole fractured bone at right angles to each other. It is often necessary to obtain *multiple oblique views* of a complex fracture in order to gain a full understanding of its configuration prior to deciding prognosis and treatment.

If the horse is to be transported to another clinic for treatment consultation with surgical colleagues prior to referral most logically takes place *at this stage* when *the fracture is stabilized* and *the radiographs have been taken*.

Emergency transport

1. Minimize distance horse has to walk.
2. Van type horsebox probably preferable to trailer as is more stable. However, it may be more difficult for the horse to enter and leave.
3. Position with good legs at front to counteract braking.
4. Confine tightly and provide support with bales. Leave head and neck loose to aid balancing.
5. Restrain foals manually.

Surgical techniques

Surgical techniques for fracture management are continually changing and improving. The advent of arthroscopy allows both the removal of small articular 'chip' fractures, e.g. in the carpus and fetlock, and the accurate reduction of major displaced articular fractures, e.g. third carpal slab fractures and displaced metacarpal condylar fractures prior to screw fixation.

Major displaced fractures usually require stabilization with some form of internal fixation device, usually screws (commonly inserted as lag screws) or combinations of screws and bone plates. Techniques for the use of external fixation in the horse have also been described. The principles governing such fixation are:

- Aseptic technique – infection remains one of the most devastating complications of equine fracture surgery and every effort should be made to attain the highest possible standards of surgical asepsis.
- Reduction – accurate anatomical reduction, particularly of articular surfaces.
- Immobilization – rigid stabilization – often by interfragmentary compression using the lag screw principle and/or ASIF dynamic compression plates.
- Minimize soft tissue damage before, during and after surgery.
- Early controlled exercise to avoid the complications of fracture disease outlined above.

It is impossible to document here the methods used for internal fixation of every individual fracture encountered in the horse but some of the commonly treated fractures are listed below:

- Sagittal and parasagittal distal phalanx fractures – lag screw.
- Sagittal and frontal plane proximal phalanx fractures – lag screws.
- Proximal sesamoid bone fractures – lag screw or wire.
- Condylar fractures of the distal third metacarpal/metatarsal bone – lag screws.
- Transverse/oblique fractures of the third metacarpal/metatarsal bone – compression plate.
- Carpal slab fractures – lag screw.
- Olecranon fractures – compression plate.
- Chip fractures of the fetlock and carpus – arthroscopic removal.

Not all equine fractures need surgery. Some minimally displaced or incomplete fractures will heal satisfactorily with conservative treatment – examples include certain 'stress' fractures seen particularly in young racehorses (e.g. third metacarpal bone, tibia, humerus, pelvis), some incomplete proximal phalangeal and lateral condylar fractures, many splint bone fractures, some accessory carpal bone fractures and non-articular third phalanx fractures.

Proximal limb bone fractures in adult horses are very difficult to reduce and stabilize adequately at surgery. Sustained traction with ropes and pulleys or an overhead hoist may aid reduction of overriding fractures. Technical advances and increasing experience will undoubtedly improve success rates in the future but euthanasia still remains the only realistic option for some equine fractures.

Fractures in smaller equines, i.e. foals/yearlings and small pony breeds, are easier to treat in mechanical terms though 'youthful exuberance' postoperatively can complicate management and disrupt fixation. Most reported cases of successful proximal longbone fracture in the horse have been in younger animals.

Aftercare

1. External support

Following fracture treatment most surgical wounds should at least be covered in the immediate postoperative period to prevent contamination. Bandaging may help to limit soft tissue swelling in response to the surgery and when combined with splints may provide some support for a fracture. Casting is appropriate to some major distal limb fractures for the recovery process, e.g. major fractures of P2, P1, Mc/Mt III, carpus and possibly distal radius and hock. Fractures proximal to these sites do not benefit from cast support and casting may be positively detrimental.

2. Recovery

Anaesthetic regimens that lead to a quiet and coordinated recovery should be used. Sedation in the recovery box may also help. Assisting recovery with ropes attached to the head collar and tail can help to stabilize horses in the standing position and prevent multiple attempts at standing which can overload implants.

3. Antibiosis

Antibiotic cover should be provided for all fracture cases where implants are used.

4. Analgesia

Horses undergoing fracture fixation usually require perioperative analgesia.

5. Confinement and exercise

Most horses undergoing fracture treatment require a period of postoperative box rest, the duration of which will vary according to the specific fracture. Exercise should start with short periods of walking in hand which are gradually increased in duration and eventually replaced with ridden walking and trotting exercise. Controlled ridden exercise is usually better than 'turning the horse out' to convalesce.

15.4 *Other bone diseases*

Osteomyelitis

Osteomyelitis is an infection involving the bone cortex and medullary cavity.

Aetiopathogenesis

Routes of infection:

- Haematogenous – usually in foals less than 4 months of age.
- Penetrating wounds
  - Traumatic or surgical.
  - Particularly in association with internal fixation of fractures where the presence of implants tends to promote the persistence of infection.
- Extension from contiguous infected focus.

Organisms are usually similar to those listed for septic arthritis, i.e. coliforms, *Staphylococci* and *Streptococci*.

Haematogenous localization usually occurs in the metaphysis or epiphysis due to sluggish blood flow within the large venous sinusoids. Infection may spread from the bone into adjacent soft tissues or into the joint.

Diaphyseal osteomyelitis is usually a consequence of open reduction and internal fixation of fractures.

Treatment

- Surgical drainage of exudate.
- Removal of infected or necrotic material.
- Stabilization – provided that implants are maintaining stability they should be left until such time as the fracture has healed at which time they should be removed.
- Antibiotic therapy.
- Bone grafting.

Prognosis

Established osteomyelitis is a very serious condition with a guarded prognosis. Infected fracture sites containing implants may still heal provided stability can be maintained. The infection will then often resolve once the implants are removed. If infection results in instability due to major implant loosening or breakage, healing will not occur and unless stability can be achieved by further intervention the animal will be permanently incapacitated.

Osteitis

Osteitis is an infection of the bone cortex.

Aetiopathogenesis

Usually a consequence of traumatic open wounds, particularly in the metacarpus/metatarsus. Such trauma exposes cortical bone, disrupts the periosteum and compromises the blood supply to the outer cortex. Such wounds are inevitably contaminated and the vascular disruption allows infection to become established. The devascularized outer cortex separates from the underlying bone to form a sequestrum and infection persists.

Treatment

Traditionally, surgical debridement and removal of necrotic and infected tissue – particularly dead bone – is performed.

Medical management with antibiotics and local wound irrigation can be successful in some cases with small sequestrae.

Physitis

There is enlargement of the physeal region of longbones in growing horses.

Aetiopathogenesis

The aetiology is unclear. It is seen in rapidly growing young horses and may be related to other developmental orthopaedic disorders including osteochondrosis.

Clinical signs

There is widening of the bone at the level of the physis. The metaphysis thus flares out adjacent to the physis, particularly at the level of the distal radius, tibia and metacarpus/metatarsus. Variable lameness/stiffness may occur. It may be seen in conjunction with other developmental orthopaedic diseases including angular limb deformities, osteochondrosis, flexural deformities and wobbler syndrome.

Radiology

Flaring of the metaphysis and epiphysis adjacent to the physis may be seen, and also irregularity of the physis and surrounding sclerosis.

Treatment

Treatment comprises reduction of energy content of ration to slow growth, ensuring correct mineral balance in ration, rest, NSAIDs.

Nutritional secondary hyperparathyroidism (bran disease, big head, osteodystrophia fibrosa)

Aetiopathogenesis

- Due to relative calcium deficiency and excess phosphate.
- Low calcium leads to increased secretion of PTH and bone resorption.
- Exclusively grain diets (e.g. bran) without hay or mineral supplementation may have such a calcium/phosphorus imbalance.
- The flat bones of the jaw and skull appear to be preferentially affected in the horse.

Clinical signs

- Symmetrical enlargement of the mandible and facial bones.
- May lead to loosening of teeth.

Treatment

Treatment consists of dietary correction and mineral supplementation.

Hereditary multiple exostoses (multiple cartilaginous exostoses, osteochondroma)

This is a rare inherited congenital condition involving multiple abnormal bony projections from long bones, ribs and pelvis. Solitary osteochondromas also occur especially on the caudal aspect of the distal radius (see carpus). They usually do not continue to grow beyond skeletal maturity of the animal. Single lesions may be amenable to surgical removal.

Tumoral calcinosis

Calcified, granular amorphous deposits occur in the subcutaneous tissues usually near joints or tendon sheaths, particularly on the lateral aspect of the stifle where it is frequently firmly attached to the joint capsule. If associated with lameness they may be surgically removed but as this may involve removing a portion of joint capsule there are associated risks of wound breakdown, poor healing and septic arthritis.

Rickets

Rickets is caused by vitamin D deficiency but is *very rare* in horses. Vitamin D is normally ingested in plant material or formed in the skin in response to sunlight. Deficiency is therefore uncommon. It results in metaphyseal flaring and bowing of the extremities but other conditions such as physitis and angular limb deformities are much more common causes of such signs.

Hypertrophic osteopathy (hypertrophic pulmonary osteoarthropathy, Marie's disease)

Aetiopathogenesis

It is classically associated with space occupying pulmonary lesions, e.g. tumours, abscesses, tuberculosis, and has also been reported in association with abdominal lesions, e.g. ovarian dysgerminoma.

Suggested disease mechanisms include neural pathways involving the vagus nerve and humoral factors such as elevated oestrogen levels.

Clinical signs

- Symmetrical limb swelling.
- Oedema.

Radiology

- Periostitis particularly at the proximal and distal ends of the long bones.

Osteoporosis

Aetiopathogenesis

Osteoporosis is usually seen as a consequence of disuse after severe protracted lameness or after application of external immobilization in the form of a cast. It occurs most dramatically in foals after casting and can result in pathological fracture if severe.

Radiology

Bones appear generally less radiodense than normal and cortices appear thin. In the distal limb the proximal sesamoid bones are often the most dramatically affected (sometimes referred to as 'ghost' sesamoids).

Treatment

Treatment comprises gradual removal of support and return to normal activity. Casts should be removed as soon as possible in foals and replaced with bandages and splints which are progressively removed to reduce the risk of pathological fracture.

Fluorosis

Aetiopathogenesis

- Ingestion of toxic amounts of fluorine in food or water – usually a result of industrial contamination via effluent or fumes.

Clinical signs

- Generalized stiffness, lameness and unthriftiness.
- Exostoses particularly on the metacarpus/metatarsus.
- Mottling of the teeth.

Radiology

- Osteoporosis and exostosis formation.

Treatment

- Removal from source of contamination.

Further reading

Butler, J.A., Colles, C.M., Dyson, S.J., Kold, S.E. and Poulos, P.W. (1993) *Clinical Radiology of the Horse*. Blackwell Scientific Publications, Oxford.

Nixon, A. (1996) *Equine Fractures*.

Stashak, T.S. (1987) *Adam's Lameness in Horses*. Lea & Febiger, Philadelphia.

Wyn-Jones, G. (1988) *Equine Lameness*. Blackwell Scientific Publications, Oxford.

16 Orthopaedics 2. Diseases of the foot and lower limbs

CONTENTS

16.1 Diseases of the foot

Cracks of the hoofwall

Classification

Vertical defects in the hoofwall occur along the direction of the lamellae. They can occur in the toe region (toe cracks), quarters (quarter cracks) and heels (heel cracks). Superficial cracks do not involve the sensitive laminae but deep cracks do. Deep cracks are often accompanied by localized infection of the dermis. Cracks can originate from the coronary band or from the solar margin and they can be partial or complete (from coronary band to solar margin).

Aetiology

- Overgrown hoofwall may lead to splitting upwards from the solar margin.
- Dry, poor quality horn and poor foot balance increase the incidence of cracks.

- Defects can be caused by tearing away of a shoe and part of the wall.
- Chronic traumatic defects in the coronary band (false quarters).
- High incidence in the toe region of Draught horses and in the medial quarter of Standardbred racehorses.

Clinical signs

- Obvious hoofwall defect with or without local discharge, heat or lameness.
- Hoof testers and unilateral nerve block are used to determine clinical significance of the crack.
- Pain associated with deep cracks is caused by irritation of the laminar and coronary dermis by differential movement of both sides of the horn defect.
- Haemorrhage from repetitive irritation.
- Purulent discharge from secondary infection of the exposed dermis.

Treatment

- Prevention with regular good foot care to eliminate foot imbalances.
- Application of oil to the hoof to prevent excessive dryness and oral administration of biotin and methionine to promote good quality horn growth.
- Groove or burn transversely down to healthy continuous horn at the proximal limit of incomplete cracks to prevent progression.
- Adequate immobilization of the crack to eliminate irritation and lameness and to allow healing from the coronary dermis down.
  - A full bar shoe with clips drawn on either side of the crack.
  - The hoofwall can be lowered either caudal to the defect (quarter cracks) or directly beneath the defect (toe cracks) to eliminate upward pressure and irritation of the coronary dermis during weight bearing.
  - Heartbar shoes and frog pads to transfer the load of weight bearing from the walls to the frog.
  - Hoof binding resins, acrylics and prosthetic repair materials. These materials should only be used after thorough debridement and elimination of infection.
  - Transversely placed nails, screws and wire, screws and metal plate, or lace of various materials (e.g. wire, polyester).

- Partial hoofwall resection for complicated cracks that prove refractory to stabilization techniques.

Prognosis

The prognosis is favourable for most cracks. However, cracks associated with chronic coronary band defects are more difficult to eliminate and have a tendency to recur.

Seedy toe/separation of the hoofwall

Definition

'Seedy toe' describes a condition in which the dermal and epidermal layers are separated in the toe region of the foot. Newly formed horn follows the line of separation and perpetuates the defect. After some time the separation is visible in the white line in the toe region and the dermal structures are exposed to ascending infection.

Aetiology

- Focal haemorrhage, seroma formation, or inflammation. This is followed by a failure of the damaged laminae to produce keratin.
- Rotation of the distal phalanx in complicated laminitis.

Clinical signs

- Presence of brown, crumbly horn-like matter along the white line in the toe region.
- Lameness in severe cases. The defect may extend as high up as two-thirds of the distance between the solar margin and the coronary band.
- Percussion of the dorsal hoofwall may produce a characteristic hollow sound.

Diagnosis

- Careful exploration of the undermined wall with a blunt radiopaque probe allows radiological documentation of the extent of separation.
- Gas shadow in the soft tissues dorsal to the third phalanx on lateromedial radiographs of the foot.

Treatment

- Regular cleaning of the defect and shoeing with wide-webbed, flat shoes to increase the base of support for the foot are sufficient in mild cases.
- In more severe cases, all separated horn must be removed from the solar margin of the toe to a level where normal interlaminar bond is present. The exposed laminae are medicated under a dressing. This allows newly formed horn to grow down in a normal direction and restores a normal interlaminar bond.

Hoofwall avulsions/separations

Aetiology

- Incomplete avulsions can be caused by complicated cracks, infection with separation of the white line, penetration of the white line by a foreign body, chronic foot imbalance, overgrown feet and improper shoe removal.
- Complete avulsions usually result from lacerations caused by sharp objects.

Clinical signs

- Moderate lameness is typical following an acute hoofwall avulsion. Severe lameness is indicative of damage to underlying bony, synovial, tendinous or ligamentous structures. Occasionally, a foreign body may lodge deep between the epidermal and dermal laminae.
- If lameness persists, the clinician should be suspicious of deep-seated soft tissue or synovial infection, or a phalangeal fracture.

Diagnosis

- Following meticulous cleaning and aseptic preparation the injury should be examined carefully for damage to structures deep to the avulsed hoofwall.
- Plain and contrast radiography should be used to identify the source of pain.

Treatment

- Avulsions without damage to coronary dermis are managed by careful debridement, removal of all loose horn, topical application of antiseptic medication and bandaging until the defect is keratinized.
- Avulsions with coronary band involvement are treated following the same principles. The coronary band must be meticulously reconstructed by suturing. If the wound is severely contaminated or has lost blood supply, delayed primary or secondary closure may be more appropriate.
- Complete immobilization of the foot in a cast for up to 4 weeks is advisable following reconstruction of acute avulsions to allow for primary healing of the coronary dermis.
- If a substantial portion of hoofwall has been excised, a full bar shoe is applied to provide stability.

Laminitis

Definition

Laminitis is not an inflammatory condition of the foot, but is a peripheral vascular disorder caused by systemic disease (or less frequently by chronic overloading of a single limb). The equine foot appears to be a target organ for vascular abnormalities. Pony breeds are predisposed to laminitis.

Pathogenesis

- It is thought that alterations in vasoactive mechanisms, induced by imbalances of vasoactive amines and/or vascular disease, ultimately lead to laminar ischaemia in the horse's foot.
- Ischaemic necrosis develops first in the epidermal, then in the dermal structures of the hoofwall. The dorsal coronary dermis, dorsal laminar dermis and dorsal solar dermis have a much less extensive collateral circulation than the palmar dermal tissues in the foot, and are therefore more susceptible to ischaemic necrosis.
- The resulting pain causes further release of catecholamines, which cause vasoconstriction and increase ischaemia in the dermal vasculature.
- The epidermal–dermal junction becomes oedematous and weakened with loss of interlaminar bond. If this damage extends over a sufficiently large area, suspensory support of the distal phalanx inside the horn capsule is lost. A combination of the forces of weight bearing, the pull of the deep digital flexor tendon (DDFT) and dorsal pressure of space occupying soft tissues (dermal congestion, oedema, seroma and epidermal hyperplasia) result in mechanical separation of the third phalanx from the hoofwall.
- If, as in most cases, mechanical separation is mainly localized in the toe region, the distal

phalanx rotates away from the dorsal hoofwall (rotation). In very severe cases in which the suspensory support is lost throughout most of the laminae, the entire third phalanx drops in the hoof ('sinking').

• Systemic changes in laminitis can be found in the cardiovascular (tachycardia, hypertension, alterations in intrinsic coagulation system) and endocrine systems (increased catecholamines, cortisol, testosterone and plasma renin, and decreased thyroxine). Renal damage (glomerulonephritis, medullary necrosis) and liver disease have also been reported.

Aetiology

The aetiology of laminitis is multifactorial, because many different predisposing factors can trigger the same vascular mechanisms:

• Nutritional carbohydrate (grain) overload.
• Obesity and ingestion of lush grass.
• Ingestion of large amounts of cold water.
• Electrolyte imbalances (Ca/P and Na/K).
• Chronic overloading of a sound limb in severe unilateral lameness.
• Strenuous and/or prolonged work on hard surfaces.
• Long-term or high dose corticosteroid administration. Steroids increase the vasoconstrictory response of the digital vasculature to circulating catecholamines and serotonin.
• High testosterone concentration has been associated with coagulopathy in the dermal vasculature and may explain why stallions appear to be at higher risk for laminitis.
• High oestrogen concentrations have been associated with laminitis in mares with anoestrus or continuous oestrus. Oestrogens are abundantly present in some grasses or legumes.
• Hypothyroidism.
• Hyperadrenocorticism.
• Systemic infections (e.g. endometritis, pneumonia, enteritis).
• Horses recovering from colic surgery are always at risk of developing laminitis.
• Cushing's disease.

Classification

The clinical presentation of laminitis can be classified into three different categories:

1. Acute laminitis: acute stage of systemic illness with accompanying lameness.
2. Chronic laminitis: residual lameness due to

structural foot changes following resolution of the acute systemic illness.
3. Chronic laminitis not associated with a clinically identifiable episode of acute systemic illness: intermittent, inconsistent lameness due to chronically distorted feet.

Clinical signs

• Animals with acute laminitis show signs of systemic disease and local signs of foot disease. Systemic signs include elevation of heart rate, increased respiratory rate, hypertension and anorexia. Fever may be present if the horse is septicaemic or toxaemic. Evidence of moderate to severe pain is present (sweating, flared nostrils, muscular tremors). Horse is reluctant to move, and if severely affected, may become recumbent.
• Laminitic ponies on lush spring pasture have a large neck crest that consists of adipose tissue. This crest tends to become firm to palpation in the early stages of the disease.
• A mild form of laminitis in racing Thoroughbreds on prolonged high levels of dietary carbohydrates (i.e. glycogen overload) is characterized by signs of indigestion, low faecal pH (<6.2), poor performance, generalized stiffness and warm feet.
• Signs indicative of foot disease are present in horses with laminitis. Most commonly, both front feet are simultaneously affected (except for cases of contralateral overload).
• A bounding digital pulse is present, often in all four limbs. The hoofwall feels abnormally warm, especially the dorsal half. Close examination may show evidence of a depression behind the proximal dorsal margin of the coronary band ('sinker') or exudative discharge from a separated coronary band (severe cases). The sole may show a convex profile just cranial to the point of the frog if the third phalanx has rotated. This same part of the sole may be discoloured by blood effusion or even show ulceration with prolapse of the solar dermis. The white line may show evidence of haemorrhage.
• Application of hoof testers or percussion over the sole (cranial to the point of the frog) and the dorsal wall, is resented.
• Animals with laminitis display a typical stance with the forelimbs stretched out in front and the hindlimbs placed beneath the body as close as possible to the centre of gravity. The gait is characterized by a typical 'heel before toe' foot placement and obvious lameness.
• Animals with chronic laminitis have local signs of foot lameness similar to those of horses with

acute laminitis. However, the feet develop long-term deformation. Rings parallel to the coronary band reflect temporary alterations in hoof growth. In laminitis, these rings tend to be closely packed in the toe region and diverge towards the heels, reflecting the discrepancy in rate of hoof growth between these different areas of the foot. The result of decreased toe growth is ultimately a 'slipper' foot. Convexity of the sole accompanied by ulceration and prolapse and necrosis of the dermis is the result of sustained pressure of the tip of the rotated third phalanx on the solar dermis and its blood supply in this area.

The dead space caused by separation and rotation between the third phalanx and the hoofwall in the toe region is gradually filled by epidermal scar tissue. This wedge of epidermal hyperplasia maintains the malalignment of both structures and can be observed as a wide and distorted white line on the solar surface of the foot.

- Secondary infection is a common feature of laminitis. These infections can range from simple subsolar abscesses to more extensive infections that can lead to septicaemia. Infection characteristically causes a sudden exacerbation of lameness.

Radiology

- Radiographs are necessary to identify the degree of phalangeal displacement, the presence of infection and chronic bony remodelling of the third phalanx.
- Third phalangeal rotation is assessed by subtracting the angle between the dorsal wall and the sole from the angle between the dorsal surface of the third phalanx and the sole. Quantification of the degree and progress of third phalangeal displacement, identified by sequential radiographs, is important prognostically.
- Sinking may be difficult to identify radiologically because the dorsal hoofwall and the third phalanx remain parallel. The presence of sinking can usually be confirmed only by comparing the different measurements on the lateromedial radiograph with published reference values (e.g. thickness dorsal wall ⩽ 18 mm).
- The presence of gas densities on foot radiographs may be indicative of local infection.
- Attention should also be paid to evidence of remodelling of the tip of the third phalanx. Fractures of the tip of the third phalanx, upwards curling of the tip due to new bone production ('Turk shoe'), irregular radiolucencies in the tip and extensive osteolysis with alterations in shape of the third phalanx justify a guarded prognosis.

- Production of new bone along the dorsal margin of the third phalanx, with or without rotation, is usually subtle and indicates the presence of laminar tearing.

Treatment

Acute laminitis should be treated as an emergency. Destruction of the laminar bed starts several hours before the first signs of lameness are apparent, and continues to progress if treatment is not initiated.

1. Removal of initiating cause:
   - Mineral oil administered by nasogastric tube will block toxin absorption from the gastrointestinal tract.
   - Animals should be removed from pasture, and fed hay and water only.
   - Systemic infections should be treated vigorously with antibiotics. Antibiotics are also advisable as prophylaxis against secondary pedal sepsis.
2. Treatment of peripheral vascular disease:
   - Acetylpromazine to reduce vasoconstriction and hypertension.
   - Isoxsuprine hydrochloride may counteract early vascular changes in laminitis.
   - NSAIDs to control digital pain and to interrupt the pain–hypertension cycle.
   - Potassium chloride is supplemented to correct depletion of potassium.
   - Sodium is removed from the diet.
   - Application of warm compresses to feet or hot tubs to counteract vasoconstriction in the digital circulation.
   - Topical application of glyceryl trinitrate ointment to the pastern to promote vasodilation in the hoof.
3. Mechanical support of the diseased laminae:
   - Nerve blocks and forced exercise must be avoided.
   - The horse should be bedded on a deep soft bed (e.g. shavings, sand, peat) that conforms easily to the shape of the sole and frog.
   - Preshaped frog pads (e.g. Theraflex, Lily pads), or plaster of Paris slippers help transfer the load of weight bearing from the walls to the frog.

In chronic laminitis, treatment is aimed at correcting the residual foot problems.

1. General management of the animal:
   - Limited intake of carbohydrates to control obesity and to prevent recurrence.

- Supplement the ration with 30 g of potassium chloride daily.
- Supplementation with oral methionine and biotin daily.

2. Corrective foot trimming:
   - Guided by good lateromedial foot radiographs.
   - Removal of excess horn in the toe region and trimming of the heels to restore normal spatial alignment between the third phalanx and the hoof.
   - Dorsal wall resection may be indicated for severely affected horses. This should never be taken lightly by the treating clinician. Once the dorsal wall is removed, the horse requires close follow-up.

3. Therapeutic shoeing for laminitis:
   - A wide-webbed, seated-out bar or egg-bar shoe of thick steel with a rolled toe, increases the base of support, minimizes the amount of pressure on the sole, and facilitates breakover of the foot.
   - A heart-bar shoe may support and immobilize the third phalanx sufficiently to prevent further rotation and allow for undisturbed revascularization of diseased laminae and restoration of the interlaminar bond.

4. Deep flexor tenotomy or inferior check ligament desmotomy:
   - This procedure may produce significant pain relief in animals with severe chronic laminitis that are unresponsive to medical treatment.
   - Tenotomy should be regarded as a salvage procedure for valuable breeding animals. The beneficial effects are only temporary and last for approximately 12 months.

Prognosis

- Most animals that develop laminitis recover with medical treatment, without the use of radical trimming or shoeing.
- If an animal with acute laminitis shows no pedal rotation by day 10, it can come off medication by day 20 and can usually be safely considered as recovered by day 60.
- The prognosis becomes unfavourable when:
  - The acute phase continues for more than ten days.
  - Digital pain is uncontrollable.
  - Blood pressure remains higher than 200 mmHg for more than a few hours.
  - Secondary infection is present.

- The third phalanx has rotated. Full athletic recovery is still possible for horses in which rotation does not exceed 5.5 degrees.
- Prognosis becomes hopeless in cases of:
  - Sinking of the third phalanx.
  - Exungulation of the hoof.

Pododermatitis

Definition

Pododermatitis is traumatic inflammation of the solar dermis with or without secondary infection.

- Subsolar bruising can occur in any portion of the solar surface of the foot.
- Corns are pressure-induced bruises in the angle of the wall and the bar.
- Chronic subsolar bruising is caused by chronic, repetitive crushing of the solar dermis and is seen most commonly in thin-soled, flat-footed horses.
- Subsolar abscesses ('pus in the foot') may be secondarily infected corns or bruises or may develop secondarily to penetrating wounds of the sole.
- 'Gravel' is a layman's term to describe a draining tract at the coronary band caused by drainage of a subsolar/submural abscess.

Aetiology

- Bruising of the dermis is caused by external pressure, either from the horn itself or from hard foreign bodies (e.g. irregular ground surface, stones, poorly fitted shoes).
- In laminitis with rotation of the third phalanx, severe bruising can be caused by downward pressure of the tip of the third phalanx.
- Thin-soled, flat-footed horses (mostly Thoroughbreds) and horses with long-toe/low-heel conformation are predisposed to solar trauma.

Clinical signs

- Varying degree of lameness. Frequently, the horse is bearing minimal weight, often on the toe only, and rests the foot continuously when standing.
- Increased warmth of the foot, with a bounding digital pulse and enlargement of the palmar and palmar digital arteries.
- Pain on percussion of the sole or walls.
- Exploration of the suspected part of the sole may reveal dark red discoloration ('dry corn') or a

seroma ('moist corn'), or lead to a sudden release of black (superficial infection) or yellow (deep necrotizing infection) pus.

- Expansion of the purulent infection may result in partial or complete undermining of the frog and solar horn. If the pus cannot escape via the sole or white line, proximal expansion can occur between the hoofwall and laminar dermis, resulting in eruption of infection between the coronary dermis and the proximal wall. Alternatively, pus may discharge at the bulbs of the heels.

Treatment

1. Removal of the shoe may be sufficient treatment.
2. Prevention by proper, regular trimming and shoeing.
3. Surgical shoes to render the horse usable:
   - Full bar shoe.
   - Set heel or dropped heel shoe.
   - Silicone rubber sole filler or leather anti-concussion pads.
4. Thinning the solar horn over the bruised site, without exposing the dermis. The horse should be rested and left barefoot on a thick, soft bed until sound. The use of NSAIDs may be appropriate in severe cases.
5. When infection is present, all the underrun horn must be removed to provide drainage and to allow topical application of medication and natural debridement of necrotic dermis. The edges of the horn defect should be thinned gradually. The foot should be medicated daily with an antiseptic solution and kept bandaged to protect it from external contamination.
6. Tetanus antitoxin or a toxoid booster should always be administered to any horse with subsolar infection.
7. In cases of 'gravel', the communicating solar abscess should be exposed to establish distal drainage. Part of the separated laminar horn may have to be removed to expose the necrotic laminar dermis. Avoid complete stripping of the wall. Proximo-distal irrigation with an antiseptic solution is useful to eliminate submural infection.

Nailbind

Definition

Nailbind is direct injury or bruising of the solar or laminar dermis by a shoe nail.

Clinical signs

The horse may haemorrhage from the nail hole and become instantly lame, but more commonly, lameness develops over a few days, as a result of intermittent trauma to the dermis during exercise. External contamination through the nail hole often results in secondary infectious pododermatitis. Nail removal may cause drainage of black purulent material from the hole.

Treatment

Treatment consists of shoe removal and widening of the nail hole to provide adequate drainage.

Keratoma

Definition

Keratoma is a localized, cone-shaped or cylindrical wedge of abnormal horn between the laminar horn and dermis.

Aetiology

- Rare tumour derived from the keratin-producing epidermal cells of the stratum germinativum of the epidermis.
- Chronic injury or irritation of the stratum germinativum by chronic hoofwall cracks, submural foreign bodies or nailbind.

Clinical signs

- Intermittently recurring purulent infections draining from the white line or coronary band. Once the keratoma has grown down the hoof, a break in the continuity of the sole allows bacteria to enter the hoof between the laminar horn and dermis.
- Acute lameness in the presence of infection. Lameness disappears with spontaneous resolution of the infection.
- Sometimes insidious, chronic, low grade lameness due to sustained pressure on the laminar dermis and third phalanx in the toe region. This may result in localized bone lysis of the third phalanx.
- Careful inspection of the white line after trimming may reveal an island of abnormal horn and widening or deformation in the white line at the toe.

- Radiography of the third phalanx reveals characteristic osteolysis along the dorsal surface of the bone.

Treatment

- Complete surgical excision by partial resection of the hoofwall.
- A bar shoe with stabilizing clips on either side of the surgically created defect in the hoofwall must be maintained for several months.
- The foot is wrapped with a sterile pressure bandage with antiseptic/astringent dressing to counteract bulging of the swollen dermis. After 2–3 weeks, a firm, dry cuticle forms and bandaging can be discontinued.
- After a firm cuticle has formed, the defect can be filled with prosthetic hoof material to protect the laminae until horn grows down to cover the defect.

Prognosis

The prognosis is favourable, but up to 12 months may be required before a normal foot has regrown.

Canker

Definition

Canker is an infectious process that results in the development of a chronic, hypertrophic, moist pododermatitis of the frog and sole, and deficient formation of solar horn.

Aetiology

- Unhygienic stabling.
- Horses in semitropical climates.
- Unknown infectious agent.
- Individual or breed predisposition, especially in Draught horses.

Clinical signs

- Characteristic foul odour.
- Caseous white exudate resembling cottage cheese.
- Ragged, filamentous appearance of frog horn.
- Usually hindlimbs affected.

- Proliferative swollen dermis covered with caseous exudate is found when loose horn is removed.
- Lameness only in advanced cases.

Treatment

- Extensive surgical debridement of all affected tissues. Debridement can cause extensive haemorrhage and is best performed with the horse under general anaesthesia and following placement of a tourniquet.
- Careful postoperative management with daily bandaging until the defect is dry and covered with normal horn.

Prognosis

Prognosis is always guarded. Treatment is prolonged and intensive, and recurrence is likely.

Thrush

Definition

Thrush is a degenerative condition of the central and collateral sulci of the frog, characterized by disintegrating horn and the presence of grey to black material in the affected areas.

Aetiology

- Unhygienic, moist stabling conditions with poor foot care.
- Infection by keratolytic organisms: multifactorial, but *Fusobacterium necrophorum* is often involved.

Clinical signs

- Black discharge in the sulci of the frog with very offensive odour.
- Lameness only when sensitive structures involved.
- Mainly hindlimbs affected.

Treatment

- Debridement of infected and separated horn. Usually must be debrided several times before infection is controlled.
- Daily topical adstringent medication under dressing. Sterile bandaging after each debridement. Continue treatment under plate shoe.

Prognosis

The prognosis is guarded to favourable. It is worse if sensitive structures are affected. Prolonged treatment is often necessary.

Penetrating wounds to the sole

Definition

These are puncture wounds through the sole or frog horn involving the dermis or the deeper structures of the foot.

Aetiology

- Standing on sharp objects, mainly nails.
- Kicking against sharp objects such as pitch fork, nail in wall, etc.

These wounds invariably become secondarily infected.

Localization and pathology

1. Puncture of solar dermis:
   - Infectious pododermatitis.
2. Puncture into digital fat cushion:
   - Heel abscess, infectious pododermatitis.
3. Puncture into third phalanx:
   - Penetration in toe region or peripheral sole.
   - Commonly bacterial osteitis with sequestration of necrotic bone fragment.
   - Fractures occur rarely and are either marginal or pathologic fractures.

The most dangerous area for penetration is the middle third of the frog and its sulci, in which case the following structures are at risk of penetration:

4. Deep digital flexor tendon:
   - Localized necrosis of tendon and severe lameness.
   - Necrosis has a tendency to spread within the tendon and erode into deeper structures.
5. Navicular bursa (penetration may occur secondary to necrosis of the DDFT):
   - Infectious navicular bursitis.
   - Navicular osteomyelitis.
   - Possible secondary infection of the DIP joint.
6. Impar ligament and DIP joint:
   - Infectious arthritis of the DIP joint.
7. Digital sheath:
   - Penetrating objects in the caudal third of the sole may enter the digital sheath.
   - Infectious tenosynovitis.

Clinical signs

- Object may still be embedded in the foot.
- Acute onset lameness that improves following removal of foreign body.
- Non-weightbearing lameness shortly afterwards due to secondary infection of the penetrated tissue. With primary fracture of the third phalanx or navicular bone, no improvement is seen following removal of the penetrating object.
- Purulent discharge from solar defect. Entry site sometimes difficult to find when sealed, especially when the frog has been penetrated.
- Often swelling and heat as far proximal as pastern and fetlock.
- Sometimes the horse displays systemic signs (e.g. septicaemia, increased temperature, anorexia).
- Sometimes stringhalt-like gait following penetration of a hind foot.

Diagnosis

- Hoof testers.
- Careful paring of sole to find site of penetration; establish direction of puncture with sterile probe after thorough cleaning.
- Synoviocentesis and synovial fluid analysis of synovial cavities that may be involved.
- Radiography:
  - If possible, radiograph the foot with object in place before removal.
  - Plain radiographs to visualize fractures, osteitis.
  - Positive contrast radiographs with radiopaque probe inside puncture; contrast agent injected via sole or intrasynovial contrast to investigate invasion of synovial structures.

Treatment

1. Acute presentation:
   - Systemic antibiotics and tetanus antitoxin (or a toxoid booster).
   - Gain maximum information on length, nature and direction of penetrating object.
   - If no synovial or tendon involvement is suspected, clean the sole thoroughly, pare widely around the site of penetration down to sensitive laminae (1–2 cm diameter), remove

all contaminated tissue, provide adequate drainage and treat with daily antiseptic dressings.

• With risk of penetration of the DDFT or a synovial cavity (middle third frog), emergency surgical debridement under general anaesthesia is warranted ('Street nail' procedure or navicular bursoscopy).

2. With established infection or confirmed synovial penetration:

• 'Street nail' procedure provides aggressive surgical debridement of infected structures and drainage through solar fenestration.

• Aftercare should consist of daily antiseptic dressings under sterile bandage. If the infection has cleared, purulent discharge ceases and the defect gradually fills with clean, pink granulation tissue.

• Navicular bursoscopy provides an alternative and less invasive approach to the navicular bursa for debridement and lavage, reducing risk of secondary complications, e.g. bursa.

Prognosis

• Always guarded.

• Poor if DDFT or synovial structures are involved. When applied to these latter cases, the 'Street nail' procedure should be regarded, at best, as a salvage procedure to achieve pasture soundness.

• Application of navicular bursoscopy to these cases gives better chance of restoring horses to athletic soundness.

• Horses presented within 7 days of injury and those with hindlimb rather than frontlimb involvement appear to have a better prognosis. Prognosis is grave if repeated debridement is necessary.

Quittor/Necrosis of the lateral cartilage

Definition

Quittor is a localized necrosis within a collateral cartilage of the third phalanx. Purulent discharge and sinus formation above the coronary band results.

Aetiology

• External trauma (lacerations, punctures, bruises from interference) to the side of the foot above the coronary band.

• Possible extension of subsolar or submural abscessation.

Clinical signs

• Chronic, suppurative draining tracts above the coronet that intermittently tend to heal and resume drainage.

• Localized pain, heat and swelling over collateral cartilage.

• Lameness occurs in the acute stage of infection.

• Extensive fibrosis and deformity of hoofwall in chronic cases.

Treatment

Treatment consists of surgical excision of the necrotic core of cartilage. Care must be exercised to avoid opening and contaminating the DIP joint.

Prognosis

The prognosis is favourable unless the collateral cartilage is extensively infected.

Lameness due to foot imbalance

Normal conformation

The weight of the horse is transmitted through the limb to the third phalanx. From the third phalanx the horse's weight is suspended, via the interlaminar bonds, from the inner surface of the hoofwall. To assure even weight distribution around the hoofwall, it is important that the foot is balanced and evenly placed around its centre of weight bearing (midpoint of the circle of laminar suspension).

Dorsopalmar imbalance – 'Long toe/low heeled foot'

• A 'long toe/low heeled foot' is a common conformational defect, especially in Thoroughbreds. Because of this inherent conformation, but also as a result of inadequate trimming of the toe, insufficient length to the branches of shoes and long intervals between shoeing, the foot tends to rock back onto the heels. Consequently, the centre of weight bearing of the affected foot is transferred towards the heels, and this increases the vertical load on the heels. The heels cannot support the extra weight, and the quarters spread, allowing the heels to collapse forward under the foot. The toe becomes long and oblique, and the foot obtains a typical 'long toe/low heel' appearance.

- This abnormal foot-shape results in tearing of the dorsal laminae and straining of the DDFT and the supporting ligaments of the navicular bone.
- Typical bilateral forelimb lameness results, especially on hard ground and when the horse is worked in circles.
- Treatment of this condition is aimed at restoring even weight distribution around the hoofwall. Shoeing the foot with a seated-out, wide-webbed, open shoe or with an egg-bar shoe provides extra length and width to give additional support to the overloaded heels.
- Severe imbalance with collapse of the heels carries a poor prognosis for long-term soundness.

Overlong feet

- Long, boxy feet are often seen in European Warmblood horses. If the foot is allowed to grow too long, the centre of weight bearing gradually moves towards the heels. This leads to excessive loading of the heels and may cause lameness.
- Treatment consists of regular trimming and shoeing with wide-webbed, open shoes that are extra long at the heels.

Lateromedial imbalance – 'sheared heels'

- 'Sheared heels' result from uneven trimming of the heels or from poor conformation. One heel (usually the medial one) strikes the ground before the other. This results in proximal displacement of this heel. The wall on this side becomes short and upright. The opposite wall expands and flares outwards.
- Continuous tearing and bruising of the sensitive laminae in the compressed heel, and breakdown of tissues that connect the heels result in lameness.
- A bar shoe is applied. The branches of the shoe are positioned and secured where the hoofwall should be. The centre line of the limb must be situated exactly over the centre of the shoe. The shoe is fitted wide on the compressed wall and tight on the expanded, flared wall. Gradually, with each shoeing, the sole is brought back perpendicular to the long axis of the limb until the ground impact is redistributed evenly over both heels.

- A bar shoe minimizes relative movement between both heels and allows the supporting structures to heal during immobilization.

Fractures of the third phalanx

Classification

Type I: non-articular fracture of palmar/plantar process.
Type II: parasagittal articular fracture from DIP joint to medial or lateral solar margin.
Type III: midsagittal articular fracture.
Type IV: fracture of the extensor process.
Type V: comminuted fractures or fractures secondary to foreign body penetration or osteomyelitis.
Type VI: non-articular marginal fractures.
Type VII: non-articular palmar/plantar process fractures in foals, originating and ending at the solar margin.

Aetiology

- Concussion with twisting as the foot lands, most commonly during flat racing on hard surface.
- Kicking unyielding objects.
- Stepping on uneven surfaces (e.g. kerb, rock, stones).
- Foreign body penetration with/without infection.
- Fractures of the extensor process may be caused by excessive tension on the extensor tendon (i.e. avulsion fracture), direct trauma or impaction of the process against the distal end of the second phalanx during hyperextension of the DIP joint.

Clinical signs

- Articular fractures cause the most severe signs: acute, severe lameness, heat, pain on hoof testers and percussion, increased digital pulses and effusion of the DIP joint.
- Horses with non-articular fractures usually present with less severe lameness, more specific response to hoof testers and may improve more quickly with rest.
- Pain from Type I fractures can be alleviated with a unilateral palmar digital nerve block (PDNB). Pain from most other types of third phalanx fracture can be alleviated only by a bilateral ASNB.

- Haemarthrosis of the DIP joint may suggest the presence of an articular fracture.
- Radiographs are necessary to confirm the diagnosis and define the fracture.
- The extensor process of both front feet may have a separate centre of ossification, which may appear radiologically as a fracture fragment. A separate centre of ossification is rarely clinically significant.
- Fractures of the extensor process may result in enlargement of the extensor process and malformation of the foot (i.e. buttress foot).
- The majority of type VI fractures occur in conjunction with remodelling of the third phalanx of horses with chronic laminitis.

Treatment and prognosis

Type I
The foot should be immobilized with a bar shoe with quarter clips or a cast, and the horse stall rested. Healing of this fracture takes 3 to 9 months depending on the size of the fragment. The prognosis for return to soundness is good.

Type II and III
- About 50% of horses treated conservatively with stall rest, foot or lower limb casts, or bar shoes with quarter clips or a full rim, return to soundness after 6 to 12 months.
- Surgical treatment by lag screw fixation usually produces better results than conservative treatment, especially in horses over 3 years of age. Time to healing is significantly shorter (3–6 months) with surgical treatment.

Type IV
Conservative treatment (i.e. rest, immobilization) is acceptable only if the fragment is non-articular. Articular fragments are best removed or stabilized with a lag screw in an attempt to avoid degenerative joint disease.

Type VI
These fractures are treated with stall rest (4 to 8 weeks) and surgical shoeing (wide-webbed shoes with anti-concussion pads).

'Pedal osteitis'

Definition and aetiology

- The term 'pedal osteitis' defines a reaction of the third phalanx, in response to a primary insult. Such potential insults to the bone are penetrating injuries to the foot with or without infection, subsolar bruising, infectious pododermatitis, laminitis, keratomas and reaction to implants. Radiological characteristics of osteitis include localized osteolysis, sclerosis, bone fragmentation, bone sequestration and new bone formation.
- The broader use of the term 'pedal osteitis' to signify a condition in its own right is incorrect. Historically, the diagnosis of this 'condition' has been based on the presence of uni- or bilateral chronic low-grade lameness of indefinable origin with radiological signs of so-called generalized demineralization of the third phalanx, widening and increase in number of the vascular channels and roughening of the solar margin of the third phalanx. It has been shown that a sufficiently wide individual variation exists in these radiological features of the third phalanx in normal horses to preclude a radiological diagnosis of 'pedal osteitis' based on these factors. The use of the term 'pedal osteitis' in this sense should therefore be discouraged.

Clinical signs

- Persistent lameness in spite of treatment of the primary condition. The character and severity of lameness are determined in part by the underlying condition (e.g. penetrating injury to the foot, subsolar bruising, infectious pododermatitis, laminitis, keratoma, implant intolerance) and in part by the amount of damage to the third phalanx.
- Horses with persistent lameness following treatment of penetrating injuries to the foot, subsolar bruising, infectious pododermatitis, laminitis, keratomas and implant surgery, should be evaluated radiologically to determine if the third phalanx shows remodelling changes.

Treatment

- Treat the primary cause.
- If a sequestrum has formed, the foot should be fenestrated to provide access for surgical debridement and drainage. Aftercare consists of daily antiseptic dressings under sterile bandage until the infection has cleared and the defect has filled.

Osseous cyst-like lesions of the third phalanx

Aetiology

The aetiology of subchondral cystic lesions (SCL) is unclear. Traumatic and developmental theories have been suggested.

Clinical signs

- The affected horse has a history of acute onset lameness (most frequently in a forelimb) that becomes chronic. Lameness tends to improve with rest but recurs with exercise.
- Improvement with PDNB, sound with abaxial sesamoid nerve block (ASNB).
- Radiographs show a circular radiolucent lesion with a sclerotic border adjacent to the subchondral bone plate of the third phalanx. The cystic lesion may or may not communicate with the joint.

Treatment

- Treatment with rest only is unrewarding.
- Surgical treatment by extra-articular debridement has been successful in selected cases.

'Sidebone'

Definition

Sidebone is a term used to describe ossification in the collateral cartilages of the foot.

Aetiology

- Common condition in heavy breeds, especially Draught horses.
- Sidebone may be associated with poorly balanced feet and uneven loading of the heels.
- Acute trauma or chronic repetitive trauma (e.g. lacerations, punctures, chronic bruising from interference) may lead to chronic inflammatory changes and osseous metaplasia of the cartilages.

Clinical signs

- Lameness, although rare, may occur in the early phase of ossification. Lameness may also be seen following local injury to an ossified cartilage.
- Prominent, hard, rigid and bony enlargement above the coronary band at the quarter.

- Radiography shows the extent of ossification. A radiolucent line is often present between the palmar process of the third phalanx and the base of the ossified cartilage, and should not be interpreted as a fracture.

Treatment

Treatment is usually unnecessary because the horse is not lame. The feet should be kept properly balanced to distribute weight bearing evenly. A bar shoe may be helpful if a lateromedial foot imbalance is present.

Fractures of the navicular bone

Incidence and location

Three types of fractures may affect the navicular bone:

- Chip fracture involving the proximal or distal borders or the wings of the navicular bone.
- Simple sagittal fracture. Occur close to the sagittal ridge.
- Comminuted fractures are uncommon. Fragments are often displaced.

Congenital non-fusion of centres of ossification of the navicular bone may be confused with fracture. The navicular bone may have two or three separate centres of ossification.

Aetiology

- Sagittal and comminuted fractures result from acute trauma to the foot such as occurs from running on hard unlevel ground, stepping on to a kerb stone or kicking at stall walls with the hindlimbs.
- Chip fractures may be avulsion fractures, located within the impar ligament or navicular suspensory ligaments.

Clinical signs

- Sagittal or comminuted fractures cause sudden onset, severe lameness.
- Walking improves greatly within 2 weeks with stall rest.
- Permanent lameness at the trot.
- Positive response to PDNB.
- Radiography confirms diagnosis. Fractures are easily confused with packing defects of the frog clefts. Always include a flexor view. The fracture

normally develops fibrous union or non-union and, therefore, remains permanently visible.

• Radiological features of a chronic fracture are remodelling along the proximal border and osteolytic changes along the fracture line often of cyst-like appearance. Because the DIP joint is involved, degenerative joint disease of the DIP joint may become established early on, in which case, the prognosis for soundness is poor.

Treatment and prognosis

• Conservative treatment using bar shoes, quarter clips, raised heels and stall rest (6 months) is generally unsuccessful.

• The only way to obtain bony union is by interfragmentary compression, using lag screw fixation. The more recent the case, the better is the prognosis for soundness.

• Pain caused by chip fracture of the extreme tip of the wing of the navicular bone, can be alleviated by a navicular suspensory ligament desmotomy.

Navicular syndrome

Definition

Navicular syndrome is a clinical manifestation (i.e. chronic palmar foot lameness) of a number of different disease processes associated with the navicular bone, the fibrocartilage of its flexor surface, the palmar part of the DIP joint, the DDFT, the navicular bursa, the ligamenta sesamoidale collateralia (navicular suspensory ligaments) and the ligamentum distale impar (distal impar ligament).

Aetiology and pathogenesis

There are two basic theories regarding the cause of the various pathological changes reported in navicular syndrome: the vascular theory and the biomechanical theory.

• The vascular theory suggests that the main nutrient arteries in the distal part of the navicular bone develop arteriosclerosis and thrombosis, which results in ischaemic necrosis and bone resorption following reperfusion. However, recent histological and morphometric data indicate that increased bone turnover occurs rather than ischaemia and necrosis and evidence of vascular thrombosis has never been found.

• The biomechanical theories are based on the presence of abnormal pressure/vibration forces between the DDFT and the flexor surface of the navicular bone, resulting in degenerative changes in the structures adjacent to the navicular bursa. Histological evidence has confirmed the presence of bone remodelling in the flexor cortex and adjacent spongiosa, similar to the changes in subchondral bone and spongiosa encountered in osteoarthritis of low-motion joints under sustained high loading (e.g. spavin). These changes include initial generalized sclerosis and thickening of the subchondral bone plate, followed by focal bone destruction with replacement by granulation tissue and fibrosis with venous hypertension in the spongiosa. The navicular bone inside a flat foot, with a long toe/low heel conformation and a broken back foot/pastern axis, may be predisposed to developing these changes.

Clinical signs

• Typically in horses 7 to 12 years old, but all ages are affected.

• Most common in Thoroughbred-cross horses and Warmbloods, rare in Arab horses or ponies.

• The onset of signs is most commonly associated with an irregular workload or a period of enforced rest.

• Lameness is insidious in onset and intermittent initially. The horse is noticed to be stiff when leaving the box or at the beginning of exercise. The horse frequently stumbles, is reluctant to work in circles, and is either reluctant to jump or rushes jumps. During the early stages of the condition, horses tend to warm out of the lameness.

• Horses can often be seen to point one foot at rest or to heap up the bedding in order to stand with the heels elevated.

• The trot is bilaterally short-strided, with a shortened cranial phase and the foot lands toe-first. Lameness is mostly bilateral, but one limb is generally more painful than the other, which results in a visible headnod.

• Lameness may switch from limb to limb when a horse is exercised in different directions in a circle or following nerve blocks.

• Lameness appears worse on hard ground.

• Distal limb flexion test generally exacerbates the lameness. Extension of the DIP joint with a wooden wedge (toe-elevation test) may also increase the severity of lameness.

• The digital arteries are often palpably enlarged without increased pulsation. Heat, pain or swelling are not present. Application of hoof testers yields no remarkable response, unless the condition is accompanied by poor foot balance.

- Regional analgesia:
  A clinical diagnosis of navicular syndrome can only be made if a horse responds favourably to at least two of the three following local analgesic techniques:
  1. Palmar digital nerve block (PDNB).
  2. Intra-articular analgesia of the DIP joint, which also eliminates sensation in the navicular bone and associated ligaments.
  3. Intrabursal analgesia of the navicular bursa.

Approximately 20% of horses positive to PDNB improve significantly more to a bursa block than to a DIP joint block. This means that a negative DIP joint block does not always exclude the diagnosis of navicular syndrome.

Radiology

The radiological criteria for diagnosis of navicular syndrome have been primarily based on the appearance of the synovial fossae along the distal border of the navicular bone, as seen on the upright pedal or high coronary projection. This approach has been widely criticized, and alternative, more reliable radiological signs to support the diagnosis of the navicular syndrome have been defined.

On the lateromedial projection:

1. An ill-defined radiolucent area in the flexor cortex (classic navicular).
2. Changes in shape (distoproximal lengthening) of the navicular bone due to peripheral new bone formation.
3. Decreased radiopacity of the flexor cortex in working horses.
4. Thinning of the flexor cortex.
5. Medullary sclerosis.
6. Loss of corticomedullary distinction.
7. Calcification of the impar ligament.
8. Calcification of other soft tissue.

On the upright pedal projection:

1. A central radiolucent area (classic sign of navicular syndrome).
2. Ill-defined radiolucency of the distal border surrounded by sclerosis.
3. Proximal or distal elongation of the navicular borders with ill-defined deposits of new bone.
4. Changes in trabecular pattern.

On the flexor view:

1. Cavitation of the flexor cortex (classic sign of navicular syndrome).
2. Alteration to the well-defined contour of the flexor cortex.
3. Decreased radiopacity of the flexor cortex.
4. Loss of a distinct interface between the cortex and spongiosa.
5. Medullary sclerosis.
6. Disruption of medullary trabecular architecture.

Diagnosis of the navicular syndrome is first and foremost a clinical diagnosis. Navicular syndrome can be diagnosed in the absence of radiological abnormalities.

Diagnosis

Diagnosis of navicular syndrome cannot be based primarily on radiological changes. Consequently it is impossible to use the radiological appearance of the distal border of a navicular bone to predict whether a horse will develop navicular syndrome.

There is a list of criteria that must be assessed for each horse if navicular syndrome is to be diagnosed. The final emphasis should lie predominantly on clinical assessment of the horse.

1. History of chronic poor performance/forelimb lameness.
2. Clinical evidence of (bilateral) forelimb lameness.
3. Response to toe-elevation test/flexion test.
4. Lack of response to hoof testers.
5. Response to palmar digital nerve block.
6. Response to DIP joint block.
7. Response to navicular bursa block.
8. Radiography.
9. Scintigraphy.

Treatment and prognosis

The wide range of response to different treatment regimens makes case selection for any of the available treatment options difficult.

1. Therapeutic foot care to encourage a more upright conformation of the foot, a straight hoof–pastern axis and downward growth of the heel:
   - Rolled toe, raised heel shoes.
   - Egg-bar shoes.
   - Wide-webbed, seated-out shoes.
   - Wedge-shape heel inserts to raise heels.

2. Medical therapy:
   - Phenylbutazone, 1 to 2 g daily, allows the horse to be exercised during treatment. Enforced rest is contraindicated for horses with navicular syndrome.
   - The β-adrenergic drug, isoxsuprine hydrochloride, increases peripheral circulation by relaxing the vascular smooth musculature. After the horse has been sound for at least 2 weeks, the drug is gradually withdrawn.
   - Intrabursal or intra-articular infiltration of corticosteroids is aimed at controlling the inflammatory bursitis or synovitis that usually accompanies navicular syndrome. The beneficial effect of the injection is somewhat short lived. Sixty percent of treated horses are sound for 2 months or more, but only 7% are sound 12 months after injection.
3. Surgical treatment:
   - Desmotomy of the suspensory ligaments of the navicular bone is performed to remove the vibratory forces between the DDFT and the flexor surface of the navicular bone. Favourable results are obtained in approximately 50% of the cases.
   - Neurectomy of the palmar digital nerves is a last resort technique to provide symptomatic relief in horses with navicular syndrome. Desensitization of the palmar structures of the foot allows the horse to exercise pain free. Unfortunately a number of neurectomy-associated complications may occur and need to be discussed with the horse's owner before surgery is undertaken. Careful foot management is required for a neurectomized horse:
     - Neuroma formation.
     - Rupture of the DDFT.
     - Exungulation of the hoof as a sequel of unattended infection.
     - Reinnervation of the desensitized site is the most common reason for recurrence of lameness. This may occur anytime between 6 months and several years following surgery.

Traumatic and degenerative arthritis of the DIP joint

Aetiology

- Subchondral cystic lesions, infectious arthritis from penetrating injuries, intra-articular fractures, sprains and luxations.

- Traumatic synovitis of the DIP joint is a significant cause of racing lameness, particularly in the American Quarter horse.
- Synovitis of the DIP joint has also been associated with navicular syndrome.

Clinical signs

- Insidious onset, mild to moderate, bilateral forelimb lameness. Most obvious on hard surfaces, on circles, and following flexion tests.
- Acute unilateral lameness with localizing signs in case of sprain.
- Frequently, effusion of the DIP joint is palpable just proximal to the dorsal part of the coronary band.
- Arthrocentesis may reveal increased fluid pressure and decreased synovial viscosity.
- Positive result to intra-articular analgesia.
- Radiological evidence of degenerative joint disease and or chronic capsulitis. Horses with synovitis of the DIP joint often do not show radiological changes. Remodelling of the synovial fossae, traditionally interpreted as the cardinal radiological sign of 'navicular syndrome' may be indicative of synovitis of the DIP joint.

Treatment

- Treat primary condition (e.g. sprain, chip fracture, subchondral cystic lesion).
- Horses with synovitis, capsulitis and degenerative joint disease can be medicated with the standard intra-articular drugs (polysulphated glycosaminoglycans, sodium hyaluronate, corticosteroids). Oral administration of anti-inflammatory drugs or glycosaminoglycan preparations may be helpful as a symptomatic treatment.
- Associated foot imbalances must be treated with corrective trimming and shoeing.

Prognosis

Horses with radiologically apparent abnormalities of the DIP joint have a poor prognosis for return to soundness.

Infectious arthritis of the DIP joint

Aetiology

- Penetrating injuries to the joint.
- Intra-articular injection (iatrogenic).

• Neurectomized horses may develop infectious arthritis from extension of an unnoticed subsolar abscess.

Clinical signs

• Severe, non-weightbearing lameness.
• Hot, painful swelling proximal to the coronary band.
• Analysis of synovial fluid to support diagnosis of infectious arthritis.

Treatment

• Treatment must consist of aggressive joint lavage in conjunction with intra-articular and systemic antimicrobial therapy. Lavage should be performed via both the dorsal and palmaro-proximal pouches of the joint.
• If severe lameness persists due to residual damage to cartilage or bone, ankylosis of the DIP joint can be attempted to obtain pasture (breeding) soundness.

Prognosis

Horses with infection of the DIP joint have a poor prognosis for return to function. Horses may be salvaged if the joint ankyloses, but ankylosis invariably results in permanent mechanical lameness.

Flexural deformity of the DIP joint

Aetiology and pathogenesis

• Flexural deformities of the DIP joint are caused by relative shortening of the musculotendinous unit of the deep digital flexor. These deformities may be congenital or acquired.
• Congenital flexural deformities of the DIP joint have been associated with intrauterine malpositioning, genetic factors and teratogenic effects. Congenital rupture of the common digital extensor tendon (CDET) may also lead to this deformity.
• Acquired flexural deformities of the DIP joint typically develop in foals of weaning age and may be a manifestation of developmental orthopaedic disease (DOD). Contributing factors are pain causing a flexion withdrawal reflex, lack of exercise, rapid growth and nutritional imbalance. Imbalance of longitudinal growth between the

skeleton and the musculotendinous unit of the deep digital flexor has been hypothesized.

Clinical signs

• Tight DDFT, detected by palpation.
• In the acute stage, the foal may only be able to walk on the tip of the toes, without heel-ground contact ('ballerina foal').
• In the subacute stage, the foot adopts a boxy appearance ('club foot', 'buck hoof') because of the lack of heel wear.
• Flexural deformity of the DIP joint can be divided into two categories:
  – Stage I in which the dorsal wall of the foot does not pass beyond the vertical.
  – Stage II in which the dorsal wall of the foot passes beyond the vertical.

Treatment

• Congenital form
  – Most improve spontaneously within first week of life.
  – Intravenous administration of oxytetracycline to promote muscle relaxation.
• Acquired form, Stage I
  – Attempt to slow down growth by dietary management.
  – Exercise/physiotherapy with judicious use of analgesic drugs.
  – Application of a toe extension and trimming of the heels. The toe needs to be protected against excessive wear and tearing of the dorsal hoofwall.
  – If the deformity is unresponsive to conservative management, desmotomy of the inferior check ligament is indicated to release some of the tension in the DDFT.
• Acquired form, Stage II
  – Inferior check ligament desmotomy.
  – DDFT tenotomy halfway down the metacarpus or at the level of the pastern.

Prognosis

Prognosis for exercise is favourable, as long as a DDFT tenotomy is not required to achieve normal posture.

16.2 *Diseases of the pastern and fetlock*

'Ringbone'

Definition

Ringbone is a bony enlargement in the pastern area. This can be caused by periostitis of the first or second phalanx or osteoarthritis of the PIP joint ('high ringbone') or DIP joint ('low ringbone'). Ringbone may be articular or non-articular.

Phalangeal periostitis

Aetiology

- Trauma, such as lacerations or brushing.
- Chronic microtrauma to ligamentous and tendinous attachments, especially with poor conformation (i.e. base narrow or base-wide; toed-in or toed-out).
- Extensor tendon strain.

Clinical signs

- Lameness only in acute stage.
- Sometimes persistent lameness if common digital extensor tendon is involved.

Treatment

- Rest and anti-inflammatory drugs.

Degenerative joint disease (DJD) of the PIP joint

Aetiology

- Usually chronic and idiopathic, with an insidious onset.
- High-speed exercise involving sudden turns and stops that occur in events such as in polo, calf roping and other rodeo events, may predispose horses to this condition.
- Less frequently, secondary to penetrating wounds, fractures or OCD.

Clinical signs

- Non-specific, chronic lameness.
- Sometimes obvious external signs, i.e. heat and pain if acute, or firm enlargement dorsal pastern if chronic.

- Lameness is exacerbated by flexion of the lower limb.
- Lameness is abolished by ASNB.
- Radiological signs of degenerative joint disease.

Treatment

- Exercise the horse if possible, using anti-inflammatory/analgesic medication.
- Intra-articular medication of the PIP joint with a corticosteroid may provide temporary relief.
- Surgical arthrodesis is usually necessary to reach a pain-free stage of ankylosis. The first and second phalanx are immobilized in compression with three lag screws or a T-plate to promote fusion.

Prognosis

Approximately 65% of surgically treated horses return to full activity. Results are better for hindlimbs than forelimbs. Complete recovery can take up to 12 months.

Subluxation of the PIP joint

Aetiology

- Dorsal subluxation:
  - Sometimes congenital in Arab horses.
  - Secondary to rupture or desmotomy of the suspensory ligament.
- Palmar subluxation:
  - Injury to palmar support structures of the pastern (four palmar ligaments and distal sesamoidean ligaments), e.g. foals jumping from heights.

Clinical signs

- Intermittent dorsal 'clicking' of pastern in Arab horses.
- Dorsal convexity or concavity of the pastern following trauma.

Treatment

- Eight weeks in cast with limb in flexion followed by 6 months of box rest.
- The PIP joint should be arthrodesed before scar tissue permanently lengthens or shortens the supporting structures.

Prognosis

Prognosis is guarded for a return to full work.

Fracture of the second phalanx

Aetiology and classification

- Fractures of the middle phalanx are most common in the hindlimbs of horses used for polo and Western performance.
- Types include chip fractures, wing (palmar/plantar process) fractures and comminuted fractures.
- Fractures of the second phalanx commonly result from sudden compression, in combination with a twisting force that occurs with sudden stops, starts or short turns.
- Comminuted fractures are more common than wing fractures. Chip fractures are rare.

Clinical signs

- Chip fractures often result in acute lameness, but lameness usually improves quickly with rest.
- Wing and comminuted fractures:
  - Acute, severe lameness.
  - Swelling, crepitus, pain.
  - Diagnosis is confirmed by radiography.

Treatment and prognosis

Chip fractures:

- Immobilization or surgical removal of the chip.
- Prognosis for return to soundness is good.

Wing and comminuted fractures:

- Immobilization in flexion using a cast, offers a good prognosis for return to breeding soundness. Some surgeons recommend the use of a full limb cast.
- Reconstructable fractures must be accurately reduced and stabilized with a single lag screw (wing fractures), or several screws and plates (comminuted fractures), to give the horse a realistic chance of returning to working soundness.
- For fractures involving the proximal articulation that cannot be accurately reduced, arthrodesis of the PIP joint may be required.
- If both the PIP and DIP joints are involved in the fracture, the prognosis for return to exercise is guarded.
- Severely comminuted fractures result in permanent lameness.

Fracture of the first phalanx

Sagittal and comminuted fractures ('split pastern')

Aetiology and classification

- These fractures propagate distally from the sagittal groove in the proximal articular surface of the first phalanx. They are caused by the screwdriver effect of the sagittal ridge of the distal end of the metacarpus/metatarsus.
- Sagittal fractures of the first phalanx may be:
  - Incomplete. The fracture extends a variable distance distally from the sagittal groove towards the medullary cavity, but does not include the lateral or medial cortex.
  - Complete, non-displaced. The fracture extends sideways from the medullary cavity to exit the lateral or medial cortex.
  - Complete displaced.
  - Comminuted, reconstructable. A continuous strut of bone remains between the fetlock joint and PIP joint.
  - Severely comminuted. No bone continuity remains between both joints. These fractures are generally unreconstructable.

Clinical signs

- Signs vary from acute, severe lameness that improves with box rest, to non-weightbearing lameness, with obvious crepitus and instability.
- Pain, heat and swelling at the pastern.
- Pain on flexion of the fetlock joint.
- Diagnosis is confirmed by radiography. Oblique radiographs are necessary to show distal propagation of the fracture line.
- The fracture line may remain invisible for several weeks following injury. In these cases bone scintigraphy will reveal fracture damage before the fracture is radiographically discernable.
- Do not use nerve blocks! Freedom from pain may turn an incomplete fracture into a comminuted one.

Treatment and prognosis

- First aid for an incomplete fracture consists of a Robert Jones bandage with lateral and medial splints. A complete fracture is best supported by a first aid cast, applied with the horse standing and the affected limb lifted off the ground by an assistant. The cannon bone and phalanges should be vertically aligned with a dorsal splint.

- Incomplete fractures can be treated by cast immobilization and/or lag screw fixation.
- Complete fractures should always be treated by lag screw fixation. Even a small displacement of fragments compromises the final outcome, because it results in permanent joint damage.
- Horses should be allowed to recover from general anaesthesia in a cast. If the fracture is not comminuted, the cast can be removed after 7–10 days.
- Horses with comminuted fractures of the first phalanx can be salvaged for breeding, using a combination of external and internal fixation, as well as cast immobilization (porcupine cast). However, if no continuous strut of bone remains between the fetlock joint and PIP joint, the prognosis for survival is guarded.

Longitudinal frontal fractures

Treatment

- Horses with incomplete, non-displaced fractures can be managed with 6 months of box rest or cast immobilization for 6 weeks followed by 6 weeks of box rest.
- Complete fractures, with or without displacement, must be accurately reduced and stabilized with lag screws.
- For fractures into the distal articulation that cannot be accurately reduced, arthrodesis of the PIP joint may be required.

Prognosis

The prognosis for athletic function depends on the degree of damage to the fetlock joint but is reasonably good.

Chip fractures

Aetiology and location

- Overextension and concussion, especially in fast gaited horses.
- Chip fractures occur at the dorsoproximal or proximal palmar/plantar articular margin of the first phalanx.
- Both dorsal and palmar/plantar fragments have also been recognized as incidental radiological findings, not associated with lameness (OCD, separate centre of ossification?).

Clinical signs

- Acute or subacute onset, moderate to severe lameness.
- Joint effusion, pain on forced flexion.
- Obvious improvement with rest, but recurrence with exercise.

Diagnosis

- Radiography is important for exact localization of the fragments. Oblique proximolateral-distomedial views may be necessary to see palmar/plantar fragments.
- Intra-articular analgesia.

Treatment

Treatment consists of removal via arthroscopy before DJD develops.

Prognosis

- The prognosis depends on the presence of concurrent damage to the fetlock joint and its supporting structures sustained during initial trauma.
- Good for return to full exercise following removal via arthroscopy, provided that no evidence of DJD is present.

Fracture of the palmar/plantar process

Location

- This type of fracture is located further abaxially along the palmar or plantar proximal articular margin of the first phalanx than the chip fracture, and tends to be larger. The lateral or medial palmar or plantar tuberosity (process) of the first phalanx is involved.
- The fracture may be articular or non-articular.
- Osteochondritis dissecans also occurs in this location.

Treatment

- Horses with non-articular fractures are managed with 3 months of box rest.
- Horses with articular fractures are candidates for removal or internal fixation of the fracture fragment.

Desmitis of the distal sesamoidean ligaments

Aetiology

Overextension of the fetlock can result in damage to any component or combination of components of the suspensory apparatus. The distal sesamoidean ligaments extend distally from the bases of the proximal sesamoid bones and form the distal attachments of the suspensory apparatus.

Clinical signs

- In the acute stage oedema, heat, pain and swelling are present dorsal to the DDFT in the region of the pastern. Normally, the distal sesamoidean ligaments cannot be palpated deep to the DDFT, but, with injury, they become palpable.
- Lameness is abolished by an ASNB.
- Ultrasonography shows enlargement and hypoechoicity of one or both of the middle and straight distal sesamoidean ligaments.
- Radiological evidence of entheseophytosis in these ligaments may also be present, but these entheseophytes are sometimes seen as an incidental finding during routine radiography of the digit.

Treatment

- Stall rest for 2–4 months and anti-inflammatory medication, followed by gradual return to exercise.
- Provide palmar foot support with egg-bar, or wide-webbed, seated-out shoes.

Prognosis

- Excellent if there is no heat or pain associated with the swelling, and the horse is not lame.
- High recurrence rate of lameness with return to exercise.

Luxation of the fetlock joint

Aetiology and classification

- Luxation is classified as:
  - Simple luxation, in which there is no tissue disruption other than rupture of the collateral ligament(s).
  - Compound luxation, in which the joint is open or the suspensory apparatus is disrupted.
- Luxation of the fetlock is usually associated with an accident in which the digit is caught (hole, cattlegrid). It can also occur during fast turning with high rotational forces on the joint (Western riding, polo).

Clinical signs

- The lateral or medial collateral ligament is disrupted or avulsed, resulting in a valgus or varus deformity of the distal limb.
- Sometimes overriding of distal end of the metacarpus/metatarsus and proximal end of the first phalanx.
- If the luxation spontaneously reduces, minimal external signs are seen. Manual reluxation and reduction of the fetlock, causing relatively little pain, may be possible (unlike fracture).

Treatment and prognosis

- Reduction and immobilization of the distal limb with a cast for 6 to 8 weeks allows most horses with simple luxation to regain pasture soundness. Open luxations are treated in a similar manner following meticulous surgical debridement and irrigation, but the risk of the horse developing secondary DJD is considerable!
- Compound luxations accompanied by suspensory breakdown or complicated fracture, may be salvaged with a surgical arthrodesis of the fetlock, but the prognosis for survival is guarded to poor.

Villonodular synovitis

Definition

Villonodular synovitis is a chronic, proliferative, hypertrophic synovitis and capsulitis in the dorsal pouch of the fetlock joint. It is caused by trauma to a normal transverse fold of synovial tissue located proximally in the dorsal pouch.

Pathogenesis

Chronic, low-grade trauma caused by repeated overextension of the fetlock.

Clinical signs

- Mainly seen in racing Thoroughbreds.

- Obvious fetlock lameness with swelling and pain on flexion.

Radiography

- Presence of a depression in the dorsodistal cortex of the metacarpus just proximal to the sagittal ridge.
- Positive contrast arthrography (filling defect) or ultrasonography is often necessary to confirm the presence of a soft tissue mass in the proximal part of the dorsal pouch of the joint.

Treatment

- Local infiltration of the mass with corticosteroids.
- Removal by arthrotomy/arthroscopy followed by 6 months of controlled rest.

Prognosis

Fifty per cent of horses regain soundness, but recurrence is possible.

Osteochondritis dissecans and subchondral cystic lesions in the fetlock joint

Location

Sites of occurrence for osteochondritis dissecans lesions in the fetlock joint are:

- The proximal end of the sagittal ridge of the distal extremity of the metacarpus/metatarsus.
- The distal end of the sagittal ridge of the distal extremity of the metacarpus/metatarsus.
- The palmar surface of the condyles of the distal extremity of the metacarpus/metatarsus.
- The proximal dorsal margin of the first phalanx.
- The proximal palmar/plantar margin of the first phalanx.

Subchondral cystic lesions in the fetlock joint are found at:

- The proximal articular surface of the first phalanx.
- The distal articular surface of the metacarpus/metatarsus.

Clinical signs

- Joint swelling, mild lameness.

- Lameness is exacerbated by flexion and abolished by intra-articular analgesia.
- Seen in young horses, mostly at the time of first introduction to exercise.
- All four fetlocks can be involved.

Treatment and prognosis

- Surgical treatment of osteochondritis dissecans lesions consists of fragment removal and debridement of abnormal subchondral bone via arthroscopy.
- Horses with subchondral cystic lesions may respond favourably to prolonged box rest. If this fails, the cyst cavity can be exposed through an extra- or intra-articular approach and debrided.

Fracture of the proximal sesamoid bone

Classification and incidence

- May be classified as apical, midbody, basilar, abaxial, or comminuted.
- Found mainly in the forelimbs of racing Thoroughbreds and the hindlimbs of Standardbreds. Sometimes occur bilaterally in young foals with osteoporosis.

Aetiology

- Acute overextension of the suspensory apparatus.
- Degenerative changes ('sesamoiditis') may be a consequence of chronic cyclical loading (bone fatigue) and predispose the sesamoid bones to fracture. Training may strengthen other components of the suspensory apparatus more than the sesamoids, making the sesamoid bones more susceptible to failure.
- Direct trauma (brushing).
- Osteoporosis in foals.

Clinical signs

- Acute, moderate to severe lameness.
- Usually only one sesamoid affected. Fracture of both sesamoids results in breakdown of the suspensory apparatus.
- The horse walks with a 'splinted' fetlock, avoids normal dorsiflexion during weight bearing.
- Horses with small chip fractures may improve dramatically with rest, but lameness recurs when exercise is resumed.

- Variable signs are swelling, effusion of the digital sheath or fetlock joint, crepitus, pain on pressure over the sesamoid bones, enlargement of a suspensory branch.

Treatment and prognosis

- Conservative treatment of horses with sesamoid bone fracture is generally unsuccessful.
- Surgical options are fragment removal or surgical reconstruction of the bone. This is advisable if athletic exercise is expected and to avoid DJD.
- Apical fractures are best removed via arthroscopy of the palmar/plantar pouch of the fetlock joint. The prognosis for return to soundness depends on the degree of damage to the suspensory ligament.
- Small basilar fracture fragments can be surgically removed. Larger fragments must be fixed to the parent bone using cancellous bone grafting or cerclage-wiring. Prognosis for return to athletic function is guarded if the basilar fragment is large, because insertion of the distal sesamoidean ligaments is lost.
- Midbody fractures are reconstructed by lag screw fixation, cerclage-wiring or cancellous bone grafting.
- Horses with an abaxial surface fracture are candidates for surgical removal only if the fracture has an articular component.

'Sesamoiditis'

Definition

The term 'sesamoiditis' is used to describe proliferative or degenerative bony changes of the proximal sesamoid bones. Two forms of sesamoiditis have been described, a periostitis form and an osteitis form.

Aetiology and pathogenesis

Periostitis form

Acute or chronic injury to the SL, distal sesamoidean ligaments and/or the palmar/plantar annular ligament of the fetlock, results in damage to the bone–ligament interface with the proximal sesamoid bones. Osseous metaplasia of scar tissue and periostitis lead to the formation of entheseophytes and changes to the contour of the bone. In this sense, 'sesamoiditis' is secondary to desmitis of the suspensory structures.

Osteitis form

The use of the term 'sesamoiditis' to describe a degenerative condition of the proximal sesamoid bones in its own right is subject to debate.

Arteriosclerosis and thrombosis of the nutrient arteries, and local ischaemic necrosis have been invoked to explain the radiological appearance of demineralization along the vascular channels within the sesamoid bones, in analogy with the vascular theory of the navicular syndrome. Equally, this theory has now been questioned. It is more likely that linear radiolucencies along the vascular channels in the proximal sesamoid bones of some horses do not indicate enlargement of vascular channels, but rather reflect the normal individual variation in their appearance. Entheseophyte formation at the insertion site of the suspensory branches, between the nutrient foramina on the abaxial surface of the bone, may also result in a false impression of decreased radiopacity and enlargement of these vascular channels.

Clinical signs

- Acute injury to the suspensory structures associated with the proximal sesamoid bones causes moderate to severe lameness with swelling, heat and pain referable to the SL. The horse moves with a 'splinted' fetlock.
- Chronic sesamoiditis produces non-specific lower limb lameness. Sometimes the suspensory structures are palpably enlarged.

Diagnosis

- Low 4-point nerve block (L4PNB) abolishes lameness.
- Radiological signs:
  - Entheseophyte formation along the non-articular surface of the bone results in change in its shape and contour.
  - Calcification within the soft tissues of the suspensory apparatus.
  - When chronic lameness is present, changes may be accompanied by a degree of disuse osteoporosis of the proximal sesamoid bones.
  - Localized areas of decreased radiopacity along the vascular channels are of questionable significance.

Treatment

- Horses with acute injuries of the SL are managed with prolonged rest and external support.

- Chronically affected horses can be managed with analgesic, anti-inflammatory drugs to control active periostitis or to allow the horse to exercise painfree.
- The use of the peripheral vasodilating drug, isoxsuprine hydrochloride, has been advocated by some clinicians to treat horses with 'sesamoiditis'.

Prognosis

The prognosis is guarded for athletic soundness and depends on the degree of damage to the SL.

Breakdown of the suspensory apparatus

Aetiology

Acute overextension of the fetlock that disrupts any or all of the components of the suspensory apparatus:

- The SL.
- The sesamoid bones.
- The distal sesamoidean ligaments.

These injuries usually occur in racehorses exercising at high speed.

Clinical signs

The fetlock drops down to the ground during weight bearing, and the pastern lies horizontal to the ground.

Diagnosis

- Radiography may be necessary to recognize accompanying bone damage (e.g. avulsion of a collateral ligament, fracture of a sesamoid bone, condylar fracture of the metacarpus/metatarsus).
- Vascular supply of the distal limb must be assessed for permanent damage. Assessment is best done after the horse has been treated for 5 to 7 days with a first aid lower limb cast, to give damaged arteries time to recover. Irreversible damage leads to ischaemic necrosis and sloughing of the limb distal to the fetlock.

Treatment and prognosis

- First aid consists of lower limb cast or splint, applied with the distal limb vertically aligned. After 5–7 days the cast is removed to examine the lower limb for damage to its vasculature.

- If the vascular supply to the distal limb is not irreversibly damaged, the limb can be re-immobilized to allow formation of fibrous tissue of sufficient strength to support the fetlock.
- The treatment of choice to salvage valuable stock for breeding is to arthrodese the fetlock joint with a dynamic compression plate and tension band wire.

Annular ligament syndrome

Aetiology and classification

The annular ligament syndrome refers to lameness caused by a restriction within the 'fetlock-tunnel' between the palmar/plantar annular ligament of the fetlock (AL) and the intersesamoidean ligament. This is almost invariably associated with thickening of the annular ligament, and can be caused by:

- Desmitis of the annular ligament.
- Chronic tenosynovitis of the digital sheath.
- Tendon swelling within the 'fetlock-tunnel'.
- Any combination of these conditions.

Clinical signs

- Persistent lameness, even after long periods of rest.
- Swelling of the digital synovial sheath, proximal and distal to the borders of the annular ligament, gives a characteristic, notched appearance to the palmar/plantar surface of the fetlock.
- Dorsiflexion of the fetlock is often reduced during weight bearing.
- Sometimes the horse is reluctant to place the heel of the foot fully on the ground.

Diagnosis

- Regional analgesia:
  - The horse is improved or sound following intrasynovial injection of local analgesics into the digital synovial sheath.
  - The horse is usually improved following an ASNB and sound following a L4PNB.
  - Sometimes the horse demonstrates residual mechanical gait restriction following regional analgesia.
- Tenography following insufflation of air into the digital sheath shows thickening of the AL.

- Ultrasonography unequivocally establishes dorsopalmar/dorsoplantar thickening of the ligament.

Treatment and prognosis

- Treatment consists of surgical decompression of the 'fetlock-tunnel' and the digital synovial sheath that is contained within it, via desmotomy of the AL.
- The horse is box rested and its limb bandaged until sutures are removed at 2 weeks. Exercise is initiated at this time and gradually increased (2 weeks walking in hand, followed by 4 weeks lunging) to avoid development of restricting adhesions within the tendon sheath.
- The prognosis for return to soundness following desmotomy is generally favourable (65–70%).

Infectious tenosynovitis of the digital synovial sheath

Aetiology

- Lacerations or punctures of the digital synovial sheath. Small puncture wounds that readily seal, may initially not be recognized as having entered the sheath.
- Injection of pharmaceutical agents into the sheath (iatrogenic).
- Occasionally septicaemia may result in infection of the sheath.

Clinical signs

- Marked lameness in most cases.
- Distension of the affected tendon sheath, sometimes difficult to localize due to generalized, painful swelling of the distal limb.
- Discharge of synovial fluid from a laceration or puncture may be present.
- Swelling, pain and lameness may not develop for some time after the initial injury, if the tendon sheath has good drainage.

Diagnosis

- Severe lameness with swelling, heat and pain of the digital sheath.
- Analysis of synovial fluid is indicated to support a diagnosis of infectious synovitis.
- Injection of sterile saline or contrast agent into the sheath may confirm communication with a wound.

- Ultrasonography is used to evaluate the integrity of the tendons within the sheath or identify the presence of foreign bodies.

Treatment

- Primary closure of an open tendon sheath shortly after injury may be contraindicated. This may trap bacteria in the sheath and produce infectious tenosynovitis. The wound should be thoroughly cleaned and is best maintained under a sterile dressing.
- Treatment of infectious tenosynovitis must consist of aggressive lavage of the sheath, in conjunction with intrasynovial and systemic broad-spectrum antimicrobial therapy.
- If the horse does not respond favourably to this treatment within a few days, surgical exploration of the sheath is advisable to debride accessible necrotic tissue and adhesions, and allow placement of indwelling fenestrated drains for continued through-and-through lavage. The drain is covered with a sterile dressing under a bulky pressure bandage, and lavage is continued twice daily for 3 to 5 days. Following removal of the drain, sodium hyaluronate can be injected into the sheath at two-weekly intervals to reduce the formation of adhesions.
- In horses with subacute or chronic infectious tenosynovitis of the digital synovial sheath, desmotomy of the annular ligament of the fetlock may give significant pain relief.

Prognosis

- Complications of infectious tenosynovitis are unresolved infection, formation of adhesions and occasionally infectious tendinitis and tendon rupture.
- Horses with penetrating wounds to the digital synovial sheath have a good prognosis for return to soundness if treatment is initiated before infectious tenosynovitis develops.
- If infection occurs and treatment is not instituted promptly, the prognosis for return to soundness is guarded.

Flexural deformity of the fetlock

Aetiology and pathogenesis

- Flexural deformity of the fetlock is caused by relative shortening of the musculotendinous units of the SDF, the DDF, the SL or any combination of these structures.

- Flexural deformities may be congenital or acquired.
- Congenital rupture of the common digital extensor tendon (CDET) may also lead to this deformity.
- Acquired flexural deformities of the fetlock develop typically in yearlings and may be a manifestation of developmental orthopaedic disease (DOD).
- The combination of growth of the distal radial physis, the position of the superior check ligament and loss of elasticity in the interosseus medius muscle may be responsible for flexural deformities of the fetlock in yearlings as opposed to flexural deformity of the DIP joint in foals.

Clinical signs

- Flexural deformity of the fetlock is characterized by a straight fetlock angle with a variable amount of dorsal knuckling of the joint.
- This deformity can be subdivided into two categories of severity:
  - Stage I in which the fetlock remains in dorsiflexion during weightbearing, with only occasional knuckling.
  - Stage II in which the fetlock is permanently knuckled forward.

Treatment

- Congenitally affected foals may correct spontaneously, or require the application of bandages and splints and intravenous administration of oxytetracycline to induce muscle relaxation.
- Limbs with flexural deformity associated with rupture of the CDET are best bandaged and supported with a PVC splint, applied to the palmar aspect of the fetlock. The splint is bent to an angle of approximately 160°.
- Mildly to moderately affected horses (Stage I) can often be treated by dietary restrictions, controlled exercise, physiotherapy in combination with analgesic drugs, and application of a bandage with a bent splint applied to the palmar aspect of the fetlock. Corrective shoes should provide a toe extension and raise the heels.
- Horses with Stage I deformity unresponsive to conservative management can be treated surgically by inferior or superior check ligament desmotomy, depending on which musculotendinous unit is primarily involved.

- Horses with Stage II deformity should be treated surgically. Both inferior and superior check ligament desmotomies followed by application of a bent palmar splint may be successful, but some horses may require tenotomy of the superficial digital flexor tendon (SDFT) or desmotomy of the SL to achieve normal posture.

Prognosis

This deformity is usually more difficult to treat than the flexural deformity of the DIP joint (see 16.1). The prognosis remains favourable if tenotomy of the SDFT or SL desmotomy is not required to regain normal posture.

Angular deformity of the fetlock

Aetiology and pathogenesis

- Angular deformity of the fetlock joint may be congenital or acquired.
- Congenital angular deformity is due to joint laxity.
- Acquired angular deformity is caused by asynchronous longitudinal growth of the distal metacarpal/metatarsal physis and is a manifestation of DOD. Because most of the growth of the distal metacarpal/metatarsal physis occurs prior to 3 months of age, correction of angular deformity of the fetlock should occur between 1 and 2 months.

Clinical signs

- Fetlock deformity is mainly of the varus type and occurs predominantly in the hindlimbs.
- Palpation to establish the presence of joint laxity.
- Radiography to assess possible involvement of the proximal physis of the first phalanx, the distal physis of the cannon bone and the presence of epiphyseal wedging.

Treatment

- Congenital form usually improves during first week of life. If joint laxity persists, the use of sleeve casts or braces may be appropriate. These foals should not be allowed free exercise.
- Conservative management consists of dietary restriction, box rest and corrective trimming of the foot.
- Foals unresponsive to conservative management are treated surgically by hemicircumferen-

tial periosteal transection or epiphyseal bridging. These procedures are best performed before the foal is 2 months old.

Prognosis

The prognosis is favourable with early recognition and management.

16.3 *Diseases of the metacarpus and metatarsus*

Condylar, metaphyseal and diaphyseal fractures of the third metacarpal/ metatarsal bone

Aetiology and classification

1. Condylar fractures:
   - These fractures occur commonly in young racehorses, especially during fast work on a hard surface.
   - Forelimbs are more frequently involved than hindlimbs.
   - Lateral condylar fracture is more common than medial condylar fracture.
   - Medial condylar fractures are more common in the hindlimb. They spiral further proximally into the metacarpus/metatarsus than do lateral condylar fractures.
2. Metaphyseal fractures:
   - Salter Harris types I and II are most common.
3. Diaphyseal fractures.

Clinical signs

- From mild lameness to non-weightbearing lameness with obvious instability.
- Avoid nerve blocks if fracture is suspected.
- Heat, pain, swelling depend on the type and age of the fracture. Horses with subacute or chronic fissure fractures may not show signs of inflammation at the fracture site.
- Metaphyseal and diaphyseal fractures are at great risk of becoming compound.

Diagnosis

1. Radiography.
   - Take all views to identify the fracture plane accurately.
   - With condylar fractures, include a flexed dorsopalmar view of the fetlock to identify palmar cortical comminution.
   - With condylar fractures, look for overlapping fracture lines in the corresponding proximal sesamoid bone.
2. Scintigraphy is useful to identify incomplete palmar cortical fractures of the metacarpal condyles.

Treatment and prognosis

- Horses with a condylar fracture should be treated by internal fixation with lag screws. The lower limb is best stabilized in a cast for recovery. The prognosis for return to exercise for horses with a condylar fracture is generally good. Horses with a chronic or displaced fracture, or a fracture with palmar comminution have a poorer prognosis for return to exercise.
- Repaired medial condylar fractures in hindlimbs are at risk of catastrophic comminution during recovery from anaesthesia. If possible, this recovery should therefore be assisted (slings, swimming pool, mats, ropes).
- A diaphyseal fracture can be reconstructed using one or two dynamic compression plates. The prognosis for survival is always guarded. The prognosis for survival becomes hopeless if the nutrient foramen is involved in the fracture.
- Horses with a metaphyseal fracture are managed by cast immobilization, with or without additional internal fixation. The prognosis for soundness is favourable, unless growth disturbances occur due to premature physeal closure.

'Bucked shins'/'sore shins'/'dorsal metacarpal disease'

Definition

These terms imply a painful condition of the dorsal aspect of the third metacarpal bone of young racehorses, caused by stress or fatigue damage to the bone.

Aetiology and pathogenesis

- During fast-gaited exercise the dorsal cortex of the third metacarpal bone suffers greater damage from compression than the rest of the cortex. If damage continues to occur regularly, the osteoclastic phase of the remodelling response exceeds the repair phase, and the bone weakens until it fails. This results in microfracture of the dorsal cortex, subperiosteal haemorrhage and callus formation.

- There are two syndromes:
  - Type I syndrome affects the dorsomedial cortex and occurs predominantly in 2 year old Thoroughbreds.
  - Type II syndrome affects the dorsolateral cortex and occurs predominantly in 3 to 5 year old Thoroughbreds.
- Both syndromes are caused by fatigue or stress damage to the bone.

Clinical signs

- The acute form of Type I dorsal metacarpal disease (DMD) causes an acute onset of painful 'shins', but the horse has no obvious lameness or radiological changes.
- The subacute form of Type I DMD is accompanied by mild lameness, variable pain on palpation, obvious dorsal swelling and radiological evidence of subperiosteal callus formation.
- Horses with Type II DMD have an incomplete, oblique fracture line in the dorsal or dorsolateral cortex of the metacarpus. Lameness is most obvious after strenuous exercise.

Treatment

- Prevention by gradually increasing the workload of immature racehorses prior to initiating fast exercise.
- Treatment of the acute form consists of 3 months of rest followed by 3 months of controlled exercise. Anti-inflammatory drugs and physical therapy are used to reduce pain and swelling.
- Treatment of horses with the subacute form Type I DMD and Type II DMD with rest and controlled exercise is often unsuccessful.
- Surgical alternatives in unresponsive horses are surgical forage of the affected area of the cortex (osteostixis), or unicortical lag screw fixation.

Proximal metacarpal/metatarsal syndrome

Definition and classification

Proximal metacarpal/metatarsal disease, proximal metacarpal/metatarsal syndrome and high suspensory disease are terms used to describe lameness referable to the proximal, palmar/ plantar third of the metacarpal/metatarsal region. Lameness in this area can be due to:

- Avulsion fractures of the proximal palmar/ plantar cortex.
- Fatigue damage and stress fractures of the proximal palmar/plantar cortex.
- Desmitis of the proximal part of the SL.

Clinical signs

- Avulsion fractures of the proximal palmar/ plantar cortex cause acute, severe lameness. Stress fractures of the proximal palmar/plantar cortex and desmitis of the proximal end of the SL more frequently cause chronic, intermittent lameness.
- Signs of focal pain can often be elicited with pressure over the proximal palmar metacarpus/ plantar metatarsus.
- Lameness can be exacerbated by localized sustained pressure.
- Sometimes the SL is palpably enlarged.
- Lameness usually improves with rest, but returns with exercise.
- Horses with a straight hock conformation are predisposed to proximal suspensory desmitis.

Diagnosis

- Radiography:
  - Subtle changes to trabecular pattern of the proximal palmar/plantar cortex.
  - Faint circular or vertical radiolucent line(s).
- Local analgesia can be used to desensitize the proximal palmar metacarpal/plantar metatarsal region (direct infiltration, ulnar nerve block, lateral palmar nerve block, subtarsal nerve block or tibial nerve block).
- Scintigraphy to identify increased bone turnover in proximal palmar/plantar cortex.
- Ultrasonography to identify changes in the proximal SL.

Differential diagnosis

- Inferior check ligament desmitis.
- Carpal tunnel syndrome.
- Carpal joint disease.
- 'High splints'.
- 'Occult spavin'.

Treatment and prognosis

- Prolonged box rest (2 to 6 months) followed by graduated return to exercise; monitor healing with ultrasonography or scintigraphy.
- Egg barr shoes to provide additional support in proximal suspensory desmitis.
- Prognosis for return to exercise is favourable, except in proximal suspensory desmitis in hindlimbs where it is poor.

'Splints'

Definition and classification

A splint is a bony enlargement involving the second or fourth metacarpal or metatarsal bones. Different types of splint are:

- *Intermetacarpal splint.* This is an exostosis between the cannon bone and a splint bone
- *Postmetacarpal splint.* This is an exostosis on the palmar/plantar or axial surface of a splint bone.
- *'Blind splint'.* This is an exostosis on the axial surface of a splint bone that remains undetectable to inspection or palpation.

Aetiology and pathogenesis

- The medial splint bone takes full axial loading from the second carpal bone, but the lateral splint bone takes only half the axial load from the fourth carpal bone. Chronic tearing and inflammation of the medial interosseous ligament may occur, when a horse is first introduced to exercise. Periostitis and osseous metaplasia of scar tissue may cause bony enlargement of the proximal third of the medial splint bone of young horses. As the horse ages, the medial splint may fuse to the cannon bone, eliminating further movement and irritation to the interosseous ligament.
- Conformational factors may exacerbate strain to the medial interosseous ligament (i.e. bench knees, carpal varus deformities), or lead to direct trauma by brushing (i.e. toed-out, base-narrow).

Clinical signs

- Hard swelling along the splint bone. Heat and pain in acute phase, quiescent in chronic phase.
- Lameness only in acute phase, usually mild, worse on hard ground and when the horse is exercised in a circle.

- Sometimes chronic lameness, due to encroachment of bony enlargement on flexor tendons or SL (very rare).

Treatment and prognosis

- Horses with acute periostitis respond favourably to rest and anti-inflammatory medication. Although an obvious lump may remain, persistent lameness is uncommon.
- In Show Horses, blemishes caused by chronic exostosis may need to be removed. Recurrence of the exostosis after surgical removal can be expected in 50% of such cases.

Fractures of the splint bone

Aetiology and classification

- Fractures of the distal third of the splint bone may occur spontaneously or may be caused by external trauma, such as kicks (especially to the lateral splint bone) or interference (especially to the medial splint bone in forelimbs). Spontaneous avulsion fractures are caused by the pull of the distal ligament of the splint bone during extreme dorsiflexion of the fetlock. Increased dorsiflexion during weight bearing is associated with desmitis of the SL. Standardbreds are affected more commonly than Thoroughbreds, and forelimbs are more frequently affected than hindlimbs.
- Proximal fractures are generally caused by kicks to the lateral aspect of a hindlimb. These fractures are usually compound and comminuted.

Clinical signs

- Acute fractures cause swelling, heat, pain and lameness.
- Often concomitant with SL desmitis.
- Lameness varies, but in spontaneous fractures, it is generally due to SL desmitis rather than fracture *per se*.
- Sometimes accompanied by generalized oedema of the lower limb.
- Sometimes an open wound is present.
- Sometimes a sequestrum forms, causing a chronic, discharging sinus.

Radiography and prognosis

- Normal healing proceeds with callus formation and remodelling.

- Sometimes distal displacement with non-union and pseudarthrosis is seen.
- Sometimes hypertrophic callus formation is seen.
- Re-fracture through callus may indicate insufficient healing of the concomitant SL desmitis.

These radiological abnormalities are rarely associated with persistent lameness, provided the suspensory ligament has healed satisfactorily.

Treatment

- Distal fractures and non-complicated proximal fractures usually heal satisfactorily with conservative management only.
- Open fractures should be treated initially as open wounds, using systemically and locally administered antibiotics, lavage, establishment of proper drainage and application of an absorbent, bulky dressing. Given this treatment, many open fractures heal without complications.
- Complicated open fractures with sequestrum formation and osteomyelitis of the splint bone should be debrided surgically. As much as the distal two-thirds of a splint bone can be safely removed, without causing instability of the remaining fragment and the adjacent joint. If less than the proximal one-third of a splint bone remains, it should be stabilized by internal fixation, except for the lateral splint bone of the hindlimb, which can be removed entirely without complications.
- Horses with proximal intra-articular fractures of a splint bone that result in joint instability should be treated by internal fixation.

Tendinitis

Definition

Tendinitis is inflammation of a tendon. It is usually caused by excessive strain. Tendosynovitis is inflammation of a tendon and its tendon sheath (cf. tenosynovitis describes inflammation of just the tendon sheath).

Aetiology

- Mechanical stress is responsible for tendinitis. Clinically apparent tendinitis may be preceded by subclinical fibrillar damage or by intratendinous degeneration.

- Injuries usually occur towards the end of an exercise, when fatigue sets in.
- The SDFT is more commonly affected because of its smaller cross-sectional area and because overextension of the fetlock joint causes more strain in the SDFT than in the DDFT.
- The usual sites of injury (at mid-metacarpal level for the SDFT and at the fetlock joint for the DDFT) are areas that are relatively avascular and acellular.

Pathophysiology

- The degree of damage varies from mild inflammation without fibrillar damage, to fibrillar stretching and slippage, to actual fibrillar rupture and, ultimately, to complete tendon rupture. The centre of the tendon is preferentially affected.
- Severe acute injuries typically are characterized by intratendinous haemorrhage, which separates and weakens remaining fibrils, oedema, fibrin, local swelling, transudation and release of hydrolytic enzymes.
- Healing occurs by production of granulation tissue and its organization into fibrous tissue. As the fibrous tissue matures, ultrasonographic examination reveals an increase in the tendon's echogenicity.
- Healing occurs by intrinsic and extrinsic mechanisms. Severe injuries rely predominantly on extrinsic repair from peritendinous connective tissue elements. Extrinsic healing is very limited for injured tendons that lie within synovial sheaths, where a physical barrier exists between the tendon and peritendinous connective tissue.

Clinical signs

- Immediate moderate to severe lameness.
- Swelling rapidly develops ('bow').
- Some injuries are not apparent for 24–48 hours.
- Some injuries cause localized heat and swelling but no lameness.
- Lameness usually improves quickly with box rest.
- The SDFT is more commonly affected than the DDFT.
- Sinking of fetlock joint occurs with severe injury to the SDFT.
- Injury to the SDFT in the region of the fetlock joint usually includes the distal branches of the SDFT. Swelling of the palmaroproximal aspect of the phalanges results, and it is difficult to distinguish this from desmitis of the distal sesamoidean ligaments.

Diagnosis

1. History and clinical signs as described above.
2. Palpation
3. Ultrasonography of tendon:
   - A core lesion is the most common finding.
   - As the injury heals, the borders of the lesion become indistinct, and the lesion more echogenic. Peritendinous oedema, which often accompanies tendinitis, disappears early in convalescence.
   - To determine when the horse is able to return to full exercise, the following criteria should be satisfied during ultrasonographic examination:
     - Good longitudinal and transverse patterns.
     - No core lesions or hypoechoic regions but homogeneous appearance.
     - Return to normal echogenicity.
     - No adhesions.

Prognosis

Prognosis for return to work depends on which structure is injured (SDFT or DDFT), the location of the injury (within or without a tendon sheath), the severity of the injury and the level of exercise expected (racing vs. hacking). Prognosis for return to previous level of exercise is always guarded.

Treatment

1. Acute tendinitis:
   - Ice-packs, cold hosing.
   - Apply pressure bandage using several layers of padding.
   - Box rest to limit further damage.
   - Experimental support exists for the use of intralesional PSGAG.
   - Shoeing with raised heels, only for DDFT injuries.
   - Tendon splitting.
   - Superior check ligament desmotomy.
2. Subacute stage:
   - Stall rest with periods of controlled hand-walking.
   - Intralesional injections (sodium hyaluronate, PSGAG).
3. Chronic stage:
   - Regime of increasing exercise.
   - Superior check ligament desmotomy.

Tendon lacerations

Clinical signs

- Wire cuts, over-reach or striking injury from other horse.
- Laceration present, although the entry wound can be deceptively small.
- Severe laceration of the DDFT causes lifting of the toe.
- Horses with lacerations of the SDFT may present with increased dorsiflexion (sinking) of the fetlock.
- Severance of both tendons as well as the SL causes total breakdown of the stay apparatus, and the fetlock rests on the ground.
- Lacerations of the long or common digital extensor tendons may cause 'knuckling' of the fetlock, and stumbling at walk and trot.
- Lacerations of the palmar/plantar aspect of the distal metacarpus/metatarsus usually involve the digital synovial sheath.

Treatment

- General principles of wound care.
- Lacerated extensor tendons usually heal without suturing. A cast or a firm bandage and shoe with a toe extension may be necessary to prevent 'knuckling'.
- Suturing of lacerated flexor tendons is recommended. The locking loop or three-loop pulley pattern is used. When apposition of the severed tendon ends is not possible, the ends are debrided and a terylene or carbon fibre implant is used. The injured limb should always be supported post-operatively with a cast for 10 to 12 weeks. Following cast removal, exercise should be resumed gradually over 3–6 months.

Prognosis

- Guarded. Horses can return to soundness if no complications occur.
- If the laceration occurs within the digital sheath, the prognosis for soundness is unfavourable.
- Unfavourable complications are infection and peritendinous adhesions.

Desmitis of the suspensory ligament

The suspensory ligament (SL) can be injured at its proximal attachment to the proximal palmar/

plantar cortex of the metacarpus/metatarsus, its main body, and its branches, which insert on the proximal sesamoid bones.

Proximal suspensory desmitis

See also section on p. 362 for more details.

Clinical signs

• Acutely affected horses often have localized oedema, heat and swelling in the palmaro-/plantaro-proximal metacarpal/metatarsal region. The medial palmar/plantar vein may be distended.
• Regional analgesia is required to localize the site of pain in chronically affected horses (direct infiltration, lateral palmar nerve block, ulnar nerve block, subtarsal nerve block or tibial nerve block).
• Radiological changes may be non-existent or include subtle changes to the trabecular pattern of the proximal palmar/plantar cortex of the cannon bone.

Ultrasonography

• Hypoechoic lesion in the proximal SL (an occasional finding in normal horses). The appearance of 'true' lesions evolves in time, as observed on repeat examinations.
• Enlargement of the SL in the dorsopalmar direction.
• Poor definition of the margins of the ligament.
• Single or multiple poorly defined focal areas of hypoechoicity, or diffuse hypoechoicity.

Treatment

• Treatment consists of box rest followed by a regime of increasing exercise (e.g. 30 days of box rest, 30 days of walking in hand, 30 days of walking and trotting). After this period, ultrasonographic appearance is reassessed. The amount of box rest is dictated by ultrasonographic appearance of the ligament and varies from 4 weeks to 9 months.
• Add support to SL with egg barr shoes.

Prognosis

The prognosis for return to exercise is about 80% for forelimbs and 20% for hindlimbs.

Desmitis of the main body of the SL

• Clinical signs are similar to those of tendinitis.
• Ultrasonography shows generalized hypoechoicity and enlargement of the ligament.

Suspensory branch desmitis

Clinical signs

• Most common injury of the SL.
• Swelling of the injured branch can be palpated. Always compare carefully with opposite branch and with the branches of the contralateral limb.

Ultrasonography

• Core lesion.
• Generalized involvement of the branch with enlargement and hypoechoicity.
• Periligamentous oedema and fibrosis.

Treatment

Treatment is similar to that for tendinitis. The degree of exercise and time for return to work should be dictated by ultrasonographic findings.

Prognosis

The prognosis is guarded because of the high incidence of recurrence and the slow, unpredictable rate of healing.

Desmitis of the inferior check ligament

Clinical signs

The signs are swelling, heat and pain in the region of the proximal palmar metacarpus.

Ultrasonography

• Ultrasonographic appearance varies from diffuse hypoechoicity to focal hypoechoic areas within the inferior check ligament. The ligament is usually enlarged.
• Echogenic extension of the inferior check ligament to the borders of the SDFT may indicate adhesion formation between these two structures.

Treatment

• Treatment comprises rest and a regime of increasing exercise dependent on ultrasonographic appearance.
• Inferior check ligament desmotomy is a possible alternative in chronic unresponsive cases.

Prognosis

• Guarded to favourable for return to previous level of exercise.
• Prognosis is worse if there is concurrent SDFT tendinitis.
• Convalescence varies from 3 to 12 months.

Further reading

Butler, J.A., Colles, C.M., Dyson, S.J., Kold, S.E. and Poulos, P.W. (1993) *Clinical Radiology of the Horse.* Blackwell Scientific Publications, Oxford.
McIlwraith, C.W. and Turner, S.A. (1987) *Equine Surgery Advanced Techniques.* Lea & Febiger, Philadelphia.
Stashak, T.S. (1987) *Adams' Lameness in Horses.* Lea & Febiger, Philadelphia.
Turner, S.A. and McIlwraith, C.W. (1989) *Techniques in Large Animal Surgery.* Lea & Febiger, Philadelphia.
Veterinary Clinics of North America: Equine Practice 5:1 (1989). *The Equine Foot.* W.B. Saunders and Co., Philadelphia.
Wyn-Jones, G. (1988) *Equine Lameness.* Blackwell Scientific Publications, Oxford.

Appendix. Differential diagnoses of lower limb lameness

1. *Acute, severe lower limb lameness*
Infectious pododermatitis ('pus in the foot')
Laminitis
Severe strain of SDFT
Severe sprain of the DIP joint or fetlock joint
Fracture of the first phalanx
Intra-articular fractures of the fetlock joint
Fracture of the third phalanx
Fracture of the navicular bone
Fracture of the second phalanx

2. *Insidious onset, low grade, uni- or bilateral forelimb lameness*
Chronic foot imbalance
Chronic subsolar bruising ('pedal osteitis')
Navicular syndrome
Traumatic synovitis of the DIP joint
DJD of the DIP or PIP joint
Low grade laminitis
Keratoma
Osseous cystic lesions of the third or second phalanx

3. *Lameness with swelling in the fetlock region*
DJD of the fetlock joint
Intra-articular fractures of the fetlock joint
Traumatic sprain of the fetlock joint
Tenosynovitis of the digital synovial sheath
Annular ligament syndrome
Desmitis of the suspensory ligament branches (and sesamoiditis)
OCD and osseous cyst-like lesions in the fetlock joint
'Low bow' (tendinitis SDFT)
Infectious arthritis of the fetlock joint
Sesamoid bone fractures
Distal sesamoidean ligament desmitis
Distal splint bone fractures
Villonodular synovitis
Tendosynovitis of the DDFT and the digital synovial sheath
Infectious pododermatitis ('pus in the foot')
Lymphangitis

4. *Lameness referable to the proximal palmar metacarpus*
Proximal suspensory desmitis
Proximal metacarpal stress syndrome
Incomplete fractures of the proximal palmar metacarpal cortex
Inferior check ligament desmitis
Proximal 'splints'

17 Orthopaedics 3. The upper limbs

17.1 *Carpus*

Anatomy

Bones

The carpus normally contains seven small carpal bones in two rows.

Proximal row:

- Radial.
- Intermediate.
- Ulnar.
- Accessory.

Distal row:

- 2nd.
- 3rd.
- 4th.

A first carpal bone is found in about 50% of horses and may be unilateral. It is usually about the size and shape of a pea and is found embedded in the medial ligament of the carpus, behind the second carpal bone. A fifth carpal bone is also occasionally seen on the lateral aspect of the carpometacarpal joint.

The carpal bones articulate proximally with the distal radius, which has three articular facets relating to the proximal surfaces of the radial, intermediate and ulnar carpal bones. The lateral aspect of the distal radius is phylogenetically the distal ulnar epiphysis and is seen as a separate ossification centre in foals. The line of fusion to the rest of the distal radial epiphysis closes radiographically before 12 months of age but often persists into adulthood as a groove on the distal radial articular surface. The epiphysis fuses with the metaphysis at 20–24 months of age. A linear, mineralized density is sometimes seen on the caudolateral aspect of the distal antebrachium – representing the vestigial distal ulna. The distal row of carpal bones articulate distally with the second, third and fourth metacarpal bones.

Joints

The articulations between the carpal bones are complex, and some consist of two or three separate facets. Altogether, there are approximately 26 separate articulations. These are divisible into three principal joint levels:

1. Antebrachiocarpal.
2. Midcarpal.
3. Carpometacarpal.

There are usually two separate synovial cavities:

1. Antebrachiocarpal.
2. Midcarpal and carpometacarpal.

The antebrachiocarpal joint moves with a rotating and gliding action. The midcarpal joint has a hinge-like action while the carpometacarpal joint is capable of very little movement. During flexion, the articular surfaces of the antebrachiocarpal and midcarpal joints become widely separated dorsally, but remain apposed at their palmar margins. The intermediate and ulnar carpal bones tend to move as one unit but the radial carpal bone is not displaced as far from the distal row of carpal bones on flexion. Its dorsodistal margin is therefore separated from the intermediate carpal bone on a flexed lateromedial radiograph.

The fibrous palmar carpal joint capsule is dense and closely attached to the palmar aspect of the carpal bones. Palmarly, it forms the smooth dorsal wall of the carpal canal. It is continued distally to form the accessory head of the deep digital flexor tendon (inferior check ligament). The carpal fascia on the palmar aspect of the carpal region forms the flexor retinaculum (transverse carpal ligament) between the free palmar edge of the accessory carpal bone and the medial aspect of the carpus. This completes the carpal canal, which contains the superficial and deep digital flexor tendons.

Traumatic arthritis, osteoarthritis (degenerative joint disease) and carpal fractures

Aetiology and pathogenesis

Equine carpal joint disease is seen most commonly as an 'occupational disease' of racehorses and occurs less commonly in horses used for other purposes. A form of traumatic arthritis/osteoarthritis (OA) appears to be the usual underlying disease entity. The majority of cases are likely to be a consequence of the chronic repetitive trauma suffered by the joint as a result of training and racing although some fractures result from a single episode of overloading of a previously normal bone. Adaptive remodelling of bone in response to training may have deleterious consequences for the integrity of the joint as a whole. Initial osteoclastic resorption may weaken the bone, predisposing to microscopic or gross fracture. Subsequent sclerosis may increase the stiffness of the bone, increasing the load on the overlying articular cartilage. Chronically accumulating damage of OA may give rise to clinical signs of uni- or bilateral forelimb lameness in its own right, as well as acting as a precursor to more acute injuries such as carpal chip and slab fractures.

Carpal OA affects the midcarpal joint more commonly than the antebrachiocarpal joint in Thoroughbred racehorses. The articular surface damage is concentrated on the medial aspect of the joint and particularly involves the radial and third carpal bones. The articular margins and surfaces on the lateral aspect of the joint often appear relatively normal both radiologically and arthroscopically. This distribution of lesions is probably a consequence of biomechanical influences, although the precise details of these remain to be elucidated.

Carpal fractures

Carpal chip fractures are frequently seen in association with OA and have been commonly considered as a potential cause of 'secondary' OA. Although this sequence of events undoubtedly occurs, the alternative scenario, that the arthrosis causes or predisposes to the fractures, may well be more common and more important, particularly with respect to distal radial carpal chip fractures. A similar role of carpal OA in predisposing to third carpal bone slab fractures has also been suggested. Such a viewpoint puts the acute injury into perspective as part of a chronic disease process and thereby establishes the limitations on the success that might be expected with surgical treatment (e.g. fracture fragment stabilization or removal).

- *Chip fractures* occur at the dorsal margins of the bones forming the antebrachiocarpal and midcarpal joints. Each individual chip fracture affects only one articular surface of the parent bone although there may be multiple chips affecting different bones, different joints and different limbs in the same horse. The most common sites are the distal margin of the radial carpal bone and the proximal margin of the third carpal bone, i.e. on the dorsomedial margin of the midcarpal joint.
- *Slab fractures* extend right through a carpal bone from the proximal to the distal articular surface. They occur most commonly in the frontal plane and primarily affect the dorsomedial aspect (radial facet) of the third carpal bone. Because they involve larger bone fragments and two articular surfaces they are a more serious injury than chip fracture and affected horses have a correspondingly more guarded prognosis for return to athletic activity. Slab fractures in the sagittal plane are occasionally seen.
- *Incomplete fissure fractures* of the third carpal bone have been described and may cause lameness with few localizing clinical signs.
- *Accessory carpal bone fractures* are seen most commonly in jumping horses and often there is a history of a fall. The fracture usually occurs in the frontal plane approximately in the middle of the bone.
- *Comminuted fractures* of one or more carpal bones cause severe disruption of the articular surfaces and often result in instability of the carpus. They are usually due to severe trauma such as falls or road traffic accidents.

Clinical signs

- Lameness localized to the carpus. This may be obvious unilateral lameness or a more insidious bilateral lameness manifested as shortening of the stride and abduction of the distal limb during protraction to reduce the necessity for carpal flexion.
- Swelling – especially carpal joint effusion in the early stages. Fibrous thickening on the dorsal aspect of the joint occurs with time and obscures the clear contours of the dorsal carpal bone margins.
- Pain on joint flexion and sometimes on palpation of the joint margins.
- Positive response to carpal flexion test.
- Restricted range of carpal flexion.
- Severe fractures may cause crepitus and instability.

Radiology

Soft tissue swelling
Soft tissue swelling may be a result of synovial effusion or thickening of the synovial membrane/joint capsule or periarticular tissues. It is useful to note on radiographs the level of maximal swelling in relation to the joints in the carpus (i.e. antebrachiocarpal joint, midcarpal joint or carpometacarpal joint) because this can help in identifying the specific carpal joint principally involved.

Entheseophytes

The carpal bones are arranged to allow for their slight displacement in a horizontal plane when the carpus is loaded. The carpal bones are linked together by ligaments which constrain this movement and absorb some of the imposed load. Overloading of this system may result in damage to the origins and insertions of the intercarpal ligaments on the dorsal aspect of the carpal bones, which results in non-articular periosteal new bone formation at the sites of these attachments, i.e. entheseophytes. Once formed, this bone tends to persist throughout the horse's life although it may remodel and become smoother in outline. Irregular, non-articular, periosteal new bone on the dorsal surface of the carpal bones in young racehorses in training may, therefore, be an indication that overloading of the carpal joints is occurring and that more serious articular surface damage may coexist. Such entheseophytes may, however, be an incidental observation without a great deal of clinical significance when seen later in life.

Osteophytes

Periarticular new bone is one of the cardinal radiological features of OA. Osteophytes may develop as a remodelling response to joint overload and damage. They may reflect an attempt to increase joint surface area and thereby reduce loading per unit surface area, and also increase joint stability. They may thus be viewed as part of the joint's adaptive response to disease. Periarticular osteophytes tend to be seen primarily on the dorsomedial aspect of the carpal joints, and remodelling of the dorsodistal margin of the radial carpal bone is particularly common.

Paramarginal subchondral bone lysis

Loss of subchondral bone cortex in a narrow strip approximately 5 mm palmar to the dorsal margin is a common radiological finding in the distal radial carpal bone of horses with OA of the midcarpal joint. It is seen as a small concave area of radiolucency in the subchondral cortical bone of the distal articular surface just palmar to the dorsodistal margin and is generally most apparent on the DLPMO projection.

Subchondral bone sclerosis

Sclerosis of the subchondral bone in the radial facet of the third carpal bone is recognized in young racehorses. This feature is best demonstrated on the dorsoproximal-dorsodistal oblique view of the third carpal bone and is seen as an increase in bone density and loss of the normal trabecular pattern. Sclerosis is probably an adaptive change in response to increased loading with training, but, by stiffening the subchondral bone, it may increase the load on the overlying articular cartilage and thereby predispose it to damage.

OA of the carpometacarpal joint

The equine carpometacarpal joint is rarely overtly affected by OA although its synovial cavity communicates with that of the frequently affected midcarpal joint. Older ponies are sometimes affected with OA of the carpometacarpal joint. The associated radiological changes bear similarities to 'bone spavin' in the hock with prominent periosteal new bone proliferation and subchondral bone lysis. Like spavin, these changes may eventually progress to fusion of the affected joints.

Treatment

1. Traumatic arthritis – see Chapter 15.
2. Osteoarthritis – see Chapter 15.
3. Fractures: Most carpal fractures can, in theory, be managed either surgically or conservatively. Surgical intervention is indicated particularly for horses with chip or slab fractures that are intended for athletic use. Surgery aims to restore articular congruency and stability so that the development of secondary OA is minimized. The limitations on this where the fractures are actually a product of existing OA have already been alluded to.

• Chip fractures are generally treated surgically by removing the fragments under arthroscopic visualization. Abnormal articular tissues, particularly soft, crumbly subchondral bone, may be debrided at the same time.
• Slab fractures are usually treated by lag screw fixation. Initial debridement and reduction may be accomplished using arthroscopic visualization.
• Accessory carpal bone fractures commonly form fibrous rather than bony unions. Techniques for lag screw repair have been described but are difficult due to the curved shape of the bone and the comminuted nature of many of the fractures.
• Comminuted fractures of one or more carpal bones usually end a horse's athletic career. Salvage for breeding or as a pet may be feasible by combining internal fixation and cast support. Comminution of multiple carpal bones is usually an indication for euthanasia.

Osteochondritis dissecans (OCD)

See Chapter 15 (p. 326).

OCD is rare in the carpus, but is occasionally seen in foals. It may be associated with disease in other joints, e.g. the proximal interphalangeal joints.

Subchondral bone cysts

See Chapter 15 (p. 326).

These have been reported in the carpus but may not be of clinical significance. They are usually managed conservatively.

Septic arthritis

See Chapter 15 (p. 327).

Angular limb deformities

The term 'angular limb deformity' refers to lateral (valgus) or medial (varus) deviation of the distal limb from the sagittal plane. Thus 'carpal valgus' refers to outward deviation of the distal limb originating at the level of the carpus. These deformities are usually seen in young foals and can be congenital or acquired.

Aetiology

● Congenital deformities – cause often unknown, but suggestions include malpositioning of the foetus in utero, prematurity/dysmaturity, genetic factors, nutritional influences on the mare, and teratogens.
● Acquired – most commonly due to physeal injury or asymmetric loading due to excessive weight bearing, e.g. as a result of overnutrition or contralateral limb injury, excessive exercise or improper foot trimming. In the case of carpal deformities, the distal radial physis is usually the site affected.

Pathogenesis

● Congenital laxity of the ligamentous support of the carpus and/or hypoplasia (inadequate ossification) of the small carpal bones may result in angular deformity. If left unsupported, the inadequately ossified bones may become crushed and deformed as the foal loads the limbs after birth.

● Acquired deformities usually develop as a result of asymmetrical growth from the distal radial physis, which may be due to excessive loading of one side of the physis.

History

Important facts to establish include:

● The age of the foal.
● If the foal was premature or smaller than normal at birth.
● If the deformity was present at birth, and if not when it first appeared.
● How the deformity has developed since it was first seen (i.e. improving, deteriorating or static).
● If there has been any associated lameness or other signs.

Physical examination

The following points in particular should be established:

● The site or sites of deformity.
● The direction of the deformity – valgus or varus.
● The degree of deviation – mild, moderate or severe.
● Evidence of instability – can the deformity be manually reduced?
● Evidence of lameness.
● Signs of inflammation – pain, heat or swelling.

Radiography

It is important to obtain dorsopalmar views centred on the carpus but including as much as possible of the distal radius and proximal metacarpus in order to be able to evaluate the degree of deformity present. This is best done using large cassettes.

Radiology

1. Morphological changes – various combinations of the following features may be seen.
   ● Irregularity of the line of the physis – often appears particularly disturbed on the convex side of the deformity.
   ● Metaphyseal and epiphyseal flaring.
   ● Wedge-shaped epiphysis.
   ● Diaphyseal remodelling with asymmetry in cortical thickness.
   ● Hypoplastic, rounded, collapsed, or subluxated carpal bones.

2. The radiographs may also be used to gain an estimate of the degree of angulation present. A piece of clear X-ray film is placed over the dorso-palmar radiograph and lines drawn down the centre of the radius and the centre of the third metacarpal bone. The intersection of these lines gives some indication of the level within the carpus at which the deformity is occurring and the degree of angulation.

Treatment

Some degree of angular limb deformity is not uncommon in neonatal foals and often improves dramatically during the first 2 weeks of life without specific treatment.

Certain management principles are helpful in dealing with angular limb deformities regardless of what other techniques are employed.

• Foals should generally be confined to a large box or small yard while the deformity is present as excessive exercise on an angulated limb tends to exacerbate asymmetric overloading of the physis, carpal bones and other joint structures.
• Limb angulation leads to asymmetric wear of the hoof. Foals with carpal valgus tend to wear the medial aspect of the hoof wall excessively. The hoof should be rasped regularly to bring it back into balance. This may be combined with the use of glue-on plastic shoes with medial (in the case of carpal valgus) or lateral (for carpal varus) extensions.
• Affected foals should not be allowed to become overweight. This may mean restricting the mare's diet to control milk production or early weaning.

Neonatal foals with deformity due to ligamentous laxity or carpal bone hypoplasia benefit from external support of the limb with either a well padded splint or tube cast for 2–4 weeks. Splints should be reset daily and casts changed after 2 weeks to reduce the chance of development of pressure sores. In foals, there is usually little to be gained by external support where there is no evidence of instability, the deformity cannot be reduced manually and the carpal bones do not appear hypoplastic radiographically.

Foals with persistent deformities due to asymmetric growth from the distal radial physis are candidates for surgical intervention if they fail to respond to the measures outlined above. Surgery aims to manipulate growth at the distal radial physis to cause limb straightening. This may involve either:

• temporary transphyseal bridging with either staples or screws and wire, or
• hemicircumferential periosteal transection.

Both techniques depend on continued growth of the bone in order to straighten the limb and there are therefore time limits after which they are likely to be much less effective. In the case of angular limb deformities of the carpus, the surgery should be undertaken before the foal is 12 weeks of age. The earlier surgery is performed, however, the more rapid and complete will be the response.

Temporary transphyseal bridging aims to slow the rate of growth on the more rapidly growing (i.e. convex) side of the physis. It is therefore performed medially in the case of carpal valgus deformity. The use of two screws (usually fully threaded, 6.5 mm diameter AO cancellous screws) with one or more figure of eight wires (18G) joining them, has certain advantages over the use of staples. The two screws can be placed independently, unlike the tines of a staple, and immediate compression across the physis is achieved as the wire(s) is tightened. There is also less risk of extrusion of the implants as the foal continues to grow. The implants must be removed as soon as the leg is straight or over-correction and deviation in the opposite direction may occur.

Hemicircumferential periosteal transection: the periosteum is postulated to exert a restraining influence on longitudinal growth of long bones. By releasing this restraint on one side of the bone, it is possible to induce asymmetric growth and thereby correct existing deformities. The transection is thus done on the side of the bone that is growing less quickly, i.e. the concave side (lateral side in the case of carpal valgus). The periosteal incision is made about 2.5 cm proximal to the physis. A simple horizontal incision is probably sufficient though many surgeons create an inverted 'T' incision and then elevate the flaps of periosteum created from the bone. In the case of carpal valgus deformities the rudimentary distal ulna is also transected at the caudal end of the horizontal periosteal incision.

Hemicircumferential periosteal transection has certain advantages over temporary transphyseal bridging:

• There is no need for a second surgery to remove implants.
• There is less risk of postoperative infection because there are no implants.
• There appears to be no risk of overcorrection.

Hemicircumferential periosteal transection and temporary transphyseal bridging may be employed simultaneously in severely affected foals.

Carpal tunnel syndrome

Aetiology and pathogenesis

This syndrome is caused by trauma or a space occupying lesion within the carpal canal leading to compression of the soft tissues within the canal (e.g. accessory carpal bone fracture, osteochondroma of the distal radius, tendinitis of the flexor tendons).

Clinical signs

- Distension of the carpal sheath with synovial fluid.
- Reduced range of carpal flexion.
- Pain on carpal flexion.
- Reduced pulse volume in the digital vessels distal to the carpus.

Treatment

- Treat the primary lesion if possible.
- Resection of the carpal flexor retinaculum.

Osteochondroma of the distal radius

This is a bony exostosis that develops on the caudal aspect of the distal radius. Its cortex is continuous with that of the distal radius and it has a cartilage 'cap'.

Aetiology and pathogenesis

There is localized abnormal growth of cartilage from an area of metaphyseal periosteum that subsequently undergoes endochondral ossification. It appears to be distinct from the condition of 'multiple exostoses', which is thought to be inherited.

Clinical signs

Signs are as for carpal canal syndrome plus palpable bony protruberance on the caudomedial aspect of the distal radius. Osteochondromas are not necessarily a cause of lameness and may thus be an incidental radiological finding.

Radiology

Radiology shows irregular exostosis on the caudomedial aspect of the distal radius.

Treatment

Treatment comprises excision of the lesion.

17.2 *Elbow*

Anatomy

The elbow is a ginglymus or hinge joint formed between the distal humerus and the proximal end of the radius and ulna.

In the foal, the distal humerus comprises separate ossification centres for the distal epiphysis and the medial epicondyle. The distal humeral epiphysis fuses to the metaphysis at 11–24 months of age. Both the radius and ulna each have a single proximal epiphysis. The proximal radial epiphysis fuses to the metaphysis at 11–24 months of age. The proximal epiphysis of the ulna initially appears quite small radiographically and well separated from the rest of the ulna. It fuses to the rest of the ulna at 24–36 months.

The elbow is restrained by collateral ligaments medially and laterally.

Ulnar fractures

These usually involve the olecranon process, and commonly the articular surface of the semilunar notch. They compromise the ability of the horse to maintain the elbow in extension during weight bearing because the fracture interferes with the triceps mechanism of which the olecranon is the insertion. They are subdivided into types according to configuration:

Type 1 – physeal fractures occurring in the young animal.
- 1a – non-articular fracture involving the growth plate only.
- 1b – Salter–Harris type II fracture involving the anconeus and proximal semilunar notch.
Type 2 – Articular fractures involving the semilunar notch.
Type 3 – Non-articular fractures involving the metaphyseal region of the olecranon.

Type 4 – Comminuted fractures which generally involve the semilunar notch and body of the olecranon.

Type 5 – Fractures of the distal olecranon/ulnar shaft that extend proximally to involve the distal semilunar notch.

Aetiology and pathogenesis

Ulnar fractures are usually due to a single episode of traumatic overloading, e.g. a kick from another horse or a fall.

Clinical signs

- Severe lameness on the affected limb, though with undisplaced fractures this may improve quite rapidly.
- Localized soft tissue swelling around the elbow.
- Horse may stand with elbow 'dropped' mimicking radial paralysis.
- Pain on manipulation of the elbow joint.
- Crepitus may be present with severe fractures but is often minimal.

Treatment

The majority of ulnar fractures are probably best treated by open reduction and internal fixation with a narrow 4.5 mm ASIF dynamic compression plate and screws. Type 1a fractures in foals may be best fixed with a pin or screw and a wire tension band as the proximal fragment is usually very small. Some undisplaced type 5 fractures may be successfully managed conservatively. If plates are used on skeletally immature horses, the implants should if possible be placed so as to avoid impeding growth at the proximal radial physis.

Subchondral bone cysts (see also Chapter 15, p. 326)

In the elbow, cysts are occasionally seen in both immature and adult horses in the proximal radius, usually on the medial aspect of the elbow joint. They are best demonstrated on a craniocaudal radiograph. They are sometimes associated with periosteal reactions at the sites of attachment of the collateral ligaments. Clinical and radiographic resolution may occur with conservative treatment. Surgical curettage via a medial extra-articular approach has been described.

Septic arthritis (see also Chapter 15, p. 327)

The elbow has been described as a predilection site for septic arthritis secondary to traumatic injuries, especially wounds caused by kicks from other horses. This may be due to the relative lack of soft tissue covering on the lateral aspect of the joint.

Capped elbow

This is an acquired subcutaneous bursa on the point of the elbow.

Aetiology and pathogenesis

It is usually due to repetitive trauma, e.g. the shoe on the affected limb hitting the elbow as the horse lies down. The small true bursa that underlies the insertion of the triceps is rarely involved.

Clinical signs

In the acute stage the condition appears as a prominent fluid swelling over the point of the elbow which may later subside to a fibrous thickening. It is not usually a cause of lameness.

Treatment

Prevent further trauma – check shoeing, 'sausage' boots. Surgical intervention is usually unnecessary and best avoided.

17.3 *Shoulder*

Anatomy

The shoulder joint is an enarthrosis (ball and socket joint) though its chief movements are flexion and extension.

The scapula has four centres of ossification

1. Body.
2. Scapular cartilage.
3. Tuber scapulae (supraglenoid tubercle) – fuses to body by 12–24 months.

4. Cranial part of glenoid cavity – fuses to body by 5 months.

The proximal humerus has three centres of ossification:

1. The diaphysis.
2. The humeral head.
3. The greater (lateral) tubercle.

These centres fuse to each other from about 3–5 months. The proximal humeral physis closes at 24–36 months.

Osteochondritis dissecans (OCD) (see also Chapter 15, p. 326)

Lesions may be uni- or bilateral and may involve only the scapula or the humerus or both. The affected articular cartilage is variable in thickness, soft and less firmly attached to the underlying subchondral bone. There are often areas of full thickness defects in the articular cartilage. The lesions are often extensive and irregular.

Clinical signs

OCD is seen most commonly in horses less than one year of age. There is mild to moderate intermittent lameness, usually with mild atrophy of the shoulder muscles.

Radiology

- Flattening of the contour of the humeral head.
- Irregular areas of subchondral radiolucency in humeral head or scapular glenoid.
- Remodelling of the joint margins particularly the caudal margin of the glenoid.

Treatment

Conservative management is directed at rest, and reduction in growth rate may be successful in mildly affected horses.

Surgical debridement under arthroscopic visualization may be undertaken in more severely affected cases.

Subchondral bone cysts (see also Chapter 15, p. 326)

These usually affect the scapular glenoid rather than the humeral head. A small lucent area in the middle of the scapular glenoid of normal horses has also been described.

Clinical signs

- Usually seen in young horses – yearlings and 2-year-olds.
- Lameness, which can be improved by intra-articular analgesia of the shoulder.

Radiology

- Seen at the junction of the middle and caudal thirds of the scapular glenoid.
- Single or multiple, with sclerotic margin.
- Vary in size and proximity to the joint – may have a visible communication.
- May move proximally (i.e. away from the articular surface) with time in association with improvement in lameness.

Fractures

Fractures involving the shoulder joint are usually fractures of the scapula rather than the proximal humerus. There is usually a history of specific external trauma such as a fall. A variety of configurations are seen but the commonest is fracture of the tuber scapulae (supraglenoid tuberosity). These may involve separation of a single discrete fragment or the fracture may be comminuted. They usually involve the articular surface of the glenoid. The tuber scapulae forms the origin of the biceps brachii muscle, and as a result, when fractured, it becomes displaced craniodistally.

Stress fractures of the caudoproximal or craniodistal humerus are occasionally seen and are probably best diagnosed by scintigraphy in the early stages.

Treatment

Horses with comminuted articular fractures are generally euthanased on humane grounds. Horses with non-articular fractures of the body of the scapula may recover with conservative treatment comprising box rest for several months. Simple fractures of the tuber scapulae have been treated surgically, with varying degrees of success, by reduction and internal fixation in young horses and by fragment excision in older animals.

Luxation

Luxation of the shoulder joint is rare. The humeral head is reported to displace either cranially or medially. Immediate reduction under general anaesthesia is suggested to be the treatment of choice. Radiographic examination is advisable because concurrent fractures may also be present.

Bicipital bursitis

The bicipital bursa surrounds the origin of the biceps brachii muscle and lies between it and the bicipital groove of the humerus. Inflammation of the bicipital bursa is an uncommon cause of lameness. The inflammation may be due to trauma or infection. There may be pain on direct palpation or on manipulation of the shoulder, particularly flexion. Treatment is rest and anti-inflammatory medication if traumatic in origin, and by lavage and antibiotic therapy if septic.

Collateral instability ('Shoulder slip', 'Sweeny')

There is traumatic damage to the suprascapular nerve, which innervates the supraspinatus and infraspinatus muscles.

Clinical signs

The following signs may appear independently or together:

- Marked atrophy of the supraspinatus and infraspinatus muscles.
- Lateral subluxation of the joint during weight bearing – the proximal humerus appears to bulge laterally as the affected limb takes weight.
- Difficulty in advancing the limb.

Treatment

Conservative treatment often produces good results. Surgical decompression of the suprascapular nerve where it crosses the cranial border of the scapula has been suggested to be useful, particularly if progress with conservative treatment is poor. However, there is still debate on the optimum time for performing such surgery.

Ossification of the biceps tendon

This has been reported as a rare cause of mild to moderate lameness. The calcification may be a result of trauma, or it may be associated with osteoarthritis of the shoulder. Treatment is usually symptomatic, and the prognosis is generally poor.

17.4 *Hock*

Anatomy

Bones

The hock is composed of six tarsal bones:

- Tibial.
- Fibular.
- Central.
- 1st and 2nd (fused).
- 3rd.
- 4th.

1. The 1st and 2nd tarsal bones of young foals may not be fused.
2. The epiphysis of the fibular tarsal bone is evident by 2 weeks – fusion occurs between 16–24 months.
3. The distal epiphysis of the tibia fuses to the metaphysis at 17–24 months.
4. The lateral malleolus of the tibia has a separate ossification centre which phylogenetically represents the distal epiphysis of the fibula – fuses to rest of epiphysis by 3 months.
5. Trochlear ridges of the tibial tarsal:
   - Lateral ridge has a longer notch at its distal end.
   - Medial ridge has a variably sized and shaped bobble at its distal end which may be present as one or occasionally several distinct fragments – these should not be mistaken on radiographs for fracture fragments.
6. The central and 3rd tarsal bones usually have dorsomedial ridge-like prominences.

Joints

There are four principal levels of articulation in the hock.

1. Tarsocrural – main hock joint where most movement occurs.

2. Proximal intertarsal (talocalcaneal-centroquartal) – communicates with tarsocrural joint.
3. Distal intertarsal (centrodistal) (communicates with tarsometatarsal in a small number of horses).
4. Tarsometatarsal.

Osteoarthritis of the small hock joints (bone spavin)

General

'Bone spavin' is a colloquial term used to refer to osteoarthritis of the intertarsal (proximal and distal) and tarsometatarsal joints. It is probably the most common cause of persistent hindlimb lameness in the horse. The disease usually affects the distal intertarsal joint primarily but the tarsometatarsal joint is also commonly affected. Osteoarthritis of the proximal intertarsal joint is less common but carries a more guarded prognosis for return to soundness. Bone spavin occurs most commonly on the dorsomedial aspect of the hock.

Clinical signs

There is uni- or bilateral hindlimb lameness usually with an insidious onset. Some affected horses may be presented because of non-specific hindlimb gait abnormalities, poor performance, or suspected back problems, particularly if the condition is bilateral. The cranial phase of the stride is shortened, causing a 'toe stabbing' gait. The limb is carried medially during protraction and lands more on the lateral aspect of the foot leading to increased wear of the toe and lateral branch of the shoe. Bilateral involvement may lead to a short, choppy hindlimb gait. There is usually a positive response to proximal hindlimb flexion – the so-called 'spavin test', though horses with other hindlimb problems may also show increased lameness in response to this manoeuvre. Bony enlargement on the medial aspect of the hock occurs in advanced disease but may not be apparent in many horses. The horse usually shows a positive response to intraarticular analgesia of the small hock joints.

Radiology

Typical radiological changes are:

- Marginal irregularity – a roughened hazy appearance to the joint margin.
- Marginal radiolucency – demineralization of the subchondral bone at the joint margin.
- Joint space may appear irregular in width and poorly defined.
- Subchondral bone erosion – seen as cyst like radiolucent areas.
- Periarticular new bone formation on the central and 3rd tarsals and 3rd metatarsal.
- Progressive joint fusion may occur in association with destructive and proliferative changes.

Some horses have pain associated with the small hock joints without accompanying radiological change (so-called 'occult spavin').

Treatment

1. Continued controlled exercise ($\pm$ NSAIDs) in the hope of achieving spontaneous ankylosis of the affected joints. Some authorities have questioned whether in fact spontaneous fusion ever actually occurs – nevertheless, controlled exercise can result in significant clinical improvement.
2. Intra-articular mediation
   - Hyaluronic acid.
   - Polysulphated glycosaminoglycans.
   - Corticosteroids.
3. Shoeing – rolled toe and slightly elevated heel.
4. Cunean tenectomy – remove 2 cm section of cunean tendon on medial aspect of hock. Postulated to relieve pressure on site of new bone formation but of debatable efficacy. (Wamberg modification – cuts through all the soft tissues on the craniomedial aspect of the hock thereby possibly destroying the nerve supply to the area.)
5. Surgical arthrodesis is performed by destroying the articular cartilage by drilling tracks across the joints. At least 60% of the cartilage should be removed. Need a minimum of 4 tracks in a pony and 5 or 6 in a larger horse. Use a 3.2 or 4.5 mm diameter drill bit. Joints to be drilled are first located with needle markers and radiographs. Postoperatively horses are box rested for 10–30 days until comfortable and then started on a programme of controlled exercise which is thought to be important in encouraging ankylosis.
6. Chemical arthrodesis by intra-articular injection of sodium monoiodoacetate has recently been described and may allow earlier return to work.

Osteochondritis dissecans

Sites

1. The distal intermediate ridge of the tibia.
2. The lateral trochlear ridge of the tibial tarsal bone.

Less commonly:

● The medial trochlear ridge of the tibial tarsal bone.
● The dorsal aspect of the medial malleolus of the tibia.

Clinical signs

● Usually young horses – Standardbreds and European Warmbloods are affected more commonly than Thoroughbreds. The disease has also been seen in Shire horses.
● Affected horses usually present with distension of the tarsocrural joint ('bog spavin').
● Lameness is variable.

Radiology

● Subchondral bone deficits and separate mineralized fragments arising from the sites outlined above.
● Some lesions are said to occur without radiological changes.

Treatment

● Surgical removal of the osteochondral fragment and curettage of the defect.
● Usually performed under arthroscopic visualization.
● Approximately 75% of affected horses can return to their intended use following arthroscopic surgery.

'Bog spavin'

1. Fluid distension of the tarsocrural joint.
2. Up to three swellings may be detectable:
   ● Dorsomedially – between the peroneus tertius and the medial malleolus, usually the largest and most obvious.
   ● Caudomedially – between the medial malleolus and the deep digital flexor.
   ● Caudolaterally – between the lateral malleolus and the tuber calcis.
3. Lameness may or may not be present.

4. Aetiology
   ● Idiopathic.
   ● OCD.
   ● Trauma $\pm$ intra-articular fractures, e.g. lateral malleolus or trochlear ridge of tibial tarsal bone.
   ● Infection – usually very painful and lame.
5. Treatment
   ● Treat underlying cause if apparent.
   ● Symptomatic local therapy, e.g. drainage and injection of sodium hyaluronate followed by bandaging (questionable efficacy and necessity if not lame).

Thoroughpin

Fluid distension of the tarsal sheath. The tendon of the deep digital flexor muscle traverses the tarsal groove formed at the back of the tarsus by the plantar surface of the sustentaculum tali and the medial surface of the tuber calcis – the deep digital flexor tendon is extremely dense at this level and is partly cartilaginous. The 'tarsal canal' is lined by a synovial membrane, the tarsal sheath. This begins 5–7 cm proximal to the level of the medial malleolus and extends distally to the upper third of the metatarsus.

Clinical signs

● Distinct swellings on either side of and ~5 cm cranial to the achilles tendon.
● The swellings vary in size – the medial one is generally the larger.
● There is sometimes a 3rd swelling on the medial aspect at the level of the tarsometatarsal joint.
● Usually unilateral.
● Swellings are cold and painless.
● Lameness is sometimes seen in association with the swellings – in which case new bone may be present on the sustentaculum tali.

Radiology

● Deposition of new bone is sometimes seen along the medial border of the sustentaculum tali in cases where there is associated lameness.

Treatment

● Drainage may provide temporary improvement but swelling often recurs.

• Horses that are lame and have sustentacular new bone have a poor prognosis for return to soundness.

Curb

Desmitis of the plantar ligament or focal damage to the superficial digital flexor tendon.

Aetiology

• Strain – especially secondary to poor conformation, e.g. sickle hocks.
• Direct trauma.

Clinical signs

• Firm swelling on the plantar aspect of the hock – approximately 10 cm distal to the point of hock.
• May be mild lameness initially.
• The head of the lateral splint bone is very prominent in some horses giving the appearance of the hock being 'curby'.

Treatment

• Rest + NSAIDs.

Prognosis

The cosmetic appearance seldom returns to normal, but the prognosis for return to soundness in a few months is good.

Displacement of the superficial digital flexor tendon from the point of the hock

• Usually lateral, but occasionally medial.
• Easily diagnosed by inspection and palpation immediately after injury but increased swelling over the next 48 hours can mask the problem.

Treatment

• The tendon usually eventually stabilizes in the displaced position, at which time the horse usually becomes pain free, though there may still be slight mechanical interference with the gait.
• Surgical replacement and repair of the supporting retinacular tissues – guarded prognosis – reluxation and wound dehiscence are not uncommon.

Gastrocnemius tendinitis

Anatomy

The gastrocnemius muscle has two heads (medial and lateral) that terminate in the mid-tibial region in a common tendon. The superficial digital flexor (SDF) tendon crosses around the medial side of the gastrocnemius tendon to become superficial just proximal to the hock. The SDF and gastrocnemius tendons are separated by a bursa that extends to the mid-tarsal level. A small bursa also lies cranial to the insertion of the gastrocnemius on the tuber calcis – there may be a communication between these bursae.

Clinical signs

• Gait:
  – Mild to moderate lameness with variable response to upper limb flexion.
  – Reduced hock flexion.
  – Lowered arc of foot flight.
  – Reduced cranial phase to the stride.
  – Reduced duration of weight bearing during the caudal half of the stride.
• Physical examination:
  – Subtle to moderate enlargement of the gastrocnemius tendon.
  – Local heat but not usually pain on palpation.
  – Enlargement of the bursa between the SDF and the gastrocnemius in some cases.
• Regional analgesia:
  – Positive response to tibial and fibular block or tibial block alone.

Ultrasound

The gastrocnemius tendon normally has a heterogeneous echogenicity proximally but becomes more uniform distally as it comes to lie cranial to the SDF tendon.

Horses with gastrocnemius tendinitis have enlargement of the tendon, poor marginal definition and localized or diffuse areas of reduced echogenicity.

Treatment

Treatment comprises box rest and controlled exercise.

Prognosis

The prognosis is generally poor – most remain lame.

Rupture of the peroneus tertius

The peroneus tertius originates from the lateral aspect of the distal femur (extensor fossa) and inserts on the dorsolateral aspect of the third metatarsal bone and fibular and 4th tarsal bones. It lies on the craniolateral aspect of the crus buried between the long digital extensor and the anterior tibialis. It mechanically flexes the hock when the stifle is flexed (part of the reciprocal apparatus).

Aetiology

- Rupture is usually a result of overextension of the hock.
- May occur if the limb becomes trapped and the horse struggles violently to free the limb.
- As a complication following the application of full hindlimb casts.

Clinical signs

- Inability to flex the hock.
- When the leg is advanced the hock remains extended – that part of the limb below the hock hangs limp as if fractured.
- The achilles tendon loses its usual tension.
- The hindlimb is readily extended caudally so that tibia and metatarsus both lie horizontal and the achilles tendon develops a flaccid curve.
- There is usually no swelling at the rupture site, and the rupture cannot be detected on palpation.
- Disruption of the peroneus tertius may be demonstrated ultrasonographically.

Treatment

- Box rest for 6 weeks.
- Good prognosis for return to soundness.

Tarsal bone necrosis and collapse

Collapse of the dorsal aspect of the central or third tarsal bones results in a flexion deformity of the hock. This condition is seen in young foals. There may be simultaneous defective ossification and collapse of carpal bones.

Aetiology

- Incomplete ossification of the tarsal bones at birth.
- Tarsal osteomyelitis.

Clinical signs

- Hock swelling, pain and angulation (sickled hocks).
- Determination of whether infection is the cause of the problem may only be possible by synovial fluid analysis in early cases.

Radiology

- Tarsal bones appear smaller than normal and rounded.
- Irregular reduction in density.
- Progressive collapse of cranial aspect of the central and third tarsal bones (wedging) with fragmentation.

Treatment

- Infection if present.
- External support with cast.

Prognosis

- Guarded prognosis for soundness.

Intra-articular fractures

These are far less common than in the carpus.

1. Lateral malleolar fractures – if the fracture is comminuted and/or the fragments are displaced they are probably best removed surgically. Horses with minimally displaced single fragment fractures can be successfully managed conservatively.
2. Slab fractures – central or third tarsal – can lag screw.

Luxations

1. Luxation of the tarsocrural joint is usually an indication for euthanasia.
   - Very difficult to reduce.
   - Usually causes severe damage to articular surfaces.

- Luxation of the more distal joints may be more treatable with elective surgical arthrodesis or cast support.

Capped hock

1. Acquired bursal distension at the point of the hock.
2. Distinct fluid accumulation or oedematous thickening.
3. Usually due to direct trauma – kicking stall walls or in trailer.
4. Not usually a cause of lameness – just a cosmetic defect.
5. Best left alone – try to prevent recurrence of trauma.
   - Avoid surgical intervention – prone to wound breakdown.
   - Drainage ± steroids or irritants
     - debatable efficacy.
     - risk of infection.

Deep capped hock

1. Swelling of the bursa lying beneath the superficial digital flexor tendon at the point of the hock.
2. Swelling appears on either side of the superficial digital flexor tendon.
3. Unlike the superficial swelling this condition produces lameness but this usually subsides with rest. See also – gastrocnemius tendinitis.

17.5 Stifle

Anatomy

Bones

1. Femur.
2. Tibia.
3. Fibula.
4. Patella.

1. The medial ridge of the femoral trochlear is much larger than the lateral. This difference in size is not apparent in the neonatal foal but develops from 2 months of age.
2. The proximal end of the medial trochlear ridge acts as a catch for the patellar fibrocartilage and the medial patellar ligament enabling the joint to be locked in extension.
3. There is a small notch at the junction between the medial trochlear ridge and the medial condyle.
4. At this site on the lateral side there is a flattened and slightly roughened area at the transition.
5. Closure of the distal femoral and proximal tibial physes occurs from 24–30 months of age.
6. Separate ossification centre for tibial tuberosity (apophysis) fuses to epiphysis at 9–12 months and to the metaphysis at 30–36 months.
7. The fibula ossifies from two or more ossification centres which are visible radiographically by 2 months. One or more residual cartilage lines separating these centres may be seen throughout life and should not be confused with fractures.

Joints

1. Femoropatellar.
2. Femorotibial
   - medial,
   - lateral.

1. The femoropatellar joint usually communicates with the medial femorotibial joint.
2. The femoropatellar joint communicates with the lateral femorotibial joint in 20–25% of horses.
3. The two femorotibial joints do not communicate with each other.

Ligaments

1. Medial and lateral collateral (femorotibial) ligaments.
2. Meniscal ligaments anchor menisci to tibia (and femur).
3. Cruciate ligaments.
4. Femoropatellar ligaments – thin.
5. Patellar ligaments
   - medial,
   - middle,
   - lateral.

A large hooked plate of fibrocartilage attaches to the medial aspect of the patella proximally and forms the origin of the medial patellar ligament. In the ordinary standing position, in which the angle of the stifle is about 135 degrees and both hindlimbs bear weight, neither stifle joint is locked. When the horse rests one limb the angle of the stifle joint of the supporting limb is increased to about 145 degrees and the fibrocartilage is hooked over the top of the medial ridge. The ridge then protrudes through the loop formed by the medial and middle patellar ligaments and the patellar fibrocartilage. This mechanism is an important part of the stay apparatus which enables the limb to support the weight of the body with the minimum of muscular effort.

Osteochondritis dissecans (see also Chapter 15, p. 326)

In this disorder there is osteochondral fragmentation from the lateral trochlear ridge of the femur.

Clinical signs

- Young horses usually <2 years old.
- Present with synovial effusion of the femoropatellar joint ± lameness.
- Commonly bilateral.
- Affected young horses (<12 months old) often have severe clinical problems and extensive radiographic changes.
- Older horses may have less severe lesions.

Radiology

- Defect in the lateral trochlear ridge ± free mineralized fragment.
- Usually involves the middle third of the lateral trochlear ridge.

Treatment

- Surgical removal of the cartilage flap and curettage of the underlying defect.
- Usually performed under arthroscopic visualization.

The prognosis is variable depending on the extent of the lesion – 64% returned to intended use after arthroscopic surgery in one large case series.

Subchondral bone cysts (see also Chapter 15, p. 326)

Clinical signs

- Generally found in young horses but can present in middle aged horses.

- Presents clinically as a persistent mild to moderate hindleg lameness. May be intermittent in nature.

Radiology

- Seen best on the caudocranial projection.
- Large circular or domeshaped cysts in the medial femoral condyle with a distinct communication with the medial femorotibial joint.

Treatment

- Conservative management (i.e. 6 months rest) may restore soundness in 20–50% of cases.
- Surgical treatment by debriding the cyst via an intra-articular approach following arthrotomy or arthroscopy has also achieved good success rates with up to 80% returning to normal work.

Upward fixation of the patella

With upward fixation of the patella the medial patellar fibrocartilage and medial patellar ligament become locked up over the proximal end of the medial trochlear ridge of the femur and do not spontaneously unlock when the horse moves forwards or unlocking is delayed.

Aetiology

- Straight-legged conformation has been suggested to predispose.
- Poor general condition or lack of fitness. Horses may start to show clinical signs when stabled.

Clinical signs

- Permanent or temporary locking of the limb in extension. Limb is held caudally.
- Intermittent catching of the patellar during motion – stifle suddenly unlocks with a jerk and sometimes an audible 'clunk'.
- Intermittent cases may be more obvious when the horse is reversed or turned toward the affected side.
- It may be possible to temporarily fix the patella by manually forcing it proximally and laterally.
- The problem may be bilateral.

Treatment

1. Mildly affected horses that are in poor condition or unfit often cease to have problems

when their general condition and fitness is improved. Young horses may similarly grow out of the problem.
2. Permanently fixed patellae may sometimes be temporarily released by
   • Suddenly startling the horse.
   • Backing the horse while pulling forward on a rope attached around the fetlock – to hyper-extend the stifle.
3. Medial patellar desmotomy – the treatment of choice for severe or persistent cases. Can be done under general anaesthesia or sedation and local analgesia. Horses should have 4–5 months rest after surgery before returning to full work.
4. Some horses develop persistent lameness following medial patella desmotomy that is associated with new bone formation or fragmentation at the distal pole of the patella. This condition has been treated successfully by debriding the lesions under arthroscopic visualization.

Patella luxation

Aetiology

1. Congenital/developmental.
   • May occur in foals especially Shetland ponies.
   • May be associated with a hypoplastic lateral femoral trochlear ridge.
   • Surgical intervention in the form of lateral retinacular release and medial imbrication. Trochlearplasty may help in some cases.
2. Acquired
   • Intermittent lateral subluxation may occur especially in young ponies.
     – Causes stifle clicking and abnormal hindlimb gait.
     – Leads to secondary osteoarthritis and joint effusion.
   • Traumatic lateral luxation may occur.
     – Patella palpable laterally.
     – Limb held semiflexed – no stability.
     – Stifle and hock collapse when weight taken.

Patellar fractures

Patellar fractures are usually a consequence of direct external trauma. Affected horses usually have local swelling over the patella and femoro-patellar joint effusion. Lateromedial and cranio-proximal-craniodistal oblique radiographs are generally the most useful to demonstrate the injuries.

Non-articular fractures may usually be managed conservatively. Articular fractures that do not impair the quadriceps mechanism (e.g. parasagittal fractures) may be managed by removal of separated fragments. Transverse articular fractures that prevent stifle extension require internal fixation and carry a guarded prognosis.

'Gonitis'

Gonitis is a non-specific term indicating inflammation of the stifle joint.

Certain traumatic stifle injuries that may occur individually or together may be considered under this heading.

Affected horses may present with hindlimb lameness, stifle pain and swelling, decreased range of movement, positive flexion test and varying degrees of positive response to intra-articular analgesia of the femorotibial joints.

Cruciate ligament injuries

1. Cruciate test – knee placed behind point of hock and shoulder behind thigh. Hands clasped around front of proximal tibia. Pull back and feel for relative movement and crepitus. Not easy or necessarily reliable – potentially dangerous to the clinician, therefore select cases to attempt such manoeuvres on carefully.
2. Radiography – new bone formation on the cranial aspect of the intercondylar eminencies, cyst like lucencies in and distal to the eminencies.
3. Arthoscopy can help to confirm the diagnosis.
4. There is no specific surgical treatment for cruciate ligament injury in the horse at present and the prognosis is poor.

Collateral ligament injuries

1. The medial collateral ligament is the more frequently affected.
2. Test – push in on stifle with shoulder and pull out on hock with one hand whilst feeling for widening of medial joint space of stifle with other hand.

3. Radiology – periarticular new bone around ligament attachments.
4. Stressed radiographs may help to demonstrate instability in acute cases.
5. Attempts at stabilization with a prosthesis have often been unsuccessful and the prognosis is generally poor.

Meniscal injury

1. May occur alone or in association with ligamentous injuries and articular fractures.
2. Arthroscopy offers the best chance of confirming the diagnosis. However, the menisci cannot be examined fully by this means.
3. Partial meniscectomy and debridement of injuries to the cranial meniscal ligaments is possible arthroscopically and initial reports of results are encouraging.

Osteoarthritis (see also Chapter 15, p. 324)

1. Comparatively uncommon as a primary disease in the stifle.
2. Radiological findings often less marked than clinical signs.

Fibrotic/ossifying myopathy

Aetiology

Traumatic injury to the semitendinosus muscle results in scarring (and in some cases subsequent calcification) with adhesions between the semitendinosus and the semimembranosus and biceps femoris muscles.

Clinical signs

The affected hindlimb is suddenly pulled downwards and backwards at the cranial limit of the stride.

The scarring or ossification of the affected muscle may be palpable as a hard area on the caudal aspect of the thigh.

Treatment

Mildly affected animals may not require treatment and be able to cope with the gait abnormality.

Surgical treatment involves tenectomy or myectomy of the semitendinosus muscle. The tenectomy procedure has fewer complications and may be preferable.

17.6 Hip

Anatomy

The hip is a ball and socket joint composed of the head of the femur and the acetabulum of the pelvis. In addition to the round ligament running from the fovea on the femoral head to the acetabular fossa as in other species, the horse also has an accessory femoral ligament that runs from the fovea medially and cranially through the acetabular notch and along the ventral surface of the pubis to insert on the prepubic tendon.

Osteoarthritis

Osteoarthritis of the hip in the horse is rare. It may occur secondary to trauma which may cause rupture of the round ligament and consequent instability (subluxation). Clinically, the horse may show outward rotation of the affected limb at rest. Crepitus may be palpable externally or on rectal examination. Scintigraphy and/or radiography may help confirm the diagnosis. The prognosis is usually poor.

Luxation

Luxation of the hip is also rare in the horse. It usually occurs as a result of trauma. The femoral head is usually displaced craniodorsally. The limb may be rotated outwards and appears shortened. The greater trochanter may appear particularly prominent and crepitus may be palpable externally or *per rectum* on manipulation. The diagnosis may be confirmed radiographically. The radiographs should be carefully scrutinized for accompanying fractures of the dorsal rim of the acetabulum.

Closed reduction under general anaesthesia may be possible in acute injury. Both open reduction and salvage by femoral head excision have also been reported.

Further reading

Butler, J.A., Colles, C.M., Dyson, S.J., Kold, S.E. and Poulos, P.W. (1993) *Clinical Radiology of the Horse*. Blackwell Scientific Publications, Oxford.

McIlwraith, C.W. and Turner, S.A. (1987) *Equine Surgery Advanced Techniques*. Lea & Febiger, Philadelphia.

Stashak, T.S. (1987) *Adams' Lameness in Horses*. Lea & Febiger, Philadelphia.

Turner, S.A. and McIlwraith, C.W. (1989) *Techniques in Large Animal Surgery*. Lea & Febiger, Philadelphia.

Wyn-Jones, G. (1988) *Equine Lameness*. Blackwell Scientific Publications, Oxford.

18 Orthopaedics 4. The vertebral column

18.1 Anatomy of the horse's back

The anatomy of the equine thoracolumbar spine involves a complex arrangement of the soft tissue structures supporting a comparatively rigid vertebral column. The equine back has been likened to a 'bow and string' arrangement, where the 'bow' is the almost rigid vertebral column and the supporting muscles and ligaments act as the 'string', maintaining the spine under tension.

There are usually 29 vertebrae in the spine (T18, L6, S5) that are held in place by a series of ligaments (Figure 1). The supraspinous ligament is the caudal continuation of the nuchal ligament and attaches at the tip of every thoracolumbar dorsal spinous process. The main muscles of the back include the largest muscle in the body, the longissimus dorsi, and the powerful gluteal muscles (Figure 2).

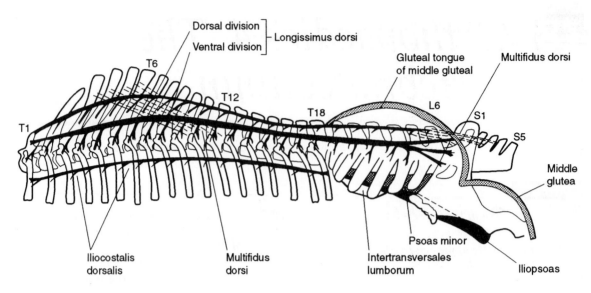

Figure 1 Ligaments of the equine thoracolumbar and sacral spine. (Reprinted from Jeffcott, L.B. and Dalin, G. (1980) *Equine Veterinary Journal* **12**, 101–108, with permission.)

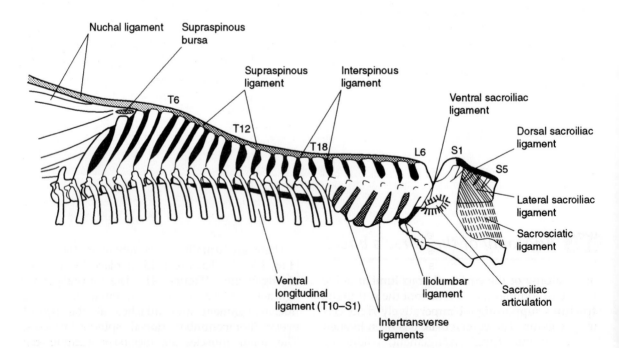

Figure 2 Epaxial muscles of the equine thoracolumbar spine (excluding the superficial layer of muscles). The multifidus dorsi forms a series of segmental muscles that lie alongside the spinous processes from T1 to S5. (Reprinted from Jeffcott, L.B. and Dalin, G. (1980) *Equine Veterinary Journal* **12**, 101–108, with permission.)

18.2 *Diagnostic approach to diseases of the horse's back*

The back of the horse is defined here as the thoracolumbar (T1 to L6) spine, sacrococcygeal (S1 to Cy2) spine and its associated structures, including the soft tissues. The most common presenting sign of back pain is loss of athletic performance.

History

The history is often of great help in determining whether one is dealing with a genuine case of back pain, or whether factors such as poor behaviour or schooling may be the underlying problem. The history is frequently long and involved; a questionnaire will help to ensure that all relevant details are obtained. Specific factors include:

- Type of work: the horse may not be suitable for the work expected of it. Certain forms of exercise may prove more problematic, e.g. jumping.
- Temperament: owners of horses with a genuine back problem frequently report that the horse has become ill-tempered, fractious or reluctant to work.
- Acute or chronic: if the problem has arisen following recent trauma, details of the accident may help localize the site of pain.
- Position of limbs: the horse may no longer straddle when urinating or defecating. There may be reluctance to bear more weight on one hindlimb (e.g. during shoeing).

Examination at rest

Stocks are useful for this part of the investigation, and the horse must be relaxed and bearing weight evenly on all four limbs.

Conformation
General condition should be noted. Abnormal curvature of the back is assessed, i.e. lordosis (ventral deviation), kyphosis (dorsal deviation) or scoliosis (lateral deviation of spine due to spinal malformation or asymmetric muscle spasm). Conformational defects (e.g. cow hocks) may predispose to hindlimb lameness.

Muscle wastage
- Differentiate from poor condition.
- Wastage may be uni- or bilateral.

- Gluteal, longissimus dorsi and thigh muscles most commonly affected.

Swellings and marks
- Assess significance of any saddle marks.
- Scars or localized soft tissue swellings.
- 'Hunter's bump' ('jumper's bump') is a prominence of the lumbar or sacral dorsal spinous processes due to poor muscling, and is often of no clinical significance in older horses.

Palpation/manipulation
- Palpate soft tissues and summits of dorsal spinous processes (DSPs) for pain, heat or swelling.
- Assess flexibility during dorsiflexion (dipping), ventroflexion (arching) and lateral bending.
- Apply pressure to both tubera coxae and tubera sacrale; pain here may indicate fracture of the ilium or a problem in the pelvic or sacroiliac region.
- Poor tail tone may indicate early cauda equina neuritis.

Examination at exercise

In hand
- The horse is walked and then trotted on a loose lead rope for lameness evaluation.
- Overt lameness or gait abnormalities should be looked for; many horses with suspected back pain suffer from hindlimb lameness. If present, this should be investigated as normal.
- Positive hindlimb flexion test(s) suggest lameness rather than back pain.
- Back pain often results in a reduced length of stride of the hindlimbs and less hock flexion.
- Turning the horse tightly in both directions may provoke longissimus dorsi spasm due to pain on lateral spinal flexion.
- There may be reluctance to move backwards, with the head being raised and back muscle spasm.

Lunging
- The horse should be exercised on both reins at trot and canter.
- Dragging and/or plaiting of hind toes, exaggerated longissimus dorsi contractions, high head carriage, tail swishing and poor hindlimb impulsion may occur. These signs may also be seen in some unfit or untrained horses.
- Signs are often more apparent on one rein.

Riding

This should be carried out, preferably by the horse's usual rider, unless the animal is considered dangerous to ride.

Observe the process of tacking-up and mounting; some horses may dip ventrally when the girth is tightened or when they are mounted. This is, however, often an acquired habit (i.e. 'cold back') and not a sign of back pain.

Assessment of gait is repeated at walk, trot and canter, on both reins.

Following a period of rest, the horse should be trotted up again; a lameness may now be apparent, or in cases of low grade exertional rhabdomyolysis ('tying up') there may be stiffness and reluctance to move.

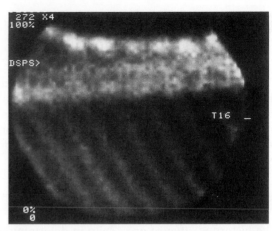

Figure 3 Image from a bone scan of the thoracic spine of an adult horse with 'kissing spines'. The bright zones at the top of the image represent areas of increased bone metabolic rate where the tips of the processes are overriding. See also Figure 5.

Aids to diagnosis

Clinical biochemistry

The blood levels of the muscle-derived enzymes, creatinine kinase (CK) and aminoaspartate transferase (AST), are measured before, immediately following, and about 12 hours after 10–20 minutes exercise (trotting and cantering). Significant rises (by more than 100–200%) suggest an exertional rhabdomyolysis.

Radiography

Powerful equipment (150 kVp/300 mAs) is required for a comprehensive radiographic examination of the thoracolumbar spine.

Sedation (e.g. detomidine or xylazine) should be used to reduce movement blur and reduce the restraint required to a minimum – this is important in optimizing radiation safety of the handlers.

Spacing of dorsal spinous processes (DSPs) from T6 to T18 can be assessed in most standing horses using mobile or portable machines.

Typical exposure values are 80 kVp/30 mAs for the DSPs of the mid-back region.

Scintigraphy

Bone scanning, using radioactive technetium labelled with methylene diphosphonate, will indicate areas of abnormal skeletal metabolic rate due to trauma (e.g. fracture), inflammation or infection. A gamma camera is used, and the examination can be carried out on standing, sedated horses, but images of better quality are obtained under general anaesthesia.

Local anaesthesia

This is most useful to confirm suspected site of pain, due to DSP impingement or overriding.

The site is localized by radiography, prepared aseptically and 5–10 ml of 2% lignocaine injected into the interspinous space using a 3.75 cm, 18-gauge needle.

Systemic analgesia

If there is doubt about the presence of pain, particularly in the chronic case, the horse may be re-exercised after a short course of a nonsteroidal anti-inflammatory agent (e.g. phenylbutazone).

Other diagnostic tests

Other tests that may be used include thermography for 'hotspots' in muscles and the 'slap test' for differentiation of low-grade proprioceptive deficits.

18.3 Disorders of the horse's back – conditions that may present as a back problem

Lameness

A wide range of conditions can be mistaken for back pain by owners. It is important to differentiate these from genuine cases of back disorders.

- Usually hindlimb lameness.
- Commonly from hock (e.g. spavin) or stifle (e.g. upward fixation of the patella).
- Locate lesion by routine work-up.

Temperamental or managemental difficulties

These include a wide range of conditions:

- Hypersensitivity of back ('cold back').
- Ill-fitting tack.
- Poor schooling and/or equitation.
- Temperamental problems.
- Lack of ability of horse to perform to owner's expectations.

Hindlimb incoordination

Horses with mild spinal cord compression/pathology in the cervical or thoracolumbar spine may present with stiffness or weakness behind resembling a back problem.

18.4 Vertebral column deformities

Lesions

These include:

- Scoliosis (lateral curvature).
- Lordosis (ventral curvature).
- Kyphosis (dorsal curvature).
- Synostosis (vertebral fusion).

Aetiology and pathogenesis

- May be congenital or acquired.
- Often becomes more pronounced with age.
- Lordosis may be due to hypoplasia of the articular facets T7 to T10 and may be complicated by crowding of the DSPs in the mid-back.
- Instability and abnormal loading may predispose to injury (e.g. vertebral fractures).

Diagnosis

- Examination, including visual inspection and palpation.
- Radiographic examination.

18.5 Soft tissue injury

Lesions

- Strain of individual muscle groups (e.g. longissimus dorsi, middle gluteal and sublumbar musculature).
- Damage to ligaments of back (e.g. supraspinous ligament, dorsal sacroiliac ligament).
- Generalized post-exercise myopathy (myositis; rhabdomyolysis) affecting back musculature.

Aetiology and pathogenesis

Exertional rhabdomyolysis follows glycogen breakdown in muscles during exercise without sufficient oxygen supply to the tissues, resulting in lactic acid accumulation and pain during or after exercise. Factors such as poor conditioning, familial predisposition, high-energy feed during a rest period and dietary mineral imbalances have been implicated. Other soft tissue lesions are frequently due to trauma, such as a fall. Unless sufficient rest is given, these lesions may become chronic.

Clinical signs

- Poor performance.
- Stiff gait.
- Back muscle spasm on palpation or exercise results in a stiff gait.
- Soft tissue swelling of affected muscle groups.
- Many affected horses show no specific signs.

Diagnosis

- A significant (at least two-fold) post-exercise rise in muscle enzymes (CK and/or AST) signifies myopathy.
- Palpation may localize sites of swelling and pain.
- Ultrasonography can be useful, but requires thorough familiarization with the normal appearance of the soft tissue structures of the back.

18.6 Fractures

Sites of fractures (Figure 4)

- Dorsal spinous processes: one or several processes may be affected.

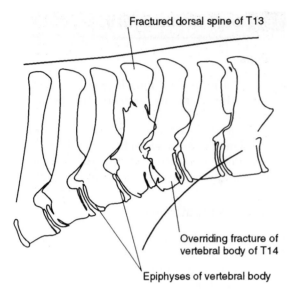

Fractured dorsal spine of T13

Overriding fracture of vertebral body of T14

Epiphyses of vertebral body

Figure 4 Diagram of a vertebral (T14) crush fracture, associated with a fracture of the T13 vertebral body, and fractured dorsal spine of T13.

• Vertebral body and neural arch: the first three thoracic and first three lumbar vertebrae and T12 (i.e. mid-point of the back) appear to be more susceptible to fractures.
• Sacral fractures with sacral nerve damage may result in local neurogenic muscle atrophy and tail paralysis.
• Coccygeal fractures may heal with permanent kinking of the tail, or tail flaccidity without perineal paralysis.

Aetiology and pathogenesis

There may be predisposing factors (e.g. lordosis; osteomyelitis, abnormal muscle spasm such as occurs in tetanus).

Multiple fractures of the DSPs at the withers (T4–T10) are usually the result of a backwards fall or somersault. Usually young animals affected (6 months to 3 years).

Other vertebral fractures are also usually due to trauma, e.g. a fall at speed.

Clinical signs

Fractures of DSPs are associated with localized pain, gross swelling and displacement of the affected summits.

Signs of vertebral body fractures vary with the degree of spinal cord damage, from mild hind-limb ataxia to acute paraplegia. Young foals are especially prone to crush-type fractures of the lumbar region.

Diagnosis

Radiography
Radiography is difficult in adults when caudal to the thoracolumbar junction due to tissue thickness and superimposition of abdominal organs, although definition of fractures in foals is usually good.

Radiographic signs of vertebral fractures include:

• Malalignment of DSP or vertebral body.
• Shortening of vertebral body due to 'crushing'-type fracture.
• Sclerosis and new bone formation in chronic cases.

Palpation
This is usually only useful if there is DSP displacement.

18.7 *Impingement and overriding of the dorsal spinous processes ('kissing spines')*

Aetiology and pathogenesis

This condition is seen most frequently in young adult Thoroughbred or TB-cross horses; rarely seen in ponies and Draught horses.

Crowding of processes occurs most commonly from T12 to T17 (i.e. beneath saddle region).

Pressure at site(s) of crowding produces bony changes, pseudarthroses (i.e. false joints) at the tips and, in some animals, pain.

Some normal horses may show marked 'kissing spines' with no apparent ill-effects. This may reflect individual variation in pain thresholds.

Clinical signs

• Usually insidious in onset (i.e. change in temperament, poor performance, reluctance to jump).
• Less commonly, acute onset seen following exacerbation by trauma.

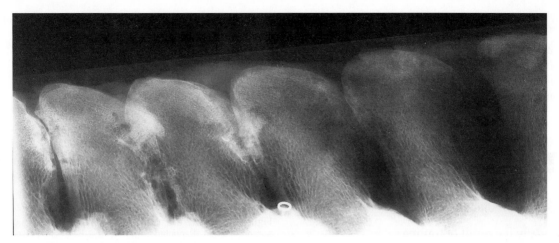

Figure 5 Post-mortem radiograph of thoracic 'kissing spines', showing marked overriding, sclerosis and bone 'cysts' at the tips of the dorsal spinous processes (same horse as in Figure 3).

● Pain is normally low-grade or not detectable by palpation, and spinal flexion in response to manipulation is restricted.
● The horse may resent flexion of back, and palpation reveals tips of DSPs close together in affected region.

Diagnosis

Radiography
● Mild cases – narrowing of interspinous spaces; sclerosis of caudal and/or cranial edges of processes.
● Advanced cases – overriding of processes, especially at tips, with sclerosis, bony remodelling and cyst-like bone lucencies (Figure 5).

Local anaesthesia
The site of pain can be confirmed by local infiltration, followed by exercise, as already described (p. 390).

18.8 *Other conditions of the spine*

Spondylosis deformans

● Formation of new bone on the ventral surface of the spine at one or several intervertebral joints.
● Predilection sites: T9–T15.
● Can occur as incidental findings. Clinical signs involve low-grade to severe pain or discomfort,
stiffness of the back, reluctance to work and impaired performance. Partial improvement with NSAID treatment.
● Diagnosis: radiography.

Osteoarthritis

● Degenerative joint disease may affect the transverse and articular processes of the caudal thoracic and lumbar spine in older horses, without clinical signs.
● If severe, may cause low-grade pain, stiffness and poor performance.
● Diagnosis: radiography; scintigraphy (bone-scanning).

Osteomyelitis

● Osteomyelitis is an infrequent cause of back disease in the horse, and occurs more commonly in younger animals and foals. Infection may occur by the haematogenous route or by extension of an abscess.
● Clinical signs vary with the site and the degree of spinal cord compression.
● Diagnosis: haematology (leucocytosis; hyperfibrinogenaemia, neutrophilia), radiography, scintigraphy. May be focal pain on clinical examination.
● Treatment: antimicrobial and anti-inflammatory agents.

Neoplasia

Tumours rarely affect the equine spine or pelvis. Multiple myeloma (plasma cell myeloma) may cause bone lysis, but other signs are usually more prominent.

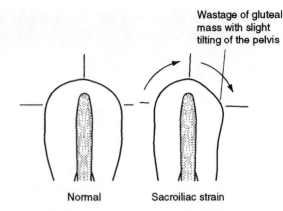

Figure 6   Diagram of a normal and a tilted pelvis subsequent to sacroiliac strain. (Reprinted from Jeffcott, L.B. (1980) *Equine Veterinary Journal* **12** (4), 197–210, with permission.)

18.9 *Sacroiliac joint disease*

Acute sacroiliac injury

- Usually the result of trauma.
- May be asymmetry of the hindquarters with the affected side dropped near midline.
- May be severe pain or crepitation on deep palpation.
- Commonly cause of lameness of hindlimb on affected side.

Chronic sacroiliac disease

Aetiology and pathogenesis

- Seen in large-framed horses with weak quarters.
- Presumed to result from low-grade instability at the joint after initial trauma.
- On post-mortem examination, the joint surface area is significantly increased by caudal or medial extensions.

Clinical signs

- Overt pain is rare; hindlimb flexion tests are usually negative.
- Gluteal wastage and lowered tuber coxae on affected side usually present (Figure 6).
- Mild hindlimb lameness or uneven gait that is best seen at slow trot.

18.10 *Treatment of back conditions*

The lack of effective conventional treatment for many cases of back pain and the frequent difficulty in coming to an accurate diagnosis has resulted in a wide range of 'alternative' therapies. Few treatment methods have been assessed objectively.

Medical treatment

Non-steroidal anti-inflammatory drugs (NSAIDs) (e.g. phenylbutazone, flunixin meglumine or meclofenamic acid) are appropriate to use in acutely painful cases, and to assist a controlled return to work. This is particularly important in chronic sacroiliac disease, where fitness and improved muscle bulk are vital to recovery.

Long-acting steroids have been injected locally into sites of 'kissing spines', with anecdotal evidence of beneficial results. Sclerosing agents have also been used.

Surgical treatment

Resection of the tips of crowded dorsal spinous processes may be carried out following a positive result to local analgesic agent infiltration. The long-term results, however, appear similar to those of conservative treatment.

Rest

A sufficient period of rest is often the most important therapy in many cases. This should be box-rest for 3 to 6 weeks in severe cases, followed by turning-out in a small paddock from 2 to 12 months.

Other treatments

Physiotherapy appears to be useful as an adjunct to a controlled programme of work. Manipulation of the back may work in some cases by altering muscle tension; however, the effect is usually temporary.

Prognosis for back conditions

In a series of 190 horses diagnosed suffering from chronic back pain, 57% recovered irrespective of the form of treatment adopted or diagnosis made. In cases of 'kissing spines', the prognosis for full recovery was reduced with increase in number of sites affected. Some horses may still perform satisfactorily despite a low-grade back problem, and complete spontaneous recovery is not uncommon.

18.11 *Pelvic fractures*

Aetiology and pathogenesis

Fractures of the pelvis are not infrequent, and result from trauma. They may occur in a bad fall, or during high speed galloping, particularly in young racehorses. Excessive abduction of the hindlimbs ('the splits') can also result in pelvic fracture.

Fracture sites are most likely to be at the ilial wing (usually in horses over 6 years of age) or shaft but may also occur at the acetabulum, pubic bone or ischium (Figure 7). Fracture of the tuber coxae is frequently caused by trauma inflicted while going through a narrow gate or doorway. The fractures are usually simple; rarely, the tuber coxae may be exposed by a wound. Fragments at the tuber ischia or tuber coxae may sequestrate.

Clinical signs

The signs vary depending on the site of injury.

Uni- or bilateral hindlimb lameness is common. Pain or crepitus may be apparent on manipulation of the limb on the affected side if the fracture is recent. When the injury is recent, there is usually associated soft tissue swelling.

In chronic cases, muscle wastage at the affected quarter is common and may be severe. Fractures of the ilial wing often result in asymmetry of the

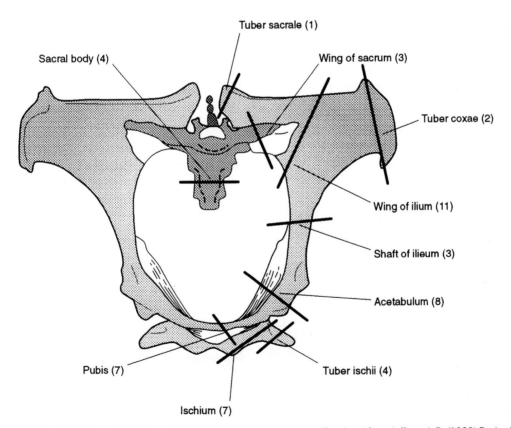

Figure 7   Diagram of the sites and incidence of 50 pelvic fractures in 41 horses. (Reprinted from Jeffcott, L.B. (1982) *Equine Practice* **3** (3), 34, with permission.)

tubera sacrale, with the affected side lower, while a fractured tuber coxae will also be visibly 'dropped'.

Deep palpation over affected areas may elicit pain. Fractures through the obturator foramen or pubic symphysis may cause a bilateral shortened hindlimb stride.

A brief period of rest may result in rapid apparent resolution of the lameness, but recurrence at increased severity is likely on return to exercise. Accurate diagnosis and prognosis are therefore essential.

Diagnosis

- Examination and palpation: rectal palpation should always be performed, but is useful mainly in displaced fractures of the pubis or acetabulum, or to detect a large haematoma.
- Radiography: ventrodorsal views, with the horse anaesthetized and in dorsal recumbency and frog-legged are required. A grid is used to reduce scatter. A method of radiography of the pelvis in the standing horse has been described, but this requires a mobile Bucky, and involves some risk to both the tube and the horse, as well as a high level of scatter radiation exposure to personnel.

A full examination of pelvic and lumbosacral regions may take six radiographs. By tipping each hip joint towards the cassette, better views of the dorsal acetabular edge and joint are obtained.
- Scintigraphy: bone scanning techniques, using either a gamma camera or point-probe technique, will readily show marked increases in bone turnover associated with fractures.
- Ultrasonography: this technique has recently proved reliable and simple to use in detecting some pelvic fractures, particularly of the ilium. Ultrasonography may also be used to monitor healing and help determine when exercise can be recommenced.

Treatment

The only surgical treatment currently undertaken for pelvic fractures is to remove tuber ischii or tuber coxae bone fragments in animals where there is sequestration or osteitis of the fragment(s).

All cases should be box-rested for a period of 1–3 months, followed by restricted exercise in a small paddock until healing has taken place. This may take up to 1 year, although for most

minimally displaced ilial fractures, 3–6 months are sufficient.

Prognosis

Horses with fractures of the tuber coxae, tuber ischii and wing of ilium carry a good prognosis for a full return to work. A poor prognosis must be given for cases of fracture through the body of the pubis, shaft of ilium or acetabulum.

18.12 *Caudal aortic or iliac artery thrombosis*

Aetiology and pathogenesis

The pathogenesis of thrombosis of the caudal aorta or iliac arteries is unknown but the migration of *Strongylus vulgaris* larvae has been implicated. Thrombosis occurs on the dorsal wall at the quadrification of the aorta and causes secondary emboli in the iliac or femoral arteries.

Signs result when an embolus obstructs a distal vessel, frequently at the popliteal artery bifurcation, and depend on the degree of obstruction. The condition may occur in all breeds and ages, but is detected more frequently in young horses performing at a high level.

Clinical signs

In the early stages, there is often the appearance of a subtle hindlimb lameness or back problem. As exercise increases, clinical signs become more apparent: stiffness in affected limb, asymmetric hindlimb gait, knuckling over or toe dragging. Signs usually resolve after 20 minutes of rest.

On palpation, the affected limb is cooler than the contralateral, particularly distally. Arterial pulsation is reduced distal to the site of obstruction. Much less frequently, horses may present with acute pain and severely lame due to sudden and extensive thromboembolism.

Diagnosis

- Rectal palpation: the terminal aorta and iliac arteries should be palpated; typically, a firmness and reduction in pulse will be detectable. Markedly occluded vessels may be enlarged and hardened. However, there may be aortic thrombosis and only peripheral embolism, with the iliac arteries unaffected.

- Ultrasonography: using a linear probe *per rectum*. Requires good familiarization with normal structures.
- Arteriography: requires specialized facilities.

Treatment

Analgesia, using NSAIDS, is indicated, particularly as controlled movement at a level below the threshold which results in clinical signs will help maintain a collateral circulation. Aspirin can help to relieve pain associated with local vasoconstriction mediated by thromboscane released from the thrombus.

Although anthelmintics have been recommended, they will not resolve an existing thrombus. Surgery in this condition is not yet feasible in horses.

Prognosis

The outlook for a return to work is relatively poor. Most cases show gradual deterioration, with the level of work requiring progressive reduction.

Further reading

Jeffcott, L.B. (1979) Radiographic examination of the equine vertebral column. *Veterinary Radiology* **20**, 135–139.

Jeffcott, L.B. (1980) Back problems in the horse – a method of clinical examination. *Veterinary Record Supplement. In Practice* **5**, 4–15.

Jeffcott, L.B. and Hickman, J. (1975) The treatment of horses with chronic back pain by resecting the summits of the impinging dorsal spinous processes. *Equine Veterinary Journal* **7** (3), 115–119.

Jeffcott, L.B. and Whitwell, K.E. (1976) Fractures of the thoracolumbar spine of the horse. *Proceedings, 22nd Annual Association of American Equine Practitioners Convention*, 91–101.

Jeffcott, L.B., Dalin, G., Ekman, S. and Olsson, S.E. (1985) Sacroiliac lesions as a cause of chronic poor performance in competitive horses. *Equine Veterinary Journal* **17** (2), 111–118.

19 Infectious diseases and parasitology

CONTENTS

19.1 Investigation of infectious disease

In equine practice most illnesses/disorders affect individual patients and so the individual, rather than the group, is often regarded as the most important unit of concern. However, from time to time equine veterinarians have to deal with outbreaks and epidemics of disease. There are some fundamental, conceptual aspects of investigating group disease which is often, but by no means always, of an infectious nature. The basis of the approach is simply a logical interpretation of biological, historical and clinical data to study the occurrence of disease within a population. The veterinarian will often subconsciously apply basic principles to a clinical scenario, but less commonly this may be performed by use of sophisticated, specialist epidemiological techniques.

The following decision-making steps may be employed when investigating an outbreak/epidemic or apparent group condition:

1. Is there an apparent increase in the incidence and/or prevalence of disease above the normal levels?

   In order to confirm that the apparent increase is real it is essential to know:
   • how new cases are being clinically defined,
   • if awareness of a condition has increased the level of reporting, rather than a true increase,
   • the rate of occurrence (i.e. incidence) and/or proportion of the group/population affected (i.e. prevalence) prior to the apparent increase.
2. If possible, confirm the diagnosis by appropriate additional tests.
3. Examine the distribution of cases within the group to establish 'risk factors'. In particular:
   • look for associations
     – when did cases occur? e.g. post-weaning, at housing etc.
     – where did cases occur? e.g. in a specific barn or pasture
     – which animals are affected, e.g. age, sex, breed, location
   • obtain rate of disease occurrence in different animal categories, e.g. in foals versus mares
   • obtain detailed information from a sample of individuals with different animal categories, e.g. duration/severity of illness in young versus old.
4. On the basis of analysis of information in 1 to 3 hypothesize why the increase in disease occurred, e.g. introduction of an animal incubating disease; change in environmental temperatures etc.
5. The purpose of going through the processes of 1 to 4 is to use the findings to formulate a control strategy. Ideally this would be by identifying the cause(s) of an increase in disease and by removing it (them) to prevent further cases. Most often control is based on:
   • initiation of immediate control measures pending confirmation of diagnosis and other investigative tests.
   • isolation/segregation of affected cases (*and* those with known direct contact prior to intervention).
   • treatment of known cases would seem logical but is not always appropriate and requires specific knowledge of the disease/condition.
   • protect high risk groups, e.g. administer hyperimmune serum to foals during rotavirus outbreak.
   • institute measures to prevent recurrence, e.g. establish quarantine protocol for new intake animals.

These comments are perhaps rather obvious but it cannot be overemphasized how easy it is to focus on the immediate clinical problem rather than to stand back and evaluate all the available information. The following information and guidelines on infectious and parasitic diseases of horses will be most useful if considered against the background of the foregoing comments.

19.2 Diagnosis of viral and bacterial infections

An accurate diagnosis is a prerequisite to specific treatment, but may be especially important in infectious diseases where there is a risk of spread to other horses. The presumptive diagnosis of viral and bacterial infections may be easy in certain diseases, being made solely on the characteristics of the history, clinical signs and physical examinations. In other cases, these characteristics may lead to a suspicion of a certain infection, which needs to be confirmed by additional information, usually in the form of laboratory tests. In other situations, such as where subclinical infection or a carrier state exists, a diagnosis may only be possible by means of laboratory examinations.

A specific diagnosis will not be required in every case of suspected infectious disease. In respiratory viral infections, for example, there may be no therapeutic benefit to be gained from knowing which virus is involved; furthermore, the results of laboratory tests may take several weeks, by which time the affected horse(s) is likely to have recovered. However, in certain situations, a specific diagnosis may be necessary (e.g. in the face of an epidemic, or when a large population of horses is at risk, or if an exotic infection is suspected). A variety of laboratory tests for the accurate diagnosis of infectious agents is available, and it is recommended that the clinician discusses the requirements for sample collection and submission with an appropriate laboratory beforehand.

Diagnosis of viral infections

The three most common methods available for the diagnosis of viral infections are virus isolation, serology and direct detection of viral antigens by immunodiagnostic methods.

1. *Virus isolation.* Samples for isolation of viruses include swabs (e.g. conjunctival, nasal, nasopharyngeal etc.), body fluids (e.g. blood, semen, tracheal aspirates, etc.) and tissues. Samples often need to be obtained in the early stages of infection and they should be collected into special transport medium which contains antibodies to prevent bacterial growth and proteins to stabilize the virus. The sample should be transported to the laboratory without delay, and may need to be kept at a low temperature (e.g. packed with ice).
2. *Serology.* A variety of serological tests is used to demonstrate serum antibodies. In many cases, the antibody titres present during the acute stage of the disease need to be compared with those in the convalescent stage 10 to 14 days later; a fourfold or greater increase in titre is generally considered significant.
3. *Detection of viral antigens.* Viral antigens may be detected in blood, secretions, scrapings and tissues by a variety of immunodiagnostic techniques, such as immunofluorescence, immunoperoxidase staining, enzyme-linked immunosorbent assay (ELISA), radioimmunoassay (RIA), PCR, etc. These methods may provide a rapid diagnosis.

Diagnosis of bacterial infections

A number of techniques similar to those used for diagnosis of viral infections may be used. The most commonly used technique in bacterial infections is culture of body fluids (e.g. nasal swabs, pus, tracheal aspirates), faeces, tissues etc. As with viral infections, the collection of the correct type of samples, and correct handling and transport of the samples, are all essential to obtain accurate laboratory results.

19.3 *Equine influenza*

The virus

The virus is an orthomyxovirus of influenza A type. Two antigenically distinct subtypes exist – A/equine/1 (H7N7) and A/equine/2 (H3N8).

Antigenic shift (major change in antigenic structure – rare) and antigenic drift (minor change in antigenic structure – commoner) can occur resulting in recurrent epizootics and the need to update commercial vaccines.

Epidemiology

A major and economically important cause of acute respiratory disease throughout the world – recorded in North and South America, Europe, Scandinavia, the former Soviet Union, the Middle East, the Far East and Africa. In North America and some parts of Europe the virus is enzootic with local outbreaks occurring regularly.

Horses of all ages are susceptible, but infection is commonest in young (2–3 years) unvaccinated horses. Infection may occur in vaccinated horses, although the severity of clinical disease and degree of viral shedding are reduced.

The extensive use of killed vaccines in Europe and North America has reduced the severity and morbidity rate of clinical disease. However, when new antigenic variants emerge, explosive outbreaks of disease can occur.

Large amounts of virus are aerosolized from affected horses due to the frequent cough. The incubation period is short (1–3 days) and virus is shed for up to 10 days.

Outbreaks are most common when large numbers of young susceptible horses are brought together at sales and shows, or for weaning and training.

Pathogenesis

Aerosolized virus is inhaled and deposits on the mucosa of the upper and lower respiratory tracts. The virus attaches to the epithelial cells and enters the cell cytoplasm where replication occurs. The epithelial lining of the entire respiratory tract is affected. Infected epithelial cells are damaged leading to inflammation, clumping of cilia and focal erosions. Secondary bacterial infections are common.

Clinical signs

- Cough (harsh and dry; sudden onset)
- Pyrexia (up to 107°F, 41.7°C)
- Lethargy
- Anorexia
- Tenderness of submandibular lymph nodes
- Serous bilateral nasal discharge (becoming mucopurulent with secondary bacterial infections)

Other signs that may be observed include tachypnoea, tachycardia, congestion of conjunctivae, epiphora, limb oedema and muscle stiffness.

In uncomplicated cases, recovery occurs in 1–3 weeks.

In some cases, secondary bacterial infection of the lower respiratory tract may give rise to bronchopneumonia with signs of dyspnoea, chest pain, reluctance to move (see Chapter 6).

In a minority of cases, myocarditis occurs causing tachycardia, arrhythmia and severe exercise intolerance.

In partially immune or vaccinated horses, the clinical signs are usually mild, or the infection may be subclinical. Performance horses may demonstrate only exercise intolerance.

Diagnosis

1. A presumptive diagnosis may be made on the basis of the clinical signs and rapid spread of disease.
2. Haematology
   - Anaemia, leucopenia and lymphopenia are seen early in the course of the infection (1–5 days).
   - Neutrophilia often occurs later as secondary bacterial infections arise.
   - Plasma fibrinogen and plasma viscosity may be elevated.
3. Virus isolation from nasopharyngeal swabs.

4. Serology – acute and convalescent serum samples demonstrate antibody rise.
5. Rapid immunological tests to detect virus antigens include enzyme and fluorescent antibody tests. An immunoassay developed to detect human influenza may also be used.

Treatment

1. Complete rest for minimum of 3–4 weeks in clean, minimum-dust environment.
2. General nursing care and provision of palatable food.
3. Antibiotic (penicillin or trimethoprim/sulphonamide) treatment is necessary only if there is significant secondary bacterial infection. If bronchopneumonia is suspected, antibiotic selection should be based on culture of transtracheal aspirate.
4. Non-steroidal anti-inflammatory drugs (NSAIDs) such as phenylbutazone are helpful in horses with high fever, depression or muscle stiffness.
5. Immunostimulants, such as mycobacterial cell wall extracts, are reported to be beneficial.
6. Bronchodilators and mucolytics may be helpful in some cases.

Control of outbreak

1. Isolate infected horses as soon as possible (as soon as a temperature rise is identified).
2. Provide adequate ventilation and minimal-dust conditions.
3. Avoid all contact between healthy and sick horses.
4. Cease exercise/training to minimize stress.
5. Maintain separate feeding, cleaning and grooming equipment, and personnel for sick horses.
6. Vaccination of healthy horses in face of the outbreak.

Prevention

1. Isolate new arrivals for 3 weeks.
2. Maintain adequate ventilation rates for all stabled horses, especially in barns.
3. Routine vaccination.
   - Current vaccines contain both influenza subtypes as either inactivated whole virus or subunit viral antigens
   - Manufacturers' recommendations vary, but most advise two primary doses 3 to 6 weeks apart, followed by a booster dose 6 months

later, a fourth dose after another 6 months and thence annually (or more frequently for high risk horses).

19.4 *The equine herpesviruses*

The viruses

Eight equid herpesviruses have been identified – equine herpesviruses (EHV) 1 to 5 occur in horses, and EHV 6 to 8 occur in donkeys.

EHV1 and 4 (formerly classified as subtypes 1 and 2 of EHV1) are associated with serious clinical disease in horses. EHV3 is associated with a mild venereal infection. EHV2 and 5 (cytomegaloviruses) are not generally considered to be of clinical significance, although EHV2 has occasionally been linked with respiratory disease in foals.

Equine herpesvirus 1 (rhinopneumonitis)

EHV1 infection is associated with respiratory disease, abortion, neonatal disease and neurological disease. The virus has a worldwide distribution.

Pathogenesis and epidemiology

Infection occurs by inhalation of virus in aerosols. The virus replicates in the epithelium of the upper and lower respiratory tracts and associated lymphoid tissue. Systemic spread by a cell-associated viraemia can occur.

The incubation period is 2 to 10 days.

Respiratory disease is commonest in young horses (up to 3 years). Older horses usually show mild or subclinical respiratory disease.

Immunity following infection or vaccination is short-lived, and horses may become reinfected on numerous occasions throughout their lives.

Latent infections by EHV1 occur, which may undergo recrudescence under conditions of stress, with the potential to cause disease or act as a source of infection to incontact horses.

Clinical signs

Respiratory disease
• Pyrexia (up to 106°F, 41.1°C)
• Serous nasal discharge (which becomes mucopurulent later)
• Coughing (variable; mild or absent)
• Depression
• Enlargement of submandibular lymph nodes

Uncomplicated cases recover in 8 to 10 days. Secondary bacterial infections may prolong the course of the disease.

Older horses show milder or subclinical disease – this may be associated with exercise intolerance or low-grade lower airway inflammation (see Chapter 6).

Abortion (see Chapter 14)
Abortion may occur due to infection of the foetus and placenta after viraemia, or due to vasculitis in the maternal endometrium.

Abortion usually occurs in late gestation (7 to 11 months). The initial respiratory infection is often subclinical.

Abortions may be sporadic or multiple (abortion 'storms').

Neonatal disease (see Chapter 20)
Foals infected in utero may be affected by severe respiratory disease, and are born ill and weak, dying within a few days. Alternatively, foals may appear normal at birth, but develop severe illness after a few days.

Neurological disease (see Chapter 11)
Neurological disease is associated with vasculitis of spinal vessels and ischaemia of the cord. It may occur in association with or in the absence of respiratory disease or abortion.

Any age group may be affected. Single, isolated cases or outbreaks may occur.

Clinical signs vary in severity, but usually have a sudden, rapid onset, with maximal severity occurring within 48 hours:

• Ataxia and paresis of hind legs.
• May progress to paraplegia or quadriplegia and recumbency.
• Urinary incontinence.
• Occasionally head tilt.

Non-recumbent horses usually recover, but full neurological function may not return for several months.

Diagnosis

Respiratory disease
• Virus isolation from nasopharyngeal swab or citrated/heparinized blood
• Serology

- Demonstration of viral antigens in nasal swabs or tracheal aspirates
- Haematology – non-specific changes

Abortion
- Virus isolation from foetal tissues/placenta
- Histopathology of foetal tissues/placenta (intranuclear inclusions)
- Demonstration of viral antigens in foetal tissues/placenta (immunofluorescence, etc.)

Neonatal disease
- Virus isolation
- Histopathology and immunofluorescence of post-mortem tissues

Neurological disease
- History and clinical signs
- Serology
- Post-mortem examination and histopathology

Treatment

Respiratory disease
- Rest for 3–4 weeks in clean, minimum dust environment
- Antibiotics as necessary to control secondary bacterial infections

Abortion
- None

Neonatal disease
- Antibiotics
- General nursing and respiratory care
- Prognosis is very poor

Neurological disease
- General nursing care
- Treatment of recumbent horses is difficult, and many cases require euthanasia due to complications of myositis, skin damage, pneumonia, etc.

Control of outbreaks and prevention

Aims:

- Minimize exposure of horses to virus.
- Maximize immune status.
- Decrease likelihood of latent virus recrudescence.

1. Isolate incoming horses for 2–3 weeks.
2. Age segregation of horses.

3. Pregnant mares should be separated from young stock, and ideally kept in small groups according to the gestational stage.
4. Horses showing clinical respiratory disease should be isolated.
5. Personnel handling infected horses should be isolated from healthy stock.
6. Bedding of infected horses should be burned.
7. Contaminated stable equipment/clothing should be disinfected.
8. Aborting mares should be kept and managed in isolation. The foetus and membranes are potential sources of infection and must be handled and disposed of carefully.
9. In cases of abortion, all mares due to foal in the same season should remain on the farm until they have foaled. Horses that leave the farm should not be allowed contact with pregnant mares.
10. In cases of neurological disease, infected horses should be isolated, and all horses on the premises should be confined until 3 weeks after the identification of the last new case.
11. Vaccination. EHV1 and 4 vaccines are available, but provide only partial and short-lived immunity. However, repeated vaccination can reduce the severity of respiratory disease and reduce the incidence rate of abortions. Two initial doses given several weeks apart are followed by regular boosters at intervals varying between 3 months and 1 year (depending on which vaccine). Unlike the recommendation for influenza, it is usually inappropriate to administer EHV1 and 4 vaccines to healthy, at-risk animals in face of an EHV outbreak.

Equine herpesvirus 4 (rhinopneumonitis)

EHV4 causes respiratory disease indistinguishable from EHV1.

The pathogenesis, clinical signs, diagnosis, treatment, control and prevention are similar to those described for the respiratory form of EHV1.

EHV4 has been linked with sporadic abortions, but has not been associated with abortion storms. It is not generally linked with neonatal disease or neurological disease.

This is a venereal infection causing small pustular vesicles on the vulva and penis, which subsequently ulcerate. The lesions persist 2 to 3 weeks.

The incubation period is 2 to 10 days.

Fertility is unaffected, but severe lesions on the penis may inhibit the stallion from covering mares.

Treatment consists of sexual rest and application of antiviral and/or antibacterial ointment to affected areas.

19.5 Equine viral arteritis (EVA)

The virus

Equine arteritis virus (EAV) is an RNA virus of the Togavirus family. Only one serotype is recognized, but there is marked variation in pathogenicity between different strains.

Epidemiology

EAV is widely distributed throughout the world, having been reported in North and South America, Europe, Africa, Asia, Australia and New Zealand. However, reports of clinical EVA are relatively few, which is explained by a high incidence of subclinical infection and confusion of the clinical disease with other viral infections such as influenza and rhinopneumonitis.

Transmission of the virus occurs via the respiratory tract (aerosolized particles) and venereally. EAV is shed in nasal secretions for up to 7 to 10 days. Stallions can transmit the virus venereally in the acute stage of the disease, and as long-term carriers.

The incubation period is 3 to 14 days.

Pathogenesis

The virus multiplies within alveolar macrophages and then passes to the bronchial lymph nodes. This is followed by viraemia and widespread distribution to many tissues. Vasculitis involving the small arteries occurs initially in the lungs and then in other tissues.

Clinical signs

Infection may result in clinical disease or be subclinical.

The clinical signs vary widely.

- Pyrexia (up to 106°F, 41°C)
- Depression and anorexia
- Limb oedema (especially hindlimbs)
- Stiffness
- Nasal or lacrimal discharge
- Conjunctivitis or rhinitis
- Periorbital/supraorbital oedema
- Ventral abdominal, scrotal, preputial or mammary oedema
- Vesicular-erosive stomatitis and hypersalivation
- Urticarial-type skin rash
- Abortion (any stage of gestation) – foetus usually partly autolysed
- Coughing, respiratory distress
- Diarrhoea
- Ataxia

Clinical disease tends to be most severe in young or old horses. Most infected horses make a full recovery, and the mortality rate is low.

Occasionally, congenital (transplacental) infections occur with newborn foals developing a rapidly progressive and fatal interstitial pneumonia and fibronecrotic enteritis.

Carrier state

A carrier state is established in 30–60% of infected stallions. The duration of the carrier state varies from several weeks to a lifetime. Carrier stallions shed the virus constantly in the semen. There is no effect on fertility.

Diagnosis

- Clinical signs
- Haematology – leucopenia and lymphopenia
- Virus isolation
  - nasopharyngeal swabs
  - conjunctival swabs
  - citrated or heparinized blood
  - placenta/foetal fluids/foetal lung and lymphoreticular tissue
- Serology (acute and convalescent samples)

Potential carrier stallions are screened by serology and virus isolation from semen.

Treatment

- Rest
- Symptomatic treatments

Prevention and control

Modified live vaccine is safe and effective in stallions and non-pregnant mares. Prevention and control depend on management practices (as described for influenza and EHV1) and selective use of the vaccine, including vaccination of the at-risk stallion population. Stallions should be vaccinated annually at least 28 days before the onset of the next breeding season. Carrier stallions should be kept in isolation and bred only to seropositive mares. Measures should be taken to prevent the spread of EAV in fresh or frozen semen used for AI.

19.6 *Equine adenovirus*

Equine adenovirus is a DNA virus which is widely distributed in the horse population worldwide. Most infections are probably subclinical. It can persist in the upper respiratory tract of adult horses in a carrier state.

Infection of foals may result in mild respiratory disease characterized by nasal discharge, coughing, conjunctivitis, pyrexia and occasionally diarrhoea.

Arabian foals affected by combined immunodeficiency syndrome (CID) (see Chapter 20) may develop severe, fatal, intersitial pneumonia (usually in conjunction with other pathogens).

19.7 *Equine picornaviruses*

The equine picornaviruses include equine rhinoviruses (ERV) 1, 2 and 3, and an acid-stable picornavirus.

The clinical significance of infection by these agents is unclear, ERV1 has been associated with acute respiratory disease (rhinitis, coughing, enlarged submandibular lymph nodes, pyrexia), but many infections by ERV1 and the other picornaviruses appear to be subclinical.

19.8 *Equine infectious anaemia (EIA)*

The virus

EIA virus (EIAV) is a lentivirus of the retrovirus family.

The virus contains reverse transcriptase, an enzyme that can convert the viral RNA genome into DNA; this complementary DNA can insert into the host DNA where it persists, protected from the host's immune defences.

Epidemiology

The virus has been identified on all continents. In Europe, it is most prevalent in the northern and central regions, and in North America it is most prevalent in the Gulf Coast and northern wooded regions of Canada.

EIAV is transmitted between horses by transfer of blood or blood products. Biting flies, especially tabanids, are the usual means of transfer, but it can also occur iatrogenically via contaminated blood, needles, surgical instruments, etc. Transplacental and colostral transmission can also occur.

Pathogenesis

EIAV replicates in macrophages in liver, spleen, lymph nodes etc. High numbers of virus are released into the circulation, which causes pyrexia. Cell-mediated and humoral immune responses clear the virus from the blood, but the virus persists within tissue macrophages.

Rapid antigenic variation allows the recurrent replication of large amounts of virus, which cause recurrent bouts of disease. Eventually, the host immune response is stimulated sufficiently to prevent bouts of viraemia.

Clinical signs

The clinical features are highly variable. Acute, subacute, chronic and subclinical syndromes are recognized. The severity of clinical signs varies according to the virulence of the strain of virus, the dose of virus, and the host response.

The *acute syndrome* is characterized by:

- Pyrexia (up to 106°F, 41.1°C)
- Thrombocytopenia
- Depression
- Anorexia
- Anaemia
- Epistaxis
- Oedema

Most horses recover from the viraemia and appear normal for several days to weeks, and then experience recurrent episodes of fever, thrombocytopenia and depression.

The frequency and severity of clinical bouts of disease decrease with time, and most horses cease to show any clinical signs after about one year.

Occasionally a *chronic disease* state occurs characterized by:

- Weight loss
- Anaemia
- Depression
- Oedema
- Death

Many infected horses have *subclinical infections* with no overt clinical signs, but they can act as a source of infection to others.

Diagnosis

1. Clinical features
2. Haematology
   - Thrombocytopenia
   - Anaemia
3. Agar gel immunodiffusion test (Coggins test) and ELISA test
4. Virus isolation is difficult

Control

Carrier horses are identified and eliminated using a serological test such as the Coggins test. Federal and State control measures operate in the USA.

19.9 *African horse sickness (AHS)*

The virus

African horse sickness viruses (AHSV) are RNA reoviruses of which there are nine serotypes.

Epidemiology

AHS is endemic in sub-Saharan Africa, but has spread elsewhere on a number of occasions, including Pakistan, the Middle East and Spain.

AHS is arthropod-borne and may spread via infected animals or by vector movement. The main vectors are *Culicoides* species of midges. Spread by contaminated needles or surgical instruments is also possible.

Clinical signs

Four syndromes are recognized:

1. Peracute or pulmonary form
   - Incubation period 3–5 days
   - Fever (up to 105°F, 40.5°C)
   - Congestion of mucous membranes
   - Dyspnoea and tachypnoea
   - Cough
   - Sweating
   - Frothy blood-tinged nasal discharge (terminally)
   - High mortality rate (95%) with death in 1–3 days
2. Subacute or cardiac form
   - Incubation period 7–14 days
   - Fever (up to 105°F, 40.5°C)
   - Congestion of mucous membranes
   - Oedematous swellings of neck, chest, lumbar and pelvic areas
   - Oedema of supraorbital fossa, eyelids, intermandibular space
   - Petechial haemorrhages on tongue and conjunctivae
   - Colic
   - Mortality rate is 50% with death in 4–8 days
3. Acute or mixed form (most common clinical form)
   - Incubation period 5–7 days
   - Clinical signs of both pulmonary and cardiac forms
   - Mortality rate 50–95% with death in 3–6 days
4. Horse sickness fever form
   - Occurs in partially immune horses and donkeys
   - Incubation period 5–14 days
   - Low grade fever (up to 103°F, 39.5°C)
   - Conjunctival congestion
   - Mild depression and inappetence
   - Recover in 5–8 days

Diagnosis

- Clinical signs
- Serology
- Virus isolation
- Necropsy

Control

Vaccination is used in endemic areas.

19.10 *Vesicular stomatitis*

The virus

The disease is caused by lyssavirus of the rhabdovirus family. Three main serotypes exist.

Epidemiology

- Endemic in central America and southern USA.
- High morbidity and low mortality.
- Virus-infected insects and plants are believed to be important means of transmission.

Clinical signs

- May be an initial fever.
- Coalescing ulcers along lips, gums and tongue.
- May be ulcers on the turbinates and nasopharynx.
- Ptyalism and reluctance to eat.
- Epistaxis.
- Dysphagia.
- Ulceration of coronary band.
- Occasionally lesions on the udder or genitalia.
- Oral ulcers heal in 1–2 weeks.
- Coronary band lesions may result in hoofwall defects or laminitis.

Diagnosis

- Clinical signs.
- Virus isolation (saliva, vesicular fluid, epithelium).
- Serology.

Treatment

- Symptomatic.
- Antibiotics to prevent secondary infections.

19.11 *Acute equine respiratory syndrome*

An outbreak of acute respiratory syndrome occurred in a training yard in Queensland in 1994. Eleven of 24 horses in the yard died as did one human (the trainer). A further 10 horses were affected on 5 other neighbouring premises, of which 3 died. The outbreak appeared to be associated with a novel virus, similar to the morbillivirus family. The incubation period was 8 to 16 days. Clinical signs included pyrexia, depression, shallow respirations, cyanotic mucous membranes and a frothy nasal discharge. Post-mortem examinations revealed severe pulmonary oedema and congestion.

19.12 *Other viral infections*

- Equine viral encephalitides (Chapter 11)
- Japanese B encephalitis (Chapter 11)
- Borna disease (Chapter 11)
- Rabies (Chapter 11)
- Rotavirus (Chapter 20)

19.13 *Salmonellosis*

Infection with *Salmonella* spp. is not uncommon in the horse and is associated with a variety of clinical scenarios from asymptomatic states to peracute enterocolitis. Equine *Salmonella* spp. infections have zoonotic importance and may also be transmitted to or acquired from other animal species. Although any equid may develop clinical salmonellosis, foals are notably more susceptible and well recognized risk factors in adult animals include recent general anaesthesia/surgery, gastrointestinal disease, antimicrobial therapy, physical exhaustion, dietary change and transportation.

Aetiology

No *Salmonella* spp. are specific or adapted to the horse and many different serotypes are sporadically isolated from equine specimens. The serotype most commonly isolated from clinical cases of salmonellosis is *S. typhimurium* with *S. agona* and *S. anatum* also fairly frequent but regarded as less pathogenic.

Pathogenesis

Clinical disease requires ingestion of large numbers of *Salmonella* spp. organisms, followed by invasion of mucosa of the ileum, caecum or ventral colon. In susceptible animals there ensues a severe fibrinous ileitis/typhilitis/colitis which constitutes a protein losing enteropathy. There is reactive mesenteric lymphadenopathy and if this immunological response is overwhelmed, bacteraemia occurs. In addition, there is endotoxaemia following absorption of intestinal bacterial endotoxins across compromised intestinal mucosa.

Clinical signs

Signs range in severity from asymptomatic carriers to peracute death.

1. Carriers/shedders
   - Usually involves non-pathogenic *Salmonella* spp.
   - Generally asymptomatic.
   - 1–5% horses are active faecal shedders; usually transient but may be protracted excretion of *S. typhimurium* after acute colitis.
   - Up to 20% of all horses are silent (non-excreting) carriers.
2. Mild infections
   - Fever
   - Anorexia
   - Dullness
   - Mild (cowpat) diarrhoea
   - Self limiting within 2–4 days
3. Acute colitis
   - Clinically indistinguishable from other acute colitides (see Chapter 3).
   - Early signs of dullness, anorexia and fever for 1–2 days.
   - Followed by moderately severe colic for next 1–2 days.
   - Diarrhoea – may be transiently mild progressing to profuse, watery.
   - Cardiovascular compromise/clinical endotoxaemia.
   - Peripheral oedema.
   - Weight loss.
4. Bacteraemia
   - Fever.
   - ± concurrent diarrhoea.
   - Septic arthritis (especially foals).
   - Sudden death (foals).

Diagnosis

- Acute colitis associated with neutropenia, hypoproteinaemia and acid–base/electrolyte imbalance but not specific for salmonellosis.
- Isolation of *Salmonella* spp. organisms: culture in specific media, e.g. tetrathionate broth, brilliant green agar; suspect *Salmonella* spp. colonies tested for H_2S production, urease activity etc.; serotype determined by slide agglutination at specialist reference laboratory.

Faeces
   - small numbers in carriers/mild infections,
   - culture of multiple sequential samples may be necessary,
   - poor isolation from rectal swab so submit large sample.

Tissues
   - use rectal biopsy or intestinal mucosa, mesenteric lymph node, liver, spleen.

PCR test has recently been described. This can be applied to faeces or environmental samples.

Treatment

- IV fluids, electrolytes, acid–base therapies.
- Anti-endotoxic NSAID protocol, e.g. 0.25 mg/kg flunixin meglumine three times daily.
- Possible hyperimmune plasma or purified endotoxin immunoglobin products.
- Monitor clinical status, plasma electrolytes/proteins, packed cell volume (PCV).
- Possible IV colloids or plasma transfusion if severe hypoproteinaemia.
- Antimicrobials – little evidence for either beneficial or detrimental effects in mild infections or acute colitis; ineffective in eliminating carrier state; indicated in foals; antimicrobial resistance common so confirm sensitivity in laboratory; consider using trimethoprim sulpha, chloramphenicol, amikacin, ampicillin or gentamicin.
- Intestinal protectants.

Prognosis

- Fifty per cent mortality in cases of acute colitis and especially foals.
- Small proportion of acute colitis cases develop chronic enteropathy with progressive weight loss and persistent diarrhoea.
- Recovered colitis cases may shed *Salmonella* in faeces for up to 4 months.
- Possible complications include laminitis, thrombophlebitis and renal failure.

Prevention and control

- Minimize stress, e.g. associated with surgery, transportation etc.
- Strict isolation of affected animals.
- Monitor in-contact animals for early signs of dullness, inapettence or fever.
- No commercially available equine vaccines but protection has been achieved using formalin killed *S. typhimurium* and *S. enteriditis*.

19.14 *Strangles*

This is a common condition that may result in upper airway constriction ('strangles') due to enlargement of the lymph nodes of the head and neck. Acute, contagious disease is caused by *Streptococcus equi* subspecies *equi* and characterized by inflammation of nasal and pharyngeal epithelium, followed by lymphadenitis, then abscessation of draining lymph nodes.

Epidemiology

Strangles is more common and severe in younger animals (foals, yearlings) but any age may be affected and predisposed by stress, e.g. weaning, transportation. It is a group disease with high morbidity of almost 100% in animals with no previous exposure. Mortality is low – about 1% – but various complications may occur. It is usually introduced by an animal incubating disease or by 'carrier' animals. Although highly contagious, spread is slow compared with respiratory viruses and requires direct contact or contaminated equipment, tack etc. Copious purulent discharges result in rapid contamination of environment, and *S. equi* organisms can survive for several months outside the host.

Pathogenesis

Streptococcus equi belongs to Lancefield's Group C, and pathogenicity is related to properties of adherence, resistance to phagocytosis and toxin/enzyme production. Infection is by inhalation or ingestion of *S. equi* organisms, which colonize upper respiratory tract/pharyngeal/palatine mucosae. The release of bacterial enzymes/toxins gives rise to rhinitis, pharyngitis and fever. This is followed by the spread of *S. equi* to local lymph nodes with resultant lymphadenitis and abscessation. In some instances there is a bacteraemia which may be associated with spread of *S. equi* to satellite lymphoid tissue. Progressive physical expansion of infected lymph nodes results in rupture either externally to the skin surface (e.g. submandibular) or internally to the guttural pouch (e.g. retropharyngeal).

Clinical signs

The incubation period is 4–10 days and clinical course about 3 weeks if untreated.

- Pyrexia – 103–105°F; often biphasic – first fever due to pharyngitis then second febrile response associated with lymph node abscessation.
- Anorexia, dullness, lethargy – improve following lymph node drainage.
- Nasal discharge; serous then mucopurulent then purulent.
- Lymphadenopathy – especially submandibular, retropharyngeal and parotid; progressive increase in size then soften and burst over 3–7 day period.
- Respiratory stertor and dyspnoea.
- Dysphagia.
- Conjunctivitis.
- Facial oedema, and/or abscessation.

Additional clinical signs occur as complications due to either local spread of infection, satellite abscessation ('bastard strangles') or immune-mediated pathology.

Common:
- Chronic nasal discharge – persistent guttural pouch empyema or sinusitis.

Rare:
- Colic/weight loss – peritonitis following rupture of abscessed mesenteric lymph nodes.
- Peripheral oedema – purpura haemorrhagica; immune-mediated vasculitis.

Very rare:
- Lameness/joint swelling – septic or immune-mediated arthritis.
- CNS dysfunction – brain/spinal cord abscess.
- Mastitis/agalactica.
- Abortion.
- Pneumonia.
- Renal failure – glomerulonephritis.

Diagnosis

- Clinical signs are generally characteristic within 7 days.
- Culture of *S. equi*; swab nasopharyngeal/draining abscess but after 7–10 days secondary infections with *S. zooepidemicus* or *Streptococcus equisimilis* are isolated more easily than causative organism; atypical isolates of *S. equi* have similar characteristics to *S. equisimilis*.

Treatment

Nursing:
- Soft foods.
- Poultice superficial lymph nodes/abscesses.
- Lance/drain mature abscesses.

- Bathe conjunctivae/abscess sinus tracts.
- Feed at floor level.
- Rest.
- Nutritional support; per stomach tube if dysphagia.
- Tracheotomy if severe dyspnoea.

Antimicrobials:
- Controversial because unsubstantiated belief that they increase complications.
- Generally not treated with antimicrobials unless life threatening or high risk of bacteraemia.
- No prophylactic benefit unless infection source removed/environment clean.
- Procaine penicillin 20 000 IU/kg twice daily, 7–10 days.

Prevention and control

- Isolation/segregation and handler hygiene should enable prevention of further spread because direct contact with infective material is necessary (compared with inhalation of aerosolized respiratory viruses).
- Thorough cleaning and disinfection of contaminated housing environments before unexposed animals enter, but within grazing environment *S. equi* remain viable for several months.
- Prophylactic antimicrobial treatments generally *not* indicated unless at very early stages of an outbreak, before the environment has become contaminated.
- No movement of animals from the premises for at least 6 weeks and all new intake animals enter only uncontaminated quarantine areas.
- Maintain separate animal groups, especially high-risk animals such as foals.
- Vaccination will at best reduce number and severity of cases. Killed whole organism or bacterial protein or bacterial enzyme vaccines are available in the USA but not UK.

19.15 *Potomac horse fever*

A common condition in regions of the USA and Canada – also known as equine ehrlichial colitis or equine monocytic ehrlichiosis. The causative agent is *Ehrlichia risticii* and infection is most typically associated with severe, acute enterocolitis but a syndrome of abortion has been recently recognized.

Epidemiology

There is regional (Eastern States) and seasonal (summer/autumn) prevalence of seropositivity and clinical disease which imply arthropod vector transmission but this has not been proven. Many animals have low-level seropositivity for antibodies to *E. risticii* but clinical disease generally occurs sporadically, i.e. many infections are subclinical. The prevalence of abortion associated with *E. risticii* infection is unknown.

Pathogenesis

The mode of transmission and route of infection have not been established but there is immediate and persistent infection of ehrlichial organisms within monocytes of the peripheral circulation. The target organ of *E. risticii* is the large intestine where it invokes an acute enterocolitis. The only directly affected tissues outside the gastrointestinal tract are the placentae of pregnant mares which can result in abortion at between 190 and 250 days of gestation.

Clinical signs

Clinical signs of Potomac horse fever are those of acute enterocolitis, but there is considerable variation of severity from anorexia/dejection/ileus to fever/marked dullness/colic/profuse diarrhoea. The clinical disease in untreated cases has approximately 5 to 10 day duration, with between 5 and 30% mortality.

- Pyrexia – often biphasic – first transient fever of 39.5°C to 41°C (due to ehrlichaemia) with a more persistent second phase 3 to 7 days later associated with obvious dullness and anorexia.
- Gastrointestinal stasis (ileus) and reduced borborygmi.
- Diarrhoea – varies from mild output to profuse, watery consistency.
- Peripheral oedema.
- Laminitis is a fairly common complication.

Diagnosis

- Isolation of *E. risticii*.
- Serology performed on paired samples but interpretation is complicated by very short timescale of antibody production – peak levels occur within a few days of infection such that a rising titre cannot always be detected if a serum sample

is not collected very early in the clinical disease. In addition, vaccination results in high titres.
- Serological methods include indirect fluorescent antibody test, enzyme-linked immunosorbent assay and competition enzyme-linked immunosorbent assay.
- Polymerase chain reaction can be used for immediate, reliable accurate diagnosis but not widely available.

Treatment

- Oxytetracycline – 6.6 mg/kg once daily for 5 days is effective if initiated early in course of disease (note: oxytetracycline is potentially causative of acute enterocolitis).
- Intravenous fluid/electrolyte therapy.
- Isolation – because of clinical similarity to acute salmonellosis and/or possible initiation of *Salmonella* spp. excretion secondary to Potomac horse fever colitis.

Prevention

- Vaccination with inactivated, partially purified, whole-cell vaccines gives fair but incomplete protection which is short-lived such that 4-monthly vaccination is required in endemic areas.
- Recovered clinical cases have a natural immunity of about 2 years' duration.

Isolation/hygiene
- Clinical cases may excrete *E. risticii* for several months; exclude healthy animals from contact with possible excretors or contaminated premises at least 6 weeks.
- Avoid crossover of equipment, tack.
- Handlers disinfect/clothing change.
- Contaminated premises steam cleaned, disinfected and vacated for 6 weeks.

19.16 *Leptospirosis*

Serological studies show that equine leptospiral infections occur worldwide but there are regional variations in both prevalence of seropositivity and the predominant serovars. Leptospirosis is rarely recognized as a clinical entity in the horse with the exception of association with anterior uveitis (see Chapter 12) and more recent implication as an infectious cause of abortion (see Chapter 14). Leptospirosis is occasionally asso-

ciated with renal disease, and with liver disease and jaundice.

19.17 *Anthrax*

Clinical disease due to *Bacillus anthracis* infection is very rare in the horse. Infection is usually rapidly fatal with signs of fever, severe colic, oedematous swelling.

19.18 *Brucellosis*

Infection with *Brucella abortus* in the horse is rare but has been associated with fistulous withers – a painful swelling of the supraspinous bursa of T2–T5 vertebrae with or without purulent discharge from a skin fistula. Affected animals may also show fever, lethargy and general stiffness.

19.19 *Tuberculosis*

Equine tuberculosis is a rare, multisystemic disease associated with signs of weight loss and neck stiffness: lesions occur in bowel, lung and cervical vertebrae.

19.20 *Ulcerative lymphangitis*

See Chapter 13.

19.21 *Glanders*

Synonyms are farcy, and enzootic lymphangitis.
    Glanders is a contagious disease caused by infection with *Pseudomonas mallei*. The disease occurs in Eastern Europe, Asia and North Africa, but is exotic to UK and USA. An acute bronchopneumonia occurs in donkeys and mules which is usually fatal, whereas in the horse a chronic cutaneous form is more common. The lesions occur on nasal mucosa, ventral abdomen, distal limbs, face and neck. Lesions are similar to ulcerative lymphangitis, consisting of subcuta-

neous nodules that ulcerate and discharge a honey-like exudate. Lymphangitis and lymphadenitis occur. Treatment is contraindicated because it may result in carrier animals.

19.22 *Lyme disease*

Lyme disease is caused by the spirochaete *Borrelia burgdorferi*. The infection has been recognized in horses in Europe, Russia, USA, China, Southeast Asia and South Africa. The organism is transmitted by ticks (*Ixodes* spp.). Serological studies indicate that exposure to the organism is common in endemic areas, but clinical disease is rare. Clinical signs associated with Lyme disease include fever, arthritis, joint swelling, lameness, muscle pain, skin lesions and neurological abnormalities.

19.23 *Equine ehrlichiosis*

Caused by *Ehrlichia equi*, the disease is a seasonal condition (autumn, winter and spring) recognized predominantly in northern California, although it has been recognized in other parts of the USA and in Europe. Tick transmission is likely, and the organism infects circulating neutrophils and eosinophils. Clinical signs include fever, depression, inappetence, limb oedema, petechiation, icterus and ataxia.

19.24 *Other equine bacterial infections*

Various other bacterial infections occur in the horse and may be associated with clinical diseases, some of which are described elsewhere in the text.

- Neonatal septicaemia (Chapter 20)
- *Rhodococcus equi* (Chapter 6)
- *Bacillus piliformis* (Chapter 20)
- *Clostridium tetani* (Chapter 11)
- *Listeria monocytogenes*
- *Actinomyces* spp.
- *Clostridium botulinum* (Chapters 11 and 20)
- *Taylorella equigenitalias* (Chapter 14)
- Also, *Ehrlichia equi* (*Rickettsia equina*)

19.25 *Investigation of parasite-associated disease*

Introduction

Although many distinct, parasitic disease states occur in equids, the majority of equine parasite infections are of mixed species of intestinal worms which are either asymptomatic or contribute to non-specific symptoms of *ill-thrift*, *anorexia*, *reduced performance* and *poor haircoat condition*. In this chapter individual parasite species infections are described in conventional terms of epidemiology, pathogenesis, clinical signs etc. but in the field it is quite rare to encounter these infections as discrete clinical entities.

History

The key points are:

- Previous confirmed parasitic diseases on the premises.
- Specific usage of anthelmintics and other parasite control measures for all animals on the premises, i.e. *not* just the affected animal.

Often parasite control is haphazard, especially in situations of shared grazing livery premises. Lack of synchronization of treatment times and/or products used are the likeliest cases of apparent failure to prevent parasitic disease but also important to consider the possibility of anthelmintic resistance. Relevant points of history for the individual clinical case suspected of parasite-associated disease are:

- Age.
- Season of year.
- Grazing – yes/no, alone/shared.
- Parasite control programme – yes/no, specific nature (see below).
- Anthelmintic dosing – frequency, products, date of last dosing and product used.

Physical examination

Few parasitic-associated diseases have characteristic physical findings other than those affecting the skin (Chapter 13).

Faecal worm egg count (FWEC)

The most common quantitative technique is the modified McMaster method. It is notoriously difficult to relate level of FWEC to worm burden and some species have particularly high fecundity, e.g. *Parascaris equorum*. Strongyle FWECs of $\leqslant 200$ eggs per gram (epg) are low and $\geqslant 1000$ epg are high whereas for *P. equorum* counts of $\geqslant 2500$ epg are considered high.

Efficacy of detection of tapeworm eggs using routine faecal flotation methods is somewhat inconsistent and relatively insensitive but may be improved by specialized centrifugation/flotation techniques.

Exclusion of parasitic disease on the basis of low or negative FWEC is a common, fundamental error: the most pathogenic stages of many equine parasites are larval, i.e. not egg laying.

Specialized flotation techniques and possibly faecal antibody estimation are required for accurate detection of *Coccidia* spp., *Cryptosporidium* spp., and *Giardia* spp.

Faecal egg count reduction test (FECRT)

The percentage of reduction of FWEC following anthelmintic dosing is calculated from the values obtained in samples on day of dosing and 10–14 days later.

Faecal larvae

Cyathostome larvae may be grossly evident as 1 cm red or white worms and if present in large numbers are evidence of clinical cyathostomosis. Larval detection can be facilitated by dilution of faeces in water and screening under microscope.

Lungworm larvae are recovered by a Baerman technique and identified using microscopy.

Haematology/blood biochemistry

Although certain parasitic diseases may result in haematological and plasma protein changes none of these have diagnostic specificity with the possible exception of hyperbetaglobulinaemia which is often associated with larval cyathostomosis.

Bronchoalveolar lavage

This is a useful technique for confirming lungworm infection (see Chapter 6).

Cytology/histopathology

In specific situations cytological examination of fluid samples and/or histopathology of affected tissues are applied to parasite-associated disease, e.g. cerebrospinal fluid (CSF) analysis (Chapter 11) or skin biopsy (Chapter 13) or rectal biopsy in cyathostomosis.

Post-mortem examination

Definitive confirmation of parasitic disease is often only made on gross pathology and/or histopathology findings.

19.26 *Control strategies for equine parasite infections*

Epidemiology of the important parasite species (typically but not invariably the strongyles) forms the basis of strategies for equine parasite control. It is important to take into account regional variations in parasite epidemiology as well as factors such as host age, group size/stocking density and introduction of new animals. In addition, management considerations such as costs, ease of sampling groups of animals and reliability of record keeping affect the decision to implement control strategies such as pasture hygiene or strategic dosing. Where possible, young stock should be grazed separately from mature animals because there is usually greater transmission of parasites within the younger groups which are more susceptible to acquiring both strongyles and ascarids.

It is impossible to make standard recommendations for every different system of horse management. Summary guidelines are included in Table 1 which can be modified according to the situation on a specific establishment. Regardless of the strategy adopted, it is considered best to *use separate drug classes for consecutive 12 month periods*, e.g. Year 1 pro-/benzimidazoles (BZ); Year 2 pyrantel; Year 3 ivermectin; Year 4 pro-/benzimidazoles etc. It may be useful to give a single boticidal drug (e.g. ivermectin) between

Table 1 Control programmes for equine parasites.

Programmes	Guidelines	Comments
1. Interval dosing	Year round pro-/benzimadozles c.4–6 weekly pyrantel c.5 weekly ivermectin c.8–10 weekly	Synchronized treatment all animals 12 month continuous use each drug class
2. Strategic dosing	Spring/summer only	Regional variations in pasture cyathostome infectivity affect timing of dosing Synchronized treatment all animals Best with set stocking
3. Selective dosing	Year round. Only treat animals positive faecal worm eggs	Monthly FWECs all animals
4. Continuous in-feed	Year round pyrantel pamoate daily in-feed	Not available in Europe
5. Pasture hygiene	Bi-weekly pasture faecal collection	Capital/labour expense high. Appropriately combined with 1, 2 or 3 above, especially 2
6. Predacious fungi	Year round daily in-feed administration	Not yet fully validated or licensed

Piperazines, phenothiazines and organophosphates available but used infrequently. Moxidectin has good efficacy against cyathostomes but not licensed in Europe or US.

November and February of each year and control of tapeworms can be achieved by dosing with double dose pyrantel twice *per annum*. It is essential to monitor the efficacy of each drug class on at least an annual basis by performing 10–14 day post-treatment FWECs which are ideally incorporated into FECRTs. Assuming accurate dosages were given and consumed, the likeliest cause of drug failure is anthelmintic resistance. Pasture larval counts are a good indicator of the efficacy of a parasite control programme but are not widely used in general practice.

Anthelmintic resistance is widespread in equine strongyles but to date is exclusively a feature of small strongyles (cyathostomes) and, of the major drug classes it has only been widely reported to BZs but also some evidence of pyrantel resistance. Almost invariably BZ side-resistance exists in resistant cyathostome populations with the possible exception of oxibendazole. However, repeated exposure of BZ-resistant cyathostomes to oxibendazole will lead to development of resistance to this drug too. For practical purposes, BZ resistance should be considered irreversible such that, following detection of resistance, BZs should either be omitted from the parasite control programme or given in combination with piperazine or phenothiazine. The practice of combination anthelmintics is not commonly used in UK but is utilized in the USA.

With resistance being virtually inevitable following prolonged, intensive dosing with anthelmintics, it is appropriate to encourage programmes which depend on limited usage of drugs wherever practicable. The pasture hygiene approach of removing faeces from pasture has the additional advantage of significantly increasing the proportional area of fields which are actually grazed.

19.27 *Strongyles*

These are colloquially known as red worms and are common equine parasites (virtually 100% prevalence small strongyle infection but previously widespread large strongyle infection now only around 5% in UK). Young animals are more susceptible but there is limited immunity so strongyle-related disease is possible at any age. There is a long-established association of colic with strongyles (especially *Strongylus vulgaris*) and more recent recognition of severe disease entity of larval cyathostomosis which usually affects animals less than 5 years old in late winter or early spring.

Aetiology/epidemiology

There are two subfamilies.

1. Strongylinae (large strongyles): *Strongylus vulgaris*, *Strongylus edentatus*, *Strongylus equinus*, *Triodontophorus* spp.
   - Direct, *migratory life* cycle (*Tridontophorus* spp. non-migratory).
   - Adult stages large intestinal.

- Prepatent periods 6–10 months.
- Seasonal variation of pasture infectivity – maximal late summer/autumn in temperate zones.

2. Cyathostominae (small strongyles/cyathostomes) – 8 genera; over 40 species of which 10 occur commonly.
   - Direct, non-migratory life cycle.
   - Adult stages large intestinal.
   - Prepatent periods 6–20 weeks.
   - Arrested larval development in large intestinal/mucosa – period of arrest maybe 2–3 years.
   - Pasture infectivity seasonal, as for large strongyles.

Pathogenesis

Larval stages rather than adults are responsible for the main pathogenic effects. Various, inter-related changes involved in pathogenesis of these effects:

- Weight loss – Protein losing enteropathy
- Colic
  - Possible involvement of strongyles in many types of colic (Chapter 2).
  - *Intestinal motility changes* with large and small strongyle infection, detailed mechanisms not known.
  - *Altered mesenteric blood flow* in *S. vulgaris* infection associated with larval migration within intestinal blood vessels gives rise to non-strangulating intestinal infarction. Precise mechanisms not known but *not* thromboembolism.
  - Peritonitis, larval migration. *S. edentatus* and *S. equinus*.
  - Colitis/typhlitis and intestinal, mucosal oedema in cyathostomosis.
- Anaemia – adult large strongyles not blood feeders but cause incidental blood loss from mucosal bites.
- Diarrhoea
  - Synchronous, mass emergence into lumen of larvae arrested in development within intestinal mucosa causes typhlitis/colitis.
  - Mucosal injury at mucosal penetration of infective larva.
  - Not marked feature of large strongyle infections.

Clinical signs

Strongylosis, i.e. mixed strongyle species infection:

- Ill-thrift/weight loss/poor body coat condition ± diarrhoea.
- Colic may be severe and occur in recurrent bouts.
- Anaemia ± lethargy ± poor performance.

Cyathostomosis:
- Weight loss: marked and progressive; may precede onset of diarrhoea.
- Diarrhoea: sudden onset; possibly severe; usually becomes chronic; less severe systemic illness than other acute colitides (Chapter 3); may be recurrent diarrhoeic bouts in older animals.
- Colic: not invariable; usually mild.
- Oedema: variable; limbs, ventral, preputial.

Diagnosis

- Faecal examination
  - FWEC *not* reliable.
  - Large numbers cyathostomes in diarrhoeic faeces/rectal scrape in cyathostomosis (note: cyathostomosis may initiate faecal excretion of *Salmonella* spp. which should be regarded as secondary/incidental).
- Blood biochemistry/haematology
  - Variable, possibly within normal ranges.
  - Hypoalbuminaemia.
  - Hyperbetaglobulinaemia on serum protein electrophoresis.
  - Neutrophilia.
- Histopathology
  - Rectal biopsy occasionally evidence of cyathostome larvae.
  - Intestinal biopsy, rarely performed in live animal but ideal for definitive diagnosis of larval cyathostomosis.
- Exploratory laparotomy
  - Non-strangulating infarction lesions grossly evident.
  - Multiple intestinal biopsies to investigate weight loss/chronic diarrhoea (Chapter 3).

Treatment

- Anthelmintic
  - Larvicidal doses; oral ivermectin 0.2 mg/kg, oxfendazole 10–50 mg/kg, fenbendazole 7.5 mg/kg on 5 consecutive days or

60 mg/kg as single dose (oral moxidectin 0.4 mg/kg – not licensed in US or Europe).
 – Repeat at 10 day intervals for cyathostomosis.
 – Possible exacerbation of colic.
• Analgesic – see Colic (Chapter 2).
• Surgery – resection infarcted bowel.
• Antidiarrhoeic – oral codeine phosphate; 1–3 mg/kg once, twice or three times daily to effect (see also Chapter 3).
• Corticosteroids – cyathostomosis – oral prednisolone 1 mg/kg once a day, before 9 a.m.

Prognosis

The prognosis is good for general strongylosis, fair for larval cyathostomosis (about 50% survive) and poor for non-strangulating infarction.

Prevention/control

This is summarized on pp. 413–414.

19.28 *Ascarids*

These are important and common parasites in animals under 2 years old.

Aetiology/epidemiology

Parascaris equorum

• Direct, migratory life cycle.
• Adult stages small intestinal.
• Prepatent period 3 months.
• Prolific egg production leading to heavy contamination of grazing/stables.
• Eggs resilient and are infective stage.

Pathogenesis

Adult stages responsible for main pathogenic effects

• Ill-thrift
 – *Not* a catabolic condition (cf. strongyle infections).
 – Reduced digestive efficiency – worms feed on intestinal content.
 – Reduced feed intake.
• Colic
 – Rare.
 – Intestinal impaction with adult worms and may lead to viscus rupture.
• Respiratory signs
 – Cough and nasal discharge during pulmonary phase of larval migration (see Chapter 6).
 – *Not* common feature unless high levels of infection.

Clinical signs

• Poor body condition or emaciation.
• Bilateral nasal discharge and coughing (rare).
• Colic (rare): may present as acute abdominal crisis.

Diagnosis

• FWEC: large, round thick-shelled eggs.

Treatment

• Anthelmintic: all classes have good efficacy against adult stages but most less effective against migrating and/or immature larvae. Proven regimens against larval stages are: fenbendazole, 10 mg/kg on 5 consecutive days; ivermectin 0.2 mg/kg; or levamisole 8.0 mg/kg (not licensed UK).
• Supportive: high quality ration.

Prognosis

The prognosis is good, but reinfection from highly contaminated environment (including stabling) is likely.

Control

Control measures are generally incorporated within the strongyle prophylaxis programme but also consider unsuitability of contaminated grazing for at least 12 months and discourage use of nursery paddocks.

19.29 *Tapeworms*

Tapeworms are common (up to 80% prevalence), and cause mainly asymptomatic infections.

Aetiology/epidemiology

Three species:

Anoplocephala perfoliata – caecum and distal small intestine (common).
Anoplocephala magna – small intestine.
Paranoplocephala mamillana – small intestine (and stomach) (rare).

- Indirect life cycle.
- Oribatid mites intermediate hosts.
- Prepatent period 6–10 weeks.

Pathogenesis

- Colic:
  - Mucosal lesions evident.
  - Possible altered intestinal motility resulting in ileocaecal disease, e.g. ileal hypertrophy or intussusception and some cases of spasmodic colic.

Clinical signs

- Asymptomatic
- Acute abdominal crisis

Diagnosis

Faecal examination:

- Flotation/centrifugation methods somewhat insensitive and inconsistent.
- Morphological differences of egg of *Anoplocephala* spp. and *P. mamillana*.

Treatment

- Anthelmintic – double dose pyrantel; embonate salt in UK, oral 38 mg/kg or pamoate salt in USA, oral 13.2 mg/kg

Prognosis

The prognosis is good. If faecal excretion of tapeworm eggs persists suspect *P. mamillana* infection.

Control

- If strong indication of specific problem on farm recommendation is double-dose pyrantel salt twice *per annum*.
- Normal dosage pyrantel salts have fair efficacy against *A. perfoliata* such that tapeworm is incidentally controlled if pyrantel in use for strongyle prophylaxis.

19.30 *Bots*

Bots are very common asymptomatic infections of equids.

Aetiology/epidemiology

There are four major species: *Gasterophilus intestinalis*, *G. nasalis*, *G. haemorrhoidalis*, *G. pecorum*.

- Stages within equine stomach are fly larvae (bots) found during winter months in temperate zones.
- Adult flies lay eggs on skin of legs (*G. intestinalis*) or head (*G. nasalis* or *G. haemorrhoidalis*).
- Self-grooming/licking causes egg to hatch to larvae which penetrate oral mucosa and migrate to stomach where persist 10–12 months.
- Larvae passed in faeces during spring and adults emerge after 1–2 months pupation on ground.

Pathogenesis

- Essentially non-pathogenic other than causing nuisance/distress when adult flies are egg laying.
- Rarely aberrant migration occurs, e.g. to the central nervous system (Chapter 11).

Clinical signs

- Mainly asymptomatic except for presence on hairs of lower limbs of eggs which appear as 2–3 mm yellow elongated structures.
- Rarely, neurological signs.

Diagnosis

Diagnosis is not required, and is made incidentally by observation of eggs on limbs, or bots within faeces or stomach.

Treatment

Treatment is not required but is commonly administered during the winter months. The drug of choice is ivermectin, oral 0.2 mg/kg. Organophosphates are also effective but toxicity and poor palatability limit usage.

Control

- *G. intestinalis* eggs can be induced to hatch by sponging with warm water or grooming or removed by clipping/shaving.
- Wintertime boticidal dosing may be incorporated into strongyle prophylaxis programme.

19.31 *Lungworm*

Donkeys are natural hosts for *Dictyocaulus arnfieldi* infection and about 30% of UK donkeys have patent, asymptomatic infections. Horses/ponies are abnormal hosts for *D. arnfieldi*: infection is very uncommon and patency rare. Lungworm infected horses/ponies show signs of chronic cough. Diagnosis suspected from historical information of grazing pastures contaminated by donkeys and confirmed by presence of large numbers eosinophils in bronchoalveolar larvae (Chapter 6). Treatment of choice is oral ivermectin at 0.2 mg/kg.

19.32 *Strongyloides westeri*

S. westeri infection is common in small intestine of foals but is usually asymptomatic. Unusual parasitic features: infection is by either ingestion of larvae in milk or skin penetration of larvae produced by free-living (i.e. non-parasitic) adult worms. Infections may be removed by anthelmintic treatments – higher dosages often required.

19.33 Oxyuris equi

O. equi (pinworm) infections commonly occur in caecum, colon and rectum and are of low pathogenicity. Adult worms infrequently cause anal pruritus during egg laying giving rise to self trauma of tailhead. Diagnosis is by identification of characteristic eggs in yellow/grey streaks of gelatinous material on perineum. Most anthelmintics are effective against these pinworms.

19.34 *Other equine parasitic infections*

Various other parasitic infections occur in the horse and may be associated with clinical disease under certain circumstances, some of which appear elsewhere in the text.

Trichostrongylus axei	*Onchocerca cervicalis* (Ch. 13)
Habronema muscae (Ch. 13)	*Parafilaria multipapillosa* (Ch. 13)
Draschia megastoma (Ch. 13)	*Echinococcus granulosus* (Ch. 3)
Habronema majus (Ch. 13)	*Fasciola hepatica* (Ch. 3)
Thelazia lacrymalis	*Eimeria leuckartii* (Ch. 3)
Micronema deletrix (Ch. 11)	*Trichomonas* spp. (Ch. 3)
Probstymaria vivipara	*Giardia* spp. (Ch. 3)
Sarcocystis neurona (Ch. 11)	*Klossiela equi*
Hypoderma spp.	*Cryptosporidium* spp. (Ch. 20)
Coccidia spp.	*Babesia* spp. (Ch. 10)
Trypanosama spp.	

Further reading

Equine Veterinary Education Manual No. 2 (1996) *Equine Exotic Diseases*. Equine Veterinary Journal Ltd, Newmarket.

Jacobs, D.E. (1986) *Colour Atlas of Equine Parasites*. Baillière, London.

Veterinary Clinics of North America: Equine Practice (1986) **2**:2 *Parasitology*. W.B. Saunders, Philadelphia.

Veterinary Clinics of North America: Equine Practice (1993) **9** (2) *Update on Infectious Diseases*. W.B. Saunders, Philadelphia.

20 *Diseases of the foal*

CONTENTS

20.1 *Prematurity*

Prematurity is defined as a foal that is delivered before 320 days gestation and has physical characteristics of immaturity.

Gestational length

- Normal gestational length varies from 320 to 360 days.
- Significant variations exist between horses, and gestational length alone is not a good indicator of readiness for birth.
- When assessing maturity, clinical appearance and gestational age must be evaluated in combination.

Definitions

1. *Prematurity*: foal less than 320 days gestation.
2. *Dysmaturity*: signs of immaturity/prematurity in foal more than 320 days gestation.
3. *Small for gestational age*: used in human medicine to describe a neonate that is small for gestational age. This suggests a derangement in normal growth patterns.

Physical characteristics of prematurity

- Small for gestational age.
- Soft/silky hair coat.
- Floppy ears.
- Increased range of joint motion; lax flexor tendons.
- Abnormal progression through normal events subsequent to foaling (e.g. standing, suckling).
- Weakness or 'floppiness'.
- Domed forehead.
- Hypothermia.
- Tachypnoea and dyspnoea.

Pathophysiology and laboratory findings

1. Immature adrenal cortical function:
   - Low cortisol levels.
   - Lack of response to ACTH.
   - Neutropenia, lymphocytosis, decreased neutrophil : lymphocyte ratios.
2. Low glycogen stores.
3. Immature renal function (not well established in the foal).
4. Pulmonary immaturity (surfactant deficiency – depends on gestational age).
5. Gastrointestinal immaturity (unable to handle oral diet; poor absorption of colostrum).
6. Susceptibility to infection; depressed immunity.

Treatment

The treatment of premature foals remains one of the most challenging cases presented to the equine practitioner.

1. Supportive care is of primary importance:
   - Maintain warm environment: blankets, lamps, heating pads, etc.
   - General nursing care.
2. Respiratory support:
   - Intranasal oxygen if hypoxaemic.
   - Surfactant treatment if deficient.
   - General nursing care – frequent turning from side to side if recumbent.
3. Cardiovascular support if necessary.
4. Nutritional support:
   - IV dextrose.
   - Enteral nutrition if gastrointestinal function is mature.
   - Parenteral nutrition if gastrointestinal function is immature.
5. Adrenocortical axis support: the use of corticosteroids is controversial.
6. Physical therapy:
   - Bandages, splints, braces, etc, as needed for musculoskeletal support.
   - Exercise should be limited if hypoplasia of the carpal or tarsal bones is present.
7. Prevention of infection:
   - Determine adequacy of passive transfer of immunoglobulins.
   - Administer colostrum or plasma if necessary.
   - Broad-spectrum antimicrobials.
8. Determine the underlying cause of prematurity if possible:
   - Infection.
   - Placental abnormalities.

Prognosis

- Survival of foals induced before 320 days is poor.
- 73% survival in spontaneous birth between 280 to 322 days gestation.
- Respiratory maturation (surfactant) is often a determining factor. Surfactant develops at approximately 290 days, but varies with the degree of maturation.

• The prognosis is guarded if the neonate does not develop a righting reflex or suckle reflex.

Prevention

Prevention is based upon good management practices, and identification of maternal problems that may influence foetal viability and/or the onset of parturition.

1. Identification and treatment of placental infection.
2. Avoid induction of parturition unless necessary, as readiness for birth is very difficult to predict.
3. Progesterone therapy of mare.
4. Steroids have been successfully used in humans and sheep to encourage foetal maturation. They have not been thoroughly evaluated in the horse, and should not be used in the face of infection.
5. Amniocentesis is being evaluated for use in the horse; monitoring foetal heart rate can give an indication of foetal well being.
6. Tocolytic drugs to delay parturition are commonly used in human medicine, but their benefits are uncertain in the horse.

20.2 *Systemic diseases involving multiple body systems*

Septicaemia

On well managed farms, morbidity associated with septicaemia is not high, but mortality is common. Secondary complications are frequent. Rapid recognition of the problem and aggressive treatment are imperative.

Aetiology

1. Systemic spread of bacteria through the bloodstream. Infection may arise in utero or postnatally.
2. Failure of passive transfer (FPT) of immunoglobulins may predispose to infection.
3. Infections are generally a result of opportunist organisms from the foal's environment, skin, or the mare's genital tract.
4. Portals of entry into the body include the respiratory tract, umbilicus, gastrointestinal tract, and placenta.

5. Gram negative infections predominate. The most common organisms vary with the geographical location. Commonly encountered bacteria include:

   • *E. coli*
   • *Klebsiella*
   • *Actinobacillus*
   • *Pseudomonas*
   • *Enterobacter*
   • *Salmonella*
   • *Pasteurella*
   • *Listeria*
   • *Serratia*
   • *Proteus*

6. Gram positive infections are less frequent. Commonly encountered bacteria include:

   • Beta and alpha-haemolytic *Streptococcus*
   • *Corynebacterium*
   • *Staphylococcus*
   • *Clostridium* spp.

Clinical signs

1. Early signs are non-specific and include depression, weakness and decreased suckling.
2. Fever, hypothermia, or normothermia may be present, depending on the severity and stage of the disease.
3. Uveitis and hypopyon.
4. Petechial or ecchymotic haemorrhages on the mucous membranes.
5. Associated infections such as pneumonia, enteritis, meningitis, omphalophlebitis, septic arthritis and osteomyelitis.
6. Severe cardiovascular collapse (shock, stupor, coma), with associated tachypnoea and tachycardia.

Diagnosis

1. Blood culture. A positive blood culture is definitive, but a negative culture does not rule out septicaemia; periods of bacteraemia may be intermittent and brief.
2. Culture of other body fluids may be beneficial, e.g. transtracheal aspirates, cerebrospinal fluid, faeces, urine, and synovial fluid.
3. History (risk factors) that may predispose to septicaemia include placentitis or vulvar discharge in the mare, maternal problems during gestation, dystocia, low birth weight, and prematurity.

4. Clinical findings: early disease may present with few, subtle signs; advanced disease may progress to shock and coma.
5. Complete blood count (haematology):
   - Leucopenia (neutropenia) is common.
   - White cell count may be normal early in the disease.
   - Differential cell counts may be more useful than total cell count, e.g. relative neutropenia or neutrophilia, presence of band forms and toxic changes.
   - Repeat cell counts are helpful.
6. Other laboratory findings:
   - Hypoglycaemia.
   - Metabolic acidosis.
   - Low plasma immunoglobulin levels (failure of passive transfer).

Treatment

1. Antibiotic therapy should be initiated as soon as possible. It is often prudent to suspect septicaemia until proven otherwise.
   - The initial choice of antibiotics should be broad spectrum with an emphasis on Gram negative spectrum.
   - Changes in therapy can be made when and if culture and sensitivity results are available.
   - Therapy should be long term in an attempt to prevent localization of infection (secondary complications).
2. Failure of passive transfer of immunoglobulins should be treated with immunoglobulin therapy (plasma).
3. Supportive care:
   - Nursing care is critical.
   - Regulate environmental temperature (provide heat source).
   - Nutritional support; hypoglycaemia is often present; glycogen and fat stores are poor in the foal.
4. Address any underlying infections.
5. Cardiovascular support if needed.

Prevention

Good management practices:

- Clean environment.
- Healthy mares.
- Check quality of colostrum and monitor for FPT.
- Umbilical hygiene.

Shock

Shock is a circulatory dysfunction that results in cell dysfunction and death. Rapid recognition and treatment of shock are important in the prevention of organ system failure. The recognition and treatment of shock in the foal do not differ significantly from the adult horse. However, cardiogenic shock, as a result of asphyxia, and septic shock as a result of infection, are relatively common in the newborn whereas they are rare in the adult horse.

Classifications

1. Distributive shock (septic, endotoxic, splanchnic and ischaemic).
   - Results in cellular damage, capillary leakage, metabolic derangements and myocardial dysfunction.
   - Secondary to sepsis, infection and strangulating intestinal lesions.
2. Cardiogenic shock: failure of the heart to act as a pump.
   - Asphyxia.
   - Metabolic (hypoglycaemia; hypocalcaemia).
   - Congenital heart disease (left to right shunts; left-sided obstructive disease; aortic stenosis; hypoplastic left heart).
   - Large patent ductus arteriosus.
3. Hypovolaemic shock.
   - Blood loss.
   - Third space loss.
   - Dehydration.
4. Asphyxia
   - Hypoxaemia.
   - Metabolic acidosis.
   - Cardiac failure.

Clinical signs

Early in the course of disease, the signs are often non-specific and difficult to recognize. Blood pressure measurements improve the recognition of shock.

1. Mucous membranes are variable in their appearance, and dependent on the underlying cause and stage of the disease.
2. Bradycardia or tachycardia.
3. Tachypnoea or irregular respiratory patterns.
4. Low blood pressure and weak peripheral pulses.
5. Decreased peripheral perfusion:
   - increased capillary refill time

- metabolic acidosis
- decreased urine output
6. Variable haematocrit.

Treatment

1. Fluid administration is the single most important treatment in any type of circulatory shock.
   - Most beneficial in hypovolaemic shock.
   - The goal of fluid therapy is to optimize the vascular volume and restore circulatory function and tissue perfusion.
   - The most appropriate fluid choice is balanced electrolyte solution containing acetate or lactate (Ringers).
   - Polyionic fluids will dilute protein and packed cell volume (PCV), but do not worsen acid–base and electrolyte imbalances.
   - Polyionic fluids remain effective in restoring vascular volume if the PCV remains greater than 20% and the total protein greater than 35 g/l.
2. Hypertonic solutions (saline) alone or in combination with colloids.
   - Smaller volume to administer.
   - May have early rapid beneficial effects.
   - Must be followed by further supportive care including isotonic saline.
3. The rate of administration of fluids is variable; in severe cases as much as 90 ml/kg should be administered rapidly.
4. Corticosteroids are controversial and not beneficial in haemorrhagic or septic shock.
5. Catecholamine therapy.
   - Increase cardiac output, arterial pressure and tissue perfusion.
   - Use is controversial in early septic shock.
6. Antibiotic therapy if associated infection exists.
7. Non-steroidal anti-inflammatories (for anti-endotoxic effects).
8. In haemorrhagic shock, whole blood replacement may be necessary if adequate response is not achieved with crystalloids only.

Asphyxia

This is a mutifactorial problem that develops secondary to impairment of tissue oxygen delivery. It is most commonly seen in the neonate shortly after birth when oxygen delivery to the tissues is interrupted.

Causes

1. Interruption of umbilical blood flow.
2. Placental insufficiency.
3. Premature separation of the placenta.
4. Diseases of the newborn such as pneumonia, congenital cardiac defects, pulmonary immaturity, septicaemia, and endotoxaemia.
5. Failure in the first few minutes after birth to develop adequate chest expansion and adequate functional residual capacity can result in airway collapse.

Pathophysiology

Two major mechanisms may result in cellular deprivation of oxygen, namely ischaemia and hypoxaemia. Ischaemia (lack of blood flow) is generally more severe than hypoxaemia, because during hypoxaemia some blood flow and oxygen delivery persists. With a lack of blood flow, anaerobic metabolites are not removed from the tissues which may result in severe local and/or cellular acidosis.

Organ dysfunction

Acidosis can result in irreversible cell damage and progressive loss of organ function.

- Cerebral necrosis, oedema and haemorrhage.
- Failure of the heart as a pump; myocardial infarcts.
- Pulmonary hypertension; respiratory failure; decreased surfactant production.
- Kidney damage: acute tubular necrosis.
- Hepatic cellular necrosis.
- Adrenal insufficiency.
- Gastrointestinal ischaemic necrosis; necrotizing enterocolitis.

Clinical signs

Signs are referable to hypoxaemia (cyanosis of mucous membranes), organ system failure and shock (see previous section on shock).

Resuscitation

1. Airway:
   - Ensure patent airway.
   - Provide intranasal oxygen.
2. Breathing: if the foal is not breathing or if breaths are infrequent or shallow, provide

mechanical ventilation with an endotracheal tube or mask (endotracheal tube is preferable).
3. Cardiovascular support and correction of metabolic disturbances (see previous section on the treatment of shock).

20.3 *Diseases of the cardiovascular system*

Examination

Physical examination

See Chapter 7.

Rate and rhythm

1. Heart rate is 60–80 immediately postpartum; it increases to 120–150 within the next several hours, then stabilizes at 80–100 beats/min within the first week of life.
2. Sinus dysrhythmias are commonly observed in ECG studies during the immediate postpartum period.
3. Various other dysrhythmias (ventricular premature contractions, ventricular tachycardia, supraventricular tachycardia) are occasionally observed in otherwise normal foals; however, they disappear within 15 minutes postpartum.
4. To determine the clinical significance of any unusual or abnormal dysrhythmias, one should take into consideration clinical, metabolic and haemodynamic findings.

Murmurs

1. Because of the foal's thin chest, the apex beat is quite prominent, and heart sounds and flow murmurs are louder than in the adult horse.
2. Holosystolic ejection-type murmurs are not uncommon in foals, and are most likely to be physiological in nature (innocent flow murmurs), rather than due to a patent ductus arteriosus (PDA).
3. Innocent murmurs may acquire unusual tones if the foal is in lateral recumbency, or is haemodynamically compromised.
4. Functional closure of the ductus arteriosus occurs shortly after birth in most foals.

Echocardiography

See Chapter 7.

Electrocardiography

See Chapter 7.

Congenital heart disease

See Chapter 7.

Ventricular septal defect (VSD)

This is the most common congenital cardiac defect in the foal.

Patent ductus arteriosus (PDA)

Functional closure of the ductus occurs shortly after birth in most foals. A left to right PDA should not be considered abnormal if it persists for a few days postpartum in an otherwise healthy foal. In some cases, a left to right PDA may become apparent a few days after birth; most of these foals have systemic disease.

Tetralogy of Fallot

Constellation of defects including VSD, pulmonic stenosis, dextroposition of the aorta with overriding, and right ventricular hypertrophy.

Tricuspid atresia

Atresia of the tricuspid valve is usually associated with a patent interatrial septum, VSD, hypoplastic right ventricle, hyperplastic mitral valve and left ventricle.

Patent foramen ovale

Anatomic closure is reported to occur between 15 days and 9 weeks postpartum. Clinical signs are rare unless associated with other cardiac defects.

Acquired cardiac defects

See Chapter 7 for more detailed descriptions.
Acquired cardiac defects are uncommon in the foal. Inflammatory or degenerative changes may be identified at necropsy.

Pericardial disease

Exudative fluid accumulates within the pericardial sac as a result of inflammation of the pericardial and epicardial surface of the pericardium. This is not a common disease in foals.

Myocardial disease

This is commonly seen secondary to viral respiratory disease. Arrhythmias are a common reflection of myocardial disease.

Supraventricular and ventricular arrhythmias

This is more common in adult horses.

Acquired heart murmurs

These may be due to aortic insufficiency, mitral insufficiency or tricuspid insufficiency.

White muscle disease

See Chapter 21.

Cor pulmonale

Right ventricular hypertrophy in response to pulmonary hypertension. See section on asphyxia above.

Congestive heart failure

Clinical signs may include jugular vein distension, ventral oedema, pulmonary oedema and ascites.

20.4 *Diseases of the respiratory system*

Examination

Respiratory rate

The respiratory rate of the neonatal foal is approximately 60–80/minute in the immediate neonatal period, and declines to 30/minute within one hour after birth.

Lung sounds

Lung sounds are very moist immediately postpartum.

Thoracic auscultation

Thoracic auscultation is not as reliable an indicator of lower respiratory disease in the neonate as in adults, because often only subtle abnormalities are appreciable on auscultation, even in the presence of very severe pulmonary disease.

An elevation of respiratory rate, increased effort, and abnormalities of breathing pattern (nostril flaring, an abdominal component to the respiratory pattern, respiratory stridor) are more appreciable than auscultatory changes in foals with respiratory disease.

Palpation

Palpation of the thorax should be performed to determine if fractured ribs are present.

Arterial blood gas analysis

Arterial blood gas analysis aids characterization and elucidation of the cause of lower respiratory disorders, and dictates the most appropriate course of therapy.

Radiography

Radiography, although not specific, may provide information regarding the type and extent of pulmonary disease.

1. Both bacterial and viral pneumonias may be characterized by alveolar and/or interstitial patterns.
2. Ventral distribution of pathological changes may be indicative of bacterial or aspiration pneumonia (bacterial or meconium).
3. A 'whispy' pattern in the mid to dorsal thorax may be seen in foals with fungal pneumonia.
4. Premature or immature foals with surfactant disorders may not exhibit signs of respiratory distress for 24 to 48 hours postpartum. Radiography in such cases often reveals a characteristic ground-glass appearance to the lungs. However, radiographic changes may not be evident in premature foals in the preclinical stages of the disorder.

Ultrasonography

Ultrasonography of the thorax is advisable in foals with suspected diaphragmatic hernias, or haemothorax due to rib fracture.

1. If possible, ultrasonography should be performed prior to radiography as it can be performed with portable equipment at the stall.
2. Because air-filled lung will float above intrathoracic intestinal contents (diaphragmatic hernia), or pleural fluid (haemothorax), the examination must be performed with the foal standing or in sternal recumbency.
3. Rib fractures can often be identified as an obvious disruption of the cortical surfaces of the rib, above but not involving the costochondral junction. Hypoechoic regions may be identified in the adjacent lung surface, representing contused lung. Homogeneous, slightly echogenic (cellular) fluid within the thorax is consistent with haemothorax. Occasionally, numerous gas echoes may be seen floating throughout the fluid, presumably as a result of lung laceration.
4. Ultrasonography, like radiography, is not specific in the identification of pulmonary parenchymal disease in the foal. Sonography of the thorax of young foals with pulmonary disease, regardless of the aetiology, often reveals the nonspecific finding of a loss of the normal reverberation artifact pattern.

Transtracheal aspirate

- Culture can identify the aetiological agent.
- Cytology can help to differentiate the type of inflammatory response.

Endoscopy

Endoscopy is indicated if upper respiratory obstruction or malformation is suspected.

Thoracocentesis

Thoracocentesis may be indicated if haemothorax, pneumothorax or pleural effusion is suspected.

- A short intravenous catheter is safer than a needle.
- Ultrasound guidance is preferable.

Respiratory distress syndrome (RDS)

Impaired alveolar gas exchange resulting in hypoxaemia and hypercapnia. Reduced lung compliance and diffuse atelectasis are identified.

Predisposing factors

1. Prematurity.
   - Pulmonary maturation occurs at approximately 290 days gestation; however, this is variable, and gestational age should not be used as an indicator of pulmonary maturation.
   - Surfactant is critical for alveolar function. Alveolar collapse and subsequent respiratory distress occurs in its absence.
2. Decreased respiratory efficiency.
   - Factors that lead to increased demand or fatigue.
   - Failure to establish functional residual capacity shortly after birth.
   - Increased vascular permeability and oedema.
   - Viral or bacterial pneumonia.
3. Dystocia or other problems at or during foaling. Premature placental separation.
4. Any condition that results in prolonged recumbency and atelectasis.
5. Reversion to foetal circulation.

Clinical signs

- Flared nostrils, increased respiratory rate and effort.
- Auscultation reveals poor air movement.
- Cyanosis may be present.
- $PaO_2 < 50$ mmHg. $PaCO_2 > 60$ mmHg.

Treatment

- Respiratory support. Oxygen therapy alone is often not sufficient, and mechanical ventilation may be necessary.
- Cardiovascular support and correction of metabolic disorders.
- Treatment of the underlying condition and surfactant replacement in premature foals.

Meconium aspiration

The foetal lung is normally protected from aspiration by the continuous movement of fluids up the trachea. During vaginal delivery, compression of the thorax and closure of the glottis help prevent aspiration.

Aetiology

• In utero asphyxia or mechanical factors during delivery may result in evacuation of meconium into the amniotic fluid.
• Deep gasping or failure of protective mechanisms can result in aspiration.
• Meconium obstructs airways, resulting in air trapping and atelectasis, and causes chemical bronchopneumonia.

Clinical signs

• Meconium stained foal with yellow-brown discoloration of the hair coat. Meconium staining does not always imply that aspiration has occurred.
• Brown tinged nasal discharge.

Treatment

• Respiratory and nursing care as needed.
• Antibiotics if secondary infection occurs.

Idiopathic tachypnoea

This syndrome is seen in Arab, Thoroughbred and Clydesdale neonatal foals. It seems to be more frequent during hot and humid weather. The pathophysiology is unknown, but may be related to a problem with the control of thermoregulation and/or respiratory rate.

Clinical signs

• Sudden onset of clinical signs in an apparently healthy foal.
• Tachypnoea and fever (38.9–42.2°C). The respiratory pattern may resemble panting, and the rate may be as high as 80 breaths/minute.

Diagnosis

• Other causes of respiratory disease must be ruled out via a complete respiratory evaluation. All other parameters should be within normal limits.
• Other causes of infection or pain must be ruled out.
• Metabolic acidosis and other causes of tachypnoea must be ruled out.

Treatment

• Temperature control – provide a cool environment; body clipping; alcohol baths.
• Antipyretics are not successful.
• Antibiotics should be used if there is any possibility of infection.
• The condition usually resolves spontaneously in days to weeks.

Upper respiratory tract (URT) disease

There are many causes of upper airway obstruction in the foal. However, the incidence is low. Many obstructions of the URT are partial, and may go unnoticed until the foal is exercised. A more thorough discussion of URT disease is found in Chapter 5.

Nasal passages and paranasal sinuses

• Deviation of the premaxilla (wry nose).
• Deviation or thickening of the nasal septum.
• Epidermal inclusion cysts.
• Paranasal sinus cysts.

Pharynx and guttural pouches

• Retropharyngeal infections.
• Persistent dorsal displacement of the soft palate.
• Pharyngeal cysts.
• Guttural pouch tympany.
• Choanal atresia.
• Pharyngeal collapse.

Larynx

Obstructive conditions involving the larynx of young foals are uncommon.

• Unilateral or bilateral paresis or paralysis.
• Rostral displacement of the palatopharyngeal arch.
• Congenital laryngeal web defect.

Trachea

• Tracheal rupture (traumatic).
• Tracheal stenosis.

Viral disease

Equine Herpesvirus 1 (rhinopneumonitis)

See also Chapter 19.

Aetiology

- In utero infection.
- Postnatal infection.

Clinical signs

- Foals may be born normal and show acute onset of respiratory disease within the first few days of life.
- Foals may be born with signs of disease: weak, dysmature, dull, depressed, tachypnoea or respiratory distress.
- Other organ systems may be involved: liver, gastrointestinal.
- Leucopenia (lymphopenia) and susceptibility to bacterial infections.

Diagnosis

- Virus isolation (inconsistent).
- Serology using paired samples.
- Histopathology: inclusion bodies, interstitial pneumonia, hypoplasia or necrosis of the thymus/spleen, hepatic pathology.

Treatment

- General nursing care.
- Antibiotics to prevent secondary bacterial infections.
- Antiviral drugs have been used in humans.

Bacterial disease

Bacterial infections are a common cause of pneumonia in the neonate and older foal. In the neonate, pneumonia is commonly associated with septicaemia.

Routes of infection

- Placenta (placentitis); aspiration during birth; umbilicus.
- Inhalation, especially in dusty, poorly ventilated environmental conditions.

Common pathogens

- Any Gram negative enteric organisms (*E. coli*, *Salmonella*, *Klebsiella*).
- *Actinobacillus*, *Pasteurella*.
- *Streptococcus*.
- *R. equi* (see Chapter 6).

Clinical signs

Variable and dependent on the severity of the infection.

- Elevated respiratory rate and fever are highly suggestive. The absence of fever should not rule out bacterial pneumonia.
- Other signs that may or may not be seen: cough, nasal discharge, depression, mucous membrane changes.
- In chronic disease: weight loss, unthriftiness, poor doing.

Diagnosis

- Clinical signs.
- Abnormal auscultation (crackles, wheezes); deep inspiration may be necessary to identify sounds; the absence of abnormal sounds does not rule out pneumonia.
- Radiology: interstitial or alveolar pattern, consolidation, abscessation.
- Ultrasonography is particularly useful for evaluating the superficial lung field.
- Transtracheal aspirates: cytology and culture.

Treatment

1. Appropriate antibiotic therapy based on culture and sensitivity.
2. Supportive care as needed which may include:
   - Intranasal oxygen.
   - Environmental temperature regulation.
   - Bronchodilators.
   - Non-steroidal anti-inflammatories.
   - Nutritional support.

Interstitial pneumonia

This is a syndrome of highly fatal, sporadic respiratory distress in foals between 2 and 8 months of age. Necropsy findings identify a bronchointerstitial pneumonia similar to that found in neonates with respiratory distress syndrome, but distinct from foals dying from severe bacterial pneumonia. The aetiology is unknown, although some possibilities include heat stress, viral disease, toxins, atypical response to bacterial disease.

20.5 *Diseases of the nervous system*

See also Chapter 11.

Examination

The neurological examination should include a complete physical examination. Systemic disease that involves the central nervous system is relatively common in the foal.

As with the adult, the neurological examination begins with assessment of the mental state, and then progresses to evaluation of head position and the cranial nerves.

Signalment and history

Critically ill neonates are often weak, depressed or recumbent. These foals must be differentiated from those with primary neurological disease.

Physical examination

When evaluating the head, it should be noted that the normal foal will often keep its head in a flexed position, and responds to stimuli with quick, jerky movements.

Cranial nerve evaluation

Evaluation of the cranial nerves is performed as in the adult horse. However, a few normal variations should be kept in mind:

- The palpebral reflex is present shortly after birth.
- The menace response does not develop until several weeks of age, however, the foal should withdraw its head from a menacing gesture.
- The pupillary light reflex can be slow in the excited foal.
- The ability to swallow can be evaluated by observing the ability to nurse. Lip and tongue tone, and recognition of the udder, are also necessary for adequate nursing. If a foal appears to be nursing but large amounts of milk are seen

coming from the mouth or nostrils, then a swallowing deficit should be considered.

Reflex testing

An advantage of the neurological examination in the young foal versus the older foal or adult horse is the relative ease of performing reflex testing. The testing of reflexes is very useful in localizing a spinal cord lesion.

1. Neonates and young foals are often hyper-reflexive (in comparison to adults) until they are several weeks of age.
2. In the pelvic limb, the patellar reflex, flexor, gastrocnemius and cranial tibial reflexes can be tested.
3. The patellar reflex is tested with the foal in lateral recumbency and the leg to be tested supported in relaxed flexion. A brisk extension of the leg (stifle) is expected when the patellar ligaments are struck with the side of the hand. This reflex involves the L4–L5 spinal segments and is mediated through the femoral nerve.
4. The pelvic limb flexor or withdrawal reflex involves the L5 to S3 spinal segments and is mediated through the sciatic nerve. Pinching the skin of the distal limb, the coronary band or the bulbs of the heel should elicit a withdrawal of the leg and/or a central recognition of pain.
5. The gastrocnemius reflex is performed by bluntly striking the gastrocnemius tendon and observing for extension of the hock. This reflex involves spinal cord segments L5 to S3 and is mediated through the tibial branch of the sciatic nerve.
6. The cranial tibial reflex is performed by holding the limb in relaxed extension and balloting the cranial tibial muscle. The expected response is flexion of the hock.
7. Reflex testing in the thoracic limbs includes evaluation of the flexor and triceps reflexes. The triceps reflex is tested by holding the limb in relaxed flexion and tapping the triceps tendon above its insertion at the olecranon. This reflex is mediated by the radial nerve through the cervical intumescence (C6–T1).
8. The flexor or withdrawal reflex of the thoracic limb is mediated through the last three cervical and first two thoracic spinal cord segments. The expected response is a flexion of the digit, carpus, elbow and shoulder. A central response to pain should be observed.

9. Thoracolumbar lesions can be localized by evaluating the cutaneous reflex along the lateral body wall.
   - Gentle pinching or poking of the skin along the lateral thorax elicits a twitching of the cutaneous trunci muscle.
   - The sensory input is carried to the spinal cord at the level of stimulation. It then travels cranially in the spinal cord white matter to the last thoracic and first cervical segments and synapses with the lower motor neurons of the lateral thoracic nerve.
   - The lateral thoracic nerve innervates the cutaneous trunci muscle. Damage to any portion of this pathway results in an absence of the cutaneous trunci reflex.
10. The perineal reflex evaluates the last sacral segments and the caudal spinal cord segments. Stimulation of the perineal area results in flexion of the tail and closure of the anus.

Gait

The gait of the foal should be examined for the presence of weakness or ataxia. The normal newborn foal will often have a choppy, springy, dysmetric gait.

Ancillary diagnostic testing

Additional ancillary testing of the neurological patient includes blood analysis, radiography, cerebrospinal fluid analysis and electrodiagnostics, as described for the adult horse in Chapter 11.

Central nervous system disorders

Neonatal maladjustment syndrome (NMS)

NMS is a loosely-used term describing a variety of clinical manifestations of CNS disturbance in the neonatal foal. Other terms used include 'wanderer', 'barker' or 'dummy foal'. NMS is the most frequent cause of CNS disturbance in the newborn foal.

Clinical signs

Clinical signs are variable and range from inappropriate nursing behaviour to seizures and coma. Foals may wander, exhibit blindness, star gaze, or infrequently produce abnormal vocalizations. Some foals may appear normal at birth, but exhibit CNS signs at 12 to 48 hours of age.

Diagnosis

Specific criteria have not been established. However, it is generally the working diagnosis for a foal exhibiting CNS signs without any other specific neurological disease.

- The history often suggests a problem during late gestation, parturition or immediately post-foaling.
- Blood analyses are non-specific. Elevated creatinine may suggest placental insufficiency.
- Sophisticated neurodiagnostic techniques (CAT scans and/or MRI scans) may be helpful if available.

Aetiopathogenesis

The aetiology is not definitely established. However, it is likely that impaired oxygen delivery, before, during or after birth, with subsequent hypoxic–ischaemic injury to the CNS is the primary cause of the syndrome.

- Intracranial haemorrhage as a result of excessive pressures during foaling may be a causative factor.
- Impaired oxygen delivery may result from placental problems before birth, problems during birth (dystocia, premature placental separation, etc.) or postpartum events.
- Most of the brain damage occurs subsequent to the hypoxia during the period of reperfusion (12 to 24 hours after the initial insult). Oxygen-derived free radicals, excitatory neurotransmitters, and intracellular calcium may be involved.

Treatment

Treatment is symptomatic and supportive:

- If present, seizures must be controlled. Diazepam is a good initial choice as it is rapidly acting, and safe. Longer acting anticonvulsants such as phenobarbitone may be necessary as diazepam's duration of activity is short.
- Anti-inflammatories (flunixin meglumine), antioxidants (vitamin E) and free radical scavengers have been recomended, but their effectiveness in the neonate has not been thoroughly investigated.

- Fluid and nutritional support (fluids should be administered cautiously as excessive fluid therapy may worsen cerebral oedema).
- Supportive care (nursing).

Prognosis

Prognosis is dependent upon the degree of hypoxic damage:

- If severe, rapid death may ensue.
- If CNS signs are not severe or can be controlled if severe, then the prognosis can be good if nursing care is adequate and secondary complications can be avoided.
- In humans, permanent mental impairment and other long-term disorders may result. With recovery in the foal, future athletic ability should not be impaired.

Developmental disorders

See Chapter 11.

- Hydrocephalus.
- Anencephaly.

Septic meningoencephalitis (bacterial meningitis)

See Chapter 11.

Viral encephalitis (EHV-1)

EHV-1 is a rare cause of diffuse cerebral disease in the neonate.

Vascular disorders

Significant vascular accidents is a term used to describe a variety of meningeal or parenchymal haemorrhages of the CNS, which can result in a variety of neurological signs depending on the location and severity. The specific aetiology is unknown, but may include metabolic disturbances, trauma, blood pressure and blood flow abnormalities. These are probably important causes of NMS.

Liver disease

See Chapter 3 and Hepatobiliary diseases section, below.

Idiopathic epilepsy

See Chapter 11.

Other causes of CNS disease

See Chapter 11.

- Toxins.
- Cataplexy–narcolepsy.
- Trauma.
- Rabies.
- Parasite migration.
- Heat stroke.
- Lightning strike.
- Leucoencephalomalacia.
- Metabolic disorders.

Cranial nerve disorders

Visual dysfunction

1. Assessment of vision
Assessment of vision in the neonate is difficult as the menace response is not easy to evaluate. Signs of blindness may include attempts to nurse from incorrect sites, and walking into obstacles.

2. Causes of blindness
- Diffuse cerebral disease can result in bilateral blindness, usually with other signs of cerebral dysfunction.
- Postictal blindness may occur subsequent to seizures.

3. Congenital stationary night blindness
This is a poorly understood condition that is most commonly seen in the Appaloosa but has been reported in other breeds.

- Visual impairment varies from poor vision during reduced light conditions during the day with blindness at night.
- A history of poor vision and an abnormal fundus allows for a presumptive diagnosis.
- Other clinical signs may include dorsal medial strabismus, mild microphthalmia and holding the head in a 'stargazing' position when attempting to visualize objects.

Other cranial nerve abnormalities

See Chapter 11.

Cerebellar disease

See Chapter 11.

Ataxia or paresis of the limbs

See also Chapter 11.

Spinal cord and vertebral trauma

1. Trauma to the vertebral column, with or without vertebral fracture, is relatively common in the foal.
2. Physical examination may identify external signs of trauma such as skin abrasions, swellings or haematomas, epistaxis and haemorrhage from the ears. However, it is not uncommon to find no external evidence of trauma. With cervical trauma, neck pain may be present.
3. Neurological signs may include varying degrees of ataxia and/or paresis to paralysis. Thoracic limb extensor hypertonia and pelvic limb paralysis (Schiff–Sherrington phenomenon) has been reported with caudal thoracic vertebral fracture.

Vertebral osteomyelitis

Aetiopathogenesis

This disorder involves the systemic spread of bacteria which localize in the vertebrae, and may result in cord compression as osteomyelitis progresses. The history often includes previous infection. A variety of organisms have been isolated: *Rhodococcus equi* is frequent in endemic areas.

Physical examination

This may identify a stiff neck, neck or back pain, and/or unthriftiness.

Neurological examination

- If spinal cord compression is present then paresis/paralysis or ataxia may be seen.
- Areas of hypo- or hyperreflexia, or patches of sweating may be seen.

Diagnosis

- Radiographs may identify bony changes. However, osteomyelitis may not be identified early in the course of the disease.
- Cerebrospinal fluid analysis may identify a neutrophilic pleocytosis.

Occipitoatlantoaxial malformation

See Chapter 11.

Paresis or paralysis of one limb

See also Chapter 11.

Plexus and peripheral nerve trauma

Aetiology

Trauma to the brachial (most common) or lumbosacral plexus occurs most frequently at birth (during difficult deliveries) but can be caused by other physical accidents.

Clinical signs

Signs include unilateral or bilateral hypotonia with depressed reflexes.

Treatment

- Anti-inflammatory drugs in the acute stage.
- Physical therapy.
- Splints may allow the foal to bear weight and prevent limb contracture and additional trauma.

Prognosis

The prognosis is dependent upon the location and severity of trauma. Spinal root injury has a worse prognosis than plexus or peripheral nerve injury.

Other diseases of the nervous system

See also Chapter 11.

Botulism (shaker foal syndrome)

See also Chapter 11.

Aetiology

- Caused by the Gram positive, anaerobic, exotoxin-producing rod, *Clostridium botulinum*.
- The exotoxin blocks the release of acetylcholine from the motor endplate at the myoneural junction producing a muscular paralysis.
- The *C. botulinum* organism is found in the soil. In the USA, the organism is particularly common in Kentucky and along the mid-Atlantic seaboard.
- The disease results from the ingestion of preformed toxin or the elaboration of toxin from the organism that has become established within the body. Necrotic lesions within the gastrointestinal tract may allow colonization; umbilical infections are another possible focus of infection.

Clinical signs

- Any age foal can be infected, but usually greater than one week of age.
- Presentation will vary with the amount of toxin ingested or elaborated.
- The toxin produces a flaccid neuromuscular paralysis.
- Affected foals are centrally bright and alert. The initial signs include a stiff gait, spending only short periods standing, and/or dysphagia (milk dripping from the sides of the mouth). The foal may progress to trembling or shaking when standing, to total paralysis. If severe, respiratory failure and rapid death may occur from diaphragmatic paralysis.

Physical examination

- Foals are bright and alert and typically afebrile.
- A flaccid neuromuscular paralysis with poor eyelid, tongue and tail tone.

Diagnosis

- Presumptive, based on clinical signs.
- Faeces can be cultured, but results are variable and generally not available before treatment must be instituted.
- Attempts to identify the toxin in peripheral blood have been unsuccessful.
- Toxin can be identified in necrotic wounds.

Treatment

- High doses of intravenous penicillin. Drugs that potentiate neuromuscular blockade (amino-glycosides, procaine penicillin, tetracycline) should be avoided.
- Good nursing and supportive care are essential. A nasogastric tube may be placed for feeding.
- Polyvalent antitoxin greatly increases the chance of survival.
- Assisted ventilation may be necessary if respiratory paralysis has developed.

Prognosis

- Dependent on the severity. If severe and treatment is not aggressive, mortality is often 100%.
- Mild cases can recover without antitoxin therapy, but antitoxin does provide the best chance for survival.
- Severe cases can have a good prognosis if therapy is aggressive (mechanical ventilation, antibiotics, nutritional support, and meticulous nursing care).

Prevention

- Vaccination of mares to provide colostral immunity is successful in endemic areas.
- If mares are unvaccinated then foals can be vaccinated early in life.

20.6 *Musculoskeletal disease*

See also Chapters 15, 16 and 17.

Examination

1. In the newborn foal, examination of the musculoskeletal system evaluates maturity and/or gestational age. Floppy ears, absence of hair or a silky hair coat, and joint laxity can indicate immaturity, prematurity or dysmaturity.
2. The skull and vertebral column should be evaluated for curvature and the calvarium its shape.
   - A domed appearance to the skull may indicate the presence of hydrocephalus, although a slight doming of the skull can be present without underlying cerebral defects, and may indicate growth retardation during gestation.
   - Curvature of the skull off midline (wry nose) and deviations of the vertebrae, scoliosis (curvature), lordosis (extension), and kyphosis (flexion) may be seen individually or in combination with other defects.

- The newborn foal should be evaluated for signs of trauma.
- Palpation of the inguinal and/or scrotal regions should be performed to rule out the presence of hernias.
  - Herniation of bowel can result in strangulation.
  - If a hernia is easily reduced, then careful monitoring and frequent reduction may be adequate.
- Palpation of the joints and physes for heat, swelling or oedema, and observation of the gait of the foal for evidence of lameness should be performed.
  - Until proven otherwise, joint effusions, with or without heat or lameness, should be presumed to be infected.
  - Arthrocentesis and identification of a total white cell count of greater than $10 \times 10^9/1$ are suggestive of infection.

Fractured ribs

Fractured ribs (dystocia or trauma at birth) are one of the more frequent injuries in the newborn foal, although brachial plexus injuries and ruptured gastrocnemius tendons/muscle are seen occasionally.

- Fractured ribs may be bilateral but usually involve one side of the rib cage only.
- A single rib may be fractured, but multiple ribs are usually involved.
- Dislocations at the costochondral junctions may occur, and are of less clinical concern as the surrounding structures are usually left undamaged.
- Multiple dislocated rib fractures are easily identified, causing pain, swelling, and/or a flail chest.
- Careful palpation of the thorax can identify individual and non-displaced fractures. Swelling or crepitus may be present. Auscultation may reveal a rubbing sound.
- Fractured ribs may be difficult to identify radiographically. Ultrasound is useful to assess whether fractures are displaced, and to monitor healing.
- The importance of identifying fractured ribs should not be underestimated as they can result in numerous life-threatening complications.

Brachial plexus injuries and tendon ruptures

Clinical signs of brachial plexus injuries will vary with the severity of injury. However, they generally result in some degree of radial nerve paralysis. The foal is unable to bear weight on the limb, and is unable to extend the carpus or digit. Rupture of the gastrocnemius muscle can occur during foaling and is identified as a swelling above the hock in the area of the gastrocnemius muscle. A complete disruption of the gastrocnemius will allow flexion of the hock when the stifle is in an extended position. Ultrasonography identifies muscle tearing.

Angular limb deformities

See Chapters 16 and 17.

Patellar luxations

Congenital patellar luxations may occur unilaterally or bilaterally. They result from varying degrees of hypoplasia of the lateral femoral trochlear ridge. Examination of the stifle, in addition to lateral luxation of the patella, may identify periarticular swelling and a squatting stance if the condition is bilateral.

20.7 *Diseases of the alimentary system*

Examination

Physical examination

1. External abdominal palpation. This can be of diagnostic benefit in small foals as impactions or other masses may occasionally be palpated.
2. Abdominal auscultation. Gastrointestinal sounds (borborygmi) can normally be heard on both sides of the abdomen. Fluid sounds may indicate enteritis. Gas distension can be confirmed by percussion with a resulting 'ping'.
3. Ballotment can be useful for determining the presence of free abdominal fluid.

Clinical pathology

Leucopenia, hypoglycaemia and metabolic acidosis are common findings in cases of enteritis.

Abdominocentesis

1. Indicated in colic or where peritonitis is suspected.
2. The technique is the same as the adult, but with special considerations:
   - The foal must be adequately restrained.
   - A standing position is preferred, although the procedure can be performed with the foal in lateral recumbency.
   - Care must be taken to prevent perforation of the bowel. The intestinal walls in the foal are thinner and more friable than the adult. Guidance with ultrasonography can be helpful.
3. Normal peritoneal fluid analysis is similar to the adult:
   - Colour – clear or pale yellow.
   - White blood cell count $<5 \times 10^9/l$.
   - Protein <25 g/l.
   NB. Caution should be used in the evaluation of peritoneal fluid to differentiate medical and surgical cases, as elevations of protein and WBC can occur in a number of conditions including surgical lesions as well as enteritis.
4. Abnormal peritoneal fluid:
   - Increased protein and WBC:
     – enteritis
     – ischaemic intestinal lesions such as intussusceptions, etc.
     – peritonitis
     – urachal or bladder infections
   - Increased RBC or haemorrhagic fluid:
     – splenic tap
     – haemoperitoneum
     – haemorrhage from vessels in the abdominal wall
   - Food material or ingesta:
     – enterocentesis
     – bowel rupture
5. Cytology is also useful to detect bacteria (which may indicate peritonitis, bowel rupture or bowel tap). Urine crystals can sometimes be seen in cases of uroperitoneum.
6. If uroperitoneum is suspected, the serum creatinine should be compared to the abdominal fluid creatinine.

Nasogastric intubation

It is important to pass a nasogastric tube and to attempt to reflux stomach contents in any foal showing signs of colic, especially with abdominal distension.

Radiography

1. Useful in cases of gastric reflux, abdominal distension, or signs of colic.
2. Abdominal radiographs are most easily taken with the foal in a standing position, although left or right lateral recumbency views are possible in small foals.
3. Abnormal radiographic findings:
   - Gas/fluid distension – ileus or intestinal displacements with resultant obstruction.
   - Free peritoneal fluid – can often see fluid lines in standing radiographs.
   - Free peritoneal gas (pneumoperitoneum) – may indicate gastrointestinal rupture.
4. Contrast studies are useful in certain cases of suspected gastrointestinal obstruction (duodenal strictures) or gastrointestinal ulceration.
   - Withhold food 4 to 12 hours or empty the stomach by nasogastric intubation prior to the study.
   - Barium sulphate suspension – 5 ml/kg via nasogastric tube.
   - Radiographs should be taken at 1, 15, and 30 minutes, then every 2 hours until the barium has passed the area of interest.
   - Barium should have left the stomach within 2 hours in a normal foal. Delayed gastric emptying can indicate pyloric outflow obstruction. However, sick foals may have delayed gastric emptying due to decreased gastrointestinal motility.
   - Barium swallow may be performed if oesophageal disease is suspected. 120 ml barium sulphate suspension (liquid or paste) via dose syringe. This is contraindicated if oesophageal perforation or dysphagia are suspected.
   - Barium enema can be useful in diseases of the distal gastrointestinal tract such as atresia coli or other obstructive lesions. 180 ml of barium sulphate suspension is administered via an enema tube, and radiographs are taken immediately.

Ultrasonography

Ultrasound examination of the abdomen is useful for the evaluation of the bladder, umbilicus, kidneys, spleen, liver and gastrointestinal tract, as well as to look for the presence of peritoneal fluid.

• Free peritoneal fluid is echolucent and easily seen around intestinal structures especially the liver and spleen. Increased echogenicity of fluid may indicate peritonitis.

• Intussusceptions can sometimes be diagnosed by ultrasound by identifying the characteristic bulls-eye appearance on cross-section.

• Small intestinal distension caused by obstruction or ileus can also be identified with ultrasound.

Endoscopy

Endoscopic examination is useful to evaluate the oesophagus, stomach and pylorus.

• For optimal visualization, withhold feed or empty the stomach via nasogastric intubation prior to the examination.

• Gastric ulcerations are common but not necessarily significant.

Faecal analysis

1. Examination for parasites or protozoa.
   • Faecal flotation – *Strongyloides westeri*, *Parascaris* and strongyles.
   • Direct faecal examination – protozoa or oocysts.
     – Normal foals older than 2 weeks should have an active faecal protozoal population.
     – Absence of faecal protozoa in foals with diarrhoea may indicate the need for transfaunation with faeces from a normal horse ('faecal cocktail').
2. Faecal cultures.
   • *Salmonella* spp. cultured using selective media.
   • Multiple cultures should be performed as shedding of the organism appears to be intermittent. Positive cultures are more often obtained from solid samples than very watery faeces.
   • Other organisms that can also be selectively cultured for include *Clostridia* spp. and *Campylobacter*.
3. Analysis for virus, especially Rotavirus.
   • Electron microscopy.
   • ELISA test.

Congenital problems of the alimentary system

Cleft palate

See Chapter 1.

Oesophageal stenosis

Congenital stenosis is very rare and considered to be secondary to persistent right aortic arch.

Atresia

See Chapter 2.

The gastrointestinal tract is incomplete. A defect may occur at the anus (atresia ani), small colon (atresia coli) or rectum (atresia recti).

Lethal white syndrome (ileocolonic aganglionosis)

See also Chapter 13.

This fatal condition is caused by lack of myenteric ganglion cells within the intestinal walls from the ileum to the rectum. It affects white foals with blue irises from overo to overo breeding. Affected foals are usually small at birth, do not pass meconium and develop signs of colic with abdominal distension within hours to one day.

Foal diarrhoea

Clinical signs

• Faeces can range from cowpie to profuse watery diarrhoea depending on the severity and cause.

• Increased borborygmi may be noticed before the onset of diarrhoea. Some cases may have decreased gut sounds.

• Depression, fever, anorexia, colic, dehydration, injected mucous membranes.

• Abdominal distension.

Laboratory data

• Increased PCV and creatinine due to dehydration.

• Neutropenia with a left shift is common in severe bacterial or viral enteritis and endotoxaemia.

- Electrolyte imbalances: hyponatraemia, hypochloraemia, metabolic acidosis.
- Hypoglycaemia.
- Low total serum protein (especially with rehydration).

Diagnosis

- Diagnosis of specific aetiology can often be frustrating but should be attempted with all cases.
- Faecal analysis, faecal cultures and blood cultures (if septicaemia is suspected) can all help.

Treatment

Primary treatment is supportive with goals of restoring/maintaining hydration, correcting acid–base imbalances, and correcting electrolyte abnormalities.

1. Intravenous fluids – balanced isotonic fluids such as lactated Ringers.
   - May need to add additional KCl if hypokalaemia exists. Carefully monitor the fluid rate: KCl administration should not exceed 0.25 to 0.5 mEq/kg/h. Cardiac dysrhythmias can arise with too rapid administration. Mild hypokalaemia is often corrected with restoration of normal hydration and does not require further supplementation.
   - Severe acidosis may require administration of isotonic bicarbonate-containing fluids. Adding bicarbonate to isotonic fluids may cause hypertonicity. If hypertonic fluids are administered too rapidly, they may cause cerebral oedema, cerebral haemorrhage and neurological signs.
   - Dextrose may be added to fluids for hypoglycaemic foals (once again, caution must be used with hypertonic solutions); alternatively, alternate 2.5% dextrose + 0.45% saline with other fluids.
2. Oral electrolyte solutions.
   - Not as effective in correcting severe electrolyte and acid–base imbalances, especially as absorption in enteritis may be variable. Some foals, especially if weaned, will be able to maintain adequate hydration and electrolyte balance if free choice electrolyte water, plain water, and a salt block with trace minerals are provided.
   - If the foal is not interested in drinking, oral fluids may be administered via nasogastric tube.

3. Nutrition/caloric intake is very important in foals. Supplementation should be considered if the foal is not nursing or eating.
4. Antibiotics.
   - May not be indicated in all cases of diarrhoea. However, very beneficial in cases of bacterial enteritis or septicaemia. Therefore broad-spectrum antimicrobial therapy is commonly used in foal diarrhoea.
   - Penicillin plus aminoglycoside combination provides good broad-spectrum coverage. Care must be taken to ensure adequate hydration when using aminoglycosides due to the potential for nephrotoxicity.
5. Intestinal protectants. Various products are available including Bismuth subsalicylate, kaolin, activated charcoal.
6. Non-steroidal anti-inflammatory agents.
   - Flunixin meglumine: indicated if signs of endotoxaemia.
   - A low dose (0.25 mg/kg) has been shown to be effective at blocking the effects of endotoxaemia. This dose also minimizes the potential for nephrotoxicity and gastrointestinal ulcers.
7. Plasma transfusion may be indicated in cases of failure of passive transfer of immunity (FPT) or if the foal develops severe hypoproteinaemia.

Aetiologies of diarrhoea

These are often difficult to diagnose and can be multifactorial. Predisposing conditions include FPT and septicaemia.

1. Foal heat diarrhoea
   - Occurs between 6 and 14 days of age. Termed foal heat diarrhoea because it often coincides with the mare's first oestrus after parturition (the 'foal heat').
   - Self-limiting diarrhoea thought to be due to normal adaptive changes in the foal's gastrointestinal tract. Also occurs in orphan foals not on mare's milk, therefore not actually related to the mare's oestrus.
   - Affected foals are not systemically ill, and no treatment is usually necessary.
   - Resolves in <1 week.
2. Nutritional causes of diarrhoea
   - Overeating or overfeeding, sudden changes in diet, or ingestion of sand or dirt can cause diarrhoea.
   - Lactose intolerance is uncommon. Usually this is a transient condition associated with

viral enteritis which may cause a temporary lactase deficiency due to intestinal mucosal damage.
3. Antibiotic-associated
   - Antibiotic administration can alter the normal microflora of the gastrointestinal tract which is thought to result in altered volatile fatty acid synthesis and subsequent colonization by pathogenic bacteria.
   - Antibiotics associated with diarrhoea include erythromycin, oxytetracycline, trimethoprim-sulphonamides, and oral penicillins.
   - There is a low incidence of antibiotic-related diarrhoeas; therefore these antibiotics should still be used if needed. If diarrhoea develops, consider discontinuing the antibiotic.
4. Infectious causes of diarrhoea
   - Bacterial.
     - *Salmonella* spp. are the most common cause of bacterial enteritis. Can cause enterocolitis with severe diarrhoea, colic, depression and fever. Concurrent septicaemia, septic arthritis, or osteomyelitis can occur.
     - *Escherichia coli* is probably not a primary cause of diarrhoea in foals, but *E. coli* is frequently a cause of septicaemia, and diarrhoea can develop secondary to this.
     - *Clostridium perfringens* A, B, and especially C, *C. welchii*, *C. sordelli* and *C. difficile* may also cause diarrhoea. Usually sporadic cases, but occasionally causes outbreaks. The diarrhoea is very severe, may be haemorrhagic, and may cause rapid death.
     - *Rhodococcus equi* can cause diarrhoea in foals 1 to 4 months of age. More commonly associated with pneumonia and lung abscesses. Can also cause septic arthritis, physitis, uveitis and abdominal abscesses.
     - Other bacteria that have been associated with diarrhoea in the foal include *Actinobacillus equuli* and *Klebsiella* spp. which are usually associated with septicaemia.
   - Viral causes of diarrhoea.
     - Rotavirus is the most common viral cause of diarrhoea in foals. Causes a profuse watery diarrhoea in foals usually <2 months of age; often several to many foals on the farm are affected within 3 to 5 days. Diarrhoea is usually profuse and watery. Severe dehydration occurs. Con-

current gastroduodenal ulcer disease has been documented although specific correlation is unknown.
     - Other viruses that have been isolated from foals with diarrhoea include coronavirus, parvovirus and adenovirus. However, little is known about the pathogenicity of these viruses in the foal.
   - Parasitic causes of diarrhoea – see also Chapter 19.
     - *Strongyloides westeri* is a nematode that may cause mild diarrhoea in the foal 1 to 4 weeks of age.
     - Heavy infestations with strongyles or *Parascaris equorum* may cause diarrhoea but is uncommon.
   - Protozoa.
     - *Cryptosporidium* may occur in immunocompromised foals. Zoonotic potential. Treatment is supportive care.

Gastroduodenal ulcers

Predisposing factors include stress, previous illness, and treatment with non-steroidal anti-inflammatory drugs.

Clinical signs

- Diarrhoea is the most common sign.
- Signs of colic/pain, bruxism (grinding teeth), salivation, dorsal recumbency.
- Fever.
- History of stress such as recent shipping or previous illness.

Diagnosis

- Often based on clinical signs.
- Faecal occult blood test; a positive test is not diagnostic, but is supportive for ulceration.
- Endoscopic examination. It may be difficult to identify ulcers due to ingesta in the stomach; the pyloric region and duodenum are difficult to visualize. Ulcers frequently occur in the stratified squamous mucosa near the margo plicatus in young foals and along the lesser curvature and cardia in older foals.
- Contrast radiographic studies may be indicated if duodenal stricture is suspected.

Treatment

1. Drugs to decrease gastric acid secretion:
   - Histamine type 2 antagonists: cimetidine and ranitidine – available in oral or IV preparations.
   - Omeprazole: acts to block HCl secretion by inhibiting the hydrogen ion pump and thereby blocking all receptor types for gastric acid secretion. Newer drug and expensive. May be indicated in cases of confirmed ulcer disease that are not responsive to other anti-ulcer medications. Capsules should be given via nasogastric tube because saliva will inactivate the drug.
2. Mucosal protectants.
   - Sucralfate. It has been suggested that sucralfate should be given 1 hour before H2 blockers because it is most effective in an acid environment, however there is a lag period between administration of H2 blockers and actual decrease in acid production. Therefore, administration of the drugs at the same time should still be effective.

Prognosis

The prognosis is good with treatment and reduction of stress, unless complications develop.

Sequelae

- Perforation of bowel – occasionally gastric or duodenal ulcers may perforate, resulting in severe peritonitis.
- Oesophageal stricture – secondary to chronic reflux oesophagitis.
- Duodenal stricture – results in delayed gastric emptying. Surgery to bypass the stricture may be indicated in severe cases.

Meconium impaction/retention

Meconium consists of the intestinal secretions, cellular debris, and digested amniotic fluid that accumulate in the intestinal tract during gestation. Normally it is completely passed during the first 24 to 48 hours of life.

Clinical signs

- Straining to defecate – usually stand with the back arched upwards, whereas foals straining to urinate will stand more stretched out.
- Tail swishing, restlessness.
- Abdominal pain. With time, abdominal distension develops.

Diagnosis

- In mild cases, diagnosis is often based on the clinical signs and response to treatment.
- Digital rectal examination may reveal firm meconium in the rectum, and rule out congenital abnormalities such as atresia.

Treatment

1. Enemas. Care must be taken not to irritate or damage the rectal mucosa. Overdistension of the rectum can result in rectal tears.
   - Warm water and saline.
   - Soapy water.
   - Commercial phosphate enemas.
2. Oral laxatives.
   - Mineral oil/castor oil via nasogasric tube.
3. IV fluids if the foal is dehydrated.
4. Surgical therapy may be required in cases with severe abdominal distension or bowel compromise.
   - Sterile saline may be infused into the bowel proximal to the impaction and then the impaction is gently massaged.
   - Enterotomy may be necessary if unable to break down the impaction or if the intestinal wall appears compromised.

Abdominal abscesses

Aetiology

Infectious agents include *Streptococcus equi*, *S. zooepidemicus* and *Rhodococcus equi*.

Clinical signs

- Depression, fever, anorexia.
- Colic – due to compressive effects on the intestines or adhesion formation.
- Peritonitis – due to inflammation or rupture of abscess.

Diagnosis

- Haematology may show neutrophilia with left shift. *R. equi* seems to frequently cause a profound neutrophilia.

• Ultrasound or radiology may be helpful in locating an abscess.

Treatment

• Medical treatment with long-term antibiotics is often unrewarding.
• If there is bowel involvement or if medical therapy is unsuccessful, surgery may be indicated to attempt resection of the abscess. Resection is ideal, but may not be possible. In these cases, debulking and establishing drainage is performed by marsupialization or drain placement.

Obstructive/strangulating lesions

Similar to adult in causing signs of colic, tachycardia and abdominal distension.
See Chapter 2.

Intussusceptions

These usually involve the small intestine – jejunojejunal or ileocaecal. Ultrasound may help diagnosis. Exploratory surgery with resection of affected area is indicated.

Hernias

These may be diaphragmatic, inguinal/scrotal, intra-abdominal (mesenteric rent) or umbilical. Inability to reduce an umbilical or scrotal hernia constitutes an emergency and surgical repair should be performed immediately to minimize bowel compromise.

Displacements and torsions

These are not common in foals, but large colon displacements and torsions can occur.

Functional obstructions – ileus

Ileus can result from electrolyte abnormalities (especially hypocalcaemia and hypokalaemia), intestinal irritation, enteritis and peritonitis. Ultrasound and radiography can be useful to determine the extent of abdominal distension. It is important to rule out mechanical obstruction as the cause of ileus. Treatment is aimed at removing the underlying cause and correcting any electrolyte imbalances. Surgery may be indicated if pain is persistent and abdominal distension is severe.

20.8 *Hepatobiliary diseases*

Examination

Physical examination and clinical signs

See Chapter 3.

Laboratory investigations

See Chapter 3.

Ultrasonography

Ultrasonography is a very useful non-invasive tool.

• The liver can be visualized on the right side of the ventral abdomen from the 6th to 15th intercostal spaces.
• Portal and hepatic vessels can normally be visualized in the parenchyma. Bile ducts are very small in normal liver and are often not seen.
• In cholestatic disease it may be possible to see distended bile ducts.
• In hepatocellular disease, inflammation or diffuse cellular infiltration results in increased echogenicity of the liver parenchyma.
• Focal hepatic diseases such as abscesses can also be diagnosed using ultrasound, appearing as masses with increased echogenicity.

Liver biopsy

See Chapter 3.

Infectious hepatobiliary diseases of the foal

Tyzzer's disease

This is an acute hepatitis in foals that is often fatal.

Aetiology

The infectious agent is *Bacillus piliformis* which is a Gram positive filamentous bacterium. Infection is thought to occur via ingestion of contaminated soil or faeces.

Clinical signs

• Usually occurs in foals 1 week to less than 2 months.

- Onset and progression of disease is very rapid over several hours to days.
- Signs commonly seen include depression, anorexia, recumbency, seizures, icterus, fever, coma, or sudden death.
- Laboratory data is suggestive of liver failure – increased liver enzymes, increased serum bilirubin, hypoglycaemia, and a neutropenia or neutrophilia.

Diagnosis

- Difficult to diagnose antemortem due to the rapid progression of the disease and the organism is difficult to culture.
- Liver biopsy may provide a diagnosis with identification of groups of parallel bacilli within hepatocytes.

Treatment

- Usually not successful.
- Intravenous antibiotics – the organism is susceptible to penicillins, oxytetracycline, streptomycin and erythromycin.
- Supportive treatment – IV fluids (with dextrose if hypoglycaemic).

Prognosis

The prognosis is very poor.

Equine herpesvirus 1

In utero infection during late gestation with EHV-1 most commonly causes abortion, but can cause interstitial pneumonia and necrotizing hepatitis in neonates. Clinical signs include weakness, depression, respiratory signs and icterus.

See Chapter 19.

Septicaemia

- Cholestasis can be associated with septicaemia or endotoxaemia. Endotoxin interferes with the normal function of bile excretion.
- Hepatitis can also develop secondary to septicaemia via haematogenous route or ascension of the bile ducts.

Liver abscesses

- Uncommon but can occur in the foal secondary to septicaemia or via ascending infection of the bile ducts.
- Clinical signs include weight loss, intermittent colic and fever.
- Ultrasonography can be very beneficial in diagnosis.

Toxic hepatobiliary disease

Iron fumarate toxicosis

Aetiology

- Administration of iron (via orally administered supplement) prior to colostrum intake. Foals are much more susceptible to iron toxicity than adults.

Clinical signs

- Usually occurs 2 to 5 days after administration of iron fumarate.
- Signs include depression, icterus, hyperexcitability, blindness, coma and death.

Diagnosis

- The liver is usually less than half the normal size.
- Histopathology shows severe necrosis, atrophy, periportal fibrosis and bile duct proliferation.

Treatment

Treatment is supportive.

Prognosis

The prognosis is poor if the foal is in liver failure.

Pyrrolizidine alkaloid toxicosis

This is very rare in foals. See Chapter 3.

Congenital hepatobiliary conditions

Portacaval shunts

These are very rare. Usually CNS signs develop at several months of age.

Biliary atresia

In this very rare condition there is lack of proper formation of the bile ducts.

Mechanical cholangiohepatitis

1. Aetiology: gastroduodenal ulcer disease can cause duodenal stricture which may occlude the common bile duct and cause cholestasis. If the stricture is distal to the opening of the common bile duct into the duodenum (hepatopancreatic ampulla), cholestasis occurs along with reflux of ingesta into the common bile duct.
2. With surgical correction of the stricture, the cholangiohepatitis should resolve unless permanent hepatic damage has occurred.

20.9 *Diseases of the urogenital system*

Examination

Physical examination

- The umbilicus should be carefully examined for any abnormalities such as urine leakage (indicating patent urachus), swelling or discharge (which may indicate umbilical infection).
- Abdominal ballotment can be useful in detecting free abdominal fluid. The bladder can often be palpated in small foals.
- The external genitalia should be examined for any abnormalities such as congenital malformations.

Serum biochemistry and electrolytes

See Chapter 8.

Urinalysis

See Chapter 8.

Radiography

1. Useful in cases of suspected ruptured bladder to look for the presence of free abdominal fluid.

2. Contrast studies can be helpful in determining the site of urinary tract disruption prior to surgery.
   - A water soluble contrast agent must be used.
   - The urinary bladder is catheterized (using aseptic techniques) and a suitable amount of contrast agent is injected to distend the bladder.
   - Lateral and ventrodorsal (if possible) radiographs are taken. Contrast material within the peritoneal cavity indicates a ruptured bladder or urachal defect. Occasionally urachal tears can occur outside the peritoneal cavity and contrast material can be seen in the subcutaneous tissue around the umbilicus.
3. Excretory urography such as an intravenous pyelogram may be useful in diagnosing ectopic ureters.
   - Caution should be used as the contrast material is potentially nephrotoxic especially if there is dehydration or impaired renal function.
   - Diatizoate salt contrast materials are the least nephrotoxic.

Ultrasonography

- Very useful in evaluating the umbilicus for infection or abscesses.
- Free abdominal fluid can be visualized, and abdominocentesis can be aided. Free abdominal fluid and lack of visualization of a fluid-filled bladder are supportive of bladder rupture. However, visualization of a fluid-filled bladder does not rule out the possibility of a rupture as some cases may involve small tears and the bladder is able to partially fill.
- The kidneys should also be evaluated especially if nephritis or congenital abnormalities are suspected.

Abdominocentesis

1. Should be performed in cases of excessive free peritoneal fluid.
2. Uroperitoneum:
   - Peritoneal fluid creatinine should be compared to serum creatinine to diagnose uroperitoneum. A ratio $> 2:1$ is highly suggestive of uroperitoneum although a normal ratio does not rule it out.
   - Increased WBC, increased total protein and/ or bacteria in cases of uroperitoneum may indicate peritonitis.

Congenital urogenital defects

Persistent cloaca

1. Congenital defect where the normal partition (urorectal septum) between the hindgut and the foetal bladder fails to form during foetal development. The result is the rectum communicates with the vagina in fillies and the urethra in colts.
2. This condition is often associated with atresia ani.
3. Diagnosis is based on clinical signs and examination. The foal will often pass some faeces with urine especially if atresia ani is also present.
4. Treatment consists of surgical closure of the defect. The prognosis in fillies is better because a rectovaginal defect is easier to repair than a recturethral defect.

Ectopic ureter

1. Uncommon congenital defect.
2. Primary clinical sign is persistent urinary incontinence which is present at birth. Foals will often develop urine scalds in the perineal region and down the backs of the legs.
3. Definitive diagnosis is by excretory urography.
4. Surgical correction is successful in some cases.

Cryptorchidism

See Chapter 8.

Patent urachus

See Chapter 8.

Omphalitis/umbilical remnant infections

Infection can occur in umbilical remnants or urachal remnants.

Clinical signs

- Swelling of the umbilicus, and occasionally purulent discharge can be expressed from the umbilicus. Lack of external swelling does not rule out umbilical remnant infection as infection/abscess can occur internally.
- Intermittent fever, leucocytosis, neutrophilia with a left shift, and increased plasma fibrinogen are non-specific signs of infection that can be seen with umbilical infections.

Diagnosis

- Can often be made on the basis of the clinical signs.
- Ultrasonography is very helpful to diagnose infections of the internal portions of the umbilical remnants and to determine the extent of infection. Any foal with signs of inflammation and infection that cannot be localized should have an ultrasound evaluation of the umbilicus.

Treatment

- Conservative therapy with long-term antibiotics is often unrewarding.
- Surgical removal of infected umbilical remnants is often the best treatment and will actually be less expensive in the long run, and provide a better chance of complete resolution of infection.

Ruptured bladder

See Chapter 8.

Primary renal disease

See also Chapter 8.

Aetiology

1. Sepsis-associated.
   - Most common cause of renal failure in foals.
   - Sepsis can cause renal failure via ischaemic damage and direct infection of the kidneys by the causative organism.
   - Common organisms involved include *Actinobacillus equuli*, *Escherichia coli* and *Klebsiella*.
2. Nephrotoxic renal failure.
   - Uncommon cause of renal failure but results from overdoses of potentially nephrotoxic drugs or administration of normal doses to a dehydrated patient.
   - Aminoglycosides can cause renal tubular damage. Gentamicin is reportedly more nephrotoxic than amikacin.
   - Non-steroidal anti-inflammatories (prostaglandin inhibition) possibly cause renal failure by inhibiting adequate blood flow resulting in ischaemic damage. They can also cause renal papillary necrosis.

3. Ischaemic renal failure. Renal failure can result from conditions causing hypovolaemia or hypoxaemia.

Clinical signs

- Depression, lethargy, anorexia, tachycardia, fever.
- Oliguria.

Diagnosis

It is important to differentiate renal failure from urinary tract disruption such as ruptured bladder or obstruction.

- Laboratory findings – azotaemia, hyponatraemia, hyperkalaemia and metabolic acidosis are commonly seen.
- Urinalysis – urine gamma glutamyl transferase:urine creatinine ratio may be elevated. Fractional excretions may be useful, but parameters are not as well established in foals. Urine cytology may reveal casts indicating renal tubular damage.

Treatment

The goals of therapy are to correct the underlying causes such as dehydration or sepsis, to correct electrolyte and metabolic imbalances, and to maintain urine output.

1. Fluid therapy. Care must be taken not to over-hydrate, especially in the oliguric patient.
   - Fluid overload can result in oedema, hypertension, CNS swelling and death.
   - Monitoring central venous pressure (CVP), urine output and PCV can be helpful. CVP may be the best indicator of fluid overloading.
   - Potassium-free fluid such as 0.9% saline is the best choice since hyperkalaemia is a common electrolyte abnormality.
2. Low dose dopamine infusion or diuretics may be used to try to improve urinary output in oliguric patients.
3. Diazepam may be indicated to control seizures.

20.10 *Endocrine/metabolic disorders*

Neonatal hypothyroidism (goitre)

See Chapter 9.

Hypoadrenocorticism

This is seen in premature or dysmature foals. The adrenocortical axis is not fully developed in premature foals.

1. Clinical signs: signs of prematurity (see beginning of chapter).
2. Diagnosis is based on clinical signs with supporting laboratory data.
   - Plasma cortisol <30 ng/ml (normal 120–140 ng/ml).
   - ACTH stimulation test: little or no response (normal: increase in plasma cortisol by 200%).
   - Often have neutropenia and lymphocytosis.
3. Treatment: steroid supplementation is controversial.

Nutritional secondary hyperparathyroidism

See Chapter 9.

20.11 *Haemolymphatic and immunological disorders*

Failure of passive transfer (FPT) of immunoglobulins

Passive transfer of maternal antibodies does not occur transplacentally in the horse. The mare's colostrum contains high concentrations of antibodies (primarily IgG). Colostrum usually contains up to five times the IgG concentration of plasma. The foal must ingest colostrum and be able to absorb the antibodies for passive transfer to occur. The foal's gastrointestinal tract is able to absorb proteins intact via specialized villus epithelial cells in the small intestine. Maximum absorption occurs within 8 hours following parturition and the specialized epithelial cells are replaced by more mature cells unable to pinocytose proteins within 24 to 36 hours.

Causes of FPT

1. Inadequate colostrum or inadequate concentration of IgG in colostrum.
   - Mares that prematurely lactate (>24 hours prior to parturition) tend to have lower IgG concentration in the colostrum.

- Premature parturition – mares foaling prior to 320 days may not have adequate colostral antibodies.
- Mares on fescue pasture during late gestation can have agalactia, thickened foetal membranes, retained placenta, and weak foals.

2. Failure of the foal to ingest and absorb colostrum within the first 12 hours. Any illness or abnormality which causes the foal to be weak can result in lack of nursing.

Clinical signs

- There are no signs specific for FPT, but these foals are predisposed to septicaemia and other infections.
- Neonatal maladjustment (dummy foals) – these foals generally do not have a suckle reflex and are unable to nurse.
- If a mare has a very distended udder, one should suspect that the foal has not nursed.

Diagnosis

1. Tests for measuring immunoglobulin levels in the foal should be performed at 24 hours of age (after antibody absorption is complete). Values < 400 mg/dl are considered diagnostic of FPT; 400 to 800 mg/dl is considered partial failure; > 800 mg/dl is considered normal.
   - Zinc sulphate turbidity test is the least expensive test available and results are available within 1 hour. However, this is not as sensitive as other tests and false positives can occur.
   - Immunoassays are commercially available. One of these is the CITE® test which registers a colour change when an enzyme combines with IgG. Results are obtained rapidly and are fairly reliable. However, this is an expensive test.
   - Radial immunodiffusion (RID) is the most accurate test available, but the results take 18 to 24 hours.
2. Measurement of IgG content of the colostrum.
   - The specific gravity of colostrum directly correlates with the IgG content. Colostrum with a specific gravity > 1.06 usually contains sufficient IgG.
   - The specific gravity can be measured with a colostrometer.

Treatment

The treatment is dependent on the reason for FPT and the age of the foal.

1. If the foal is < 18 to 24 hours old:
   - Frozen colostrum can be administered via bottle or nasogastric tube. At least 1 litre of colostrum should be administered within the first 12 hours of life, divided into several feedings. Frozen colostrum should not be microwaved.
   - Lyophilized IgG is an oral IgG supplement. Variable absorption has been reported so the IgG levels should be measured.
   - Plasma can be administered orally, but it is not considered to be as effective as intravenous administration.
2. If the foal is > 24 hours old or if colostrum is not available:
   - Plasma transfusion.
   - Approximately 20 to 40 ml/kg plasma is necessary to raise IgG levels to > 400 mg/dl. If the foal is already sick, additional amounts will be necessary.
   - Ideally the plasma should be cross-matched if commercial cell-free plasma from anti-RBC negative donors is not being used.
   - Serum IgG levels should be tested at least 1 to 3 hours following administration and additional plasma should be administered if the IgG levels are still low.
   - Caution should be taken not to cause fluid overload, especially in sick or very small foals.

Prevention

- Mares should be removed from pastures that contain fescue grass or hay that contains fescue early in gestation.
- The colostrum should be checked on every mare. Stickiness is a better indicator of good quality than colour or thickness. It is best to measure the specific gravity.
- The foal should be watched to ensure that it stands and nurses within a reasonable time after birth.
- If there is any doubt, the foal's serum IgG levels should be measured.
- Large breeding farms should establish a colostrum bank; 200 to 400 ml of colostrum can be taken from a normal mare without jeopardizing her foal's IgG levels. Also mares that die or lose their foals should be milked out and the colostrum frozen.

Combined-immunodeficiency (CID)

See Chapter 10.

Neonatal isoerytholysis (isoimmune haemolytic anaemia)

This condition occurs when a mare develops antibodies against the foal's erythrocytes. This can occur if the foal inherits paternal RBC antigens that the mare does not have and if the mare has previously been exposed to these antigens (usually this exposure occurs during a previous pregnancy because foetal blood and maternal blood do not mix except for some leakage at parturition). After the foal nurses and absorbs colostral antibodies, severe haemolytic disease occurs.

Clinical signs

- Usually normal at birth. Signs develop from 8 hours to 4 days following parturition.
- Weakness, icterus, increased heart and respiratory rates.
- Seizures can occur if the anaemia is severe.

Diagnosis

- Haematology (complete blood count) shows very low RBC cell count; PCV is usually 10 to 20%; WBC may be increased (stress response); plasma is icteric.
- Haemoglobinuria.
- Minor cross-match (foal's RBC + mare's serum) – positive agglutination is supportive of a diagnosis of neonatal isoerythrolysis.

Treatment

1. If the foal is less than 24 hours old at the time of diagnosis, it should not be allowed to nurse the mare until 24 to 48 hours of age.
2. Blood transfusion:
   - A transfusion should be considered if the anaemia is severe (PCV <15%) or if the foal is weak and shocked.
   - Sources of blood for transfusion include the mare's blood (RBCs must be washed to remove any antibodies); other donors should be cross-matched with the foal's blood prior to transfusion. If unable to cross-match, a gelding donor is less likely to cause a reaction.
   - 20 to 30 ml/kg of packed red blood cells will usually raise the PCV to 15–20%.
   - Transfused red blood cells have a very short-half life (2 to 4 days), therefore the PCV needs to be closely monitored as further transfusions may be needed.
3. Plasma transfusions may be necessary if serum IgG levels are low.
4. Broad-spectrum antibiotics should be given to protect against opportunist infections.

Prevention

- Blood-typing of mares: alloantigens Aa and Qa are responsible for most cases; therefore mares without these alloantigens are more likely to be at risk.
- Testing during late gestation: the mare's serum can be tested against samples with known alloantigens. If there are any significant reactions, colostrum should be withheld from the foal and a supplemental colostrum (free of alloantibodies) should be given.
- Testing at the time of birth: the foal can be tested at the time of birth, and colostrum withheld until the test results are known.

20.12 *Miscellaneous conditions*

Steatitis (yellow fat disease)

Steatitis is a rare disease seen primarily in pony and donkey foals, usually between 1 and 6 months of age. The aetiology is uncertain, but might be associated with selenium and/or vitamin E deficiency.

Clinical signs include pyrexia, inappetence, depression, tachypnoea and weakness. Firm, indurated subcutaneous plaques are palpable over the body, and the ligamentum nuchae is thickened, hard and painful. Other signs that may be present include hyperlipaemia, ventral oedema and diarrhoea. There is no effective treatment.

Further reading

Koterba, A.M., Drummond, W.H. and Kosch, P.C. (1990) *Equine Clinical Neonatology*. Lea & Febiger, Philadelphia.

Mair, T.S., Freestone, J., Hillyer, M.H., Love, S. and Watson, E.D. (1995) The Endocrine system. In *The Equine Manual* (Eds. A.J. Higgins and I.M. Wright), Chapter 11. W.B. Saunders, London.

Rossdale, P.D. and Ricketts, S.W. (1980) *Equine Stud Farm Medicine*, 2nd Edition. Baillière Tindall, London.

Sojka, J.E. and Levy, M. (1995) Evaluation of endocrine function. *Veterinary Clinics of North America, Equine Practice. Clinical Pathology* **11** (3), 415–436.

Vaala, W.E. (1994) Perinatology. *Veterinary Clinics of North America. Equine Practice* **10** (1).

21 *Muscle disorders and performance problems*

CONTENTS

21.1 *Examination of the muscular system*

Physical examination

• The horse should be evaluated initially from a distance. Symmetry, size and shape of the muscle groups should be assessed.
• The various muscle groups and pairs of muscles are palpated to give an impression of tone, sensitivity, asymmetry or atrophy. The horse should be given time to relax so that apprehension to palpation does not elicit a false impression.

• The horse is walked and examined for evidence of lameness, weakness or pain associated with movement. The differentiation of weakness caused by muscular or nervous disease can be difficult.

Clinical pathology

Three enzymes are routinely measured in the evaluation of muscular disease:

• Creatinine phosphokinase (CPK).
• Lactate dehydrogenase (LDH).
• Aspartate aminotransferase (AST).

1. Creatinine phosphokinase:
   - CPK is found predominantly in skeletal and cardiac muscle and in the brain.
   - When the muscle cell wall is disrupted, CPK is released from the cytoplasm and enters the extracellular fluid.
   - Elevated serum CPK is usually caused by myopathy rather than neuropathy, since CPK activity in nervous tissue is not sufficient to elevate serum levels.
   - Elevated serum levels of CPK can be a sensitive indicator of muscle damage. Serum levels increase within hours of an insult to muscle.
   - Training, transport and strenuous exercise can cause a mild elevation in serum CPK, whereas diseases such as exertional rhabdomyolysis or nutritional muscular dystrophy may cause CPK levels of thousands to hundreds of thousands of IU/l.
2. Lactate dehydrogenase:
   - Serum LDH activity is tissue non-specific, although muscle, liver and erythrocytes may be the major source of high activity.
   - Elevations of serum LDH can be seen in horses with exertional rhabdomyolysis and other causes of myodegeneration, myocardial necrosis and in association with liver disease.
   - To differentiate the source of LDH, it is helpful to separate it into its isoenzyme forms by electrophoresis.
3. Aspartate aminotransferase:
   - Serum AST (SGOT) has high activity in skeletal muscle, liver, red blood cells and other tissues.
   - AST is used to detect general cellular damage, and is not muscle specific.
4. Interpretation of enzyme levels:
   - Levels of CPK peak in 6 to 12 hours and AST levels peak in 12 to 24 hours.
   - The half-life of CPK is 1 to 2 days, and for AST it is 7 days.
   - Therefore, elevated CPK levels indicate active muscle damage. If CPK decreases or is normal and AST is high this indicates that myonecrosis is not continuing. If the injury is not progressive, CPK will return to normal in 24 to 48 hours.
   - Collection and storage of blood samples are important. Ideally, samples should be transported to the laboratory immediately. Separation of the serum or plasma should be done as soon as possible since RBC lysis can lead to release of AST and LDH.

Muscle biopsy

Percutaneous muscle biopsy allows examination of myofibres, neuromuscular junctions, nerve branches, connective tissue and blood vessels. Biopsies should be obtained from both normal and abnormal muscle tissue. Standardized sites from the gluteus medius and semitendinosus muscles are most common. Samples for biochemical analysis are frozen in liquid nitrogen. Samples for histological analysis are frozen in freon or isopentane suspended in liquid nitrogen.

Electromyography

Electromyography and nerve conduction velocities are used most commonly to investigate neuromuscular diseases rather than primary muscle disorders.

21.2 *Congenital/familial disease*

Myotonia

Myotonia is a skeletal muscle disorder primarily affecting the Quarter horse, characterized by a period of involuntary contraction of muscles following stimulation or voluntary motion.

Aetiology/pathogenesis

- The mode of inheritance is unknown.
- The pathophysiology is thought to involve abnormalities in sarcolemmal chloride conductance.

Clinical signs

- Primarily affects young horses less than 1 year of age.
- Primarily affects the extensor muscles of the pelvic limbs resulting in a stiff gait.
- Bilateral focal enlargement of the proximal caudal thigh and rump muscles gives the impression that the horse is overdeveloped or is 'double muscled'.
- Percussion of affected muscles induces a prolonged contraction resulting in raised lumps or 'dimpling' which lasts for a minute or more with eventual slow relaxation.

- Clinical signs usually do not progress beyond 6 to 12 months of age, but can involve multiple organ systems.

Diagnosis

- Tentatively based on clinical signs, age and breed.
- Definitive diagnosis is based on an EMG examination. The high frequency crescendo–decrescendo repetitive electrical bursts produce a characteristic 'dive bomber' sound.

Treatment

- Treatment cannot be recommended since the pathophysiology is unknown.
- Phenytoin, quinine and procainamide can provide symptomatic relief in humans but have been unsuccessful in horses.

Prognosis

- Variable, depending on the severity of the clinical signs.
- Euthanasia may be indicated in cases that progress to fibrosis and pseudohypertrophy.

Hyperkalaemic periodic paralysis (HYPP)

A familial disorder which affects pure and crossbred Quarter horses. Affected horses experience intermittent episodes of muscle tremors and weakness which may result in collapse.

Aetiology and pathogenesis

- HYPP is inherited as an autosomal dominant trait.
- The gene responsible has been identified in descendants of the stallion Impressive.
- The pathogenesis involves an altered permeability of muscle membranes to sodium and potassium by affecting the sodium ion channel. An uncontrollable influx of sodium causes depolarization of muscle fibres resulting in uncontrollable muscle twitching and weakness.

Clinical signs

- Recurrent episodes of muscle weakness, tremors and collapse.

- Usually less than 4 years of age. HYPP has been recorded as young as 2 months and as old as 15 years.
- Males are overrepresented.
- Signs often begin with stiffness, sweating and muscle fasciculations.
- Some horses 'dog-sit'; some become recumbent.
- Occasionally episodes are accompanied by respiratory noises due to paralysis of the larynx and pharynx.
- Horses remain bright and alert and respond to noise and painful stimuli.
- During episodes of clinical disease there is an increase in PCV/total protein and hyperkalaemia (serum potassium 5.0 to 12.3 mEq/l).
- Clinically normal between and after episodes cease.

Diagnosis

- DNA blood test available at the University of California – Davis is the most reliable and effective way of identifying carriers of the HYPP gene.
- HYPP can be tentatively diagnosed on the basis of the clinical signs and signalment.
- Potassium chloride challenge test – involves administering 90–150 mg/kg of potassium chloride dissolved in water and given via nasogastric tube following an overnight fast. A positive result is characterized by signs of HYPP in 2–4 hours. Known affected horses do not always test positive at the lower doses.

Note: It is recommended to start with the low dose and increase by 25% daily. Horses receiving the test should not be left alone because it can cause life-threatening hyperkalaemia. Once a horse demonstrates signs of HYPP, treatment should begin.

Treatment

Prior to treatment, blood samples are obtained for potassium levels and muscle enzymes.

Mild attacks (trembling but no recumbency):
- Exercise the horse by walking or lunging. This stimulates adrenaline, which aids in the replacement of intracellular potassium.
- Feed grain because the carbohydrates will supply glucose which will stimulate insulin release which promotes potassium uptake by cells.

- Acetazolamide orally. This carbonic anhydrase inhibitor will increase potassium excretion by the kidneys.

Severe attacks (horse is recumbent and unable to rise):
- Insert an intravenous catheter.
- Calcium gluconate 23%: 150 ml added to 1 to 2 litres of 5% glucose per 500 kg body weight. The majority of affected horses will stand immediately following this treatment.
- If there is no response to calcium gluconate, administer 1 litre of 5% sodium bicarbonate IV (1 mEq/l).
- If there is no response, give 3 litres of 5% dextrose IV and monitor the potassium levels.
- Once diagnosed, most cases can be managed with dietary and exercise modifications. Decrease or eliminate alfalfa to decrease potassium levels and replace with oat or grass hay or pasture turnout.
- Pasture or paddock exercise is preferred to stall rest.
- If conservative treatment is ineffective, oral acetazolamide can be administered two to three times a day.
- Affected horses should not be bred.

21.3 *Myopathy with physical causes*

Postanaesthetic myoneuropathy

Pathophysiology

- Affected horses are usually large and well-muscled, and have been exposed to prolonged or deep anaesthesia on a hard surface.
- Muscle compression and prolonged immobility result in muscle ischaemia and hypoperfusion.
- A history of gaseous anaesthesia, mechanical ventilation and mean arterial pressures of less than 65 mmHg for an extended period of time.
- A localized form ('compartmental syndrome') is associated with damage within osteofascial compartments.
- The generalized form is thought to be due to the combination of the compartmental syndrome, muscle sensitivity to anaesthesia, stress, lowered blood pressure and use of muscle relaxants.

Clinical signs

This disorder primarily affects the triceps, quadriceps, hindlimb extensors, longissimus muscles, masseter and gluteal muscles.

1. Localized form:
   - Lateral recumbency affects the triceps, deltoid and hindlimb extensors.
   - Dorsal recumbency affects the longissimus and gluteals.
   - Affected muscles can be flaccid or hard, hot and painful on deep palpation and are swollen.
   - The horse is weak and unable to support its weight on the affected limb. It may have a dropped elbow appearance or knuckling of both hind fetlocks.
   - Signs may first appear 30 to 60 minutes after standing.
   - There is usually recovery within 24 hours if only a single muscle group is involved.
2. Generalized form:
   - The front limbs, pectorals and/or hindlimbs can be affected.
   - Generalized weakness or paresis.
   - Restlessness, anxiety, sweating or colic.

Diagnosis

1. History and clinical signs.
2. Elevated levels of CPK, AST and LDH.
3. Sometimes there is myoglobinuria.

Treatment

1. Mild cases:
   - Phenylbutazone or flunixin meglumine
   - Dimethyl sulphoxide (DMSO) IV or topically to affected muscles.
2. Severe generalized acute rhabdomyolysis:
   - Goals are to prevent further muscle damage, acute renal failure secondary to myoglobinuria, provide analgesia and relieve stress.
   - NSAIDs.
   - Xylazine, detomidine or romifidine.
   - Butorphanol.
   - Meperidine.
   - Acepromazine.
   - Fluid therapy with balanced electrolyte solution is indicated to prevent acute renal failure and to maintain normal electrolyte and acid/base balance.
   - Mannitol may be indicated in the severely affected horse.
   - Glucocorticoids may be indicated in the acute phase to reduce inflammation and

muscle damage by stabilizing cell membranes and preventing lipid peroxidation of cellular membranes.

Prevention

● Proper padding and positioning under general anaesthesia; pull lower forelimb forward and separate hindlimbs.
● Anaesthesia should be maintained on the lightest plane possible and mean arterial pressures maintained greater than 70 mmHg.
● Dantrolene sodium orally 1 to 2 mg/kg 1 to 2 hours prior to surgery may aid reduction of myopathy.

Exertional rhabdomyolysis

Other terms for this disorder are azoturia, 'Monday morning disease', 'tying up', paralytic myoglobinuria and myositis.

Aetiology

● Numerous predisposing factors which act alone or in combination.
● The classical description is the draught horse in work that is rested for the weekend and maintained on full feed. Then when the horse returns to work, it suffers an attack of the disease.
● A rapid or sudden increase in work intensity or duration.
● Highly strung mares and fillies are affected more than colts.
● Tends to be an increased incidence in certain breed lines and families of horses.
● Hypothyroidism may play a role.
● Respiratory tract viral infections predispose to myopathy in some horses.

Pathogenesis

● Not known; originally thought to be a result of increased lactate production in the muscle.
● Metabolic alkalosis is common.
● Disruption of the blood supply to the affected muscles is thought to lead to local hypoxia in fast twitch fibres. These fibres are more susceptible to ischaemia because they are larger than the slow twitch fibres, and have fewer associated capillaries.
● Fast twitch fibre pathology is evident by light microscopy.

● Diet, environment and exercise can alter fluid and electrolyte balance which can alter blood flow causing the disease.
● Vitamin E and selenium deficiencies are inconsistently implicated.

Clinical signs

● Signs vary, depending on the extent of muscle degeneration.
● Commonly see a stiff or stilted gait and reluctance to move.
● Pain may be elicited by deep palpation of the back and hindlimb musculature.
● Tachycardia, tachypnoea and pyrexia are sometimes seen.

Diagnosis

● Clinical signs.
● Increased serum levels of CPK, AST and LDH.
● Pigmenturia/myoglobinuria.
● Fluid and electrolyte imbalances: dehydration, hypochloraemia, hypocalcaemia.

Treatment

● Goals are to limit further muscle damage, to maintain fluid and electrolyte balance and to prevent acute renal failure.
● Further exercise or movement is contraindicated in most cases.

1. Mild cases:
   ● Phenylbutazone or flunixin meglumine.
   ● Meclofenamic acid.
   ● Acepromazine to increase peripheral blood flow.
   ● Rest for 3 to 5 days.
   ● Vitamin E and selenium orally or IM.
2. Severe cases:
   ● Intravenous fluids to prevent renal failure.
   ● Corticosteroids (dexamethasone).
   ● Phenylbutazone or flunixin meglumine.
   ● Xylazine if very painful.
   ● Rest for 6 to 8 weeks before returning to training.
3. Chronic intermittent cases:
   ● Dantrolene – questionable efficacy.
   ● Phenytoin. Must be withdrawn 7 days prior to racing. Side effects may include drowsiness, ataxia and rarely seizures.
   ● Assessment of electrolyte metabolism and appropriate dietary supplementation.

Fibrotic and ossifying myopathy

See Chapter 17.

21.4 *Myopathy of infectious origin*

Clostridial myonecrosis

Aetiology and pathophysiology

- Most clostridial infections are a result of intramuscular injections affecting the cervical, pectoral and caudal hindlimb muscles.
- Local muscle necrosis, trauma or concurrent infection provide low oxygen tension which is optimal for growth of clostridial organisms.
- Introduction of spores or organisms is usually by hypodermic needles.
- Clinical signs are seen when the spores become vegetative exotoxin-producing organisms.
- *Clostridium chauvoei*, *septicum* and *perfringens* type A are most commonly isolated.

Clinical signs

- Muscle swelling, lameness, stiff gait or reluctance to lift the head, and head oedema, depending on the muscles affected.
- Affected muscles are warm to the touch with gas accumulation (crepitus).
- Laryngeal hemiplegia due to recurrent laryngeal nerve damage.
- Pyrexia, tachycardia, tachypnoea and decreased capillary perfusion.

Diagnosis

- History of intramuscular injection within the last 24 to 48 hours.
- Culture, cytology and Gram stain.

Treatment

- Antibiotics: potassium penicillin; procaine penicillin; chloramphenicol; metronidazole.
- Surgery involves fasciotomy and debridement of the affected area.
- Basic supportive care; intravenous fluids, analgesics, wound management.

Prognosis

- *Clostridium chauvoei*, *septicum* – poor prognosis; patients often die.
- *Clostridium perfringens* – highest survival rate.

Corynebacterium pseudotuberculosis abscesses

See also Chapter 13.

These abscesses are also referred to as pigeon-breast, Colorado strangles and dry land distemper.

Aetiology

- The bacteria responsible for this disease is *Corynebacterium pseudotuberculosis*. It also causes ulcerative lymphangitis and contagious acne.
- Seen in the late summer and fall in western USA.
- There is a possible association with cutaneous habronemiasis and onchocerciasis.

Clinical signs

- Large abscesses of the pectoral muscles and less frequently of the axilla, ventral abdomen and limbs.
- Abscesses are thick walled and progressively increase in size.
- There may be ventral oedema.

Diagnosis

- Clinical signs and culture.

Treatment

- May spontaneously rupture or can be surgically incised and flushed daily.
- Antibiotics – penicillin.
- Applications of vaseline to the skin to prevent serum burn.

21.5 *Myopathy of metabolic origin*

Hypocalcaemic tetany

See Chapter 11.

Synchronous diaphragmatic flutter

This condition is referred to as 'thumps'. It is seen in association with fluid and electrolyte abnormalities, caused by endurance riding, exercise, transport and digestive disorders.

Aetiology and pathogenesis

- Diets high in calcium may predispose horses to synchronous diaphragmatic flutter.
- Several conditions may incite the condition: extensive exercise, transit or lactation tetany, trauma, digestive disorders and frusemide treatment.
- Metabolic acidosis with hypochloraemia, hypokalaemia and hypomagnesaemia.
- Fluid and electrolyte abnormalities may disrupt normal membrane potentials of the phrenic nerve. This allows the phrenic nerve to discharge in response to atrial depolarization.

Clinical signs

- Major clinical signs are the result of the synchronous contraction of the diaphragm with the heartbeat.
- Unilateral or bilateral twitch of the flank. This twitch can result in the characteristic 'thumping' noise.

Treatment

- Usually a transient disorder which resolves when acid–base and electrolyte abnormalities are corrected.
- Respond quickly to intravenous calcium solutions.
- See treatment for hypocalcaemia (Chapter 11).

Malignant hyperthermia

Malignant hyperthermia is a generalized condition in which there is progressive hyperthermia, hypercapnia and muscle rigidity associated with certain anaesthetic agents or muscle relaxants.

Aetiology

- Agents implicated are inhalation anaesthetics (halothane), suxamethonium (succinylcholine) and local anaesthetics with an amide structure.
- Tends to be a genetic predisposition.

- Associated anaesthetic factors are difficult induction, increased $PaCO_2$ levels, anaesthesia time greater than 2 hours and metabolic acidosis.

Pathogenesis

- It is suggested that there is a defect in the sarcoplasmic reticulum which allows high levels of calcium to remain in the sarcoplasm.
- This defect results in continuous muscle contraction with heat production due to the energy needed to sustain the contractions.

Clinical signs

- Muscle stiffness, fasciculations.
- Progressive rise in body temperature (42.2°C, 108°F).
- Tachycardia, sweating and variable breathing patterns.
- Severe cases may develop metabolic and respiratory acidosis.

Diagnosis

- Based on clinical signs, especially if receiving inhalational anaesthesia.

Treatment

- Discontinue anaesthesia as soon as possible.
- Decrease body temperature with the use of alcohol baths, ice baths or cool IV fluids.
- Support cardiac and respiratory function as needed.
- Dantrolene sodium 2 to 3.5 mg/kg IV can help alleviate signs.

21.6 *Myopathy of nutritional origin*

Nutritional myodegeneration

Termed white muscle disease or nutritional muscular dystrophy. A myodegenerative disease that can affect cardiac and skeletal muscle of foals, and occasionally adults.

Pathogenesis

- Highly reactive oxygen free radicals are byproducts of normal cellular metabolism.

• Oxygen free radicals can react with unsaturated fatty acids and form toxic lipid peroxidases which can disrupt cell membranes and proteins which lead to a loss of cell integrity.
• Vitamin E is an antioxidant which scavenges free radicals preventing cell disruption.
• Selenium is a component of glutathione peroxidase which converts hydrogen peroxide and lipoperoxidases into water and less harmful alcohols.
• Vitamin E and selenium deficiency allows these toxic events to occur leading to myodegeneration.

Clinical signs

1. Acute myocardial degeneration:
   • Foals display difficulty rising, tachycardia, tachypnoea, dyspnoea.
   • Death usually occurs within 24 hours despite therapy.
   • Lesions are found in the heart, diaphragm and intercostal muscles.
2. Skeletal form:
   • Foals display muscle stiffness and weakness.
   • Tachycardia, tachypnoea, dyspnoea and failure to suckle.
   • Affected muscles may be swollen and painful on palpation.
   • Adults show signs of diffuse muscular involvement, stiff gait and weakness.
   • Depression, difficulty eating, head and neck swelling and myoglobinuria.

Diagnosis

• Cases usually occur in selenium deficient areas.
• Clinical signs.
• Laboratory findings:
  – increases in CPK, AST and LDH,
  – hypochloraemia,
  – hyperkalaemia,
  – hyponatraemia,
  – myoglobinuria.
• Necropsy
  – bilateral symmetrical myodegeneration,
  – affected muscles have pale streaks.
• Vitamin E and selenium levels.

Treatment

• Cardiac form: Supportive treatment, but condition is usually fatal.
• Skeletal form: Vitamin E/selenium supplementation. Selenium administered parenterally, vitamin E administered orally. Injectable combi-

nations do not provide adequate levels of vitamin E, as vitamin E is poorly absorbed from IM sites.

21.7 *Ionophore antibiotic toxicity*

These antibiotics include monensin, lasalocid and salinomycin. They are often used in the control of coccidiosis in poultry and ruminants, and as growth promoters in ruminants.

Pathophysiology

These antibiotics complex with various cations and are transported across cellular membranes. This disrupts normal ionic gradients resulting in cellular dysfunction.

Clinical signs

Horses can suffer from an acute clinical disease or a delayed toxicity with cardiovascular effects.

1. Acute toxicity:
   • Anorexia, colic, hypovolaemic shock, ataxia, weakness, cardiovascular dysfunction.
   • Death can follow in 24 to 48 hours.
2. Chronic toxicity:
   • Exercise intolerance and cardiovascular dysfunction, usually atrial fibrillation.
   • Signs may not be seen for weeks or months.
   • Azotaemia, haematuria, haemoglobinuria, myoglobinuria.
   • Increases in CPK, AST and LDH.
   • Increased hepatic enzymes and total serum bilirubin.

Diagnosis

• Clinical signs.
• History of exposure.
• Rule out other conditions.

Treatment

• Basic supportive therapy.
• Mineral oil or activated charcoal via stomach tube to decrease intestinal absorption.
• Fluid therapy.
• Vitamin E and selenium may be beneficial.

21.8 *Atypical myoglobinuria*

Myopathy that resembles exertional rhabdomyolysis clinically and pathologically, but that occurs in unworked or minimally worked horses. The disease has been recognized sporadically in the UK. Atypical myoglobinuria often occurs as an outbreak on the same property, and primarily affects young horses kept outdoors. Adverse climatic conditions appear to predispose to the onset of disease. The clinical course is short and often severe. Many affected horses become recumbent, and there is a high mortality rate. The clinical features, diagnostic features and treatment are similar to exertional rhabdomyolysis.

21.9 *Performance problems*

Poor performance can be defined as a suboptimal level of performance or the inability of a horse to perform at a previous level of exercise. Special attention must be given to the systems responsible for performance: the respiratory, cardiovascular, musculoskeletal and haematopoietic systems.

Diagnostic evaluation

History

An accurate history should include age, sex, breed, intended use and training programme. Performance history should include details of the previous level of exercise, the onset of problems (training, competition, racing), whether poor performance is consistent or intermittent, any associated respiratory noise or lameness. Most horses either perform badly throughout exercise or develop exercise intolerance and finish poorly.

Clinical examination

A thorough physical examination is indicated with special attention to the respiratory, cardiovascular and musculoskeletal systems. Auscultation of the heart to detect murmurs and arrhythmias. The lung fields should be auscultated with and without a rebreathing bag. The chest is percussed. The horse should be evaluated for any subtle lameness.

Diagnostic tests

- Haematology, plasma biochemistry.
- Electrocardiography.
- Endoscopy.
- Transtracheal wash/bronchoalveolar lavage.
- Muscle biopsy.
- Exercise testing.
- Radiology.

21.10 *Causes of poor performance/ exercise intolerance*

See Table 1.

21.11 *Thermoregulatory problems*

Pathophysiology

Working muscle requires a tremendous increase in metabolic rate. Since only a portion is utilized, the rest accumulates as heat which is removed by the vascular system. The vascular system removes the heat from the core to the skin where heat exchange can occur. Heat dissipation occurs via four mechanisms: radiation, convection, conduction and evaporation. The first three require a favourable heat gradient between the horse and the environment to be effective. Evaporation is the most important mechanism for the exercising horse to dissipate heat. A racehorse can lose 10 to 15 litres of sweat in a race and an endurance horse may lose 10 to 15 litres per hour. Heat associated illnesses are usually seen in horses exercising in a hot, humid environment where there is a competing demand for heat dissipation.

Heat stroke

Aetiology

Heat stroke usually occurs in horses that are transported in poorly ventilated trailers or horses that are overworked during hot, humid weather. The major contributing factor to heat stroke is dehydration due to sweat loss which compromises the horse's ability to lose heat. Other contributing factors are long hair coat, obesity, heavy

Table 1 Causes of poor performance

Respiratory causes

Obstructive upper airway diseases
Laryngeal hemiplegia
Epiglottic entrapment
Arytenoid chondritis
Guttural pouch infections
Aryepiglottic fold entrapment
Tracheal stenosis, stricture, collapse
Arytenoid chondroma
Ethmoid haematoma
Nasal polyps
Pharyngeal and subepiglottic cysts
Rhinitis, nasal granuloma

Lower airway diseases
Exercise induced pulmonary haemorrhage
Chronic obstructive pulmonary disease (COPD)
Viral infections; EHV-1, rhinovirus, reovirus, adenovirus
Bacterial pneumonia
Pleuritis
Pulmonary abscessation
Interstitial pneumonia

Cardiovascular causes
Atrial fibrillation
Heart block
Ventricular premature beats
Congestive cardiac failure
Mitral insufficiency
Tricuspid insufficiency
Ruptured chordae tendinae
Pulmonic stenosis
Endocarditis
Myocarditis
Pericarditis
Cor pulmonale
Aortoileofemoral arteriosclerosis or thrombosis

Metabolic/systemic causes
Anaemia
Fluid and electrolyte abnormalities
Anhidrosis
Heat exhaustion
Generalized granulomatous disease
Thyroid adenoma/adenocarcinoma
Hyperparathyroidism
Liver disease
Myeloproliferative disease
Diarrhoea
Neoplasia

Musculoskeletal causes
Exertional rhabdomyolysis
Degenerative joint disease
Fracture
Osteochondrosis, bone cysts
Tendinitis, desmitis
Hoof imbalance
Back problems
Sacroiliac problems
Chronic sarcocystosis
Other causes of pain or lameness

General causes
Obesity
Unfit horse
Poorly trained horse
Genetically slow horse

Neurological causes
Equine protozoal myelitis
Equine cervical vertebral malformation

blanketing, extensive skin damage or anything that can affect sweat evaporation.

Clinical signs

- Tachycardia.
- Tachypnoea.
- Pyrexia ($>40°C$).
- Restlessness, depression, disorientation, collapse or death.
- Sweating may be profuse but usually less than expected.
- Skin hot to touch.

Treatment

1. Control body temperature:
   - Cold water or alcohol bath.
   - Provide good ventilation – fans.
2. Restore hydration:
   - Intravenous lactated Ringers solution.
   - 0.9% NaCl + 10–15 mEq KCl/l.
3. Antipyretics:
   - Dipyrone.
   - Phenylbutazone.
   - Flunixin meglumine.

Anhidrosis

See Chapter 9.

21.12 *Exhausted horse syndrome*

Equine fatigue or exhaustion is the inability of a horse to maintain a given level of exercise.

Aetiology and pathophysiology

Can involve brief maximal exercise (racing) or prolonged submaximal exercise (endurance).

- Involves a combination of impairment of excitation–contraction coupling, loss of energy production, depletion of energy substrates (glycogen) and fluid and electrolyte imbalances.
- Exercise leads to an increased metabolic rate and increased use of energy which results in increased generated heat. In this case sweating is the primary way of thermoregulation. This can cause fluid losses of 20 to 40 litres or more.
- Equine sweat is hypertonic and contains sodium, potassium, chloride and magnesium. These electrolytes tend to be slightly decreased in serum but serum levels do not necessarily reflect the total body losses.
- The energy consumed can deplete gycogen stores while blood glucose is usually within normal limits.
- The decrease in chloride, potassium and magnesium can alter membrane potentials and neuromuscular transmission, cause gastrointestinal stasis, cardiac arrhythmias, muscle spasms and cramps.
- Thirst is suppressed in the exhausted horse for two reasons. First the hypothalamus is only responsive to blood osmolarity which is hypotonic due to the hypertonic sweat being lost. Secondly intestinal motility is decreased in exhausted horses; this often leads to small intestinal distension causing pain and this decreases the desire to drink.

Clinical signs

- Pyrexia.
- Tachycardia, tachypnoea.
- Dehydration.
- Decreased or absent borborygmi.
- Concentrated or absent urine.
- Increased capillary refill time.
- Increased jugular filling.
- Muscle cramps/spasms.
- Cardiac abnormalities.
- Synchronous diaphragmatic flutter may be present.

Diagnosis

- History and clinical signs.
- Serum electrolytes: hypokalaemia, hypocalcaemia, hyponatraemia.
- Mixed respiratory and metabolic alkalosis, or purely metabolic alkalosis.
- Bicarbonate may be normal or increased.

Treatment

Goals are to restore circulating blood volume, correct electrolyte abnormalities, provide a metabolizable source of energy and to prevent acute renal failure. This can be accomplished with oral or intravenous fluids.

1. Intravenous fluids:
   - Polyionic solutions, e.g. lactated Ringer's solution.
   - 0.9% NaCl + 10–15 mEq KCl/l.
   - dextrose 5% or 50% can be added to lactated Ringer's solution to provide 50–100 g/h.
   - If needed, calcium solutions (calcium borogluconate) 100–300 ml of 20% solution can be given slowly.
2. Oral fluids:
   - Should be isotonic or hypotonic.
   - 5 to 8 litres at a time; can be repeated every 30–60 minutes.
   - Isotonic fluids: 1 tablespoon NaCl, 1 tablespoon Lite salt per gallon of water.
   - Hypertonic fluids should be avoided because they draw fluid in from the depleted intracellular fluid.
3. Analgesics if needed (xylazine or detomidine).
4. Non-steroidal anti-inflammatory drugs can be used but have the potential to produce toxicity in dehydrated animals.
5. Glucocorticoids are controversial due to the possibility of inducing laminitis.
6. Phenothiazine derived tranquillizers should not be used, because they may cause collapse and death.

Further reading

Arighi, M., Baird, J.D. and Hulland, T.J. (1984) Equine exertional rhabdomyolysis. *Compendium on Continuing Education for the Practicing Veterinarian* **6**, S726.

Brown, C.M., Kaneene, J.B. and Walker, R.D. (1988) Intramuscular injection techniques and the development of clostridial myositis or cellulitis in horses. *Journal of the American Veterinary Medical Association* **193**, 668.

Cox, J.H. and De Bowes, R.M. (1990) Episodic weakness caused by hyperkalemic periodic paralysis in horses. *Compendium on Continuing Education for the Practicing Veterinarian* **12**, 83.

Harris, P. (1989) Equine rhabdomyolysis syndrome. *Veterinary Record Supplement. In Practice* **11**, 3.

Hodgson, D.R. (1985) Myopathies in the athletic horse. *Compendium on Continuing Education for the Practicing Veterinarian* **10**, S551.

Hodgson, D.R. and Rose, R.J. (1994) *The Athletic Horse. Principles and Practice of Equine Sports Medicine.* W.B. Saunders, Philadelphia.

22 Metabolic diseases and toxicology

CONTENTS

22.23 *Heavy metals*

Lead
Selenium
Zinc
Arsenic
Other heavy metals

22.24 *Anthelmintics*

Carbon tetrachloride
Phenothiazine

22.25 *Petroleum products*

22.26 *Feed-associated poisonings*

Ionophores
Antibiotics
Blister beetle (cantharidin) poisoning
Aflatoxin

22.1 *Calcium metabolism*

Calcium is one of the most abundant minerals in the body. Ninety-nine per cent of calcium (Ca^{2+}) stores are in the bones and teeth; these serve as reserves.

Calcium is essential for neuromuscular activity, cell membrane permeability, muscle contraction, and blood clotting.

Calcium exists in three forms within the intravascular compartment: complexed, protein-bound and ionized.

Complexed calcium

Calcium complexes with phosphate, citrate and sulphate.

Protein-bound calcium

- Represents 40–50% of total calcium.
- Binds with albumin.
- Serum protein level (especially albumin level) should be considered when interpreting the results of blood calcium estimations.

Ionized calcium

- Ionized calcium is the biologically active form.
- This represents 40–60% of the total calcium stores.
- Alkalosis increases protein-binding of calcium, thereby reducing the concentration of ionized calcium.
- Acidosis decreases protein-binding thereby increasing the concentration of ionized calcium.

22.2 *Calcium homeostasis*

Parathyroid hormone (PTH)

See chapter 9.

- Produced by the parathyroid gland.
- Secretion is stimulated by hypocalcaemia.
- Causes an increase in the production of vitamin D [1,25-$(OH)_2$D].

Calcitonin

- Produced by C-cells of the thyroid gland.
- Secreted in response to hypercalcaemia.
- Inhibits renal resorption of calcium and resorption of calcium from the bone.

1,25-Dihydroxycholecalciferol

- Vitamin D [1,25-$(OH)_2$D].
- Stimulates absorption of calcium in the small intestine.
- Hypocalcaemia causes an increase in PTH and 1,25-dihydroxycholecalciferol which stimulates an increase in intestinal absorption of calcium and an increase in bone resorption.

22.3 *Hypercalcaemia*

Serum calcium is more than 3.5 mmol/l in hypercalcaemia.

Renal failure

See Chapter 8.

- Both acute and chronic renal failure may cause hypercalcaemia, but present in less than 50% of renal disease cases.
- Possibly due to a decrease in renal excretion of calcium due to a decrease in glomerular filtration rate, renal epithelial death, and decreased gastrointestinal absorption due to decreased 1,25-dihydroxycholecalciferol.
- Possibly due to a subnormal parathyroid hormone activity.

Plant toxicity

1. Wild jasmine (*Cestrum diurnum*):
   - Found in Texas and Florida.
   - Toxic all year round.
   - Clinical signs of toxicity are weight loss and progressive lameness.
   - Dystrophic calcinosis of the elastic tissues of the heart, arteries, tendons and ligaments.
   - Contains a steroidal glycoside that acts like vitamin D.
   - Causes an increase in intestinal absorption beyond that which can be physiologically accommodated.
2. Other plants that cause similar syndromes:
   - *Solanum malacoxylon* (South America).
   - *Solanum sodomauim* (Hawaii).
   - *Trisetum flavescens* (Germany).

Other causes of hypercalcaemia

1. Excessive or rapid administration of intravenous calcium.
2. Neoplasia (pseudohyperparathyroidism – see Chapter 9).

22.4 *Hypocalcaemia*

Lactation tetany/transport tetany/idiopathic hypocalcaemia

See Chapter 11.

Synchronous diaphragmatic flutter

See Chapter 21.

Blister beetle (cantharidin) toxicosis

Poisoning occurs by horses eating alfalfa contaminated by the blister beetles. The toxin (catharidin) is contained in the lymph of the beetles.

Hypocalcaemia is frequently seen with this condition. The pathophysiology is unknown. Clinical signs vary with the dose of toxin, and include anorexia, colic, depression, straining to urinate and diaphragmatic flutter. Therapy is symptomatic.

Other causes of hypocalcaemia

- Malignant hyperthermia (see Chapter 21).
- Pancreatic disease.
- Exertional rhabdomyolysis (see Chapter 21).
- Oxalate toxicity.
- Acute renal failure (see Chapter 8).
- Tetracycline therapy.
- Furosemide therapy.
- Excessive sodium bicarbonate administration.

22.5 *Phosphorus metabolism*

Phosphorus is stored in the bones and teeth, in close association with calcium. Intracellular phosphorus is utilized as adenosine triphosphate (ATP), the primary form of energy in the cell. Phosphorus in the extracellular fluid is an essential part of acid–base balance. Phosphorus is regulated by dietary factors, vitamin D, parathyroid hormone and calcitonin. Young horses have a higher serum concentration of phosphorus than adults.

22.6 *Hyperphosphataemia*

Secondary nutritional hyperparathyroidism

See Chapter 9.

22.7 *Hypophosphataemia*

1. Seen with chronic renal failure (see Chapter 8).
2. Seen with excessive ingestion of *Brassica* spp. (turnips, swedes, rape).

3. Also seen with chronic wasting states, starvation, and with deficient dietary sources.

22.8 *Sodium metabolism*

Sodium represents 90% of the positive ions of the extracellular fluid. Rapid, major changes in sodium concentrations can lead to neurological signs. The normal serum range is 130–140 mEq/l.

Plasma sodium levels provide information about the relative amounts of water and electrolytes in the extracellular fluid, and, by inference, on the state of intracellular hydration.

22.9 *Hypernatraemia*

Causes

- Dehydration.
- Aggressive administration of hypertonic fluids.

It may result in haemoglobinaemia and haemoglobinuria.

If hypernatraemia is longstanding, correction must be slow; rapid correction can lead to severe cerebral oedema.

22.10 *Hyponatraemia*

In hyponatraemia the serum concentration is less than 110 mEq/l.

It can occur with colic, renal disease, iatrogenic/idiopathic water overloading, aggressive enema administration and uroperitoneum in foals.

22.11 *Magnesium metabolism*

The normal serum concentration is 0.9–1.2 mmol/l. Approximately 80% of magnesium is diffusible, with 35% of serum magnesium bound to protein.

22.12 *Hypermagnesaemia*

This is rare. It may be associated with CNS depression and cardiac depression.

Causes

- Can occur as a result of overzealous oral administration of epsom salt as a cathartic.
- May also occur in renal disease, liver disease and after glucose ingestion.

22.13 *Hypomagnesaemia*

The serum magnesium is less than 0.6 mmol/l in hypomagnesaemia. It can cause central nervous system irritability (hyperresponsiveness), which can lead to nervousness, muscle tremors, ataxia and seizures.

Causes

- Grass tetany.
- Catharidin toxicosis.
- Endurance exercise.
- Renal disease with high urine output.

22.14 *Potassium metabolism*

The plasma concentration of potassium is largely dependent upon renal function, and will not necessarily reflect potassium state of the body cells. Normal serum potassium is 4.2 mmol/l.

22.15 *Hyperkalaemia*

Causes

- Frequently present with uroperitoneum.
- Transfer of potassium from intracellular to extracellular fluid:
  - haemolysis,
  - muscle damage with reduced renal excretion,
  - acidosis.
- Reduced renal excretion.

Hyperkalaemia causes peaking or 'tenting' of the T waves of an ECG.

Hyperkalaemic periodic paralysis

See Chapter 21.

22.16 *Hypokalaemia*

Hypokalaemia is caused by a decrease of oral intake, increased loss via gastrointestinal tract, or shifts between the intra- and extracellular compartments due to acid/base imbalance.

Specific causes

- Frequently seen in horses with gastrointestinal disturbances (colic, diarrhoea, equine monocytic erhlichiosis).
- Can be seen with renal tubular acidosis.
- Polyuria.
- Alkalosis.

22.17 *Free fatty acids metabolism*

See Chapter 9.

22.18 *Acid/base balance*

Protein metabolism results in the formation of hydrogen ions (H^+). This represents fixed acid. Carbohydrate and fat metabolism results in the formation of CO_2. This represents volatile acid.

The body maintains a homeostasis by buffering the acids produced via metabolism.

- A buffer can accept hydrogen ions to minimize change in pH.
- The bicarbonate–carbonic acid system is used to monitor acid/base in the horse.
- Bicarbonate is the primary buffer of the extracellular fluid.
- Proteins and phosphate are the primary buffers of the intracellular fluid.

Acid/base disturbances arise from either metabolic or respiratory imbalances. In decreasing order of frequency, acid/base disturbances include:

- Metabolic acidosis.
- Respiratory acidosis.
- Metabolic alkalosis.
- Respiratory alkalosis.

These disturbances are considered either primary or compensatory.

Collection of blood for blood gas analysis

A 2 to 5 ml syringe should be precoated with lithium heparin (1000 U/ml). All excess heparin should be removed from the syringe to avoid dilution of the sample. All air bubbles should be removed from the syringe, and the needle must be capped with a rubber stopper. If the sample is exposed to air, PCO_2 is decreased, pH is increased and PO_2 is increased.

Common sites for collection of arterial blood include carotid, facial, transverse facial, submandibular and greater metatarsal arteries. The greater metatarsal artery is used only in the anaesthetized horse to avoid self-injury.

Sites in the foal include greater metatarsal, brachial, radial, carotid, facial and femoral arteries.

The arterial pulse should be palpated, and the area disinfected. A 20-gauge needle (adults) or 25-gauge needle (foals) should be used for arterial puncture. After the artery has been punctured, the artery should be compressed for 5 minutes to avoid haematoma formation.

The sample should be analysed as soon as possible (within 30 minutes or less), otherwise the sample can be stored on ice for up to 2 hours until analysed.

Metabolic acidosis

Both pH and bicarbonate concentrations are reduced.

- Seen in normal horses in response to exercise (transient).
- Frequently seen in:
  - hypovolaemic shock,
  - surgical colic involving strangulated bowel (compartmentalization of fluid),
  - diarrhoea,
  - endotoxic shock.
- Sometimes seen in:
  - peritonitis,
  - ruptured bladder,
  - renal failure,
  - renal tubular acidosis.

The compensatory respiratory response is an increase in respiratory rate to lower PCO_2. This response starts immediately, and is at maximal effect within hours.

Treatment

- Diagnosis and treatment of the underlying disease that has caused the metabolic acidosis is frequently all that is needed to restore normal acid/base balance.
- In severe acidosis, therapy with $NaHCO_3$ is necessary. A general rule of thumb is to provide half of the base deficit rapidly, and the other half slowly over 24 hours. The dose of $NaHCO_3$ is calculated as:

$NaHCO_3$ needed =
    $0.4 \times$ body weight (kg) $\times$ base deficit

Respiratory acidosis

This is uncommon. It causes a decreased pH with an increase in PCO_2.

It may be seen in association with a severe decrease in ventilatory efficiency:

- Upper airway obstruction.
- Pneumonia.
- Pleuritis.
- CNS depression (CNS disease or drugs).
- Respiratory distress syndrome.

The metabolic compensatory response is renal retention of bicarbonate. This response starts immediately but does not reach maximal effect for several days.

This condition is a result of poor ventilation, not deficient bicarbonate, therefore *bicarbonate therapy is contraindicated.*

Treatment

- Rapid diagnosis and treatment of any underlying cause of alveolar hypoventilation.
- Any obstruction of ventilation (i.e. airway obstruction, pleural fluid, pneumothorax) must be removed.
- Oxygen therapy is indicated in acute respiratory distress. O_2 therapy can lead to a decrease in ventilation as hypoxaemia becomes the key driving force of ventilation in longstanding hypercapnia.

- Mechanical ventilation may be necessary. Arterial blood gases should be monitored to properly adjust ventilation rate and depth.

Metabolic alkalosis

Metabolic alkalosis causes an increase in both pH and bicarbonate concentration. Decreased circulating fluid volume, chloride or potassium depletion all lead to the impairment of renal bicarbonate excretion.

1. Occurs in conditions that cause excessive amounts of gastric reflux:
   - duodenitis–proximal jejunitis,
   - ileus,
   - gastrointestinal obstruction (most of these cases are in fact associated with a metabolic acidosis).
2. Also seen in endurance horses after massive sweating.
3. Can be seen with excessive bicarbonate administration.

Treatment

- Diagnosis and treatment of the underlying disease.
- Renal bicarbonate excretion is linked to H^+, and loss of H^+ leads to renal inability to excrete bicarbonate. Administration of fluids containing chloride and potassium will allow renal excretion of excess bicarbonate.

Respiratory alkalosis

- Rare. Caused by hyperventilation.
- Occasionally seen with hypoxaemia, fear, pain.
- Treatment is by removal of underlying cause.

22.19 *Toxicology*

Basic therapy of poisonings:

1. Prevent further exposure.
2. Establish a tentative diagnosis of the cause/poison involved.
3. Delay further absorption.
4. Administer specific antidotes/treatments.
5. Hasten elimination of absorbed poison.
6. Administer supportive therapy.

Emergency treatment:

1. Begin treatment promptly.
2. Retain samples for analysis – blood, urine, faeces.
3. Keep the horse warm and comfortable during therapy.

In cases of ingested poisons, gastric lavage may be attempted (either in the conscious horse or under general anaesthesia) to prevent further absorption of toxin. Alternatively, a laxative mineral oil may be administered to speed emptying of the gastro-intestinal tract. Activated charcoal should be administered by nasogastric tube (250–500 g in 2–4 litres water) to adsorb toxin in the digestive tract; this dose may be repeated in 12 hours.

In cases of skin exposure, the coat should be washed with a mild detergent and plenty of water.

22.20 *Toxic plants*

Plants containing pyrrolizidine alkaloids

A large number of plants contain pyrrolizidine alkaloids. Most of these plants are unpalatable, and horses will only eat them when other forage is scarce, or when the plant is baled in hay or pelleted, or when the plant has been killed by herbicides.

This group of plants include:

- Ragworts (*Senecio* spp.): *S. jacobaea* (stinking willie), *S. vulgaris* (common groundsel).
- Fiddleneck (*Amsinckia* spp.).
- Rattleweed (*Crotalaria* spp.).
- Hound's tongue (*Cynoglossum officinale*).
- Salivation Jane (*Echium lycopsis*).

Toxicity usually occurs from chronic ingestion of the plants over periods of weeks to months. The alkaloids damage the liver, and result in weight loss and inappetence, followed by specific signs of liver damage and hepatic encephalopathy.

See Chapter 3 (liver disease).

Castor bean (*Ricinus communis*)

Castor bean is grown in southern USA. The seeds contain a phytotoxin, ricin. The seeds may be eaten when mixed with other feedstuffs.

Acute toxicity is characterized by anaphylaxis and shock. Signs include incoordination, sweat-ing, muscle spasms, tachycardia, tachypnoea, diarrhoea and colic. Death occurs within 36 hours, and is preceded by convulsions.

Plants producing CNS dysfunction

1. Locoweed and Darling pea (*Astragalus* spp., *Oxytropus* spp., *Swainsona* spp.) – see Chapter 11.
2. Yellow star thistle (*Centaurea soltitialis*) and Russian knapweed (*C. repens*) – see Chapter 11.
3. Birdsville (*Indigophera enneaphylla*) – see Chapter 11.
4. Water hemlock, cowbane (*Cicuta* spp.). Signs occur 10 to 60 minutes after ingestion. Pupillary dilation, muscles fasciculations, laboured breathing, ataxia, convulsions and death.
5. Oleander (*Nerium oleander*). Found in southern USA. Horses only eat the plant when it is wilted. Toxicity causes depression, profuse diarrhoea, colic, heart arrhythmias and murmurs, sweating, muscle tics, coma and death.
6. White snakeroot (*Eupatorium rugosum*). Found in midwest USA. Signs of toxicity include reluctance to move, sluggishness, stiffness, ataxia. Death occurs after about 2 days.
7. Yew (*Taxus* spp.). Contains an alkaloid, taxine. Toxicity usually occurs when horses are given access to trimmings or debris after storms. The horse is extremely susceptible to yew toxicity, and one mouthful can be fatal. Death occurs rapidly (within 5 minutes) and there are rarely any other clinical signs.
8. Bracken fern (*Pteridium aquilinum*). Horses usually consume bracken in late summer, when other forage is scarce, or when it is used as bedding. The toxic agent is thiaminase, which results in myelin degeneration in peripheral nerves. The plant is usually consumed over a period of several months prior to the onset of clinical disease. Signs include weight loss, weakness, progressive incoordination and staggering, muscle tremors, cardiac arrhythmias, recumbency, clonic convulsions and opisthotonus. Death occurs within 2 to 10 days. Treatment with thiamine hydrochloride IV or IM is often successful if begun early in the clinical disease.
9. Horsetail, marestail (*Equisetum arvense*). The plant is usually consumed in hay. Toxicity and clinical signs are similar to bracken fern.
10. Hemlock (*Conium maculatum*). Horses usually

consume the plant in the spring when it is palatable. Toxicity is due to alkaloids, especially conine. Signs occur about 2 hours after ingesting the plant, and include posterior incoordination, trembling, recumbency and coma. Death occurs in severe cases.

11. Nightshades (*Solanum* spp.). Nightshades are not normally consumed by horses, unless it is present in hay. Clinical signs include depression, dyspnoea, muscle tremors, weakness, paralysis, colic and diarrhoea.

12. Caley pea (*Lathyrus hirsutis*). Toxicity usually occurs following ingestion of the plant in baled hay. The clinical disease is characterized by incoordination without paresis. Residual signs may be seen for years, and the horse may develop a stringhalt-like gait (see Chapter 11).

13. Ryegrass, Bermuda grass and Dallas grass – see Chapter 11.

Plants containing cyanogenic glycosides

A large number of plants contain glycosides that release hydrogen cyanide and hydrocyanic acid on hydrolysis in the gastrointestinal tract. These include hydrangeas (*Hydrangea* spp.), flax (*Linum* spp.), various cherries (*Prunus* spp.), and Sudan grass (*Sorghum* spp.). Cyanide blocks cytochrome oxidase, which prevents oxygen uptake by tissues. Clinical signs are due to tissue anoxia despite adequate blood oxygenation. Signs include dyspnoea, trembling, ataxia and recumbency. Death occurs from respiratory arrest.

Treatment includes IV administration of sodium nitrite and sodium thiosulphate. Sodium thiosulphate can also be given orally to fix free cyanide in the stomach.

Sorghum grass ataxia is described in Chapter 11.

Plants containing cardiac glycosides

Ingestion of milkweeds (*Asclepias* spp.), azaleas and rhododendrons (*Rhododendron* spp.) and foxglove (*Digitalis* spp.) may result in sudden death. Clinical signs may be observed, including anorexia, colic and diarrhoea.

Oak (*Quercus* spp.)

Acorn poisoning is occasionally encountered in the UK at the end of long, dry summers. Acorns and oak contain tannic acid and other tannins. Toxicity results in renal failure and gastrointestinal damage. Clinical signs include depression, anorexia, weakness, colic, constipation followed by diarrhoea, incoordination and dysphagia. Death from stomach rupture has been reported. There is no specific treatment.

Maple (*Acer* spp.)

Toxicity is most commonly caused by red maple (*Acer rubrum*). Horses usually ingest the plant in the form of wilted leaves. Clinical signs include anorexia, depression, methaemoglobinaemia and weakness. This is followed in 24 hours by haemolysis, anaemia, Heinz body formation, haemoglobinuria, icterus, cyanosis and respiratory distress. Severely affected horses become comatose after 4 to 5 days, and often die. Mildly affected horses usually recover after 7 to 14 days.

Treatment of methaemoglobinaemia with methylene blue is not highly effective but may be tried.

Black walnut (*Juglans nigra*)

Black walnut is used in the furniture industry. Poisoning occurs when horses are bedded on shavings containing a large proprtion of black walnut. Clinical signs are usually seen about 24 hours after exposure. Signs include depression, laminitis, reluctance to move and severe oedema of the legs.

Wild jasmine (*Cestrum diurnum*)

See p. 462.

Plants causing photosensitization

Photosensitization results from the interaction of light with photodynamic chemicals, resulting in cellular damage in the skin. Primary photosensitization occurs following the ingestion of plants containing photodynamic substances; these substances reach the skin following absorption from the alimentary tract. Secondary photosensitization occurs in association with liver damage. Liver dysfunction can result in the accumulation of phylloerythrin, a photodynamic breakdown product of chlorophyll.

Primary photosensitivity has been associated with the ingestion of St Johnswort (*Hypericum perforatum*), clovers (*Trifolium* spp.), vetches (*Vicia* spp.) and buckwheat (*Fagopyrum* spp.). Clinical signs are seen several days after ingestion. Erythema and oedema of the unpigmented areas of skin occurs, followed by blistering and sloughing of the skin. The affected areas are painful, and the horse may seek out shade. Horses will make a full recovery if kept out of the sun and removed from the source of the plant.

22.21 Insecticides

Chlorinated hydrocarbons

Toxicity is usually seen within an hour of exposure. Clinical signs include apprehension, hyperexcitability, muscle spasms, hyperaesthesia, and repeated tonic–clonic seizures. Seizures may last several hours, and the horse may die or recover slowly.

There is no specific therapy.

Organophosphorus and carbamate insecticides

See Chapter 11.

22.22 Rodenticides

Warfarin and other anticoagulants

Produce coagulation system defects by antagonizing vitamin K. Clinical signs include epistaxis, bloody diarrhoea, subcutaneous haematomas and lameness due to haemarthrosis. Occasionally, massive haemorrhage into the abdomen or thorax may result in sudden death.

Treatment involves replacing inhibited coagulation factors (blood transfusion) and administering vitamin K_1.

Strychnine

Strychnine antagonizes inhibitory spinal cord neurons, which results in convulsions and seizures. There is acute onset of seizures that may resemble tetanus. The seizures rapidly worsen ending in death in less than one hour. Rigor mortis occurs rapidly. There is no specific therapy.

ANTU (alpha-naphthylthiourea)

ANTU increases the permeability of lung capillaries causing pulmonary oedema. Death occurs within hours.

Arsenic

Arsenic poisoning can occur by exposure to a number of different pesticides, rodenticides, defoliants and drugs. The toxicity of arsenic varies with the formulation.

Arsenic is a heavy metal that produces digestive tract irritation within hours of ingestion. Signs include colic with excessive peristaltic activity, diarrhoea (which becomes bloody), dehydration, cardiovascular collapse and death.

Dimercaprol (BAL) is the specific antidote. Sodium thiosulphate may be used as an alternative.

22.23 Heavy metals

Lead

See Chapter 11.

Selenium

Poisoning occurs in areas with high selenium levels in soil, and may be acute, subacute or chronic. Acute toxicity causes depression, diarrhoea, laboured breathing, recumbency and death. Death may occur within several hours. Subacute toxicity results in liver and CNS dysfunction with signs of depression, blindness, weakness, paralysis and death. Chronic toxicity results in weight loss, hair loss from the mane and tail, and cracking at the coronary bands.

There is no specific therapy. Approximately 50% of chronic cases recover if they are removed from the source of selenium.

Zinc

Toxicity usually occurs from environmental contamination of pastures around lead and zinc mines, zinc smelters, etc. Toxicity is usually seen in foals and yearlings. Signs include enlargement of the epiphyses of long bones, lameness or stiff gait, weight loss and ill-thrift. There may be an association with the development of osteochondritis dissecans.

Arsenic

See p. 468.

Other heavy metals

- Cadmium – nephrotoxic.
- Copper – hepatotoxic and haemolysis.
- Mercury – gastrointestinal tract irritation, CNS and kidney damage.

22.24 *Anthelmintics*

Carbon tetrachloride

Carbon tetrachloride has a peculiar odour, and is rarely ingested by horses. Ingestion of large quantities causes liver damage (centrilobular necrosis and fatty infiltration) and kidney damage. Clinical signs include depression, weakness, ataxia, diarrhoea, collapse and death.

Phenothiazine

Signs of toxicity are seen within hours of drug administration, and include anorexia, depression, staggering hindleg gait, colic, jaundice and haemoglobinuria. Photosensitization may also occur.

22.25 *Petroleum products*

Ingestion of petroleum products (kerosene, fuel oils, crude oil and partially refined petroleum products) causes blistering of the mouth, salivation, colic and diarrhoea. Skin exposure causes hair loss and local irritation. Inhalation of droplets of petroleum products results in coughing, sneezing and dyspnoea.

22.26 *Feed-associated poisonings*

Ionophores

See Chapter 21.

Antibiotics

Severe, and often fatal, colitis has occurred in horses after feeding lincomycin, tylosin, tetracycline and neomycin. The toxicity probably involves overgrowth by pathogenic bacteria, but the precise identity of these bacteria is uncertain. Clinical signs are usually observed 24 to 48 hours after exposure to contaminated feedstuffs.

Blister beetle (cantharidin) poisoning

See p. 462.

Aflatoxin

Aflatoxins are a group of mycotoxins produced in grains by *Aspergillus* spp. They cause acute hepatotoxicity, and the clinical disease is characterized by anorexia, fever, lethargy, tachycardia, tachypnoea and diarrhoea. Jaundice may also be seen. Coagulation defects and bleeding tendencies may occur if the horse survives the acute stage of toxicity.

Further reading

Clarke, M.L., Harvey, D.G. and Humphreys, D.J. (1981) *Veterinary Toxicology*, 2nd edition. Baillière Tindall, London.

Galey, F.D. (1992) *Current Therapy in Equine Medicine 3* (Ed. R.E. Robinson), Section 8. Toxicology. W.B. Saunders, Philadelphia.

Madigan, J.E. and Dybdal, N. (1990) Endocrine and metabolic diseases. In *Large Animal Internal Medicine* (Ed. B.P. Smith), Chapter 39. C.V. Mosby, St Louis.

Oehme, F.W. (1987) *Current Therapy in Equine Medicine 2* (Ed. R.E. Robinson), Section 16. Toxicology. W.B. Saunders, Philadelphia.

Index

Numbers in italic refer to tables or illustrations; numbers in bold refer to main discussion in a string of numbers